Springer

Tokyo
Berlin
Heidelberg
New York
Barcelona
Budapest
Hong Kong
London
Milan
Paris

M. Nagai (Ed.)

Brain Tumor
Research and Therapy

With 166 Figures, Iucluding 17 in Color

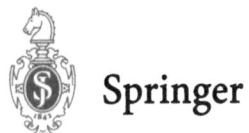

Springer

Masakatsu Nagai, M.D., Ph.D.
Professor and Chairman
Department of Neurosurgery
Dokkyo University School of Medicine
Mibu, Tochigi, 321-02 Japan

Printed on acid-free paper

Library of Congress Cataloging-in-Publication Data
Brain tumor : research and therapy / M. Nagai, (ed.).
    p. cm.
    Based on the 3rd Japanese Conference on Brain Tumor Research and
Therapy, held at Nasu, Japan, Nov. 1994.
    Includes bibliographical references and index.
    ISBN 978-4-431-66889-3   ISBN 978-4-431-66887-9 (eBook)
    DOI 10.1007/978-4-431-66887-9
    1. Brain—Cancer—Congresses. I. Nagai, M. (Masakatsu), 1930–
. II. Japanese Conference on Brain Tumor Research and Therapy (3rd
: 1994 : Nasu-machi, Japan)
    [DNLM: 1. Brain Neoplasms—congresses. WL 358 B8132 1995]
RC280.B7B695   1995
616.99'481—dc20
DNLM/DLC
for Library of Congress   95-45947
                                                CIP

© Springer-Verlag Tokyo 1996

Softcover reprint of the hardcover 1st edition 1996

Typesetting: Best-set Typesetter Ltd., Hong Kong

Preface

The title of this monograph, *Brain Tumor Research and Therapy*, is the name of the Conference itself, which had its inaugural meeting in the United States in 1975 and has since progressed to the international scale. In Japan, the first conference of its kind was organized by Dr. Takao Hoshino and me and was held at Nikko in 1980, hence its name, the Nikko Conference on Brain Tumor Research and Therapy. Though it started as a small, closed meeting, the conference has grown considerably, and in 1992 it was reorganized as the Japanese Conference on Brain Tumor Research and Therapy and was opened to all neurosurgeons and neuropathologists interested in the study of brain tumor problems and who are participating in this field.

The main purpose of the Conference on Brain Tumor Research and Therapy is the candid and informed discussion of the most up-to-date developments in basic research and clinical treatment of brain tumors. The 3rd Japanese Conference on Brain Tumor Research and Therapy was held at Nasu (Tochigi Prefecture), Japan, in November 1994. It was a great honor to welcome many distinguished guests from overseas who kindly attended each session and made valuable contributions.

This volume comprises 46 selected papers from 13 special lectures and 145 presentations focusing on four main subjects. Part I includes a comprehensive review and reevaluation of the fundamental problems concerning classification and grading of brain tumors. In parts II and III, advances in brain tumor cell biology and neurooncology are described using the terminology of molecular biology and molecular genetics. Part IV is composed of basic and clinical studies on biological response modifiers (BRM) therapies, including gene therapy, which might become the leading method of treatment for malignant brain tumors in the twenty-first century.

Nearly fifty years ago, in *Death Be Not Proud*, John Gunther described precisely the details of the treatment of his son Johnny who was suffering from glioblastoma multiforme. How far have the current therapeutic methods progressed since his time? Malignant glioma still remains one of the most grim, intractable, and lethal tumors. The editor sincerely hopes that this book will serve as a bridge between current molecular biological research on central nervous system tumors and the development of epoch-making therapies against them.

I gratefully acknowledge the endeavors of all authors contributing to this volume and the help of the staff of Springer-Verlag, who cooperated efficiently to enable the prompt publication of this edition.

Masakatsu Nagai

Contents

Preface V
List of Contributors XIII

Part I. Reevaluation of Classification and Grading of Brain Tumors

Section 1. General Considerations and Statistics

Histopathological Classification of Brain Tumors According to the
Revised WHO Classification: Current State and Perspectives
W. Wechsler and G. Reifenberger 3

Histological Aspects of Certain Benign Brain Tumors: Review of
Current Topics
A. Hirano, K. Sugiyama, and J.F. Llena 21

The Statistical Analysis of Prognostic Factors for Brain Tumors
K. Nomura, N. Yamaguchi, and S. Watanabe 29

Section 2. Glial Tumors

Evaluation of Histological Grading Systems of Astrocytic Tumors
N. Kawano, H. Oka, T. Suwa, and K. Yada 39

Histological and Radioimaging Study of Malignant Change in Low-Grade
Astrocytoma
M. Tamura, T. Shibasaki, S. Horikoshi, A. Zama, H. Kurihara, N. Ono,
and S. Ishiuchi 45

Clinicopathological Study of Mixed Oligoastrocytoma
Y. Shimada, O. Kubo, Y. Tajika, H. Hiyama, S. Atuji, and K. Takakura 51

Metallothionein in Gliomas
H. Nitta, Y. Hayashi, Y. Okada, O. Tachibana, M. Mouri, T. Yamashima, and
J. Yamashita 61

Section 3. Meningioma

Histological Grading of Meningioma Based on MIB-1 Immunoreactivity
J. Hirato, Y. Nakazato, and M. Hirato 69

Incidental Meningiomas in Autopsy Cases in Computed Tomography and
Magnetic Resonance Imaging Era
K. Sugiyama, A. Hirano, J.F. Llena, T. Uozumi, K. Kurisu, K. Harada,
E. Taniguchi, and T. Nishi 79

Clinicopathological Study of Malignant Meningiomas
J. Mizuno, H. Nakagawa, K. Hara, and Y. Hashizume...................... 89

Part II. Dynamic Aspects of the Biology of Brain Tumor Cells

Section 1. Cell Motility

Expression of L1CAM in Brain Tumors: Immunohistochemical
Study Using Anti-L1CAM Antibodies
S. Izumoto, N. Arita, T. Ohnishi, S. Hiraga, T. Taki, and T. Hayakawa 103

Expression and Biological Functions of L1 Cell Adhesion Molecule
in Malignant Glioma Cells
T. Ohnishi, S. Izumoto, N. Arita, S. Hiraga, T. Taki, and T. Hayakawa 109

The Role of Urokinase-Type Plasminogen Activator in the Invasion
and Proliferation of Malignant Brain Tumors
S. Takano, Y. Yoshii, T. Nose, B. Landau, and S. Brem 119

Section 2. Cell Kinetics

Stemline Study Based on the Nuclear Characterization and Image
Cytometry in Resected Brain Tumors
Y. Yoshii, A. Saito, K. Tsuboi, S. Takano, Y. Komatsu, H. Tsurushima,
and T. Nose 127

Efficiency of Glioma Score in Glioma Patients Using
Proliferating Potential with MIB-1 Monoclonal Antibody
T. Maeda, K. Saruta, S. Ito, H. Sawa, and I. Saito 141

Part III. Molecular Neuro-Oncology and Its Impact on the Clinical Management of Brain Tumors

Section 1. Molecular Biology and Genetics

Molecular Analysis of Phosphorylated Tyrosine-Binding Proteins in the
Transduction of Proliferation and Differentiation Signals
K. Nagashima, S. Tanaka, S. Ota, H. Hasegawa, and M. Matsuda 151

Gene Alterations in Glial Tumors
C.D. James 161

A Model for the Molecular Pathogenesis of Astrocytic Gliomas
O.D. Wiestler and A. von Deimling 173

Molecular Genetics of Oligodendroglial Tumors
G. Reifenberger, J. Reifenberger, L. Liu, C.D. James, W. Wechsler,
and V.P. Collins 187

Section 2. Expression of Oncogene and Growth Factor

The Correlation Between *flg* Gene Expression and the Progression of Glioma
Y. Komatsu, K. Tsuboi, Y. Yoshii, and T. Nose 203

Expression of trk Proto-Oncogene Product in Medulloblastoma
T. Kokunai, A. Kawamura, H. Sawa, I. Izawa and N. Tamaki. 211

Differential Expression of FGF Receptor-1 and FGF Receptor-2
Is Associated with Malignant Progression of Gliomas
F. Yamaguchi, R.S. Morrison, H. Saya, J.M. Bruner, H. Takahashi, and
S. Nakazawa 221

Point Mutations of Epidermal Growth Factor Receptor Transcripts in
Primary Human Malignant Gliomas
N. Sugawa, Y. Nakagawa, and S. Ueda 233

Expression of Vascular Endothelial Growth Factor in Human Brain
Tumors In Vivo
K. Ikezaki, K. Samoto, T. Inamura, T. Shono, M. Fukui, M. Ono, and
M. Kuwano 237

Section 3. Tumor Suppressor Gene

Studies of Retinoblastoma and *p53* Gene Mutations in Human Astrocytomas
T. Tsuzuki, S. Tsunoda, T. Sakaki, N. Konishi, Y. Hiasa, H. Hashimoto,
T. Yabuno, and M. Nakamura 247

Immunohistochemical Assessments of P53 Protein Accumulation and
Tumor Growth Fraction During the Progression of Astrocytomas
K. Watanabe, N. Ogata, K. von Ammon, Y. Yonekawa, M. Nagai, H. Ohgaki,
and P. Kleihues 255

Homozygous Deletion of the p16 Gene in Malignant Glioma
S. Izumoto, N. Arita, T. Ohnishi, S. Hiraga, T. Taki, and T. Hayakawa 263

Detection of Binding Proteins of Merlin, the NF2 Tumor Suppressor
Gene Product
H. Takeshima and H. Saya 269

Mutations and Loss of Heterozygosity of the von Hippel-Lindau
Tumor Suppressor Gene in Sporadic Central Nervous System
Hemangioblastomas
S. Ito, H. Kanno, K. Kondo, T. Shuin, M. Yao, M. Hosaka, S. Fujii,
and I. Yamamoto 277

Section 4. Apoptosis

Anti-Fas Antibody Induces Apoptosis in Cultured Glioma Cells by
Activation of the Sphingomyelin Pathway
T. Shiraishi, S. Nakagawa, K. Toda, S. Kihara, Y. Ju, and K. Tabuchi 283

Induction of Apoptosis in Malignant Glioma Cells by Anti-Fas Antibody
C. Park, O. Tachibana, Y. Okamoto, Y. Hayashi, T. Yamashima,
and J. Yamashita 293

Part IV. Advances of Novel Therapeutic Approaches — BRM Therapy and Gene Therapy—on Malignant Brain Tumors

Section 1. BRM Therapy (Basic and Clinical Studies)

Monocyte Chemoattractant Protein-1 (MCP-1) Derived from
Brain Tumors: Its Significance and Clinical Application
J. Kuratsu, H. Takeshima, T. Nishi, K. Sato, K. Yoshizato, S. Yamashiro,
Y. Ushio, and T. Yoshimura 305

Experimental Analysis of Proto-Oncogene and Histocompatibility
Antigen Gene Expression During Brain Tumor Progression
T. Yamasaki, K. Moritake, Y. Akiyama, M. Fukuda, and S. Nagao 315

Suppressed Expression of T-Cell Costimulatory Molecules B7 and B70 in
Human Glioblastomas In Vivo
M. Tada, A.-C. Diserens, M.-F. Hamou, R. Jaufeerally, E.G. van Meir,
and N. de Tribolet 327

Clinical Trials with Interferon-Alpha as a Chemosensitizer in Gliomas
J.C. Buckner 339

Evaluation of Interferon Therapy on Malignant Gliomas
M. Nagai, S. Okuhata, K. Watanabe, J. Narita, C. Ochiai, and T. Arai 349

Clinical Results of Specific Targeting Therapy Against Patients with Malignant
Glioma
M. Hishii, T. Nitta, M. Ebato, K. Okumura, and K. Sato 363

Structural Analysis of Anti-Cancer Antibody, CLN-IgG and Anti-Idiotypic
Antibody, Idio-No. 3, for the Study of Idiotope Image Transmission:
An Insight into Antigen-Specific Human Monoclonal Antibody Therapy
H. Hagiwara and Y. Aotsuka 371

Clinical Effect of CLN-IgG on Glioma and Its Correlation with the
Induction of Antianti-Idiotypic Antibody in the Serum
M. Nagai, J. Narita, K. Watanabe, M. Endoh, C. Ochiai, and H. Hagiwara 381

Section 2. Gene Therapy (Basic Studies)

Gene Therapy for Central Nervous System Tumors
S. Dee, J. Fick, and M.A. Israel 389

Application of the Apoptotic Gene to Gene Therapy of Malignant Gliomas
A. Asai, C. Kitanaka, A. Sugiyama, K. Mishima, and Y. Kuchino 397

Experimental Therapy for Malignant Brain Tumors Using Genetically
Engineered Herpes Simplex Virus Type 1
T. Mineta, S.D. Rabkin, and R.L. Martuza 409

Investigations of Retroviral-Mediated Gene Therapy for Malignant Glioma:
Transduction with HTK-Bearing Retroviruses Sensitizes Glioma Cells to
Ganciclovir
Y. Miyao, K. Shimizu, M. Tamura, M. Yamada, K. Tamura, H. Kishima,
K. Nakahira, T. Yoshimatsu, K. Mikoshiba, K. Ikenaka,
and T. Hayakawa 415

Cytokine Gene Therapy of Malignant Glioma by Means of DNA/Liposomes
J. Yoshida, T. Wakabayashi, M. Mizuno, T. Takaoka, S. Okamoto, H. Okada,
K. Harada, and K. Yagi 423

Analysis of *sdi-1* Gene Functions in Human Malignant Gliomas
K. Harada, K. Kurisu, K. Sugiyama, T. Sadatomo, O. Niwa, and T. Uozumi ... 435

Antisense DNA Approach to the Growth of Human Glioma Cells
S. Yoshida, R. Tanaka, and R. Yamanaka 441

Index 449

List of Contributors

Akiyama Y. 315
Aotsuka Y. 371
Arai T. 349
Arita N. 103, 109, 263
Asai A. 397
Atuji S. 51

Brem S. 119
Bruner J.M. 221
Buckner J.C. 339

Collins V.P. 187

de Tribolet N. 327
Dee S. 389
Diserens A.-C. 327

Ebato M. 363
Endoh M. 381

Fick J. 389
Fujii S. 277
Fukuda M. 315
Fukui M. 237

Hagiwara H. 371, 381
Hamou M.-F. 327
Hara K. 89
Harada K. 79, 423, 435
Hasegawa H. 151
Hashimoto H. 247
Hashizume Y. 89
Hayakawa T. 103, 109, 263, 415
Hayashi Y. 61, 293

Hiasa Y. 247
Hiraga S. 103, 109, 263
Hirano A. 21, 79
Hirato J. 69
Hirato M. 69
Hishii M. 363
Hiyama H. 51
Horikoshi S. 45
Hosaka M. 277

Ikenaka K. 415
Ikezaki K. 237
Inamura T. 237
Ishiuchi S. 45
Israel M.A. 389
Ito, Satoyuki 141
Ito, Susumu 277
Izawa I. 211
Izumoto S. 103, 109, 263

James C.D. 161, 187
Jaufeerally R. 327
Ju Y. 283

Kanno H. 277
Kawamura A. 211
Kawano N. 39
Kihara S. 283
Kishima H. 415
Kitanaka C. 397
Kleihues P. 255
Kokunai T. 211
Komatsu Y. 127, 203
Kondo K. 277
Konishi N. 247

Kubo O. 51
Kuchino Y. 397
Kuratsu J. 305
Kurihara H. 45
Kurisu K. 79, 435
Kuwano M. 237

Landau B. 119
Liu L. 187
Llena J.F. 21, 79

Maeda T. 141
Martuza R.L. 409
Matsuda M. 151
Mikoshiba K. 415
Mineta T. 409
Mishima K. 397
Miyao Y. 415
Mizuno J. 89
Mizuno M. 423
Moritake K. 315
Morrison R.S. 221
Mouri M. 61

Nagai M. 255, 349, 381
Nagao S. 315
Nagashima K. 151
Nakagawa H. 89
Nakagawa S. 283
Nakagawa Y. 233
Nakahira K. 415
Nakamura M. 247
Nakazato Y. 69
Nakazawa S. 221
Narita J. 349, 381

Nishi, Tohru   79
Nishi, Toru   305
Nitta H.   61
Nitta T.   363
Niwa O.   435
Nomura K.   29
Nose T.   119, 127, 203

Ochiai C.   349, 381
Ogata N.   255
Ohgaki H.   255
Ohnishi T.   103, 109, 263
Oka H.   39
Okada H.   423
Okada Y.   61
Okamoto S.   423
Okamoto Y.   293
Okuhata S.   349
Okumura K.   363
Ono M.   237
Ono N.   45
Ota S.   151

Park C.   293

Rabkin S.D.   409
Reifenberger G.   3, 187
Reifenberger J.   187

Sadatomo T.   435
Saito A.   127
Saito I.   141
Sakaki T.   247
Samoto K.   237
Saruta K.   141
Sato, Kiyoshi   363
Sato, Kyoichi   305

Sawa, Hideki   211
Sawa, Hiroki   141
Saya H.   221, 269
Shibasaki T.   45
Shimada Y.   51
Shimizu K.   415
Shiraishi T.   283
Shono T.   237
Shuin T.   277
Sugawa N.   233
Sugiyama A.   397
Sugiyama K.   21, 79, 435
Suwa T.   39

Tabuchi K.   283
Tachibana O.   61, 293
Tada M.   327
Tajika Y.   51
Takahashi H.   221
Takakura K.   51
Takano S.   119, 127
Takaoka T.   423
Takeshima H.   269, 305
Taki T.   103, 109, 263
Tamaki N.   211
Tamura K.   415
Tamura, Masakazu   415
Tamura, Masaru   45
Tanaka R.   441
Tanaka S.   151
Taniguchi E.   79
Toda K.   283
Tsuboi K.   127, 203
Tsunoda S.   247
Tsurushima H.   127
Tsuzuki T.   247

Ueda S.   233
Uozumi T.   79, 435
Ushio Y.   305

van Meir E.G.   327
von Ammon K.   255
von Deimling A.   173

Wakabayashi T.   423
Watanabe K.   255, 349, 381
Watanabe S.   29
Wechsler W.   3, 187
Wiestler O.D.   173

Yabuno T.   247
Yada K.   39
Yagi K.   423
Yamada M.   415
Yamaguchi F.   221
Yamaguchi N.   29
Yamamoto I.   277
Yamanaka R.   441
Yamasaki T.   315
Yamashima T.   61, 293
Yamashiro S.   305
Yamashita J.   61, 293
Yao M.   277
Yonekawa Y.   255
Yoshida J.   423
Yoshida S.   441
Yoshii Y.   119, 127, 203
Yoshimatsu T.   415
Yoshimura T.   305
Yoshizato K.   305

Zama A.   45

Part I
Reevaluation of Classification and Grading of Brain Tumors

Section 1. General Considerations and Statistics

Histopathological Classification of Brain Tumors According to the Revised WHO Classification: Current State and Perspectives

Wolfgang Wechsler and Guido Reifenberger

Abstract. The first edition of the World Health Organization (WHO) international histological classification of tumors of the central nervous system was the result of a collaborative effort coordinated by Professor Klaus-Joachim Zülch in cooperation with 10 experts from 9 countries. This edition of the so-called Blue Book was published under WHO auspices in 1979. To keep the classification up to date, meetings were convened in Houston, Texas, USA (1988), and in Zurich, Switzerland (1990). At the latter meeting an expanded board of 26 experts from 13 countries formulated a consensus report for a revised classification. This revised classification, consisting of definitions, explanatory notes, and an extended panel of representative photomicrographs, was published in 1993 by P. Kleihues, P.C. Burger, and B.W. Scheithauer. Like the first edition, the revised classification is based on histopathological tumor typing and tumor grading. However, a number of changes have been included in the new edition. The monstrocellular sarcoma has been deleted because immunohistochemistry for glial fibrillary acidic protein (GFAP) has clearly documented the astrocytic nature of this neoplasm. Several new tumor types have been added, including most notably the pleomorphic xanthoastrocytoma, the central neurocytoma, the dysembryoplastic neuroepithelial tumor, and the desmoplastic infantile ganglioglioma. Ependymomas and meningiomas appeared with new histological subtypes. The term primitive neuroectodermal tumor (PNET) has been introduced to designate the small-cell malignant tumors of childhood, the most frequent example of which is the cerebellar medulloblastoma. Based on immunohistochemical and molecular genetic data, several tumor types have been moved from one tumor group to another; for example, the glioblastoma is no longer listed under the poorly differentiated and embryonal tumors but is regarded as the most malignant type among the astrocytic neoplasms. The essentials of the new WHO classification are discussed in this chapter. Particular emphasis will be placed on the impact of immunohistochemistry and molecular genetics for the differential diagnosis and grading of brain tumors. It is hoped that further advances in the field of molecular genetics will not only provide new tools for the improvement of diagnostic accuracy but also rational guidelines for better therapeutic strategies.

Key words. Brain neoplasms—Classification—Grading—Immunohistochemistry—Molecular genetics

Department of Neuropathology, Heinrich-Heine-University Düsseldorf, D-40225 Düsseldorf, Germany

Introduction

The history of brain tumor classification, as so many fields of pathology, commenced in the middle of the nineteenth century with the work of the German pathologist Rudolph Virchow (1821–1902). In his lectures entitled "Die krankhaften Geschwülste," Virchow described the neuroglia and related it to brain tumors. He was the first who separated the gliomas from the "psammomas," the "melanomas," and the other "sarcomas" of the nervous system [1]. The second milestone in brain tumor classification was reached more than half a century later with the fundamental work of Bailey and Cushing [2]. For the first time, the gliomas were systematically subclassified on a histogenetic basis and the concept of brain tumor grading, that is, the relation of certain histopathological characteristics to patient outcome, was introduced. Later in the twentieth century, hallmarks of brain tumor classification were the monographs of individual scientists with outstanding expertise such as Penfield [3], del Rio Hortega [4], Kernohan and Sayre [5], Zülch [6], Russell and Rubinstein [7], and Rubinstein [8]. However, the classifications used by these authors differed considerably in conceptional approaches, in the histological criteria used for classification, and in the applied nomenclature. Furthermore, the preference for different classification systems in different countries, for example, the Kernohan system in the English-speaking countries and del Rio Hortega's system in the Portuguese- and Spanish-speaking world, greatly complicated comparisons of scientific and therapeutic results at an international level.

It was against this background that the World Health Organization (WHO) Collaborating Centre for the Histological Classification of Tumors of the Central Nervous System was established in 1970 at the Max Planck Institute for Brain Research in Cologne, Germany, to prepare a unified classification of tumors of the central nervous system. Under the leadership of Professor Klaus Joachim Zülch, an international committee of neuropathologists from nine countries, among them Professor Lucien J. Rubinstein from the United States of America and Professor Yoichi Ishida from Japan, studied 230 cases that were reviewed at meetings in 1974 and 1976. At those meetings, a consensus classification of central nervous system tumors was worked out that was reviewed by a second group of pathologists and finally published by the WHO in 1979 as part of the series "International Histological Classification of Tumors" [9]. This so-called Blue Book, edited by Professor Zülch under the title "Histological Typing of Tumors of the Central Nervous System," was not designed as a comprehensive textbook but rather as a brief outline of the consensus classification supplemented by definitions and explanatory notes as well as a series of histopathological pictures. Its international character was stressed by including the classification in four different languages: English, French, Russian, and Spanish. Thus, the major intention of the WHO classification was to promote the adoption of a uniform terminology of central nervous system tumors and thereby facilitate and improve communication among neuropathologists, neurosurgeons, radiation therapists, and medical oncologists at an international level.

The Revised WHO Classification of Tumors of the Central Nervous System from 1993

Enormous advances have been made in basic, experimental, and clinical neurooncology since the publication of the first WHO classification of central nervous system tumors in 1979. New tumor entities have been described, and the development and widespread availability of immunohistochemical methods has greatly enriched the diagnostic tools and thereby significantly improved diagnostic accuracy. Furthermore, the advent of molecular genetics in brain tumor research has provided a number of important new insights concerning the development and progression of these tumors. To keep the WHO classification up to date and to further promote its international use, meetings were convened in 1988 in Houston, Texas, USA [10], and in 1990 in Zürich, Switzerland. At the latter meeting an expanded board of 26 experts from 13 countries from all over the world, including Professor F. Ikuta and Professor Y. Ishida from Japan, extensively discussed all tumor types including a number of new entities (see following), and formulated a consensus report for a revised classification. This revised classification, the second edition of the Blue Book, was published in 1993 by P. Kleihues, P.C. Burger and B.W. Scheithauer [11]. Like the first edition, the revised classification is based on histopathological tumor typing and an optional WHO grading scheme ranging from grade I (benign) to grade IV (malignant). It includes definitions and explanatory notes as well as a significantly extended panel of representative photomicrographs. In addition, a morphology code according to the International Classification of Diseases for Oncology (ICD-O) and Systematized Nomenclature of Medicine (SNOMED) was added to the tumor entities.

A number of changes have been included in the revised edition. The monstrocellular sarcoma has been deleted because immunohistochemistry for glial fibrillary acidic protein (GFAP) has clearly documented the astrocytic nature of these neoplasms. Therefore, such a tumor is now considered as a variant of glioblastoma, that is, a giant cell glioblastoma with a sarcomatous component [12]. Several new tumor types have been added to the classification, including most notably the pleomorphic xanthoastrocytoma (PXA) and the central neurocytoma, but also rare tumors such as the dysembryoplastic neuroepithelial tumor (DNT) and the desmoplastic infantile ganglioglioma (DIG). Ependymomas and meningiomas appeared with new histological subtypes. In addition to the deletion or introduction of certain tumor types, a number of important conceptional changes have been included. Examples are (1) the introduction of the term primitive neuroectodermal tumor (PNET) to designate small-cell malignant tumors of childhood, the most frequent example of which being the cerebellar medulloblastoma; (2) the transfer of the glioblastoma from the group of "poorly differentiated and embryonal tumors" to the astrocytic tumors; and (3) the creation of a group of "neuroepithelial tumors of uncertain origin" comprising the astroblastoma, the polar spongioblastoma, and gliomatosis cerebri. An excellent introduction to the revised WHO classification with supplementory comments and explanations has been published by the editors [12]. In our contribution, we would like to present the conceptional improvements and new achievements by comparing tumor types and tumor groups between the two editions. We also discuss some perspectives of brain tumor classification in the light of recent developments concerning the immunohistochemistry and molecular genetics of these tumors.

Tumors of Neuroepithelial Tissue

Comparison between the first and second edition reveals a number of minor and major changes in the group of "tumors of neuroepithelial tissue," which forms the first major category in both editions. Minor changes can be noted for the oligodendrogliomas and mixed gliomas, which are no longer listed together under the heading of oligodendroglial tumors but form two separate groups. The new group of "mixed gliomas" consists of oligoastrocytomas (WHO grade II), anaplastic (malignant) oligoastrocytomas (WHO grade III), and other mixed gliomas. The separation of the mixed gliomas from the group of oligodendroglial tumors is a point of discussion. With respect to the molecular alterations associated with these tumors, our recent studies demonstrate that the vast majority of oligodendrogliomas has lost genetic information on 19q and 1p. In contrast, mixed gliomas revealed a more heterogeneous pattern of genetic alteration, either loss of alleles on 19q and 1p or loss on 17p or other clonal alterations [13]. However, other authors have reported results suggesting that oligodendrogliomas and mixed gliomas share similar genetic alterations, that is, loss of alleles on 19q and 1p [14,15], which would imply that mixed gliomas (oligoastrocytomas) are genetically more closely related to oligodendrogliomas than to astrocytomas.

With regard to the histopathological classification of oligodendrogliomas and mixed gliomas, certain problems may arise in the differential diagnosis between such tumors. In our experience there is no differential diagnostic problem so long as the astroglial tumor part is geographically separated from the oligodendroglial component. For such tumors the diagnosis of mixed oligoastrocytoma is straightforward and appropriate. However, in cases with diffuse intermingling of both components the situation may become more complicated, particularly in the anaplastic variants, because anaplastic oligodendrogliomas are well known to "often contain a significant admixture of neoplastic astrocytes" [11]. In addition, both anaplastic oligodendrogliomas and anaplastic oligoastrocytomas can further develop into highly malignant gliomas that morphologically may be indistinguishable from glioblastoma (WHO grade IV). This possibility is recognized by the new WHO classification. However, in contrast to the astrocytic tumors (see following), the borderline between anaplastic oligodendrogliomas and anaplastic mixed gliomas of WHO grade III on the one hand and the WHO grade IV glioblastomas on the other hand is not precisely defined. Therefore, the classification leaves some space for diagnostic subjectivity in the differential diagnosis of anaplastic oligodendroglioma, anaplastic mixed glioma, and glioblastoma.

Similar to the oligodendrogliomas and mixed gliomas, the ependymal tumors and choroid plexus tumors have been separated in two distinct groups in the revised edition. The cellular and clear cell variants were added to the group of ependymal tumors. Concerning the choroid plexus tumors, the rare malignant variants are now designated as choroid plexus carcinomas, which is in accord with the generally accepted use of the term carcinoma for malignant epithelial tumors. The group of "pineal parenchymal tumors" has been supplemented by an intermediate form of pineal tumor called mixed pineocytoma/pineoblastoma. This is in line with the observation that many pineal parenchymal tumors do not fit precisely into either the pineocytoma or the pineoblastoma category. Although the WHO classification does not ascribe a certain malignancy grade to the mixed pineocytoma/pineoblastoma, one would assume that the biological behaviour of such lesions reflects the pineoblastoma component.

With regard to the other groups of neuroepithelial tumors, including the astrocytic, neuronal, mixed neuronal-glial, and embryonal tumors, major conceptional changes as well as a number of new entities were introduced in the new edition. We therefore discuss these groups in more detail in the following sections.

Astrocytic Tumors

The changes within the astrocytic tumor family have to be considered of paramount importance. They consist in the transfer of the glioblastomas from the old group of "poorly differentiated and embryonal tumors" to the group of astrocytic tumors. In addition, a new entity, the pleomorphic xanthoastrocytoma [16], was included in this group. More importantly, however, the diagnostic criteria with regard to the distinction between the diffuse astrocytomas of WHO grade II, the anaplastic astrocytomas of WHO grade III, and the glioblastomas of WHO grade IV have been revised. The histopathological criteria for the differentiation between astrocytomas (WHO grade II) and anaplastic astrocytomas (WHO grade III) are (1) increased cellularity, (2) pleomorphism, (3) nuclear atypia, and (4) mitotic activity. In contrast to the first edition, vascular proliferation and necrosis are no longer allowed in anaplastic astrocytomas but are regarded as the essential criteria for the diagnosis of glioblastoma (WHO grade IV). This more stringent use of the criteria for anaplasia facilitates the classification and grading of astrocytic tumors. However, certain tumors that according to the former classification were diagnosed as anaplastic astrocytomas must now be classified as glioblastomas. This might lead to considerable problems when comparing experimental or therapeutic studies based on either the first or the revised WHO classification system. Furthermore, there is some inconsistency inasmuch as necrosis and vascular proliferation are still allowed in WHO grade III anaplastic oligodendrogliomas and anaplastic mixed gliomas.

Glioblastoma

The inclusion of the glioblastoma in the astrocytic tumor group is in line with the presence of at least a fraction of tumor cells with astrocytic differentiation in most of these neoplasms. In addition, it is well known that astrocytomas and anaplastic astrocytomas may progress to glioblastomas on recurrence. However, individual glioblastomas may evolve from oligodendroglial or, extremely rarely, from ependymal tumors, but even in such tumors at least some astrocytic tumor cells are usually present. Without doubt, certain cases of glioblastoma may be so poorly differentiated that one might have great difficulty in finding histological evidence for astrocytic differentiation. However, in our experience immunohistochemistry for GFAP or S100 protein invariably detects at least small fractions of immunoreactive tumor cells in these tumors, indicating their glial nature. The view that glioblastoma is essentially the most malignant astrocytic tumor type is further supported by molecular biological studies on the development and progression of astrocytic tumors, which have been excellently reviewed by several authors [17–19].

With respect to the further subtyping of glioblastomas on the basis of molecular genetic alterations, several studies have recently provided evidence for genetic heterogeneity in these tumors [20–22]. All three studies analyzed molecular genetic alterations known to be common in glioblastomas, that is, allelic loss on chromosome 10, 17p, and *EGFR* gene amplification. Rasheed et al. [22] additionally looked for *p53* mutations and amplification of certain other cellular oncogenes. Von Deimling et al. [20] first proposed a molecular genetic subdivision of glioblastomas by distinguishing tumors with loss of alleles on 17p but no *EGFR* amplification ("glioblastoma type 1") from those without 17p abnormalities but *EGFR* amplification ("glioblastoma type 2"). However, there was also a large group of glioblastomas without any of these alterations as well as individual cases with both abnormalities, 17p loss and *EGFR* amplification [20]. The "type 1" glioblastomas preferentially occurred in younger patients (average age, 40.5 years), while "type 2" glioblastomas preferred older patients (average age, 56.3 years). It was speculated that at least some "type 1" glioblastomas might represent tumors that had developed by progression from lower grade astrocytomas ("secondary glioblastomas") while the majority of "type 2" tumors probably represent glioblastomas arising de novo ("primary glioblastomas") [20]. In this study, loss of alleles on chromosome 10 was not used as a discriminating factor for subdividing glioblastomas. Leenstra et al. [21], however, suggested a subdivision into four groups: "type 1", only 17p loss; "type 2", only 10 loss; "type 3", 17p and 10 loss; and "type 4", 10 loss and EGFR amplification. These authors claimed a prognostic relevance of their subtyping; patients with "type 1" tumors did survive significantly longer than patients with tumors of "types 2–4." However, they used the old classification system according to Kernohan and Sayre [5] and included grade III and IV anaplastic astrocytomas in their molecular analysis. As 4 of 7 "type 1" tumors but only 4 of 27 "type 2–4" tumors in their series were grade III and the mean age of the patients with "type 1" tumors was significantly lower than in the other groups, it appears to be not too surprising that the type 1 patients did survive longer.

In essence, the major and common finding of the studies cited is that glioblastomas with 17p alterations or p53 mutations tend to occur preferentially in younger patients, less than 45 years in age [20–22]. Mean survival in this group might therefore be better. However, one must keep in mind that glioblastomas have grossly rearranged genomes comprising multiple amplification sites as well as numerous gains and losses of genetic information. These can be elegantly visualized with modern molecular cytogenetic methods such as comparative genomic hybridization [23,24]. Furthermore, recent studies have provided strong evidence for the existence of alternative molecular mechanisms that may result in similar effects on cell cycle regulation and cellular proliferation. For example, the amplification and overexpression of MDM2 can cause the functional inactivation of wild-type p53 protein by complex formation, thus representing an alternative mechanismus to p53 gene mutation or loss [25]. Another example is the amplification of CDK4 which appears to be an alternative mechanism to the homozygous deletion of the MTS1 (p16) tumor suppressor gene in malignant gliomas [26,27]. In conclusion, the "molecular subclassifications" of glioblastomas that have been suggested so far must be regarded as rather preliminary. Future studies analyzing in greater detail the molecular alterations in large and well-controlled series of tumors are needed, and it is hoped that such investigations will eventually provide new prognostically and therapeutically relevant parameters.

Pleomorphic Xanthoastrocytoma (PXA)

This tumor type was first described by Kepes et al. in 1979 as "a distinctive meningeal glioma of young subjects with relatively favorable prognosis" [16]. Despite some discussions related to the histogenesis of these neoplasms [28,29], PXA is now generally accepted as a clinicopathological entity and numerous additional cases have been reported since 1979 (for review see [30]). The WHO classification defines the PXA as "an astrocytoma with a mixture of pleomorphic tumor cells, ranging from ordinary fibrillary astrocytes to giant, multinucleated forms. The latter typically contain lipid vacuoles; thus they are xanthomatous, but express GFAP." These tumors develop preferentially within the cerebral hemisphere of children and young adults and show a predisposition for a superficial and leptomeningeal growth. The superficial and leptomeningeal tumor areas usually exhibit a dense reticulin network because of the pericellular basement membranes. Reactive lymphocytic infiltrates are common. As far as tumor grading is concerned, PXAs usually have a favorable prognosis (WHO grade II), but progression to anaplastic astrocytomas (WHO grade III) or even glioblastomas (WHO grade IV) may occur. Unusual variants such as the epitheloid form [31], the angiomatous form [32], or a PXA as a component of a ganglioglioma [33] have been described.

Neuronal and Mixed Neuronal-Glial Tumors

This group has considerably enlarged by the introduction of new tumor entities. These new tumor types are fairly rare cerebral neoplasms; nevertheless, they are well characterized both morphologically and biologically. Most of them are slowly growing neoplasms with some lesions lying at the borderline between developmental disturbances and benign neoplasms.

Dysembryoplastic Neuroepithelial Tumor (DNT)

Dysembryoplastic neuroepithelial tumors were first described in 1988 by Catherine Daumas-Duport and co-workers [34]. DNTs are benign (WHO grade I), predominantly supratentorial and intracortical lesions with a preferential location temporal and frontal. They occur in young patients with intractable partial seizures and are curable by surgical resection. Histopathologically, DNTs are mixed glial-neuronal neoplasms with multinodular architecture and a heterogeneous cell composition, with oligodendrocytes being more frequently involved than astrocytes. With regard to differential diagnosis, DNTs may be mistaken for oligoastrocytomas or oligodendrogliomas, particularly in cases in which the neuronal component is less obvious. Furthermore, they have to be differentiated from "ordinary" gangliogliomas as well as so-called pure protoplasmic astrocytomas [35]. A cerebellar tumor morphologically similar to DNT has recently been reported [36]. Detailed immunohistochemical, ultrastructural, and cell kinetic findings in DNTs as well as so-called simple and complex forms of this lesion were summarized by Daumas-Duport in 1993 [35].

Desmoplastic Infantile Ganglioglioma (DIG)

This new tumor type was first described as a clinicopathological entity in 1987 by Vandenberg et al. [37]. DIGs are rare, usually large, firm, and partially cystic tumors arising superficially within the cerebral hemispheres in children younger than 2 years. Histologically they are characterized by "a dense fibrous stroma containing an admixture of neuroepithelial cells displaying astrocytic and neuronal differentiation" [11]. Despite the usually large tumor size at clinical presentation as well as the possible presence of primitive, mitotically active neuroepithelial cells, cellular pleomorphism, and cellular atypia, DIGs grow slowly and prognosis after surgical resection appears to be favorable. Thus, histopathologically DIGs correspond to WHO grade I. Taratuto et al. [38] first described six cases of closely related tumors without a neuronal tumor cell population. This tumor type is now designated "desmoplastic cerebral astrocytoma of infancy" [39] or "infantile desmoplastic astrocytoma" [40]. Whether desmoplastic infantile gangliogliomas and desmoplastic cerebral astrocytomas of infancy are distinct entities or only variations of one tumor type remains to be elucidated.

Central Neurocytoma

This tumor entity was characterized first in 1982 by Hassoun et al. and designated "central neurocytoma" [41]. In the meantime, more than 100 cases have been reported in the literature [42]. Central neurocytomas are intraventricular tumors composed of uniform round cells with immunohistochemical and ultrastructural features of neuronal differentiation. They develop typically in the region of the foramen of Monro. Before recognition of their neuronal nature, these tumors had been misdiagnosed either as ependymomas, that is, the "ependymoma of the foramen of Monro" [43], or oligodendrogliomas. The peak incidence lies between 20 and 40 years. Some cases may exhibit evidence for additional glial differentiation [42]. Anaplasia is rare and therefore prognosis is usually favorable (corresponding to grade I).

Embryonal Tumors

In 1973 Hart and Earle proposed the name "primitive neuroectodermal tumor" (PNET) for medulloblastoma-like tumors of the cerebral hemispheres in children [44]. Rorke discussed the relation of cerebellar medulloblastoma to primitive neuroectodermal tumors and suggested using the term PNET for different embryonal central nervous system tumors including medulloblastoma, ependymoblastoma, neuroblastoma, and pineoblastoma [45]. The conceptual basis for this suggestion was the assumption that PNETs are derived from a common progenitor cell population, precursor cells of the subependymal matrix layer in the cerebrum or the external granular cell layer in the cerebellum. Whether this hypothesis is true, however, remains to be investigated further. The WHO classification therefore tried to avoid a controversy concerning the terminology of PNET and a compromise solution was accepted. Accordingly, the term PNET was reserved as a "generic term" for cerebellar medulloblastomas and for those tumors morphologically indistinguishable from the cerebellar medulloblastomas that are located in other sites of the brain or in the spinal cord. Well-established entities of embryonal tumors such as ependymoblastoma, neuroblastoma, and medulloepithelioma were retained. Primitive polar spongioblastoma and gliomatosis cerebri were, however, moved to the new group of "neuroepithelial tumors of uncertain origin" (see following).

Neuroepithelial Tumors of Uncertain Origin

In this newly formed category three rare lesions were grouped: astroblastoma [46], polar spongioblastoma [47], and gliomatosis cerebri. The precise histogenesis of these lesions is still a matter of discussion. Furthermore, it is well known that astroblastic features may occur in circumscribed areas of "ordinary" gliomas, a finding that does not justify the diagnosis of an astroblastoma. The same applies to spongioblastic differentiation that may focally be present in oligodendrogliomas, pilocytic astrocytomas, or medulloblastomas. Thus, some experts of the WHO working group did not accept astroblastoma and polar spongioblastoma as true clinicopathological entities.

The precise origin of gliomatosis cerebri is also still unknown. However, it has been stressed that the phenotype of these lesions may vary considerably, that is, astrocytic or oligodendrocytic differentiation may occur. Malignant dedifferentiation into glioblastoma is also possible. The histopathological differential diagnosis between diffuse gliomas and gliomatosis cerebri is difficult and usually cannot be established by a single biopsy. The diagnosis of gliomatosis cerebri requires a diffuse and widespread involvement of several cerebral lobes. On occasion, the basal ganglia, the brainstem, and even the cerebellum and the spinal cord may be additionally affected. Modern neuroradiological techniques such as computed tomography (CT) and nuclear magnetic resonance (NMR) imaging are therefore required for a diagnosis intra vitam.

Tumors of Cranial and Spinal Nerves

With respect to the classification of nerve tumors, the term schwannoma was preferred to neurilemmoma or neurinoma in the revised edition because these tumors
are predominantly composed of Schwann cells. Cellular, plexiform, and melanotic
variants of schwannoma were included. Among the neurofibromas, solitary and
plexiform subtypes are listed. Schwannomas and neurofibromas are benign neo
plasms and are therefore graded as WHO grade I. The malignant forms of nerve tumors
corresponding to WHO grade III or IV are designated as "malignant peripheral nerve
sheath tumors" (MPNST). Three rare subtypes are distinguished: epitheloid,
melanotic, and MPNST with divergent mesenchymal or epithelial differentiation.

Tumors of the Meninges

The histogenesis and classification of tumors of the meninges has always been of
paramount interest for neuropathologists. Because of their richness in morphological
details and high variability of phenotype, meningeal tumors cover a particularly
broad spectrum of tumor types and variants. Bailey and Bucy [48] described 8 types
with benign behavior and one malignant sarcomatous neoplasm. Cushing and
Eisenhardt [49] differentiated 9 types with 11 variants, that is, 20 subtypes. In the first
edition of the WHO classification, five main categories had been separated, the majority of tumors belonging to the large group of meningiomas. The revised WHO classification summarizes among the "tumors of meningothelial cells" four groups:
meningioma, atypical meningioma, papillary meningioma, and anaplastic (malignant) meningioma. The large meningioma group consists of 11 variants, among them
a number of newly recognized subtypes such as microcystic, secretory, clear cell,
chordoid, lymphoplasmacyte-rich, and metaplastic meningiomas.

The hemangiopericytic meningiomas of the first edition are no longer considered
as belonging to the meningothelial tumors because these neoplasms are undis-
tinguishable from hemangiopericytomas occurring in other parts of the body.
Hemangiopericytomas ultrastructurally lack the interdigitating processes and well-
developed desmosomes typical of meningiomas and are immunohistochemically
negative for epithelial membrane antigen (EMA) (for review see [40]). Furthermore,
recent molecular genetic and cytogenetic studies have provided evidence that
hemangiopericytomas, in contrast to the majority of meningiomas, do not show loss
of genetic information on chromosome 22 [50] but are characterized by chromosomal
translocations involving most frequently the long arm of chromosome 12 [51,52].
Together, these data clearly separate the hemangiopericytomas from the meningiomas. Thus, the new WHO classification lists these tumors under the heading of
"mesenchymal, nonmeningothelial tumors." However, although hemangiopericytomas have a definite tendency for local recurrence and metastasis, their inclusion
in the group of malignant neoplasms together with chondrosarcoma, malignant
fibrous histiocytoma, rhabdomyosarcoma, and other sarcomas is debatable. The biological behavior of these tumors obviously covers a wide spectrum ranging from
relatively benign tumors that may readily be cured by surgical removal to frankly
malignant neoplasms [53].

An important advance in the new classification is the introduction of a new
meningioma type with intermediate biological behavior, the atypical meningioma. In
contrast to the ordinary meningiomas of WHO grade I, these tumors are character-

ized by histological signs of increased growth activity such as high mitotic activity, increased cellularity, higher nuclear/cytoplasmic ratio, uninterrupted patternless or sheetlike growth, and foci of necrosis. Clinically, these tumors show an increased tendency to recurrence [54]. Histopathological recognition of atypical meningiomas is therefore of great importance and such patients should be followed up more closely after surgery. In our experience immunohistochemical staining for the proliferation-associated antigen Ki-64 using the MIB1 monoclonal antibody on paraffin sections pretreated by microwave cooking can be of considerable help for the recognition of increased proliferative activity in meningiomas and thereby facilitate their grading.

In summary, the revised WHO classification of central nervous system tumors offers significant improvements in the group of tumors of the meninges. It provides a detailed specification of meningioma subtypes (variants), some of them with physiological specification, and a better approach to tumor grading of meningiomas. It remains to be shown whether other parameters such as the expression of certain receptor molecules or the demonstration of certain molecular genetic alterations may become of additional relevance for the differential diagnosis or grading of meningeal tumors. Mutation or deletion of the neurofibromatosis type 2 (NF2) gene on chromosome 22q12 has been observed in approximately 60% of all meningiomas [55,56]. Interestingly, fibroblastic and transitional types are preferentially affected while meningotheliomatous meningiomas only rarely demonstrate loss of 22q and NF2 alterations [55,56]. In atypical and malignant meningioma, an increased incidence of allelic losses on chromosomes 1p, 10, and 14q has been observed, suggesting that these chromosomal regions contain so far unknown tumor suppressor genes associated with the progression of meningiomas [57–60].

A further novelty in the classification of meningeal tumors is the introduction of the group of "mesenchymal, non-meningothelial tumors" (for review, see [61]). In the old classification, the tumor types combined in this group had been listed among various headings such as "meningeal sarcomas," "xanthomatous tumors," and "other malformative tumors and tumor-like lesions." The new group of mesenchymal, nonmeningothelial tumors is subdivided into benign neoplasms, that is, osteocartilaginous tumors, lipoma, fibrous histiocytoma, and others, and malignant neoplasms, including hemangiopericytoma, chondrosarcoma, malignant fibrous histiocytoma, rhabdomyosarcoma, meningeal sarcomatosis, and other types of sarcomas. The classification of these tumors follows that of the WHO classification of soft tissue tumors [62].

The group of primary melanocytic lesions has been extended by the inclusion of diffuse melanosis and melanocytoma. These two benign lesions need to be distinguished from malignant melanomas and meningeal melanomatosis. A further novelty in the revised WHO classification is that the capillary hemangioblastoma, a tumor arising either in the setting of von Hippel–Lindau syndrome or, more often, as a solitary sporadic lesion, has been moved from the "tumors of blood vessel origin" to a new category of "tumors of uncertain origin." This reflects the fact that despite extensive immunohistochemical and electron microscopic studies, the nature and origin of the "principal" or "stromal cells" in capillary hemangioblastomas are still uncertain. Different studies have characterized these cells as showing phenotypes as diverse as undifferentiated mesenchymal [63] to neuroendocrine [64] and even fibrohistiocytic [65]. The molecular genetic alterations underlying the growth of capillary hemangioblastomas are also poorly understood at present. The recent identification and cloning of the von Hippel–Lindau (VHL) tumor suppressor gene [66] in conjunction with the finding of mutations or deletions of the VHL gene in sporadic capillary hemangioblastomas [67] and other neoplasms associated with von Hippel–

Lindau disease [68–70] suggest a loss of function of the *VHL* gene as a critical step in the development of these tumors. In addition, there are studies showing that the characteristic proliferation of capillary vessels may be caused by the production and secretion of vascular endothelial-derived growth factor (VEGF), a potent angiogenic factor, by the stromal cells [71,72]. Thus, there is evidence that the stromal cells in capillary hemangioblastomas represent the actual tumor cells and that the proliferation of capillary vessels in these tumors might be a secondary event, probably induced by secretion of angiogenic growth factors such as VEGF by the stromal cells. With respect to the important differential diagnosis of capillary hemangioblastoma versus metastatic renal cell carcinoma, immunohistochemistry for EMA is of great help because capillary hemangioblastomas are EMA negative while renal cell carcinomas express this antigen on their tumor cells [73].

Other Tumor Groups

The nomenclature of malignant lymphomas of the central nervous system was updated in the new WHO classification. Old terms such as "reticulosarcoma" or "reticulum cell sarcoma" were abandoned. Most primary central nervous system lymphomas, occurring either sporadically or in immunosuppressed patients, are in fact high-grade non-Hodgkin's lymphomas of B-cell origin. Immunohistochemistry for leucocyte common antigen (LCA) as well as for B- and T-cell markers is of great help for the differential diagnosis toward other malignant tumors and reactive or inflammatory lesions. It is recommended to classify central nervous system lymphomas according to either the National Cancer Institute Working Formulation [74] or to the Kiel classification [75]; however, in many cases precise subclassification according to these classification systems for systemic non-Hodgkin's lymphomas may be difficult [76,77].

The classification of intracranial germ cell tumors follows the criteria of the WHO for "histological typing of testis tumors" [78]. A further change is the transfer of the craniopharyngeomas from the old group of "other malformative tumors and tumor-like lesions" to the new category of "tumors of the sellar region." Two subtypes, the "classical" adamantinomatous craniopharyngeoma and the less frequent papillary variant, are recognized.

Survey and Comments

In summary, comparing the first edition of the WHO "Histological Typing of Tumors of the Central Nervous System" from 1979 with the revised edition from 1993 it is evident that the second edition will continue the objective to propose a uniform nomenclature for central nervous system neoplasms with an increasing acceptance at the international level. According to the authors, the WHO classification should serve as a "reliable guideline in day-to-day surgical pathology and as a unifying basis for the evaluation of brain tumor therapy trials" [12]. The changes introduced reflect the progress in brain tumor research at both the cellular and the molecular level that had been achieved during a period of only 14 years. Based on new achievements concerning immunohistochemistry and molecular genetics, it became evident that the old tumor group of "poorly differentiated and embryonal tumors" including glioblastomas, medulloblastomas, polar spongioblastomas, and gliomatosis cerebri" is obsolete. The highlights of the new edition are the transfer of the glioblastomas to the astrocytic tumors, the inclusion of PXA, the streamlining of embryonal tumors without overemphasizing the concept of primitive neuroectodermal tumors, the extension of the group of neuronal and mixed neuronal-glial tumors by inclusion of several well-characterized new entities (DNT, DIG, central neurocytoma), and the modernization of the histological typing and grading of meningeal tumors. However, one has to keep in mind that, like the first Blue Book, the revised edition represents a compromise solution and in certain aspects has a provisional character. In addition, some rare lesions such as gliofibroma [79-81] or the atypical teratoid/rhabdoid tumors (for review, see [40]) were not included. Nevertheless, the revised WHO classifications represents a significant advance compared to the former classification system, and we strongly support their general use by neuropathologists and pathologists around the world.

Tumor Grading

In the first edition of the WHO classification, in addition to describing histological evidence of differentiation or anaplasia, the biological behavior of central nervous system (CNS) tumors had been characterized by a tumor grading system ranging from grade I (benign) to grade IV (malignant). This WHO grading system was a malignancy scale ranging across a wide variety of neoplasms of the central nervous system. It is now widely used, particularly in European countries. An increasing acceptance can be noted in Japan and in the United States and Canada.

As in the first edition, editors and participants of the revised version hold the view that this grading system should be continued on an optional basis. The use of the term "WHO grade I-IV" or "WHO grading system" was advocated to avoid any confusion with other grading systems. The WHO grading is based on cytological and histological features. WHO grade I lesions generally include tumors with a minimal proliferative potential and the possibility of cure following surgical resection alone. Typical examples are the pilocytic astrocytomas, subependymomas, myxopapillary ependymomas, and a variety of neuronal and mixed neuronal/glial tumors as well as the meningiomas. Tumors of WHO grade II are those with low mitotic activity but a tendency for recurrence because of diffusely infiltrative growth. The well-differentiated astrocytomas, oligodendrogliomas, mixed gliomas, and ependymomas are typical examples of WHO grade II tumors. WHO grade III is reserved for neoplasms with histological evidence of anaplasia, generally in the form of increased mitotic activity, increased cellularity, nuclear pleomorphism, and cellular anaplasia. The designation WHO grade IV was assigned to mitotically active and necrosis-prone highly malignant neoplasms that are associated with a rapid pre- and postoperative evolution of the disease, for example, the glioblastomas and the majority of embryonal neoplasms. Possible problems with the grading of gliomas, particularly of the high-grade tumors, have already been mentioned. The differences in use of the criteria for anaplasia between anaplastic astrocytomas on the one hand and anaplastic oligodendrogliomas and anaplastic mixed gliomas on the other hand should be further discussed. Another problem in the day-to-day routine diagnostic work in our experience is the size of the tumor piece received for neuropathological examination. In particular, the increasing use of stereotactic biopsy frequently provides the neuropathologist with only very small tumor pieces. In view of the well-known regional heterogeneity of malignant gliomas, it is absolutely essential that the neuropathologist be informed about all the relevant clinical and neuroradiological data before coming to a conclusion about the histological findings. The WHO grading system is illustrated in Table 1.

Table 1. World Health Organization (WHO) grading system of central nervous system tumors (modified after [12]).

Tumor type	WHO grade I	WHO grade II	WHO grade III	WHO grade IV
Subependymal giant cell astrocytoma	X			
Pilocytic astrocytoma	X			
Astrocytoma		X		
Pleomorphic xanthoastrocytoma		X	X	
Anaplastic astrocytoma			X	
Glioblastoma				X
Oligodendroglioma		X		
Anaplastic oligodendroglioma			X	
Oligoastrocytoma		X		
Anaplastic oligoastrocytoma			X	
Subependymoma	X			
Myxopapillary ependymoma	X			
Ependymoma		X		
Anaplastic ependymoma			X	
Choroid plexus papilloma	X			
Choroid plexus carcinoma			X	X
Gangliocytoma	X			
Ganglioglioma	X	X		
Anaplastic ganglioglioma			X	
Desmoplastic infantile ganglioglioma	X			
Dysembryoplastic neuroepithelial tumor	X			
Central neurocytoma	X			
Paraganglioma of the filum terminale	X			
Olfactory neuroblastoma			X	
Pineocytoma		X		
Mixed pineocytoma/pineoblastoma			X	X
Pineoblastoma				X
Medulloblastoma				X
Other primitive neuroectodermal tumors (PNETs)				X
Medulloepithelioma				X
Neuroblastoma				X
Ependymoblastoma				X
Schwannoma	X			
Neurofibroma	X			
Malignant peripheral nerve sheath tumors (MPNST)			X	X
Meningioma	X			
Atypical meningioma		X		
Papillary meningioma		X	X	
Anaplastic meningioma			X	
Hemangiopericytoma		X	X	
Hemangioblastoma	X			
Craniopharyngeoma	X			

It should be noted that certain types of tumors may occur with different degrees of anaplasia, which underlines the importance of adding the WHO grade to the diagnosis.

Summary and Perspectives

Between 1979 and 1993, within a period of only 14 years, brain tumor research made enormous progress both at the clinical level, with the tremendous advances in neuroimaging and the development of new sophisticated neurosurgical techniques, as well as at the laboratory level. In neuropathology, the development and widespread application of immunohistochemical methods that can be reliably applied to routinely processed material has provided a powerful new tool not only for research purposes but, even more importantly, for the daily diagnostic work. Immunohistochemistry for differentiation antigens greatly facilitates differential diagnosis and thereby improves diagnostic accuracy (for review, see [82]). The demonstration of certain antigens such as the proliferation-associated antigen Ki-67 may help in assessing the tumor growth fraction and provide additional information for the grading of brain tumors [82,83]. In addition, immunohistochemistry allows the visualization of overexpression or pathological accumulation of key molecules related to the neoplastic process, such as the epidermal growth factor receptor or the p53 tumor suppressor gene product, which might be of some relevance as additional prognostic indicators [84].

Cytogenetic and molecular biological methods have revealed important new insights in the molecular alterations underlying the development and progression of different types of brain tumors. Preliminary data point to the potential usefulness of certain molecular abnormalities as prognostic parameters. It is hoped that future molecular genetic studies will soon provide new tools for the improvement of diagnostic accuracy as well as rational guidelines for better therapeutic strategies. So far as the revised edition of the WHO classification is concerned, some impacts of the ongoing "molecular genetic revolution in neuro-oncology" could already be noted as changes in the tumor classification, for example, the consideration of glioblastoma as the most malignant type among the astrocytic tumors and the separation of the hemangiopericytoma from the meningioma group.

In this review, we have presented the essentials of the new WHO classification. We emphasized the impact of immunohistochemical methods for differential diagnosis and tumor grading. In addition, recent achievements in the molecular biology and genetics of central nervous system tumors have been briefly discussed insofar as they might be relevant for brain tumor classification. Apart from these basic concepts, it is necessary to keep on facilitating and improving communication among clinicians, neuropathologists, and basic scientists working in the various fields of neurooncology. We believe that the revised WHO classification of tumors of the central nervous system can be regarded as a milestone in this respect.

References

1. Virchow R (1864/1865) Die krankhaften Geschwülste. Achtzehnte Vorlesung: Psammome, Melanome, Gliome. Verlag von August Hirschwald, Berlin, pp 106–169
2. Bailey P, Cushing H (1926) A classification of the tumors of the glioma group on a histogenetic basis with a correlated study of prognosis. Lippincott, Philadelphia

3. Penfield W (1932) Cytology and cellular pathology of the nervous system. Hoeber, New York
4. del Rio Hortega P (1945) Nomenclatura y clasificación de los tumores del sistema nervioso. López and Etchefoyen, Buenos Aires [Arch Histol (B Aires) 3:5–63]
5. Kernohan JW, Sayre GP (1952) Tumors of the central nervous system. Armed Forces Institute of Pathology, Washington, DC
6. Zülch KJ (1956) Biologie und Pathologie der Hirngeschwülste. Handbuch der Neurochirurgie, vol III. Springer, Berlin Göttingen Heidelberg
7. Russell DS, Rubinstein LJ (1959) Pathology of tumors of the nervous system. Arnold, London
8. Rubinstein LJ (1972) Tumors of the central nervous system. In: Atlas of tumor pathology, 2nd series, Fasc 6. Armed Forces Institute of Pathology, Washington, DC
9. Zülch KJ (1979) Histological typing of tumors of the central nervous system. International histological classification of tumors, no. 21. World Health Organization, Geneva
10. Fields WS (1989) Primary brain tumors—a review of histological classification. Springer, Berlin Heidelberg New York Tokyo
11. Kleihues P, Burger PC, Scheithauer BW (1993) Histological typing of tumors of the central nervous system, 2nd edn. International histological classification of tumors. Springer, Berlin Heidelberg New York Tokyo
12. Kleihues P, Burger PC, Scheithauer BW (1993) The new WHO classification of brain tumors. Brain Pathol 3:255–368
13. Reifenberger J, Reifenberger G, Liu L, James CD, Wechsler W, Collins VP (1994) Molecular genetic analysis of oligodendroglial tumors shows preferential allelic deletions on 19q and 1p. Am J Pathol 145:1175–1190
14. von Deimling A, Louis DN, von Ammon K, Petersen I, Wiestler OD, Seizinger BR (1992) Evidence for a tumor suppressor gene on chromosome 19q associated with human astrocytomas, oligodendrogliomas, and mixed gliomas. Cancer Res 52:4277–4279
15. Kraus JA, Koopmann J, Kaskel P, Maintz D, Brandner S, Schramm J, Louis DN, Wiestler OD, von Deimling A (1995) Shared allelic losses on chromosomes 1p and 19q suggest a common origin of oligodendroglioma and oligoastrocytoma. J Neuropathol Exp Neurol 54:91–95
16. Kepes JJ, Rubinstein LJ, Eng LF (1979) Pleomorphic xanthoastrocytoma: a distinctive meningocerebral glioma of young subjects with relatively favorable prognosis. Cancer 44:1839–1852
17. Collins VP, James CD (1993) Gene and chromosomal alterations associated with the development of human gliomas. FASEB J 7:926–930
18. Wong AJ, Zoltick PW, Moscatello DK (1994) The molecular biology and molecular genetics of astrocytic neoplasms. Semin Oncol 21:139–148
19. Batra SK, Rasheed BKA, Bigner SH, Bigner DD (1994) Oncogenes and anti-oncogenes in human central nervous system tumors. Lab Invest 71:621–637
20. von Deimling A, von Ammon K, Schoenfeld D, Wiestler OD, Seizinger BR, Louis DN (1993) Subsets of glioblastoma multiforme defined by molecular genetic analysis. Brain Pathol 3:19–26
21. Leenstra S, Bijlsma EK, Troost D, Oosting J, Westerveld A, Bosch DA, Hulsebos TJM (1994) Allele loss on chromosome 10 and 17p and epidermal growth factor gene amplification in human malignant astrocytoma related to prognosis. Br J Cancer 70:684–689
22. Rasheed BKA, McLendon RE, Herndon JE, Friedman HS, Friedman AH, Bigner DD, Bigner SH (1994) Alterations of the TP53 gene in human gliomas. Cancer Res 54:1324–1330
23. Schröck E, Thiel G, Lozanova T, du Manoir S, Meffert MC, Jauch A, Speicher MR, Nürnberg P, Vogel S, Jänisch W, Donis-Keller H, Ried T, Witkowski R, Cremer T (1994) Comparative genomic hybridization of human malignant gliomas reveals multiple amplification sites and nonrandom chromosomal gains and losses. Am J Pathol 144:1203–1218
24. Muleris M, Almeida A, Dutrillaux AM, Pruchon E, Vega F, Delattre JY, Poisson M, Malfoy B, Dutrillaux B (1994) Oncogene amplification in human gliomas: a molecular cytogenetic analysis. Oncogene 9:2717–2722
25. Reifenberger G, Liu L, Ichimura K, Schmidt EE, Collins VP (1993) Amplification and over-expression of the MDM2 gene in a subset of human malignant gliomas without p53 mutations. Cancer Res 53:2736–2739

26. Reifenberger G, Reifenberger J, Ichimura K, Meltzer P, Collins VP (1994) Amplification of multiple genes from chromosomal region 12q13–14 in human malignant gliomas: preliminary mapping of the amplicons shows preferential involvement of CDK4, SAS, and MDM2. Cancer Res 54:4299–4303

27. Schmidt EE, Ichimura K, Reifenberger G, Collins VP (1994) CDKN2 (p16/MTS1) gene deletion or CDK4 amplification occurs in the majority of glioblastomas. Cancer Res 54:6321–6324

28. Paulus W, Peiffer J (1988) Does the pleomorphic xanthoastrocytoma exist? Problems in the application of immunological techniques to the classification of brain tumors. Acta Neuropathol (Berl) 76:245–252

29. Paulus W, Peiffer J (1991) History, histology, histochemistry and histiocytic histogenesis of the pleomorphic xanthoastrocytoma. Brain Tumor Pathol 8:67–71

30. Kepes JJ (1993) Pleomorphic xanthoastrocytoma: the birth of a diagnosis and a concept. Brain Pathol 3:269–274.

31. Iwaki T, Fukui M, Kondo A, Matsushima T, Takeshita I (1987) Epithelial properties of pleomorphic xanthoastrocytomas determined in ultrastructural and immunohistochemical studies. Acta Neuropathol (Berl) 74:142–150

32. Sugita Y, Kepes JJ, Shigemori M, Kuramoto S, Reifenberger G, Kiwit JCW, Wechsler W (1990) Pleomorphic xanthoastrocytoma with desmoplastic reaction: angiomatous variant. Report of two cases. Clin Neuropathol 9:271–278

33. Lindboe FL, Cappelen J, Kepes JJ (1992) Pleomorphic xanthoastrocytoma as a component of a cerebellar ganglioglioma. Case report. Neurosurgery (Baltimore) 31:353–355

34. Daumas-Duport C, Scheithauer BW, Chodkiewicz JP, Laws ER, Vedrenne C (1988) Dysembryoplastic neuroepithelial tumor: a surgically curable tumor of young patients with intractable partial seizures. Neurosurgery (Baltimore) 23:545–556

35. Daumas-Duport C (1993) Dysembryoplastic neuroepithelial tumors. Brain Pathol 3:283–295

36. Kuchelmeister K, Demirel T, Schlörer E, Bergmann M, Gullotta F (1994) Dysembryoplastic neuroepithelial tumor of the cerebellum. A case report (abstract). Clin Neuropathol 13:256

37. Vandenberg SR, May EE, Rubinstein LJ, Herman MM, Perentes E, Vinores SA, Collins VP, Park TS (1987) Desmoplastic supratentorial neuroepithelial tumors of infancy with divergent differentiation potential ("desmoplastic infantile gangliogliomas"). Report on 11 cases of a distinctive embryonal tumor with favorable prognosis. J Neurosurg 66:58–71

38. Taratuto AL, Monges J, Lylyk P, Leiguardia R (1984) Superficial cerebral astrocytoma attached to dura. Report of six cases in infants. Cancer 54:2504–2512

39. Vandenberg SR (1993) Desmoplastic infantile ganglioglioma and desmoplastic cerebral astrocytoma of infancy. Brain Pathol 3:275–281

40. Burger PC, Scheithauer BW (1994) Tumors of the central nervous system. In: Atlas of tumor pathology, 3rd Series, Fasc 10. Armed Forces Institute of Pathology, Washington, DC

41. Hassoun J, Gambarelli D, Grisoli F, Pellet W, Salamon G, Pellissier JF, Toga M (1982) Central neurocytoma. An electron-microscopic study of two cases. Acta Neuropathol (Berl) 56:151–156

42. Hassoun J, Söylemezoglu F, Gambarelli D, Figarella-Branger D, von Ammon K, Kleihues P (1993) Central neurocytoma: a synopsis of clinical and histological features. Brain Pathol 3:297–306

43. Zülch KJ (1986) Brain tumors. Their biology and pathology, 3rd edn. Springer, Berlin Heidelberg New York Tokyo, pp 258–270

44. Hart NM, Earle KM (1973) Primitive neuroectodermal tumors in children. Cancer 32:172–188

45. Rorke LB (1983) The cerebellar medulloblastoma and its relationship to primitive neuroectodermal tumors. J Neuropathol Exp Neurol 42:1–15

46. Bonnin JM, Rubinstein LJ (1989) Asroblastomas: a pathological study of 23 tumors, with a postoperative follow-up in 13 patients. Neurosurgery (Baltimore) 25:6–13

47. Russell DS, Cairns H (1947) Polar spongioblastomas. Arch Histol Norm Patol 3:423–441

48. Bailey P, Bucy PC (1931) The origin and nature of meningeal tumors, Cancer Res 15:15–54

49. Cushing H, Eisenhardt L (1938) Meningiomas, their classification, regional behaviour, life history and surgical end results. Thomas, Springfield
50. Ruttledge MH, Xie YG, Han FY, Peyrard M, Collins VP, Nordenskjöld M, Dumanski JP (1994) Deletions on chromosome 22 in sporadic meningioma. Genes Chromosomes & Cancer 10:122–130
51. Sreekantaiah C, Bridge J, Rao U, Neff J, Sandberg AA (1981) Clonal chromosomal abnormalities in hemangiopericytoma. Cancer Genet Cytogenet 54:173–181
52. Herath SE, Stalboerger PG, Dahl RJ, Parisi JE, Jenkins RB (1994) Cytogenetic studies of four hemangiopericytomas. Cancer Genet Cytogenet 72:137–140
53. Enzinger FM, Weiss SW (1995) Soft tissue tumors, 3rd edn. Mosby, St. Louis, pp 713–729
54. Maier H, Öfner D, Hittmair A, Kitz K, Budka H (1992) Classic, atypical, and anaplastic meningioma: three histopathological subtypes of clinical relevance. J Neurosurg 77:616–623
55. Ruttlege MH, Sarrazin J, Rangaratnam S, Phelan CM, Twist E, Merel P, Delattre O, Thomas G, Nordenskjöld M, Collins VP, Dumanski JP, Rouleau GA (1994) Evidence for the complete inactivation of the NF2 gene in the majority of sporadic meningiomas. Nature Genet 6:180–184
56. von Deimling A, Wellenreuther R, Kraus JA, Lenartz D, Schramm J, Louis DN, Gusella JF, Wiestler OD (1994) Involvement of the NF2 gene in meningiomas (abstract). Clin Neuropathol 13:241–242
57. Bello MJ, de Campos JM, Kusak ME, Vaquero J, Sarasa JL, Pestana A, Rey JA (1994) Allelic loss at 1p is associated with tumor progression of meningiomas. Genes Chromosomes & Cancer 9:296–298
58. Lindblom A, Ruttledge M, Collins VP, Nordenskjold M, Dumanski JP (1994) Chromosomal deletions in anaplastic meningiomas suggest multiple regions outside chromosome 22 as important in tumor progression. Int J Cancer 56:354–357
59. Griffin CA, Hruban RH, Long PP, Miller N, Volz P, Carson B, Brem H (1994) Chromosome abnormalities in meningeal neoplasms: do they correlate with histology. Cancer Genet Cytogenet 78:46–52
60. Rempel SA, Schwechheimer K, Davis RL, Cavenee WK, Rosenblum ML (1993) Loss of heterozygosity for loci on chromosome 10 is associated with morphologically malignant meningioma progression. Cancer Res 53:2386–2392
61. Jellinger K, Paulus W (1991) Mesenchymal, non-meningothelial tumors of the central nervous system. Brain Pathol 1:79–87
62. Weiss SW (1994) Histological typing of soft tissue tumors, 2nd edn. Springer, Berlin Heidelberg New York
63. Frank TS, Trojanowski JQ, Roberts SA, Brooks JJ (1989) A detailed immunohistochemical analysis of cerebellar hemangioblastoma: an undifferentiated mesenchymal tumor. Mod Pathol 2:638–651
64. Becker I, Paulus W, Roggendorf W (1989) Histogenesis of stromal cells in cerebellar hemangioblastomas. An immunohistochemical study. Am J Pathol 134:271–275
65. Nemes Z (1992) Fibrohistiocytic differentiation in capillary hemangioblastoma. Hum Pathol 23:805–810
66. Latif F, Tory K, Gnarra J, Yao M, Duh FM, Orcutt ML, Stackhouse T, Kuzmin I, Modi W, Geil L, Schmidt L, Zhou F, Li H, Wei MH, Chen F, Glenn G, Choyke P, Walther MM, Weng Y, Duan DSR, Dean M, Glavac D, Richards FM, Crossey PA, Ferguson-Smith MA, Le Paslier D, Chumakov I, Cohen D, Chinault AC, Maher ER, Linehan WM, Zbar B, Lerman MI (1993) Identification of the von Hippel–Lindau disease tumor suppressor gene. Science 260:1317–1320
67. Kanno H, Kondo K, Ito S, Yamamoto I, Fujii S, Torigoe S, Sakai N, Hosaka M, Shuin T, Yao M (1994) Somatic mutations of the von Hippel–Lindau tumor suppressor gene in sporadic central nervous system hemangioblastomas. Cancer Res 54:4845–4847
68. Crossey PA, Foster K, Richards FM, Phipps ME, Latif F, Tory K, Jones MH, Bentley E, Kumar R, Lerman MI, Zbar B, Affara NA, Ferguson-Smith MA, Maher ER (1994) Molecular genetic investigations of the mechanisms of tumourigenesis in von Hippel–Lindau disease: analysis of allele loss in VHL tumours. Hum Genet 93:53–58

69. Shuin T, Kondo K, Torigoe S, Kishida T, Kubota Y, Hosaka M, Nagashima Y, Kitamura H, Latif F, Zbar B, Lerman MI, Yao M (1994) Frequent somatic mutations and loss of heterozygosity of the von Hippel–Lindau tumor suppressor gene in primary human renal cell carcinomas. Cancer Res 1994:2852–2855

70. Gnarra JR, Tory K, Weng Y, Schmidt L, Wei MH, Li H, Latif F, Liu S, Chen F, Duh FM, Lubenski I, Duan DR, Florence C, Pozzatti R, Walther MM, Bander NH, Grossman HB, Brauch H, Pomer S, Brooks JD, Isaacs WB, Lerman MI, Zbar B, Linehan WM (1994) Mutations of the *VHL* tumour suppressor gene in renal carcinoma. Nature Genet 7:85–89

71. Morii K, Tanaka R, Washiyama K, Kumanishi T, Kuwano R (1993) Expression of vascular endothelial growth factor in capillary hemangioblastoma. Biochem Biophys Res Commun 194:749–755

72. Plate K, Wizigmann-Voos S, Breier G, Risau W (1994) Evidence for a paracrine growth regulatory mechanism in human hemangioblastoma (abstract). Clin Neuropathol 13:264

73. Hufnagel TJ, Kim JH, True LD, Manuelidis EE (1989) Immunohistochemistry of capillary hemangioblastoma. Immunoperoxidase-labeled antibody staining resolves the differential diagnosis with metastatic renal cell carcinoma, but does not explain the histogenesis of the capillary hemangioblastoma. Am J Surg Pathol 13:207–216

74. National Cancer Institute sponsored study of classification of non-Hodgkin's lymphomas 1982. Summary and description of working formulation for clinical usage (1982). Cancer 49:2112–2135

75. Lennert K, Feller AC (1991) Histopathology of non-Hodgkin lymphomas (according to the updated Kiel classification), 2nd edn. Springer, Berlin Heidelberg New York

76. Grant JW, Isaacson PG (1992) Primary central nervous system lymphoma. Brain Pathol 2:97–109

77. Braus DF, Schwechheimer K, Müller-Hermelink HK, Schwarzkopf G, Volk B, Mundinger F (1992) Primary cerebral malignant non-Hodgkin's lymphomas: a retrospective clinical study. J Neurol 239:117–124

78. Mostofi FK (1977) Histological typing of testis tumors. International histological classification of tumors, no. 16. World Health Organization, Geneva

79. Friede RL (1978) Gliofibroma: a peculiar neoplasia of collagen forming glia-like cells. J Neuropathol Exp Neurol 37:300–313

80. Schober R, Bayindir C, Canbolat A, Urich H, Wechsler W (1992) Gliofibroma: immunohistochemical analysis. Acta Neuropathol (Berl) 83:207–210

81. Cerda-Nicolas M, Kepes JJ (1993) Gliofibromas (including malignant forms), and gliosarcomas: a comparative study and review of the literature. Acta Neuropathol 85:349–361

82. Wechsler W, Reifenberger G (1991) Immunohistochemistry in brain tumor classification. In: Paoletti P, Takakura K, Walker MD, Butti G, Pezzotta S (eds) Neuro-oncology. Kluwer, Netherlands, pp 11–19

83. Wechsler W, Reifenberger G (1989) Application of immunohistochemistry for tumor grading in human neuro-oncology. In: Fields WS (ed) Primary brain tumors—a review of histologic classification. Springer, Berlin Heidelberg New York, pp 133–141

84. Chozick BS, Pezzullo JC, Epstein MH, Finch PW (1994) Prognostic importance of p53 overexpression in supratentorial astrocic tumors. Neurosurgery (Baltimore) 35:831–838

Histological Aspects of Certain Benign Brain Tumors: Review of Current Topics

Asao Hirano, Kazuhiko Sugiyama, and Josefina F. Llena

Abstract. Histological features of certain mostly new entities of brain tumors are reviewed here. These include central neurocytoma, subependymal giant cell astrocytoma, pleomorphic xanthoastrocytoma, desmoplastic infantile ganglioglioma, meningoangiomatosis, and aggressive papillary tumor of the temporal bone. All these entitles were reported to have favorable outcomes following surgical removal.

Key words. Brain tumor—Histology—Electron microscopy—Immunohistochemistry

Introduction

The World Health Organization published the second edition of the International Histological Classification of CNS (central nervous system) Tumors in 1993 [1]. Several new entities such as central neurocytoma, pleomorphic xanthoastrocytoma, desmoplastic infantile ganglioglioma, dysembryoplastic neuroepithelial tumors, and paraganglioma of the filum terminale were included in the new edition. Several excellent reviews of these entities have been published [2–9].

In this chapter, we briefly review our experience at Montefiore and present highlights of the histological features of these tumors, as well as certain aspects of additional entities such as subependymal giant cell astrocytoma, meningo-angiomatosis, and aggressive papillary tumor of the temporal bone. It has been reported that all these tumors have a favorable prognosis after their surgical resection.

Central Neurocytoma

Almost 20 years ago, a large tumor mass of approximately 7 cm at its largest diameter was removed from the cerebellar vermis of an 18-month-old boy [10]. There was clear evidence of neuronal differentiation as documented by the presence of numerous synaptic vesicles in many cell processes and of occasional complete synapses in the tumor tissue. This unusual case was presented in 1978 at the International Congress

Division of Neuropathology, Department of Pathology, Montefiore Medical Center, The University Hospital for the Albert Einstein College of Medicine, Bronx, NY 10467, USA

of Neuropathology in Washington, DC [10], and published in *Acta Neuropathologica* in the same year [11]. The tumor cells were in many ways quite similar to the descending granule cells seen during development, but an important difference was the absence of Purkinje cells, the usual postsynaptic mates of the granule cells. Other neuronal and glial elements were also absent. A noteworthy histological feature of the tumor was a certain resemblance to the desmoplastic variant of medulloblastoma [12]. However, the latter lacks definite neuronal differentiation. The synaptic vesicles in cell processes of the tumor were mostly clear, round, and measured approximately 40–50 μm in diameter. Dense core vesicles were only occasionally seen. It is of interest that despite the absence of postsynaptic mates, presynaptic specializations were found frequently. These were termed "unattached presynaptic terminals" [13]. This case was reported as a cerebellar neuroblastoma [10,11], and similar cases have been reported by others [14] since its original description.

Hassoun et al. in 1982 [2] reported two cases of a primary tumor in the region of the foramen of Monro and septum pellucidum in young adults. The tumor is often calcified and is located primarily within the ventricular cavity, obstructing ventricular flow. Histologically it mimics oligodendroglioma, but neuronal differentiation of the tumor cells is evident as is demonstrated by the electron microscopic identification of synapses, clear presynaptic vesicles, and dense core vesicles, as well as by the immunohistochemical detection of synaptophysin [2]. In one of the six cases of central neurocytoma diagnosed in our institution (NS 88-171), both clear and dense core synaptic vesicles were seen in the cell processes. Although this tumor is also sometimes referred to as cerebral supratentorial or intraventricular neurocytoma, the term central neurocytoma has been generally used [2]. The tumor has also been reported in the fourth ventricle and inside the brain parenchyma and the spinal cord [2,14,15]. A comprehensive up-to-date review based on 127 published cases was presented by Hassoun et al. in 1993 [2]. The origin of the tumor cells of central neurocytoma is unknown and the nature of the transmitter substance involved remains to be investigated.

Subependymal Giant Cell Astrocytoma

In addition to central neurocytoma, two other benign tumors develop in the region of the foramen of Monro; one is subependymoma [16] and the other is subependymal giant cell astrocytoma. The latter tumor is composed mainly of large plump astrocytes. It may present additional histological features that may be deemed to be malignant as in our two 1990 cases. The first case was an 11-year-old boy with a family history of tuberous sclerosis. Although there was no neurological symptom, bilateral papilledema was found on routine ophthalmological examination and a large circumscribed intraventricular mass was identified by computed tomography (CT). The second case was a 4-year-old boy with no family history of tuberous sclerosis. This patient underwent partial resection of a large tumor in the region of the foramen of Monro in May 1990 and then total tumor removal in October 1990. The histological features of both cases were those of typical subependymal giant cell astrocytoma. However, in addition there were areas of focal necrosis associated with pseudopallisading, occasional endothelial proliferation, and sporadic mitosis. Although these findings would suggest a malignant tumor, the clinical course of the two patients has been uneventful. Similar cases were reported by Chow et al. in 1988 [17] and by Shepherd et al. in 1991 [18].

Pleomorphic Xanthoastrocytoma

This rare variant of astrocytoma was described by Kepes et al. in 1979 and reviewed by Kepes in 1993 [3]. It occurs in children or young adults and involves superficial areas of the cerebral hemispheres, especially the temporal lobe. The tumor is often associated with a cyst. As its name implies, this pleomorphic astrocytoma exhibits various froms, ranging from the usual fibrillary astrocytes to giant multinucleated forms. The giant cells typically contain lipids and express glial fibrillary acidic protein (GFAP). The tumor shows an intimate relationship with the meninges; it stains with reticulin because of the presence of basal lamina overlying the subpial astrocytes that face the subarachnoid space. Despite histological features of pleomorphism, nuclear atypia, and bizarre multinucleated giant tumor cells, macroscopically the tumor is usually well demarcated and in general has a relatively favorable prognosis. Necrosis and endothelial proliferation are usually absent, and mitotic figures are rare. The development of malignancy has been reported in a minority of pleomorphic xantho-astrocytomas [3]. It is thought that pial astrocytes are the most likely cells originating the tumor, of which 14 cases have been reported in Japan [19].

Our first experience with this type of tumor was a consultation case of the late Professor Yoichi Ishida who visited our laboratory on September 1, 1980. The patient was a 37-year-old man who had seizures and very slowly progressing difficulties with walking since the age of 17. A well-circumscribed cystic mass (approximately 3 cm in diameter) was removed from the right temporal lobe of the patient. The histology was identical to that described by Kepes in 1979 as "xanthomatous lesions of the central nervous system" [20]. It should be mentioned in this context that one of our rather early experiences with this tumor was a patient who was operated on in 1967 with the diagnosis of glioblastoma (NS 5936). To our surprise, the patient was alive and well in August 1983. This prompted a new review of the slides, and at that time the diagnosis of pleomorphic xanthoastrocytoma was made. Two subsequent cases, a 3-year-old girl (NS 85-118) and a 19-year-old boy (NS 86-3), are illustrated in the *Color Atlas of Neuropathology* [21].

Dysembryoplastic Neuroepithelial Tumor

Uncommon supratentorial lesions affecting adolescents and young adults with a long history of partial complex seizures were reported from several institutions in 1988 (see [22]). The name dysembryoplastic neuroepithelial tumor (DNT) has been used in the International Histological Classification of Tumors [1] to describe the characteristic clinicohistological features of the new entity, which were first described and reviewed by Daumas-Duport et al. Several studies of this entity and related subjects have been published recently from various institutions [6–9,23–25].

Meningoangiomatosis

Meningoangiomatosis is a rare benign intracranial lesion associated with von Recklinghausen disease. As its name indicates, it is composed of meninx and vasculature admixed with altered cerebral cortex producing the characteristic localized histological features. Meningoangiomatosis may also occur in patients with no family history of von Recklinghausen disease, such as case 1 of Halper et al. [26]. One of the most interesting histological features of the lesion are Alzheimer's neurofibrillary changes in the affected neurons in the tumor. Although "Alzheimer's neurofibrillary changes" is one of the best known terms in neuropathology, these types of changes are rarely found in neurooncology. We have seen them only once in a cerebral cortical tuber of a patient with tuberous sclerosis [27]. At the request of Dr. Scheithauer of Mayo Clinic, we carried out an electron microscopic study of the tissue of case 1 reported by Halper et al. in 1986 [26] and confirmed the light microscopic findings of Alzheimer's neurofibrillary tangles in this case. As far as we are aware, no further fine structural analyses of such meningoangiomatosis changes have been reported.

We describe next some additional ultrastructural features of meningo-angiomatosis. The cells composing this tumor are endothelial cells, pericytes, smooth muscle cells, fibroblasts, astrocytes, and neurons. These cells are well differen-tiated and contain their respective intermediate filaments. The astrocyte processes display remarkably well-formed, thin, sheathlike expansions that contain compact bundles of glial filaments. Numerous Alzheimer's neurofibrillary tangles are evi-dent in neurons. The individual filaments display both constricted forms with peri-odic narrowings and straight forms without regular constrictions, identical to those reported in Alzheimer's disease and other conditions. All filaments are within the neuron, and unlike advanced lesions in certain neurodegenerative diseases with cell loss, no extracellular neurofibrillary tangles are seen in meningo-angiomatosis.

The intraganglionic filaments may run in the same direction or may be distributed randomly among the other neuronal organelles. The abnormal neurons are found very close to large extracellular spaces that contain large numbers of collagen fibers. However, a thin astrocytic cell process is always identified between the neuron and the collagen-rich extracellular space, and no neuron is exposed directly to the extracellular space. The external plasma membrane of the astrocytes facing connec-tive tissue is always covered by a basal lamina. Thus, the normal mature central nervous system appearance is clearly maintained in such a complex pathological tissue as that of meningoangiomatosis. Amyloid, one of the essential elements of Alzheimer's disease, is absent in this condition. The coexistence of glial fibrils and Alzheimer's neurofibrillary tangles in the same astrocyte, reported by Nakano et al. [28] in an atypical case of Alzheimer's disease with extraordinarily prolonged clinical course, has not been observed in this entity. The results of an immunohistochemical study of Alzheimer's neurofibrillary tangles in one meningoangiomatosis case have been reported [29].

Desmoplastic Infantile Ganglioglioma

We became aware of the rare new brain tumor entity called desmoplastic cerebral astrocytoma of infancy, which was first described by Taratuto et al. in 1984, through the fifth edition of Rubinstein's *Pathology of Tumours of the Nervous System* [30]. In their original report, Taratuto et al. [31] described six cases of superficial cerebral astrocytoma attached to the dura of infants. This generally massive and grossly cystic tumor has a predilection for the frontoparietal region. The remarkable feature of this tumor is its apparently favorable course after resection. Its recognition has been, by and large, facilitated by the use of the GFAP stain that readily rules out the possibility of a fibrosarcoma. Furthermore, expression of immunohistochemical neuron markers such as neurofilaments and synaptophysin has been demonstrated with frequency, denoting neuronal differentiation in addition to glial components. Thus, VandenBerg et al. proposed the term desmoplastic infantile ganglioglioma in 1987 [32].

Our experience with this entity was gained by reviewing stained slides of a case that was presented in 1993 by Sugiyama et al. at the clinicopathological session of the 11th meeting of the Japanese Society of Brain Tumor Pathology. The patient was a 2-month-old girl with a large frontoparietal mass and prominent hydrocephalus. The histology of the tumor was that of a typical desmoplastic infantile ganglioglioma, that is, a mixed neuronal and astrocytic neoplasm with a prominent desmoplastic component. In addition to GFAP-positive glial cells, there were neurons that reacted with antineurofilament protein antibody. Reticulin staining was strongly positive in the tumor tissue. The patients is doing well and had no recurrence 2 years after surgery.

One case of desmoplastic infantile ganglioglioma was presented at the slide session of the 69th annual meeting of the American Association of Neuropathologists held at Salt Lake City, Utab, in 1993 (case 8). Another case presented at the same meeting was reported recently in *Acta Neuropathologica* [33]. A review of the subject and the follow-up of 22 cases of desmoplastic infantile ganglioglioma was presented by VandenBerg in 1993 [5], who confirmed the good prognosis of this condition. Another Japanese case was reported in 1994 [34].

Aggressive Papillary Tumor of the Temporal Bone

A petrous bone tumor was recently removed at Montefiore Medical Center from each of three patients who had a clinical history of hearing loss and facial palys. A destructive lesion involving the region of the unilateral petrous bone was observed in these patients. The preoperative diagnosis in two patients (NS 90-49, a 19-year-old girl, and NS 90-125, a 40-year-old woman) was that of a jugular glomus tumor. In the third patient (a 37-year-old woman), a schwannoma at the cerebellopontine angle was suspected before her first operation (NS 93-87), and a petrous bone tumor was removed from the same location at the second operation (N 93-179). The histology of the three tumors was identical, with features of a well-developed papillary adenoma instead of a paraganglioma or schwannoma. The basal portion of the cuboidal or low columnar epithelium was marked by an ample, pale, vacuolated cytoplasm and the nuclei located toward the apical region. The keratin and cytokeratin reactions were positive, and a strong reaction for vimentin was noted in the basal half of the epithelium. The blood vessels were fenestrated and the microvilli were short and stubby. No cilia were identified and mitoses were absent.

These histological features are identical to those reported recently as typical of aggressive papillary tumor of temporal bone [35]. This primary tumor has a slow growth rate and is histologically benign, not metastasizing elsewhere. The tumor destroys the posterior temporal bone and may extend into the intracranial posterior fossa, as occurred in our third patient. It has been postulated that the tumor originates from the endolymphatic sac [36]. Aggressive papillary tumors of the temporal bone have usually been treated by otolaryngologists, but participation of neurosurgens has promoted its recognition as a neuropathology entity. Thus, a case report was published for the first time in a Japanese neurosurgical journal by Kuroiwa et al. in 1993 [37].

Acknowledgments. The authors are grateful to Dr. Fritz Herz for his valuable criticism during the preparation of this manuscript.

References

1. Kleihues P, Burger PC, Scheithauer BW (1993) Histological typing of tumours of the central nervous system, 2nd edn. Springer, Berlin, pp 1–112
2. Hassoun F, Soylemezoglu F, Gambarelli D, Figarella-Branger D, von Ammon K, Kleihues P (1993) Central neurocytoma: a synopsis of clinical and histological features. Brain Pathol 3:297–306
3. Kepes JJ (1993) Pleomorphic xanthoastrocytoma: the birth of a diagnosis and a concept. Brain Pathol 3:269–274
4. VandenBerg SR (1993) Desmoplastic infantile ganglioglioma and desmoplastic cerebral astrocytoma of infancy. Brain Pathol 3:275–281
5. VandenBerg SR (1992) Current diagnostic concepts of astrocytic tumors. J Neuropathol Exp Neurol 51:644–657
6. Daumas-Duport C (1993) Dysembryoplastic neuroepithelial tumors. Brain Pathol 3:283–295
7. Hirose T, Scheithauer BW, Lopes MBS, VandenBerg SR (1994) Dysembryoplastic neuroepithelial tumor (DNT): an immunohistochemical and ultrastructural study. J Neuropathol Exp Neurol 53:184–195
8. Raymond AA, Halpin SFS, Alsanjari N, Cook MJ, Kitchen ND, Fish DR, Steven JM, Harding BN, Scaravilli F, Kendall B, Shorvon SD, Neville BGR (1994) Dysembryoplastic neuroepithelial tumor. Features in 16 patients. Brain 117:461–475
9. Leung SY, Gwi E, Ng HK, Fung CF, Yam KY (1994) Dysembryoplastic neuroepithelial tumor. A tumor with small neuronal cells resembling oligodendroglioma. Am J Surg Pathol 18:604–614
10. Shin WY, Laufer H, Hirano A, Zimmerman HM (1978) Fine structure of a cerebellar neuroblastoma. In: Abstracts, 8th international congress of neuropathology, Washington DC, USA, p 690
11. Shin W-Y, Laufer H, Lee Y-C, Aftalion B, Hirano A, Zimmerman HM (1978) Fine structure of a cerebellar neuroblastoma. Acta Neuropathol 42:11–13
12. Russell DS, Rubinstein LT (1989) Pathology of tumours of the nervous system, 5th edn. Williams and Wilkins, Baltimore, pp 261–263
13. Hirano A, Shin W-Y (1979) Unattached presynaptic terminals in a cerebellar neuroblastoma in the human. Neuropathol Appl Neurobiol 5:63–70
14. Russell DS, Rubinstein LJ (1989) Pathology of tumours of the nervous system, 5th edn. Williams and Wilkins, Baltimore, pp 265–266
15. Coca S, Moreno M, Martos JA, Rodriguez J, Barcena A, Vaquero J (1994) Neurocytoma of spinal cord. Acta Neuropathol 87:537–540
16. Hirano A (1992) Guide to neuropathology, 3rd edn. Igaku-Shoin, Tokyo, p 300
17. Chow CW, Klug GL, Lewis EA (1988) Subependynal giant-cell astrocytoma in children: an unusual discrepancy between histology and clinical features. J Neurosurg 68:880–883
18. Shephered CW, Scheithauer BW, Gomez MR, Altermatt HJ, Katzmann JA (1991) Subependymal giant-cell astrocytoma: a chemical, pathological and flow cytometric study. Neurosurgery 28:864–868
19. Kawano N (1992) Pleomorphic xanthoastrocytoma: some new observations. Neuropathology 11:323–328
20. Kepes JJ (1979) "Xanthomatous" lesions of the central nervous system: definition, classification and some recent observations. In: Zimmerman HM (ed) Progress in neuropathology, Vol 4. Raven, New York, pp 179–214
21. Hirano A (1988) Color atlas of pathology of the nervous system, 2nd edn. Igaku-Shoin, Tokyo, p 123
22. Hirano A (1994) Benign intracranial cysts and certain congenital neoplasms. Brain Tumor Pathol 11:51–58

23. Plate KH, Wieser H-G, Yasargil MG, Wiestler OD (1993) Neuropathological findings in 224 patients with temporal lobe epilepsy. Acta Neuropathol 86:433–438
24. Armstrong DD (1993) Neuropathology of temporal lobe epilepsy. J Neuropathol Exp Neurol 52:433–443
25. Matsuda K, Hirano A (1994) Neuropathology of epilepsy. In: Asakura T (ed) Recent surgical therapy of epilepsy. Igaku-Shoin, Tokyo, pp 12–15
26. Halper J, Scheithauer BW, Okazaki H, Laws ER Jr (1986) Meningo-angiomatosis: a report of six cases with special reference to the occurrence of neurofibrillary tangles. J Neuropathol Exp Neurol 45:426–446
27. Hirano A, Tuazon R, Zimmerman HM (1968) Neurofibrillary changes, granulovacuolar bodies and argentophilic globules observed in tuberous sclerosis. Acta Neuropathol 11:257–261
28. Nakano I, Iwatsubo T, Otsuka N, Kamei M, Matsumura K, Mannen T (1992) Paired helical filaments in astrocytes: electron microscopy and immunohistochemistry in a case of atypical Alzheimer's disease. Acta Neuropathol 83:228–232
29. Goates JJ, Dickson DW, Horoupian DS (1991) Meningoangiomatosis: an immunohistochemical study. Acta Neuropathol 82:527–532
30. Russell DS, Rubinstein LJ (1989) Pathology of tumours of the nervous system, 5th edn. Williams and Wilkins, Baltimore, p 124
31. Taratuto AL, Monges J, Lylyk P, Leigurada R (1984) Superficial cerebral astrocytoma attached to dura. Report of six cases in infants. Cancer 54:2505–2512
32. VandenBerg SR, May EE, Rubinstein LJ, Herman MM, Perentes E, Vinores SA, Collins VP, Park TS (1987) Desmoplastic supratentorial neuroepithelial tumors of infancy with divergent differentiation potential ("desmoplastic infantile gangliogliomas"). Report on 11 cases of a distinctive embryonal tumor with favorable prognosis. J Neurosurg 66:58–71
33. Aydin F, Ghatak NR, Salvant J, Muizelaar P (1993) Desmoplastic cerebral astrocytoma of infancy. A case report with immunohistochemical, ultrastructural and proliferation studies. Acta Neuropathol 86:666–670
34. Tadokoro M, Ozawa T, Abe M, Shinagawa T, Sakurai T, Taguchi Y (1994) A case of desmoplastic infantile ganglioglioma. Brain Tumor Pathol 11:93–98
35. Poe DS, Tarlov EC, Thomas CB, Kveton JA (1993) Aggressive papillary tumors of temporal bone. Otolaryngol Head Neck Surg 108:80–86
36. Heffner DK (1989) Low-grade adenocarcinoma of probable endolymphatic sac origin: a clinicopathologic study of 20 cases. Cancer 64:2292–2302
37. Kuroiwa T, Moriwaki K, Nagasawa S, Ohta T (1993) Primary adenomatous tumor of the middle ear: a case report. Neurol Surg (Tokyo) 21:463–466

The Statistical Analysis of Prognostic Factors for Brain Tumors

Kazuhiro Nomura[1,2], Naohito Yamaguchi[3], and Show Watanabe[3]

Abstract. The study population consisted of cases diagnosed as astrocytoma (AS), malignant astrocytoma (MA), and glioblastoma multiforme (GM) in the supratentorial region and listed by the Brain Tumor Registry of Japan from 1978 to 1987. Prognostic factors (PFs) for survival were analyzed by the Kaplan–Meier (KM) method, Cox proportional hazards (Cox) model, regression tree (RT) analysis, and others. The PFs examined here were histological types (AS, MA, and GM), location of tumor (A, cerebral lobes; B, ventricles or para-ventricles; C, basal ganglia or rostral brainstem region), size of tumor (5 cm or less compared to larger than 5 cm), and clinical grade (better, those with less than severe clinical signs; worse, those with disturbance in consciousness or in the respiratory center). All the PFs showed significant association with survival in univariate analysis by the KM method. The largest relative contribution was histological type (58%, log rank statistics contribution) and the second largest was age (52%). The Cox model was also applied separately to each of three histological types to evaluate the joint effects of these three PFs and revealed that three explanatory variables, except tumor location A compared to B, showed significant associations with the survival in all histological types. The results of regression tree analysis revealed that all the cases were first classified by age, 50 years or younger compared to older than 50 (920 in log rank score), followed by histological type (584) for age 50 or younger, and clinical grade (102) for age over 50 years. Significant survival difference among terminal groups classified by regression tree analysis would suggest that clinical treatment trial design for malignant glioma patients should be categorized to several more homogeneous patient subgroups.

Key words. Prognostic factor—Regression tree analysis—Astrocytic tumor—Brain tumor

[1] Department of Neurosurgery, National Cancer Center Hospital, Chuo-ku, Tokyo, Japan
[2] The Committee of Brain Tumor Registry of Japan, Chuo-ku, Tokyo, Japan
[3] Epidemiology Division, National Cancer Center Research Institute, Chuo-ku, Tokyo, Japan

Introduction

Several prognostic variables could be identified as statistically significant for brain tumors [1]. They are mainly age at diagnosis, histological grade of tumor, and performance status before and after operation. On the other hand, the T(N)M classification of brain tumor has been proposed by International Union Against Cancer (UICC) for all kinds of brain tumors pathologically determined. However, it is obvious that this classification could not apply to all kinds of brain tumor. No neurooncologist would believe that extraaxial tumors, such as meningioma, schwannoma, and others, could be discussed on the same basis of prognostic factors as intraaxial tumors such as gliomas. This is because the location, but not the extent of tumor in T(N)M classification, would be the most important prognostic factor for extraaxial tumors such as meningioma and other, different prognostic factors would exist for other tumors of this category. From this point of view, we chose astrocytic tumor in the supratentorial region for the trial of the T(N)M classification. Because the Brain Tumor Registry of Japan had already collected data on more than 53000 patients with brain tumors between 1969 and 1987, it was possible to analyze the multivariant factors for selected supratentorial astrocytic tumors. This chapter presents the results of the determination of prognostic factors for making suitable T(N)M classifications.

Material and Methods

Study Subjects

The study population consists of cases registered to the Brain Tumor Registry of Japan. The cases included were those diagnosed as having astrocytoma, malignant astrocytoma, or glioblastoma multiforme during the period from 1978 to 1987, because computed tomography (CT) scanning became popular in Japan after 1975. We restricted the current analysis to patients with tumors located in the lobe, ventricle, or deep brain regions of the supratentorial location. A total of 4864 cases were identified in the brain tumor database, of which 1621 cases were astrocytoma, 995 malignant astrocytoma, and 1966 glioblastoma multiforme. We excluded 282 cases because of inadequate information about birth date, date of diagnosis, or date of observation.

Prognostic Factors

The prognostic factors examined in the present analysis were histological type (astrocytoma, malignant astrocytoma, glioblastoma multiforme), location of tumor (A, B, or C), size of tumor (5 cm or less versus larger than 5 cm), and clinical grade (better versus worse). Category A of tumor location consists of tumors in the frontal, temporal, parietal, and occipital lobes. Category B consists of tumors in the third ventricle, lateral ventricle, and pineal region. Category C consists of tumors in corpus callosum, septum pellucidum, rostral brainstem, basal ganglia, and aqueduct. Clinical grades were classified according to patient status (1, no sign or symptom; 2, subjective complaints only; 3, focal signs and symptoms; 4, signs and symptoms of intracranial hypertension; 5, conscious disturbance; 6, coma; 7, disturbance of respiratory center);

a tumor was classified into the "worse" clinical grade if the patient had disturbance in consciousness or disturbance in the respiratory center. Those patients with tumors with less severe clinical signs were classified into the "better" clinical grade. Age at diagnosis was dichotomized to 50 years or younger.

Statistical Methods

Distribution of survival functions were estimated by the Kaplan–Meier method [2] for various subgroups of cases. The log rank and Wilcoxon test statistics were calculated to test the difference between two or more survival functions [3]. The joint effects of more than one prognostic factor were evaluated by the forward stepwise procedure, in which covariates are added to the set of explanatory variables so far as the improvement log rank statistic was significant at the 5% significance level [4]. The relative contribution of each covariate to the joint effect chi-square was evaluated by the linear regression method, in which the overall log rank score for the joint effect was modeled as linear combinations of covariates [4]. The Cox proportional hazards model was also applied to the data to evaluate the magnitude of effects of prognostic factors [5]. The cases were classified in terms of survival by the regression treelike method [6]. The best combination of prognostic factors was identified as that by which the survival functions were differentiated most efficiently. In this method, a group of cases was further split into daughter groups by a prognostic factor for which the goodness-of-split statistic was the largest and significant at the 5% level among prognostic factors yet to be considered. We adopted the marginal log rank score as the goodness-of-split statistic [7]. All the prognostic factors are dichotomized or trichotomized in advance on the basis of clinical practice. Accordingly, a group of cases was divided into three daughter groups if any pair of the three categories exhibited a significant log rank score. The splitting procedure was terminated when none of remaining prognostic factors showed significant log rank score at the 5% level.

Results

All the prognostic factors showed significant associations with the survival cases in univariate analysis by the Kaplan–Meier method (results not shown). The histological type showed the largest log rank score of 1143.7 with 2 degrees of freedom (df), followed by age group, 1002.9 with 1 df, and then clinical grade, 344.7 with 1 df. Furthermore, the effects of all the factors were statistically significant when the joint effects were evaluated by the forward stepwise procedure. The relative contribution to this overall log rank statistic was the largest for the histological type, by which 58% of the total log rank statistic could be explained (Table 1). The second largest contribution was made by age, the proportion being 52%. The contribution of the combination of histological type and age amounted to 85%. The risk ratio to most favored group in survival by the analysis based on the Cox proportional hazards model was also applied to histological types, tumor location, age, tumor size, and clinical grade using the stepwise selection procedure. The results are shown in Table 2. In histological types, glioblastoma showed the highest value of 3.2 as compared to astrocytoma with a 95% confidence interval of 2.91–3.54, followed by malignant astrocytoma at 2.0 (CI = 1.81–2.25). For other prognostic factors, tumor location showed a value of 1.79 (CI = 1.58–

Table 1. Relative contribution of prognostic factors to the joint-effect log rank statistic.[a]

Model	Histology	Age	Clinical grade	Size of tumor	Location of tumor	Number of factors	Contribution (%)
1					X	1	1.1
2				X		1	2.5
3			X			1	17
4		X				1	51.5
5	X					1	58.4
6				X	X	2	3.7
7			X		X	2	17.8
8			X	X		2	18.7
9		X			X	2	53.9
10		X		X		2	54
11	X			X		2	59.8
12	X				X	2	61
13		X	X			2	64.1
14	X		X			2	70.8
15	X	X				2	85.4
16			X	X	X	3	19.5
17		X		X	X	3	56.6
18	X			X	X	3	62.6
19		X	X	X		3	65.8
20		X	X		X	3	66
21	X		X	X		3	71.7
22	X		X		X	3	73
23	X	X		X		3	87
24	X	X			X	3	89
25	X	X	X			3	95.7
26		X	X	X	X	4	67.9
27	X		X	X	X	4	74
28	X	X		X	X	4	90.8
29	X	X	X	X		4	96.7
30	X	X	X		X	4	98.8
31	X	X	X	X	X	5	100

X, Prognostic factors included in the model.
[a] The two best models are displayed for each model with different numbers of independent variables.

Table 2. Survival analysis of astrocytic tumors based on Cox proportional hazards model with stepwise selection procedure.

	Risk ratio	95% CI
Astrocytoma	1.00	
Malignant astrocytoma	2.02	1.81–2.25
Glioblastoma multiforme	3.21	2.91–3.54
Lobes, Ventricles, and pineal region	1.00	
Brainstem	1.79	1.58–2.02
Age 50 years or younger	1.00	
Age greater than 50 years	2.28	2.11–2.47
Size $\leq$ 5 cm	1.00	
Size > 5 cm	1.17	1.09–1.26
Clinical grade, better	1.00	
Clinical grade, worse	1.77	1.60–1.95

CI, confidence interval.

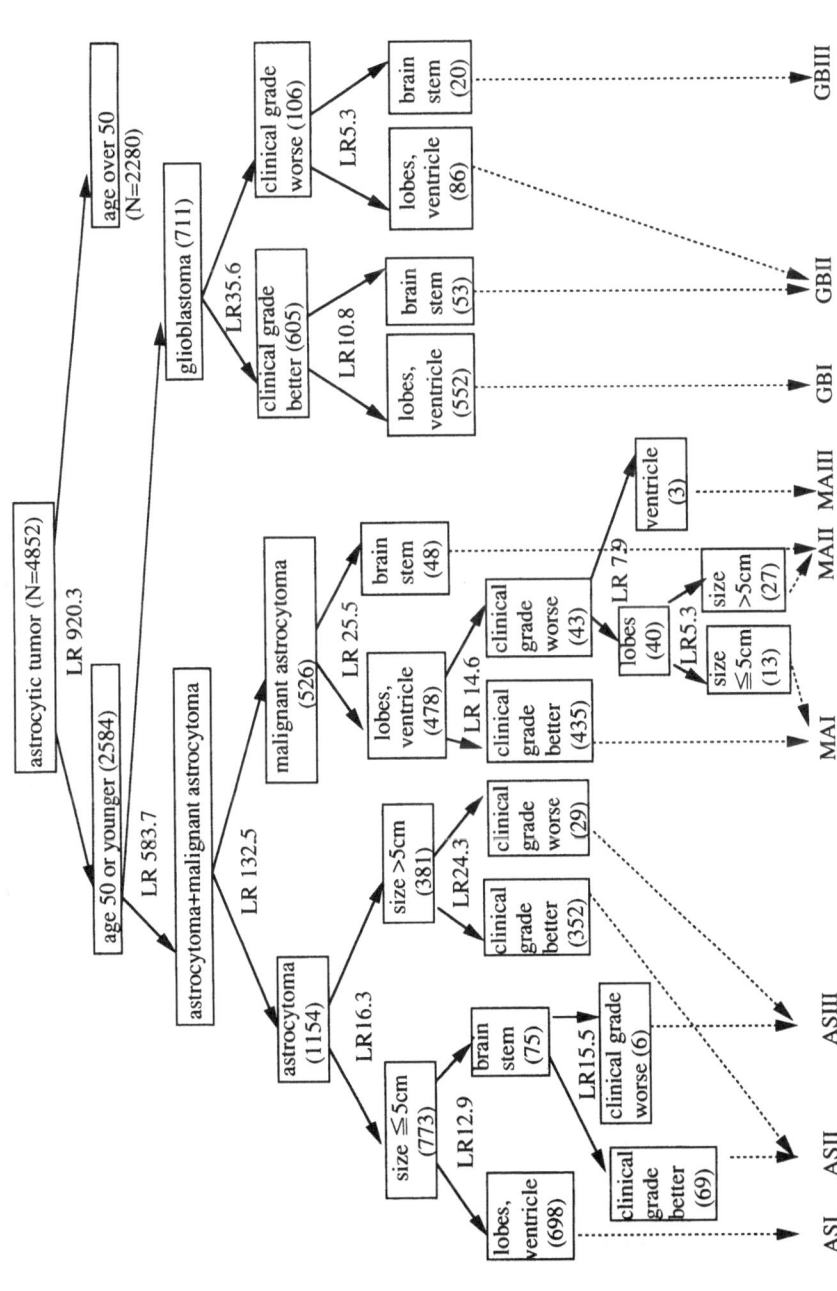

Fig. 1. Regression tree of prognostic factors (50 years or younger age group)

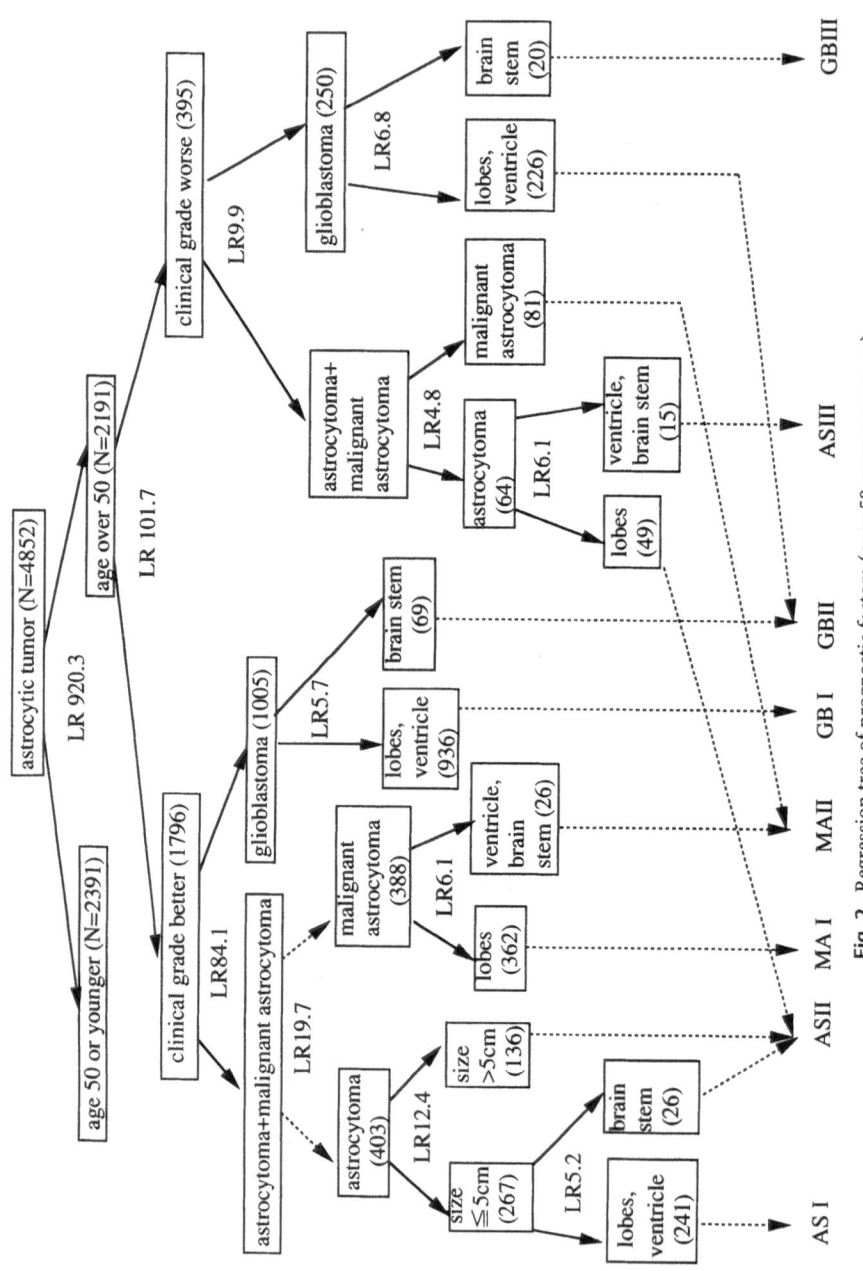

Fig. 2. Regression tree of prognostic factors (over 50 years age group)

2.02), age that of 2.28 (2.11–2.47), size a value of 1.17 (1.09–1.28), and clinical grade was 1.77 (1.6–1.95) versus each standard group, respectively.

Regression Tree Analysis

The result of regression tree analysis is shown in Figs. 1 and 2. All the cases were first classified by age, 50 years or younger or over 50, which showed the largest log rank score of 920.3. Therefore, the result of the analysis would be described by classifying two age groups.

Patients Aged 50 Years or Younger

The most significant split was by histological type (Fig. 1). An additional split among astrocytomas of this age group was created by the tumor size. Thereafter, astrocytoma cases with a tumor size of 5 cm or less were classified significantly by tumor location A and B versus C, and that of location C was divided into two clinical grades, better or worse. On the other hand, among astrocytoma cases with tumor size larger than 5 cm, only clinical grade created an additional split with median survival time (MST) of 5 years for better clinical grades and 1 year and 4 months for worse clinical grades, respectively. Accordingly, astrocytoma was classified into five prognostic groups.

Malignant astrocytoma was classified by location after split of age. The location A and B were merged into one category because the log rank scores for comparisons of A versus B were not statistically significant. Those located in the A and B clinical grade showed significant association with survival. The tumor size further was significant only in the cases with worse clinical grade and location A. Of those located in C, the tumor size as well as clinical grade did not show any significant association with survival. Thus, malignant astrocytoma was classified into five prognostic groups.

Glioblastoma multiforme was first classified by the clinical grade. Those with either clinical grade were further classified by the tumor location, A and B versus C. Therefore, glioblastoma multiforme was split into four prognostic groups in this age group.

Patients Older Than 50 Years

For this age group (Fig. 2), patients were first classified by clinical grade and then by histological type. Cases with astrocytoma of better clinical grade were further classified by tumor size. Thereafter, for cases with tumor size of 5 cm or less, location was split A + B versus C, while for those with tumor size of more than 5 cm, this was the last branch. The cases with worse clinical grade split in two categories, location A versus B and C as a last branch. For malignant astrocytomas and glioblastomas, the cases with better clinical grade split A versus B and C. Malignant astrocytoma in this category showed no significant subclassification when analyzed by the factor of tumor size or tumor location. Therefore, in cases with age of more than 50 years, astrocytoma, malignant astrocytoma, and glioblastoma split into five, three, and four prognostic groups, respectively.

Discussion

Brain tumors are mainly classified as extraaxial and intraaxial by their location. In this classification, meningioma, schwannoma, and pituitary adenoma belong to the former category and glioma to the latter. This original location of the tumor is significantly related to prognosis of the patients, as the 5-year survival rate of patients with extraaxial brain tumors was 95%, while those with intraaxial tumors was 38% [8]. For these extraaxial tumors, it is not useful to classify them into stages such as T(N)M, they should be classified by other independent factors. On the other hand, patients with intraaxial tumors, especially gliomas, could not be cured by surgical resection only because of infiltration into normal brain tissue, and thus the staging system of T(N)M classification could be applied to such cases.

It is well known that glioma is pathologically classified into more than ten different kinds of tumors. Each of these shows different characteristics of infiltration into the normal brain tissue. Glioblastoma shows rapid growth and develops early in regions far distant from the site of origin in the brain. Oligodendroglioma is mostly well localized in the early stage of the disease. In this sense, the glioma itself would be divided into two categories, astrocytic tumor and nonastrocytic tumor. The former constitutes astrocytoma, anaplastic (malignant) astrocytoma, and glioblastoma, and the latter oligodendroglioma, ependymoma, choroid plexus papilloma, and other relatively rare glial tumors. In this classification, astrocytic tumor accounts for the highest frequency of gliomas, and a large number of cases could be analyzed for prognostic factors in a short time.

This chapter has presented the results of computer analysis of the prognostic factors on astrocytic tumors. Tumor location is very important, even for astrocytic tumor, whether infratentorial or supratentorial. It is well known that patients with infratentorial astrocytoma show much better prognosis than those with supratentorial, and thus we could not discuss these tumors together. Therefore, we considered only supratentorial astrocytic tumors to avoid such complications.

Prognosis of the tumor was first studied by univariate analysis. Histological type, age, and clinical grade showed a significant difference ($P < 0.0001$) between factors in each of these categories. Patients with tumors in the ventricle system showed better prognosis than those with tumors in other regions. This means that tumors in the ventricles did not always indicate the poorer prognostic factor, as was suggested in the T(N)M classification on brain tumors. The result of regression tree analysis (Figs. 1 and 2) showed that astrocytic tumors of the group aged 50 years or younger were divided into three categories depending on the degree of pathological malignancy, astrocytoma, malignant astrocytoma, and glioblastomas. In the case of astrocytoma, which means well-differentiated astrocytoma, the size of tumor was related to the prognosis directly (see Fig. 1), but in other tumors diagnosed as malignant astrocytoma, the size of tumor became the less important prognostic factor, shown as log rank value of 5.3, even in the cases in which tumor location in the lobes was limited.

Glioblastoma did not show any significant difference by the factor of tumor size. However, for malignant astrocytoma and glioblastoma, clinical grade was the next important prognostic factor, followed by pathological grades. This indicated that clinical grade could show a much more exact extent of tumor in these infiltrative tumors than findings from modern imaging systems (CT or MRI), which could not determine the exact prognosis. On the other hand, astrocytic tumors of age over 50

Table 3. Survival and classes by regression tree analysis of prognostic factors.

Class		Histology	Size	Locations	Clinical grade	MST
Age 50 years or younger						
AS	I	Astrocytoma	≦5 cm	A + B	—	>10 yr
AS	II	Astrocytoma	≦5 cm	C	Better ⎫	
		Astrocytoma	>5 cm	—	Better ⎭	5 yr
AS	III	Astrocytoma	≦5 cm	C	Worse ⎫	
		Astrocytoma	>5 cm	—	Worse ⎭	1 yr 5 mo
MA	I	Malignant astrocytoma		A + B	Better ⎫	
		Malignant astrocytoma	≦5 cm	A	Worse ⎭	3 yr 2 mo
MA	II	Malignant astrocytoma		C	— ⎫	
		Malignant astrocytoma	>5 cm	A	Worse ⎭	1 yr 2 mo
MA	III	Malignant astrocytoma		B	worse	3 mo
GB	I	Glioblastoma		A + B	Better	1 yr 4 mo
GB	II	Glioblastoma		C	Better ⎫	
		Glioblastoma		A + B	Worse ⎭	11 mo
GB	III	Glioblastoma		C	Worse	3 mo
Age more than 50 years						
AS	I	Astrocytoma		A + B	Better	1 yr 9 mo
AS	II	Astrocytoma		C	Better ⎫	
		Astrocytoma		—	Better ⎬	1 yr
		Astrocytoma		A	Worse ⎭	
AS	III	Astrocytoma		B + C	Worse	4 mo
MA	I	Malignant astrocytoma		A	Better ⎫	
		Malignant astrocytoma		B + C	Better ⎭	1 yr 1 mo
MA	II	Malignant astrocytoma		—	Worse	7 mo
GB	I	Glioblastoma		A + B	Better	10 mo
GB	II	Glioblastoma		C	Better ⎫	
		Glioblastoma		A + B	Worse ⎭	5 mo
GB	III	Glioblastoma		C	Worse	3 mo

AS, astrocytoma; MA, malignant astrocytoma; GB, glioblastoma multitorma; MST, median survival time; A, cerebral lobes; B, ventricle and paraventricle; C, mainly basal ganglia and rostral brain stem (see text for details).

were first divided by clinical grades followed by histological malignancies (log rank value = 84.1 and 9.9). Thereafter, astrocytoma of better clinical grade split into two categories by tumor size, while that of worse clinical grade into categories by tumor location (see Fig. 2).

Malignant astrocytoma and glioblastoma just showed a significant difference by categories of tumor locations. Although the regression tree analysis method ensures that two categories divided from the same parent indicates significant difference, it is possible that a terminal branch from the distinct parents may have similar survival profiles. This possibility was tested among the terminal 24 branches by the Wilcoxon test to determine whether sufficiently homogeneous outcome existed to merit merging selected groups. As shown in Table 3, the 14 terminal branch groups in patients aged 50 or younger (12 in patients aged over 50 years) were amalgamated into nine (eight) classes, ranging in size from 20 (15) to 698 (936) patients. The median survival time of these patient classes ranged from 3 months (3 months) to more than 10 years (1 year and 9 months) (Table 3).

In summary, significant survival difference among terminal groups classified by regression tree analysis would suggest that clinical treatment trial design for malignant glioma patients should be categorized to several more homogeneous patient subgroups. Without such subclassifications, any new approach and clinical trial treatment, radiotherapy, or chemotherapy may be under- or overestimated concerning their effect because of the influential power of the pretreatment variables for patient survival [9].

Acknowledgments. This research was supported in part by a Grant-in-Aid for Cancer Research from the Ministry of Health and Welfare, Japan, and grants from the Brain Foundation in Japan. (Permission for the publication of date herein was granted September 9, 1994, by the committee of the Brain Tumor Registry of Japan.)

References

1. Sandberg-Wellkeim M, Malmström P, Strömblad L-A, et al (1991) A randomized study of chemotherapy with procarbazin, vincristine and lomustine with and without radiation therapy for astrocytoma grade 3 and/or 4. Cancer 68:22–29
2. Kaplan EL, Meier P (1958) Nonparametric estimation from incomplete observations. J Am Stat Assoc 53:457–481
3. Kalbfleisch JD, Prentice RL (1980) The statistical analysis of failure time data. Wiley, New York, pp 16–19
4. SAS Institute (1985) The LIFETEST procedure. In: SAS User's Guide: Statistics. SAS Institute, Cary, pp 529–557
5. Cox DR (1972) Regression models and life tables (with discussion). J R Stat Soc 34:187–220
6. Segal MR (1988) Regression trees for censored data. Biometrics 44:35–47
7. Segal MR, Bloch DA (1989) A comparison of estimated proportioal hazards, models and regression trees. Stat Med 8:539–550
8. The Brain Tumor Registry of Japan (1992) 5-Year relative survival rate (1979–1983). Neurol med chir 32(special issue):478–479
9. Curran WJ Jr, Scott CB, Horton J, et al (1993) Recursive partitioning analysis of prognostic factors in three radiation therapy oncology group malignant glioma trials. J Natl Cancer Inst 85:704–710

Section 2. Glial Tumors

Evaluation of Histological Grading Systems of Astrocytic Tumors

Nobuyuki Kawano, Hidehiro Oka, Tomonari Suwa, and Kenzoh Yada

Abstract. To determine the clinical correlation of histological grading systems of astrocytic tumors, we examined Kernohan's grading system (the 1979 WHO [World Health Organization] grading system), Burger's grading system (the 1993 WHO grading system), and Daumas–Duport's grading system. Each grading system was applied to our cases, and its clinical correlation was evaluated by Kaplan–Meier's survival curve. Subjects of the study, who were all adult (>15 years old), had astrocytic tumors that excluded mixed glioma, gliosarcoma, and pleomorphic xanthoastrocytoma. Thirty-eight of 157 intracranial astrocytic tumors, all located in the cerebral hemisphere, were selected. Our results indicated that the Daumas–Duport grading system and that of Burger were simple and easy to use, and showed good clinical correlation. Kernohan's grading system, however, had poor clinical correlation.

Key words. Brain neoplasm—Astrocytoma—Glioblastoma—Pathology—Grading system

Introduction

In the past, several histological grading systems of astrocytic tumors have been proposed (Table 1) [1–9], and many institutes seem to use different grading systems at present. Because of the differences among these grading systems, it is difficult to evaluate the clinical results from different institutes; such evaluation may improve the methods of treatment of gliomas. A common international histological grading system undoubtedly is needed. However, few studies have tried to evaluate the clinical correlation of each grading system with identical series of patients. Thus, we undertook a study to determine which grading system correlates well with clinical outcome and has practical usefulness.

Department of Neurosurgery, Kitasato University School of Medicine, Sagamihara, Kanagawa 228, Japan

Table 1. Histological grading systems proposed in the past.

Author	Year	Steps of grading	Nomenclature of graded tumor
Kernohan [1,2]	1949, 52	4	Gr.I–II: astrocytoma; III–IV: glioblastoma
Ringertz [3]	1950	3	Astrocytoma, intermediate, glioblastoma
WHO [4][a]	1979	4	Gr.I–II: astrocytoma; III: anaplastic a.; IV: glioblastoma
Burger [5,6][b]	1982	3	Astrocytoma, anaplastic a., glioblastoma
Nelson [7][c]	1983	3	Astrocytoma, anaplastic a., glioblastoma
Daumas-Duport [8]	1988	4	Gr.1–4
WHO revised [9]	1993	3(4)	Astrocytoma, anaplastic a., glioblastoma

Each grading system has been placed chronologically from the top, with the most recent at the bottom. WHO, World Health Organization; Gr., grade; a., astrocytoma.
[a] This system basically follows the Kernohan system.
[b] Brain Tumor Study Group, USA.
[c] Radiation Therapy Oncology Group, USA.

Table 2. Histological criteria of Kernohan grading system [1,2].

Parameter/Grade	I[a]	II[a]	III[b]	IV[c]
Tumor cells	Almost normal astrocytes	Some large astrocytes	Many atypical astrocytes	Many anaplastic cells
Cell density	Slightly increased	More than grade I	—	Marked
Pleomorphism	Scarce	Some	Considerable	Prominent
Giant cells	None	None	Some	Common
Mitosis	None	None	Some	Numerous, one per field
Necrosis	None	None	Common	Common
Endothelial and adventitial proliferation	None	None	Some	Prominent

[a] Corresponds to astrocytoma of WHO [4].
[b] Corresponds to anaplastic astrocytoma of WHO [4].
[c] Corresponds to glioblastoma of WHO [4].

Table 3. Histological criteria of the grading system of Burger [5,6][a].

Parameter	Astrocytoma	Anaplastic astrocytoma	Glioblastoma
Cellularity	Low	Moderate	Moderate to high
Pleomorphism	None	Moderate	Moderate to high
Necrosis	None	None	Present
Endothelial proliferation	None	None	Present

[a] The new WHO grading system of 1993 [9] is consistent with this system.

Materials and Methods

Subjects were carefully selected; the astrocytic tumor cases that met the following conditions were used in the study. Tumors were of supratentorial hemispheric location in adult (>15 years of age) patients and histologically excluded special

Table 4. Histological criteria of the grading system of Daumas-Duport [8], popularly called the St. Anne–Mayo or Rochester system.

Sum of parameters[a]	Grade
0	1
1	2
2	3
3,4	4

There are four histological parameters: necrosis, nuclear atypia, mitosis, and endothelial proliferation.

subtypes such as mixed glioma, gliosarcoma, and pleomorphic xanthoastrocytoma. Surgical specimens of all cases contained enough tumor tissue for the study. Thirty-eight cases from 157 intracranial astrocytic tumors provided the subjects of the study.

Histological examination was performed in all cases, which were classified into histological grades of malignancy in the following three grading systems: Kernohan's grading system [1,2] (=WHO 1979 [4]), which has been used widely as an international grading system; Burger's grading system [5,6], representing three-tiered grading systems and similar to the revised WHO classification published in 1993 [9]; and the recently proposed Daumas–Duport grading system [8] because the authors claimed it has simplicity and high reproducibility. The histological criteria of each grading system are summarized in Tables 2–4. Survival curves of the Kaplan–Meier method [10] were used to evaluate the clinical correlation of each histological grading system.

Results

Kernohan Grading System

In the grading process of Kernohan's system [1,2], we found difficulty in distinguishing between grade III and grade IV, because in both grades necrosis can be seen commonly in Kernohan's criteria. In the study, grade III and grade IV were separated according to the quantity of necrosis and mitosis observed.

Figure 1 shows the clinical correlation of each histological grade. In our study, there were no cases classified as grade I. The survival curves of grade III and IV patients were closely similar, and the grade II survival curve was located far from those of grades III and IV; this seemed to be a problem in this grading system.

Burger Grading System

Histological grading was easy for examiners when using this grading system [5,6], probably because there were considerably fewer histological parameters for grading criteria than in Kernohan's system, and also because of its three-tiered grading system. Figure 2 shows the result, which exhibits the good clinical correlation found in this grading system.

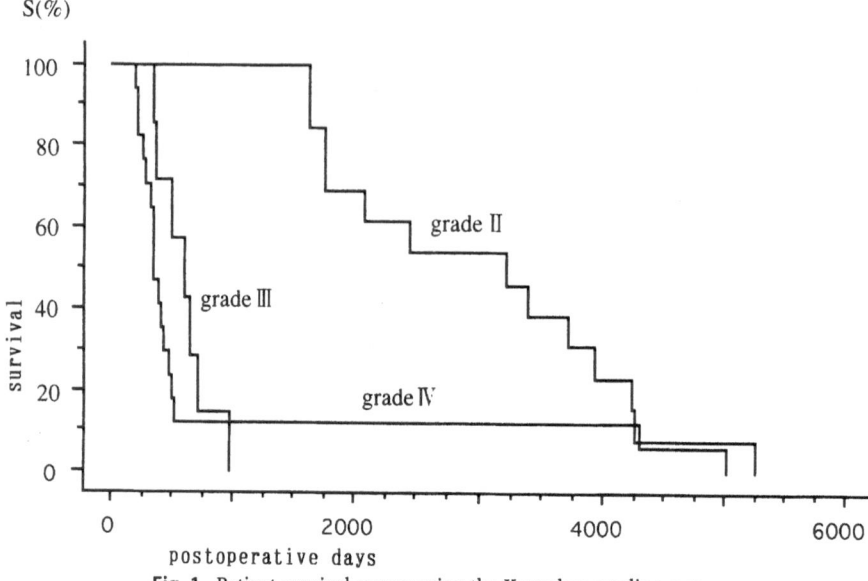

Fig. 1. Patient survival curves using the Kernohan grading system

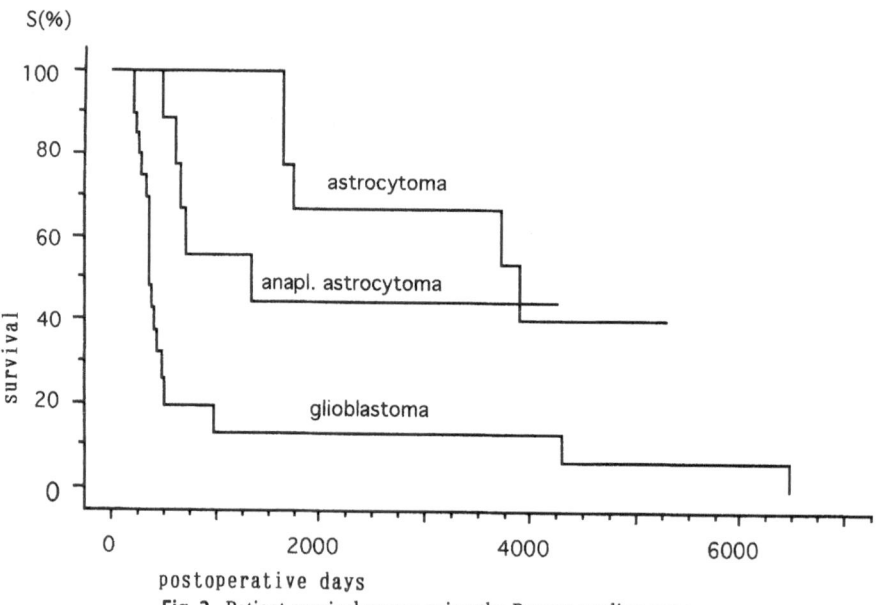

Fig. 2. Patient survival curves using the Burger grading system

Daumas–Duport Grading System

Grading work with the Daumas–Duport system [8] was easy because the examiner's task was merely to judge "present" or "not present" for each histological parameter in the tumor tissue. The grade was automatically decided by simply adding positive parameters. The result is shown in Fig. 3. Survival curves of each grade

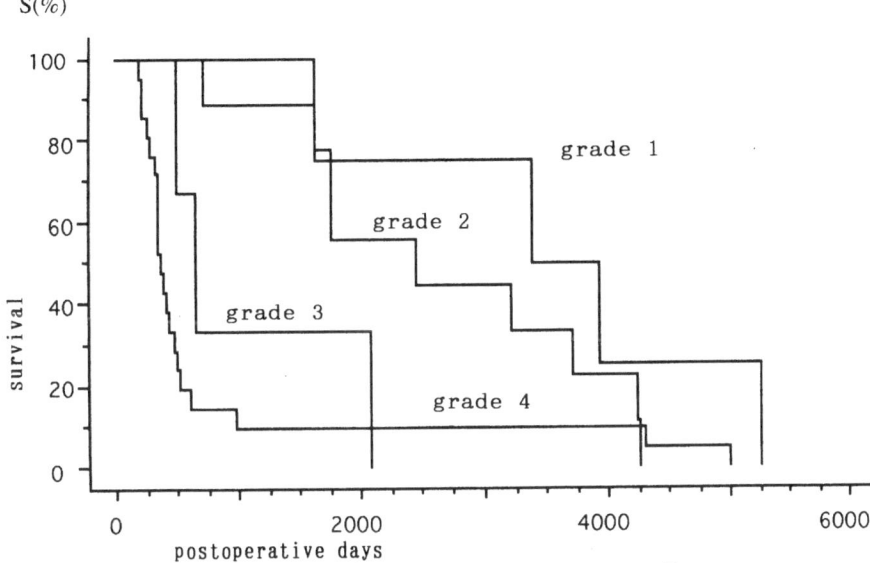

Fig. 3. Patient survival curves using the Daumas–Duport grading system

are spaced equally far apart; that is, graded patients showed orderly graded survival curves.

Discussion

Kernohan's grading system [1,2], which was adopted as the 1979 WHO grading system [4], has been criticized by Nelson et al. [7] and by Scanlon and Taylor [11] as showing no difference of survival between grade III and grade IV. Our study supports these results. The explanation may be that because both grade III and IV contain areas of necrosis in Kernohan's system, pathologists may have a difficult time in discriminating grade III from grade IV. Furthermore, the large number of histological parameters in this grading system gives examiners another complicated task.

Probably because of the reasons described, the simple three-tiered grading proposed by Ringertz [3] and by Burger et al. [5,6] and the four-tiered grading system with fewer histological parameters proposed by Daumas–Duport et al. [8], have been welcomed by pathologists. It is interesting to note that Daumas–Duport et al. rejected the use of cellularity from their criteria because cellularity is influenced by the thickness of the specimen and is likely to be judged subjectively.

What is necessary for an ideal histological grading system? First, good clinical correlation, and second, the grading system should be simple and easy for pathologists to use. The latter factor naturally improves objectivity and reproducibility of the grade considering the judging process of pathologists. From this standpoint, of the three grading systems evaluated in this study the Burger and Daumas–Duport grading systems are recommended. The new 1993 WHO grading [9] system, which essentially adopts a three-tiered grading system similar to that of Burger et al., offers better clinical correlation than the earlier version.

References

1. Kernohan JW, Mabon RF, Svien HJ, Adson AF (1949) A simplified classification of the gliomas. Proc Staff Meet Mayo Clin 24:71–75
2. Kernohan JW, Sayre GP (1952) Tumors of the central nervous system. Armed Forces Institute of Pathology, Washington, DC, pp 22–42
3. Ringertz N (1950) "Grading" of gliomas. Acta Pathol Microbiol Scand 27:51–64
4. Zulch KJ (1979) Histological typing of tumours of the central nervous system. No. 21 of international histological classification of tumours. World Health Organization, Geneva
5. Burger PC, Vogel FS (1982) Surgical pathology of the nervous system and its coverings, 2nd edn. Wiley, New York, pp 226–266
6. Burger PC, Vogel FS, Green SB, Strike TA (1985) Glioblastoma multiforme and anaplastic astrocytoma. Cancer 56:1106–1111
7. Nelson JS, Tsukada Y, Schoenfeld D, Fulling K, Lamarche J, Peress N (1983) Necrosis as a prognostic criteria and malignant supratentorial, astrocytic gliomas. Cancer 52:550–554
8. Daumas-Duport C, Scheithauer B, O'Fallon J, Kelly P (1988) Grading of astrocytomas: a simple and reproducible method. Cancer 62:2152–2165
9. Kleihues P, Burger PC, Scheithauer BW, Sobin LH (eds) (1993) Histological typing of tumours of the central nervous system. In: International histological classification of tumours of WHO. Springer, Berlin
10. Kaplan EL, Meier P (1958) Nonparametric estimation from incomplete observations. J Am Stat Assoc 53:457–481
11. Scanlon PW, Taylor WF (1979) Radiotherapy of intracranial astrocytomas: analysis of 417 cases treated from 1960 through 1969. Neurosurgery 5:301–308

Histological and Radioimaging Study of Malignant Change in Low-Grade Astrocytoma

Masaru Tamura, Takashi Shibasaki, Satoru Horikoshi, Akira Zama, Hideyuki Kurihara, Nobuo Ono, and Shougo Ishiuchi

Abstract. Potential indicators for malignant change in low-grade astrocytoma were examined in 17 patients with low-grade astrocytoma (excluding pilocytic astrocytoma) treated surgically; 7 patients showed recurrence and 3 had a second operation. The histology and bromodeoxyuridine labeling index (BrdU-LI) of the tumor specimens were examined. Positron emission tomography (PET) and single photon emission computed tomography (SPECT) were also used to assess the tumors. The primary tumors were 16 fibrillary and 1 protoplasmic astroytomas, with BrdU-LIs of less than 1% except 1 case of 3%. Recurrent operation revealed 2 glioblastomas and 1 anaplastic astrocytoma, with BrdU-LIs of 19%, 9%, and 4%, respectively. PET of the primary tumors showed low glucose and high amino acid metabolism, and low regional cerebral blood flow and oxygen uptake at the lesion. SPECT studies showed low accumulation of ^{201}Tl chloride (^{201}Tl) and ^{123}I-isopropyl iodoamphetamine. PET of the recurrent tumors showed high glucose and amino acid metabolism. SPECT showed high accumulation of ^{201}Tl. Malignant change was recognized in the recurrent tumors, both histologically and by imaging, but no prediction about which primary low-grade astrocytoma would show malignant transformation could be made.

Key words. Astrocytoma—Bromodeoxyuridine—Recurrence—Positron emission tomography—Single photon emission computed tomography

Introduction

Low-grade astrocytomas, World Health Organization (WHO) grade 2, involve a significant risk of malignant progression. More than 70% of low-grade astrocyomas have showed anaplasia at recurrence, and nearly half of them progressed to frank glioblastoma [1]. This study investigated the potential indicators for identifying whether individual low-grade astrocytoma would progress into anaplastic astrocytoma or glioblastoma. The histological characteristics and bromodeoxyuridine labeling index (BrdU-LI), and positron emission tomography (PET) and single photon emission computed tomography (SPECT) scans of a series of primary and recurrent lesions, were retrospectively examined.

Department of Neurosurgery, Gunma University School of Medicine, Maebashi 371, Japan

Clinical Materials and Methods

Seventeen patients with low-grade astrocytoma (excluding pilocytic astrocytoma) were treated at Gunma University Hospital between January 1988 and December 1993. Seven patients showed recurrence, and 3 of these patients underwent a second operation.

PET studies were performed with $C^{15}O_2$, $^{15}O_2$, [^{18}F]fluorodeoxyglucose ([^{18}F]FDG), and [^{11}C]methionine ([^{11}C]Met) using a PCT-H1 (Hitachi, Tokyo, Japan). The steady-state inhalation methods using $C^{15}O_2$ and $^{15}O_2$ were used to measure the regional cerebral blood flow (rCBF) and regional cerebral metabolic rate for oxygen (rCMRO$_2$), respectively, and [^{18}F]FDG and [^{11}C]Met to measure the glucose and amino acid metabolism, respectively. Doses of 200–300 MBq [^{18}F]FDG and 450–600 MBq [^{11}C]Met were administered intravenously on different days, and distributions of the radiotracers in the brain were measured after 60 min ([^{18}F]FDG) and 20 min ([^{11}C]Met). The uptake at the lesion was compared visually with the contralateral corresponding region or with the region surroundign the tumor.

Simultaneous SPECT studies were performed with 111 MBq isopropyl [^{123}I]iodoamphetamine ([^{123}I]IMP) and 111 MBq [^{201}Tl]chloride (^{201}Tl) using a HEADTOME SET031 (Shimadzu, Kyoto, Japan) by changing the energy window levels of the SPECT device to 128–192 keV for ^{123}I and 56–86 keV for ^{201}Tl to image the radioisotope distributions. SPECT images were taken at 15 min (early image) and 3–4 h (delayed image) after tracer injection and were evaluated visually.

BrdU (200 mg/m^2) dissolved in 100 ml saline was injected during surgery before tumor removal, after receiving informed consent, in 14 patients at the primary operation and all 3 patients at the second operation. The surgical specimens were fixed in 10% buffered formaldehyde or 70% ethanol. Specimens were classified histologically according to the WHO [2] and St. Anne/Mayo systems [3] using formaldehyde-fixed, paraffin-embedded tissue with hematoxylin and eosin staining. The proliferative activity was measured by immunohistochemical staining using avidin–biotin–peroxidase complex (ABC) (Vectastain ABC kit, PK 4002, Vector, Burlingame, CA, USA) with anti-BrdU monoclonal antibody (Becton-Dickinson, Mountain View, CA, USA) at 1:20 dilution using ethanol-fixed, paraffin-embedded tissue. The BrdU-LI was calculated as the number of positively stained nuclei per 500 tumor cells.

Results

Table 1 summarizes the clinical courses of patients with tumor recurrence. The primary tumor was removed when located in an accessible region, but only biopsy was carried out for tumors in anatomically important regions of the brain. Radiation therapy (32–52 Gy) was given postoperatively. Tumor recurrence was recognized after 9–70 months. Second tumor removal was performed in three patients with localized recurrence. Chemotherapy using a combination of cis-diaminedichloroplatinum (II), cis-diamine[1,1-cyclobutanedicarboxylato]-platinum, methyl-6-[3-(2-chloroethyl)-3-nitrosoureido]-6-deoxy-α-D-glucopyranoside, etoposide (VP-16), and interferon-β, plus conventional radiotherapy or γ-knife surgery, was given. Five patients have since died, and two are still alive.

Histological examination of the tissue specimens obtained at the first operations showed 16 fibrillary astrocytomas and 1 protoplasmic astrocytoma, classified as grade

Table 1. Clinical summary of recurrent astrocytomas.

Case no.	Age, sex	Tumor site	For primary tumor		Time to relapse (mo)	For recurrence		Outcome (mo)
			Surgery	Radiation (Gy)		Surgery	Radiation/ chemotherapy	
1.	54, F	Parietal	Subtotal	50	21	Partial	CDDP, MCNU, TNF	8, D
2.	41, F	Frontal	Subtotal	32	19	Partial	60 Gy/CDDP, MCNU	11, D
3.	33, M	Frontal	Partial	44	16	Partial	50 Gy/CDDP, MCNU, IFN, CBDCA, Et	18, D
4.	61, F	Basal ganglia	Biopsy	50	9	(−)	50 Gy/CBDCA, Et	6, D
5.	23, M	Cerebellum	Biopsy	50	15	(−)	γ-Knife	7, D
6.	31, F	Temporal	Subtotal	50	24	(−)	54 Gy/CDDP, MCNU	6, A
7.	28, M	Midbrain	Biopsy	52	70	(−)	γ-Knife	4, A

A, alive; CDDP, cis-diaminedichloroplatunum (II); CBDCA, cis-diamine [1,1-cyclobutanedicarboxylato]-platinum; D, dead; Et, etoposide; IFN, interferon-β; MCNU, methyl-6-[3-(2-chloroethyl)-3-nitrosoureido]-6-deoxy-α-D-glucopyranoside; TNF, tumor necrosis factor.

Table 2. Histology and proliferative potential of recurrent astrocytomas.

Case no.	Primary tumor			Recurrent tumor		
	WHO designation	St. Anne/ Mayo grade	BrdU-LI	WHO Designation	St. Anne/ Mayo grade	BrdU-LI
1.	Fibrillary astrocytoma	2	3%	Glioblastoma	4	9%
2.	Fibrillary astrocytoma	2	<1%	Glioblastoma	4	19%
3.	Fibrillary astrocytoma	2	<1%	Anaplastic astrocytoma	3	4%
4.	Fibrillary astrocytoma	2		No surgery		
5.	Fibrillary astrocytoma	2		No surgery		
6.	Fibrillary astrocytoma	2	<1%	No surgery		
7.	Fibrillary astrocytoma	1	<1%	No surgery		

BrdU-LI, bromodeoxyuridine labeling index; WHO, World Health Organization.

1 or 2 (St. Anne/Mayo system). The proliferative potential was examined in 14 cases, showing BrdU-LIs of less than 1% in 13 cases and 3% in 1 case (case 1). Table 2 summarizes the histology and BrdU-LI of the recurrent tumors. The 3 recurrent tumors that were removed were 2 glioblastomas and 1 anaplastic astrocytoma. Examination of proliferative potential found higher BrdU-LI in the recurrent lesions than in the primary ones.

Table 3 summarizes the PET and SPECT studies of the recurrent cases. PET studies of the primary lesion showed hypermetabolism of amino acids in two of two patients examined, low glucose metabolism in four of four patients, low rCBF in five of five

Table 3. PET and SPECT studies of recurrent astrocytomas.

Case no.	Primary tumor						Recurrent tumor			
	PET				SPECT		PET		SPECT	
	[11C]Met	[18F]FDG	C15O2	15O2	201Tl	[123I]IMP	[11C]Met	[18F]FDG	201Tl	[123I]IMP
1.	NE	—	—	—	—	—	+	NE	+	+
2.	NE	—	—	—	—	—	NE	NE	+	—
3.	+	NE	—	—	—	—	NE	+	+	—
4.	NE	—	NE	NE	—	—	NE	NE	+	—
5.	NE	NE	NE	NE	NE	NE	NE	+	NE	NE
6.	+	—	—	—	—	—	NE	+	+	—
7.	NE	NE	—	—	—	—	NE	+	—	—

+, high uptake; —, low uptake; NE, not examined; [11C]Met, [11C]methionine; [18F]FDG, [18F]fluorodeoxyglucose; [123I]IMP, [123I]isopropyl iodoamphetamine; PET, positron emission tomography; SPECT, single photon emission computed tomography; 201Tl, [201Tl]chloride.

patients, and low $rCMRO_2$ in five of five patients. Delayed SPECT images showed low accumulation of 201Tl and [123I]IMP in all six patients examined. PET studies at the time of recurrent lesion showed hypermetabolism of amino acids in one patient examined and high glucose metabolism in four of four patients. Delayed SPECT images showed high accumulation of 201Tl in five of six patients and high accumulation of [123I]IMP in one of six patients.

Discussion

The prognosis of astrocytomas correlates well with histological malignancy and BrdU-LI [3–7]. Patients with low-grade astrocytoma excluding the pilocytic type have a median survival of 4 years [3] to 5 [8] years. In particular, St. Anne/Mayo grade 1 is associated with a longer survival time than grade 2 [3]. The median survival time of patients with Kernohan's grade 1 astrocytoma is 8.7 years and with grade 2 is 2.8 years [8]. In our series, 4 of 17 patients with low-grade astrocytoma had St. Anne/Mayo grade 1, and case 7 was the only patient with recurrence after 70 months. The other 3 patients are still alive at 2, 5, and 6 years with no sign of recurrence. There may therefore be adequate reason for separating low-grade astrocytoma into grades 1 and 2 according to Kernohan's [9] and/or the St. Anne/Mayo system [3].

The BrdU-LIs of low-grade astrocytoma are usually less than 1% [4] or a mean of 1.2% [7], but some appear to have the same proliferative potential as anaplastic astrocytoma with a BrdU-LI of 1%–5% [4,7]. In our series, case 1 showed a BrdU-LI of 3% and recurred at 21 months, becoming a glioblastoma with a BrdU-LI of 9%. Four of the other 13 cases in which BrdU-LI when examined was less than 1% resulted in recurrence. The possibility of early recurrence cannot be predicted from the BrdU-LI alone.

PET studies demonstrated hypermetabolism of amino acids, hypermetabolism of glucose, low rCBF, and low $CMRO_2$, and SPECT showed low accumulation of 201Tl and [123I]IMP in the primary lesions; these data are all well correlated with low-grade glioma. In contrast, PET studies showed high glucose and amino acid metabolism, and SPECT studies revealed high accumulation of 201Tl in the recurrent lesions, which indicated high-grade glioma [10,11]. The PET and SPECT studies also could not predict early recurrence of low-grade astrocytoma. Quantitative measurements using

PET with [^{18}F]FDG and [^{11}C]Met have not been examined as an indication of malignant transformation.

Conclusion

More precise histological diagnosis (Kernohan's grades 1 and 2, St. Anne/Mayo grades 1 and 2), measurement of proliferative potential (BrdU-LI, Ki-67), and quantitative analysis of glucose and amino acid metabolism in combination may allow prediction of malignant change of low-grade astroctytoma.

References

1. Russell DS, Rubinstein LJ (1989) Pathology of tumours of the nervous system. Arnold, London, pp 95–161
2. Kleihues P, Burger PC, Scheithauer BW (1993) Histological typing of tumours of the central nervous system, 2nd edn. In: World Health Organization international histological classification of tumours. Springer, Berlin, pp 11–16
3. Daumas-Duport C, Scheithauer B, O'Fallon J (1988) Grading of astrocytomas. Cancer 62:2152–2165
4. Hoshino T, Nagashima T, Murovic JA (1986) In situ cell kinetics studies on human neuroectodermal tumors with bromodeoxyuridine labeling. J Neurosurg 64:453–459
5. Hoshino t, Prados M, Wilson CB (1989) Prognostic implications of the bromodeoxyuridine labeling index of human gliomas. J Neurosurg 71:335–341
6. Labrousse F, Daumas-Duport C, Batorski L (1991) Histological grading and bromodeoxyuridine labeling index of astrocytomas. Comparative study in a series of 60 cases. J Neurosurg 75:202–205
7. Fujimaki T, Matsutani M, Nakamura O (1991) Correlation between bromodeoxyuridine-labeling indices and patient prognosis in cerebral astrocytic tumors of adults. Cancer 67:1629–1634
8. Westergaard L, Gjerris F, Klinken L (1993) Prognostic parameters in benign astrocytomas. Acta Neurochir (Wien) 123:1–7
9. Kernohan JW, Sayre GP (1952) Tumors of the nervous system. In: Atlas of tumor pathology, Section X-Fascicle 35. U.S. Armed Forces Institute of Pathology, Washington, DC, pp 22–42
10. Tamura M, Shibasaki T, Horikoshi S (1991) Malignancy of glioma estimated by PET-^{18}FDG, PET-^{11}C-methionine, and SPECT-^{201}thallium. In: Tabuchi K (ed) Biological aspect of brain tumors. Springer, Heiddberg Berlin New York Tokyo, pp 158–163
11. Tamura M, Shibasaki T, Horikoshi S (1994) Small gliomas: metabolism and blood flow. Neurol Med Chir (Tokyo) 34:91–94

Clinicopathological Study of
Mixed Oligoastrocytoma

Yukie Shimada, Osami Kubo, Yasuhiko Tajika, Hirohumi Hiyama,
Shouko Atuji, and Kintomo Takakura

Abstract. Mixed oligoastrocytoma was categorized into mixed glioma by the Would
Health Organization (WHO) classification, and its clinical behavior has not been well
investigated. The therapy and histology of mixed oligoastrocytoma were previously
investigated in studies on oligodendroglioma, but there have been few reports on
radiotherapy and chemotherapy for mixed oligoastrocytoma. We diagnosed mixed
oligoastrocytoma in 20 patients by immunohistochemical examination, assessed the
proliferative ability of mixed oligoastrocytoma in these cases using MIB-1, a monoclonal antibody for proliferation marker Ki67. We also investigated the prognosis of
these patients. The 20 patients with mixed oligoastrocytoma included 11 men and 9
women ranging from 1 to 54 years in age (mean age, 39 years). Of the 20 patients, 7
received radiotherapy only, 1 received chemotherapy only, 8 received both radiotherapy and chemotherapy, and 4 received neither treatment. Currently, 12 have
survived for 1–13 years; 6 patients had recurrence with death ensuing in 2 of the 6.
Malignant transformation was documented histologically in 5 of the 6 patients with
recurrence. The 20 patients were divided into a recurrence group and a nonrecurrence
group; Furthermore, mixed oligoastrocytoma was classified into type A, in which the
lesion had oligodendroglial components and astrocytic components that were relatively separate, and type B, a lesion in which oligodendroglial components and astrocytic components were present in a diffused and composite form.

Key words. Mixed oligoastrocytoma—MIB-1-positive rate—prognosis

Introduction

Mixed oligoastrocytoma has traditionally been classified histologically as a variant of
oligodendroglioma, and immunohistochemical examination and histological characterization of mixed oligoastrocytoma have been performed as part of studies on
oligodendroglioma. Accordingly, mixed oligoastrocytoma has only been reported to
be poorly differentiated in general, and few reports have been published about radio
therapy and chemo therapy for this disease and the correlation between the degree of
malignancy and growth factor-related antigen [1–7]. No pathological investgation nor
statistical analyses have been performed on mixed oligoastrocytoma, even after this

Department of Neurosurgery, Neurological Institute, Tokyo Women's Medical College, Shinjuku-ku,
Tokyo, 162 Japan

disease was categorized as mixed glioma by the new World Health Organization (WHO) classification. We recently diagnosed mixed oligoastrocytoma in 20 patients by means of immunohistochemistry, assessed the proliferative ability of mixed oligoastrocytoma in these cases by using MIB-1, a monoclonal antibody for proliferation marker Ki67. We also investigated the prognosis of these patients.

Materials and Methods

This study was performed on 20 patients with mixed oligoastrocytoma who were seen at our hospital in the period from 1979 to 1994. These patients, 11 men and 9 women, ranged from 4 months to 54 years in age, with a mean age of 39 years. Of the 20 patients, 19 underwent neurosurgery for tumor resection; in the other patient (1) only biopsy was performed, and the natural course of the disease was then monitored. In all cases, the tumor location was a supratentorial lesion. The resected tumor specimens were fixed in 20% formalin, for embedding on both hematoxylin and eosin (H & E-stained) sections and glial fibrillary acidicprotein (GFAP-stained) sections. Mixed oligoastrocytoma was diagnosed when cells containing perinuclear halos and showing the typical honeycomb structure were present and when both proven oligodendroglioma and astrocytoma were present in one preparation. Immunohistochemical examination was performed by the peroxidase-antiperoxidase (PAP) technique using GFAP, nevrofilament protein (NSE), and S-100, and by the enzyme-labeled antibody technique vimentin (Dako, Copenhagen, Denmark), and anti-Leu 7 antibody (Becton and Dickinson, Osaka, Japan), according to the avidin biotin complex (ABC) method. The paraffin sections were deparaffinized, placed in $0.01M$ acetic acid buffer solution, and heated in a microwave oven to activate antigenicity. With these specimens, immunohistochemical staining was performed by the ABC method, using the monoclonal antibody MIB-1 to Ki67 antigen expressed in the nucleus of proliferated cells, and the number of positive cellls was counted. Intranuclear-stained cells were counted at a magnification of $\times 400$ in a site yielding the apparent highest positive rate, and the MIB-1-positive rate was determined as the percentage of the total number of positive nuclei to total tumor cells. The tumor was resected in 19 of the 20 patients; 17 of them underwent radiotherapy, and 12 of 17 patients were also treated with chemotherapy, mainly using nimustine hydrochloride nitrosourea (ACNU). These patients were followed up postoperatively. Survival curves were generated by Kaplan-Meier's method. The log rank test and generalized Wilcoxon test were applied to examine the homogeneity of the survival curve between groups. All the patients investigated are listed in Table 1.

Table 1. Case history information for 20 patients in study of mixed oligoastrocytoma.

Prognosis	Recurrence	6[a]
	Nonrecurrence	12
	Unknown	2
Sex	Male	11
	Female	9
Age	4 mo – 54 yr	(median, 39 yr)

[a] Number of cases.

Results

Histology

Tumor preparations stained with H & E and with GFAP were examined by light microscopy. Both oligodendroglioma, which showed the typical honeycomb structure (Fig. 1), and an astrocytic component of greater than about 20% were observed in the same preparation, and mixed oligoastrocytoma was thus defined and neurocytoma ruled out using electron microscopy. In the immunohistochemical examination, the tumor tissue preparations were positive for GFAP and S-100 in all patients; only 1 patient was positive for NSE. Several patients were positive for myelin basic protein (MBP), all were negative for Leu 7, and several were positive for vimentin.

Comparison Between Types A and B of Mixed Oligoastrocytoma

The location of oligodendroglioma and astrocytoma, and their relative proportions when mixed, were determined by H & E staining. Lesions having the oligodendroglial component and the astrocytic component separately were defined as type A, and lesions having both components diffusely were defined as type B (Table 2). Histologically, a cluster of cells having round nuclei of similar size that were not stained with GFAP represented oligodendroglioma, and a cluster of GFAP-stained cells represented astrocytoma. Thus, specimens consisting of GFAP-positive

Table 2. Definition of mixed oligoastrocytoma types.

Type A: Oligodendroglial components are separated from astrocytic parts
Type B: Oligodendroglioma and astrocytoma are diffusely mixed

and GFAP-negative cell clusters were type A lesions (Fig. 2), and specimens consisting of diffused GFAP-positive and GFAP-negative cells were type B lesions (Fig. 3).

Table 3 lists ten patients as having type A lesions, including grade II as defined by the Would Health Organization (WHO), with recurrence. In one of the two patients with recurrence, the tumor remained grade II and was not malignant at the time of recurrence. The other patient with a recurrent tumor did not undergo resection but was examined only by biopsy, and the natural course of the disease was then monitored. Ten patients were classified as type B; four of the type B patients had recurrence, and three died. The mean survival time was 108 months in the type A group and 70 months in the type B group. The MIB-1-positive rate was 4.0% in the type A group and 5.7% in the type B group (Table 3). The 5-year survival rate was 100% in the type A group and 90% in the type B group; the 10-year survival rates were 100% and 74%, respectively; and the 15-year survival rates were 100% and 36%, respectively. The survival rate was higher in the type A group , although no significant difference was shown between the two groups by the log-rank test (Fig. 4).

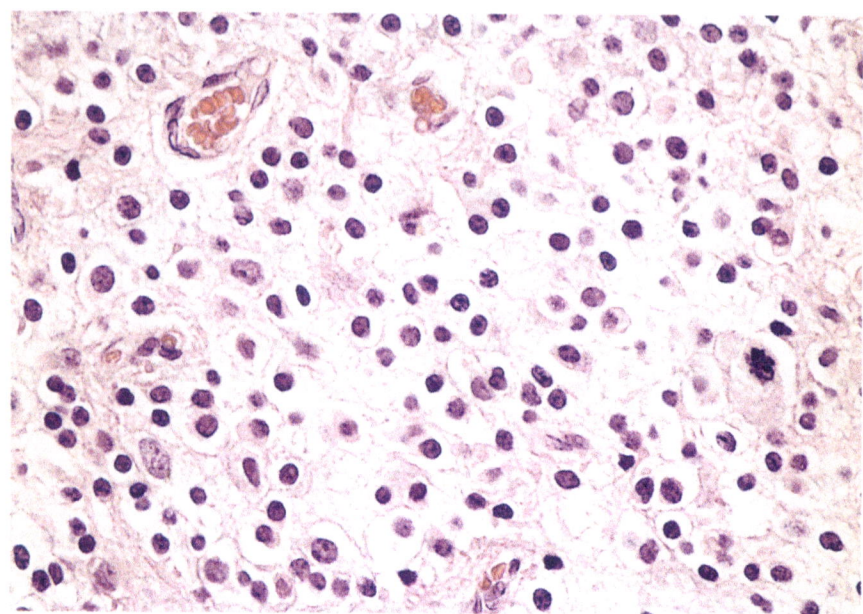

Fig. 1. Oligodendroglial Component of mixed oligoastrocytoma: typical honey comb structure. Hemotoxylm and eosin (H & E), ×400

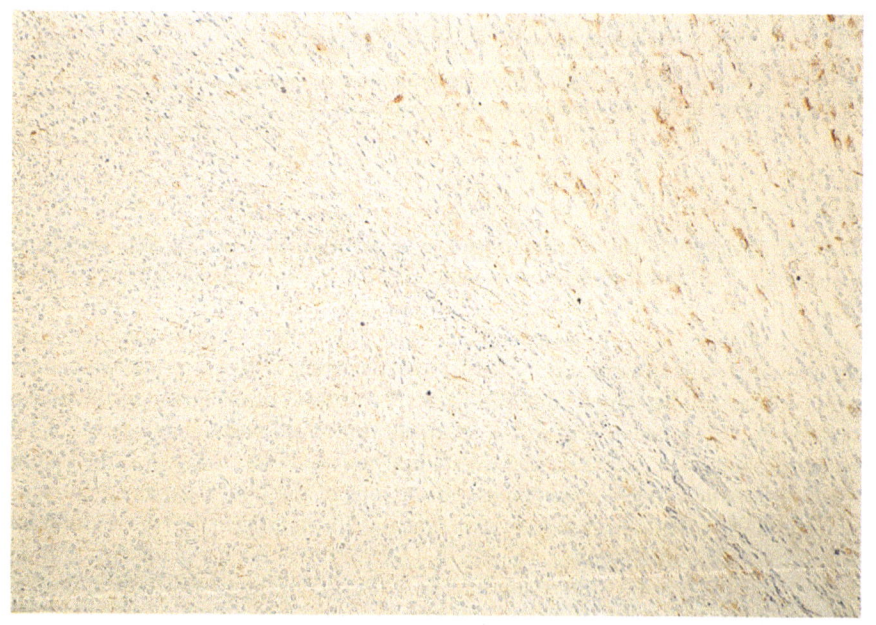

Fig. 2. GFAP-positive (astrocytic component, A, *right side*) and GFAP-negative cell clusters (oligodendroglial component, O, *left side*) cells indicated type A mixed oligoastrocytoma. GFAP, glial fibrillary acid protein. ×20

Table 3. Comparison of type A and type B cases of mixed oligo-astrocytoma.

Type	Number of cases	MIB-1 (%)	Recurrence (n)	Median survival time (mo)
A	10	4.0	2	117
B	10	5.7	4 (3 deaths)	72

MIB-1, monoclonal antibody for proliferation marker Ki67.

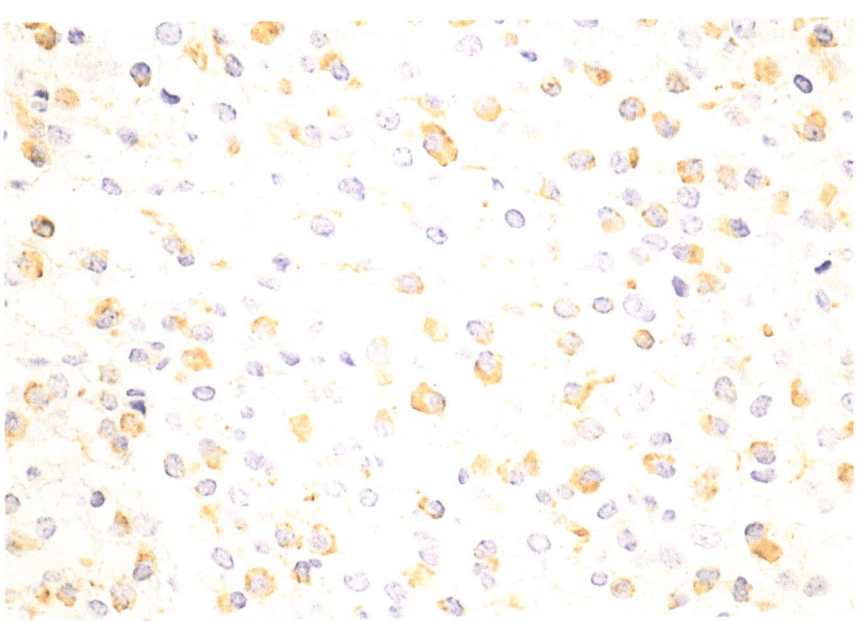

Fig. 3. Diffused GFAP-positive and GFAP-negative cells defined type B oligoastrocytoma. ×20

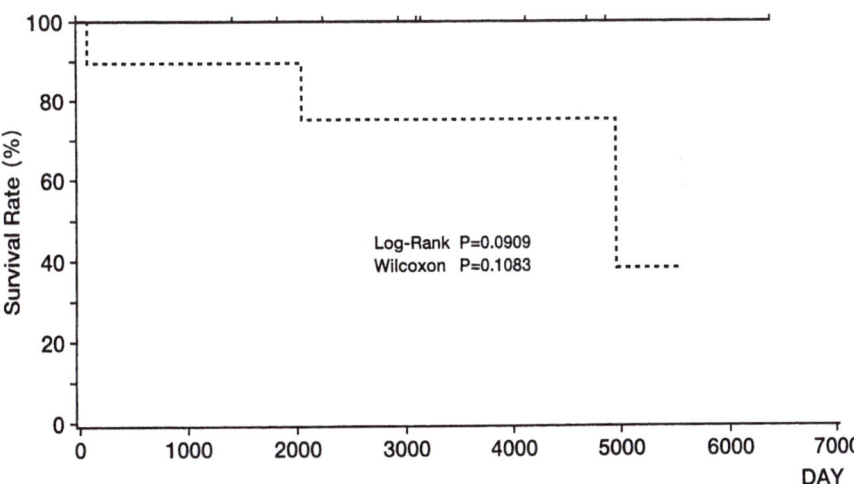

Fig. 4. Difference in survival rate between type A patients (*solid line*) and type B patients (*dashed line*) was not significant by the log-rank test

Factors Related to Prognosis

Analysis of Patients with No Recurrence

Eleven patients are currently surviving without recurrence of their tumor, including 8 in the type A group and 3 in the type B group (Table 4). The areas of oligodendroglioma and astrocytoma occurred in almost equal proportions in 8 of the 11 patients. The MIB-1-positive rate was 4.5% in the overall lesions, 5.5% in the oligodendroglial components, and 4.3% in the astrocytic components; 9 of the 11 patients received radiotherapy and 7 received chemotherapy. The median survival time was 99 months as of December 1994.

Analysis of Patients with Recurrence

Lesions recurred in 6 of the 20 patients, and 2 died. Four of these 6 patients underwent radiation after surgery for the first lesions, and only 2 underwent chemotherapy (Table 5). The mean time until recurrence was 62.7 months; it was about 56 months in

Table 4. Examination of the 11 patients with no recurrence.

Case	Type	O:A	MIB-1 (%)	MIB-1 (%) (0)	MIB-1 (%) (A)	Radiation	Chemotherapy	Survival time (mo)[a]
1	A	1:1	4	2	6	−	−	138
2	A	1:1	1	1		+	−	77
3	B	1:1	4	2	6	+	+	67
4	A	O > A	5	5		+	+	105
5	A	1:1	5	5		+	+	106
6	A	1:1	0.2	1	5	+	+	99
7	A	1:1	5	7	4	+	−	162
8	A	O > A	13	25	2	−	+	62
9	A	O > A	2	2		+	+	156
10	B	1:1	3	3	3	+	−	95
11	B	1:1	7	7		+	+	17
Mean			4.5%	5.5%	4.3%			

O, oligodendroglioma; A, astrocytoma.

[a] Median survival time, 99 months.

Table 5. Treatment and prognosis of patients with recurring lesions.

Case	Type	MIB 1% (1)	(2)	Radiation	Chemotherapy	t_1	t_2	Prognosis	Pathology (2)
1	A	0	15	−	−	47	49	Alive[a]	G3
2	B	2.8	5.8	+	−	43	73	Dead	G3
3	B	20.0	10.8	+	+	110	165	Dead	G2
4	A		4.2	−	−	78	213	Alive	G2
5	B	9.9	61.7	+	−	54	84	Alive	G4
6	B	0	20.0	+	+	86	115	Alive	G3
Mean		6.5	20.0						

(1), First operation; (2), second operation; t_1, time from first operation to recurrence (mo); t_2, survival time (mo).

[a] Median Survival time, 100 mo; mean of t_1, 74 mo.

the 4 patients treated with radiation alone after surgery. Histological examination of the resected specimens after recurrence revealed malignant transformation in 5 of the 6 patients. The mean MIB-1-positive rate was 6.5% after the first operation and 20.5% after the second operation. A high MIB-1-positive rate was seen in 5 patients. In the patients with recurrence, the median survival time was 100 months; death ensued in 2 patients. Of the 6 patients experiencing recurrence, 2 were of the type A group and 4 of the type B group; thus, recurrence was more frequent in the group with type B lesions. Figure 5 shows a case diagnosed as type B by means of GFAP staining in the lesion at the first operation that changed to an anaplastic malignancy after recurrence, with a marked change in the MIB-1-positive percentage from 9.9% (left side of Fig. 5) to 62% (right side of Fig. 5). Of the 20 patients, the 1 whose tumor was not resected and 2 who were not followed up do not appear in the above analysis.

Comparison Between the Recurrence Group and the Nonrecurrence Group

In the 6 patients experiencing recurrence, type B patients outnumbered type A; in the 11 patients with no recurrence, type A patients outnumbered type B (Table 6). The MIB-1-positive rate was higher in the recurrence group than in the nonrecurrence group, 6.5% versus 4.5%. The median survival time was 100 months in the recurrence group and 99 months in the nonrecurrence group, believed to result from the shorter follow-up period in the nonrecurrence group. The mean age at the onset of the disease was 33 years in the recurrence group and 52 years in nonrecurrence group. Chemo-

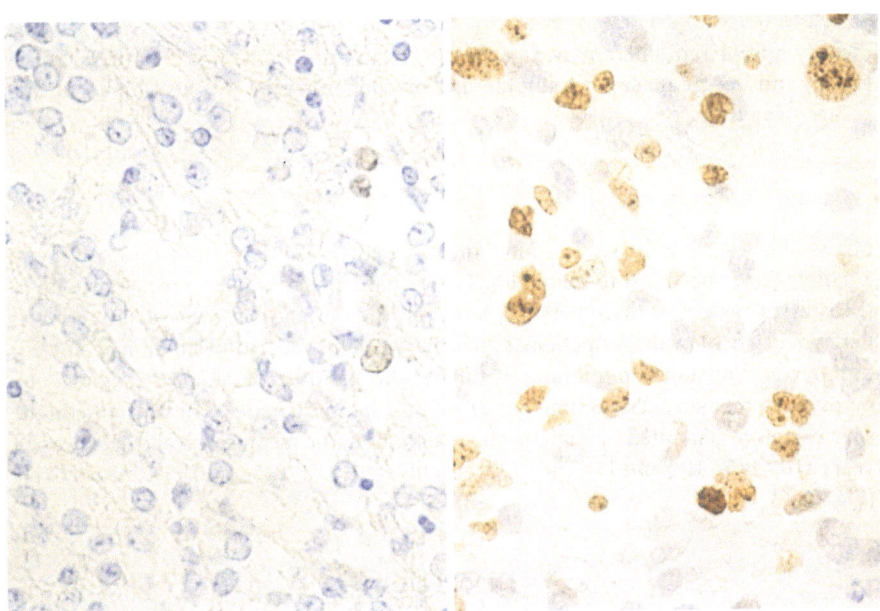

Fig. 5. This case was diagnosed as a type B tumor at the time of the first surgery (*left side*); at the time of the second for recurrence (*right side*), the malignancy had changed to anaplastic with the MIB-1-positive percentage increasing from 9.9% to 62%. ×400

Table 6. Comparison of recurrence group and nonrecumrrence group.

Number of cases	Prognosis	Type	MIB-1 (%)	Median survival time (mo)	Median age (yr)	Radiation (%)	Chemotherapy (%)
Recurrence, 6	Death (2)	A < B	6.5	100	33	66	33
Nonrecurrence, 11	All survived	A > B	4.5	99	52	82	64

Of the 20 patients, the 1 whose tumor was not resected and 2 who were not followed up are excluded.

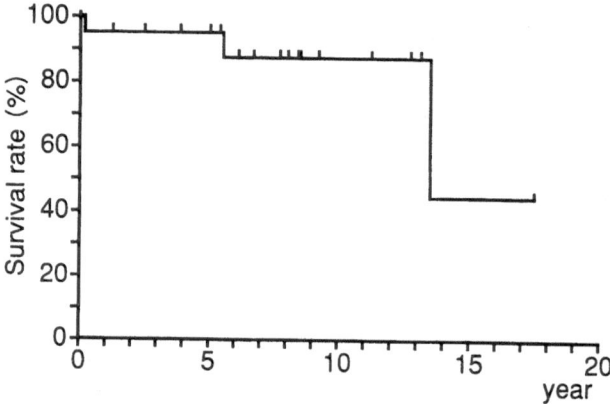

Fig. 6. Rate of survival (%) versus time in years for 20 cases of mixed oligoastrocytoma

therapy and/or radiotherapy was performed in more patients in the nonrecurrence group, and the frequency of radiotherapy or chemotherapy was also higher in the recurrence group.

Survival Time

Mixed oligoastrocytoma recurred in 6 of 20 patients, resulting in death in 2 of them; 2 patients have been lost to follow-up. Twelve patients have had no recurrence up to the present time; 1 of these persons, however, died of another disease. Surgery was performed on 19 of the 20 patients; the other patient underwent no craniotomy for tumor resection but was monitored during the natural course after diagnosis by biopsy. The median survival time was 91 months in the 20 patients overall, and on the survival curve generated by Kaplan-Meier's method, the mean survival period was 14 years and the 5-, 10-, and 15-year survival rates were 95%, 88%, and 45%, respectively (Fig. 6).

Discussion

Although the diagnosis of oligodendroglioma per se is generally determined by elimination, in this study oligodendroglioma was diagnosed when the typical honeycomb structure was observed on light microscopy in a preparation stained with

H & E and then GFAP, and mixed oligoastrocytoma was diagnosed when both oligodendroglioma and astrocytoma were present in the same section of a resected specimen. Furthermore, neurocytoma was ruled out using electron microscopy.

Edward et al. [2] evaluated the prognosis of mixed oligoastrocytoma based on age when the radiation component was predominant as a tumor component, and reported that the median survival time was 6.3 years in patients with grade I or II mixed oligoastrocytoma; also the 5-and 10-year survival rates was lower in their series. In our series, the survival rate was not modified by a difference in age (Fig. 7). In the series studied by Edward et al., multivariate analysis demonstrated a significant difference between patients aged less than and more than 37 years. Because we investigated only 20 patients in our study, a significant difference may be documented with an extended follow-up in the future. We divided mixed oligoastrocytoma into type a (lesions in which oligodendroglioma and astrocytoma were present separately) and type B (lesions containing diffused oligodendroglial components and astrocytic components). The MIB-1-positive rate was slightly higher for type B; the recurrence rate was also higher and the median survival time shorter for type B. Because such a classification of mixed oligoastrocytoma has not been reported previously, further investigation is needed to clarify the histological differences between types A and B so as to understand the implications of such differences.

Comparison between patients with recurrence and those without recurrence indicated a slightly higher MIB-1-positive rate in the resected first-operation tumor specimens of the patients with recurrence; the MIB-1-positive rate was also higher in the resected tumor specimens from patients with recurrence.

All the patients of this series were considered to have histological grade II lesions according to the WHO classification. However, in the 10-year postoperative course postoperative radio- or chemo therapy was considered to be important, and the results of this study also suggested that the postoperative nonrecurrence period and survival time can be extended by using postoperative therapies such as chemotherapy and radiotherapy. The median postoperative survival time in the 20 patients is 8 years

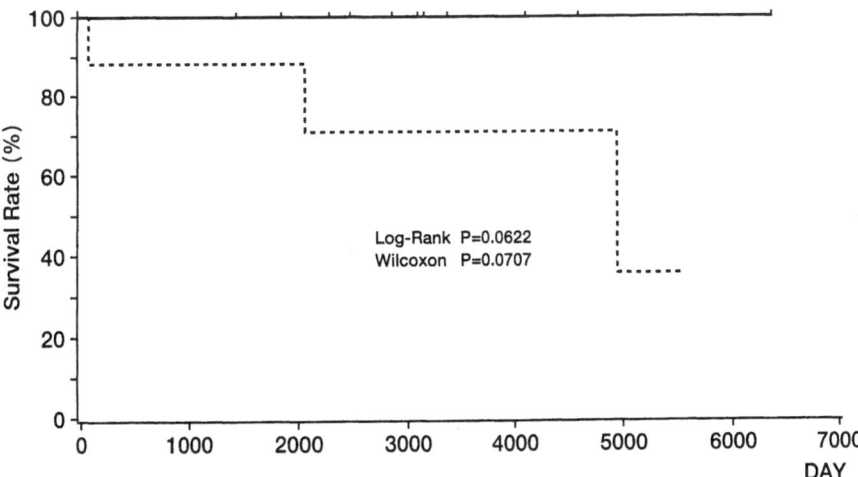

Fig. 7. Rate of survival (%) versus time in days for patients aged less than 45 years (*solid line*) and those aged 45 years or more (*dashed line*)

at present; this short survival time is ascribed to the short follow-up period of this study and is expected to extend with prolongation of the follow-up period. Thus, further studies appear to be warranted on mixed oligoastrocytoma in a larger scale so that the histological profile of this disease can be better clarified and the factors related to malignant transformation can determined.

References

1. Kubo O, Tajika Y, Tajika T, Toyama T, Sakairi M, Katahira M, Kitamura K (1988) Clinikopathological study of oligodendroglioma with special reference to immuno-histochemical investigation (in Japanese). No Shinkei Geka (Neurol Surg) 16:1029–1035
2. Shaw EG, Scheithauer BW, O'Fallon JR, Davis DH (1994) Mixed oligo-astrocytomas: a survival and prognostic factor analysis. Neurosurgery (Baltimore) 34:577–582
3. Glass J, Hochberg FH, Gruber ML, Louis DN, Smith D, Rattner B (1992) The treatment of oligodendrogliomas and mixed oligodendroglioma-astrocytomas with PCV chemotherapy. J Neurosurg 76:741–745
4. Montine TJ, Vandersteenhoven JJ, Aguzzi A, Boyko OB, Dodge RK, Kerns BJ, Burger PC (1994) Prognostic significance of Ki-67 proliferation index in supratentorial fibrillary astrocytic neoplasms. Neurosurgery (Baltimore) 34:674–679
5. Carincross JG (1992) Aggressive oligodendroglioma: a chemosensitive tumor. Neurosurgery (Baltimore) 31:78–82
6. Shibata T, Burger PC, Kleihues P (1988) Cell kinetics of oligodendroglioma and oligo-astrocytoma: Ki67 PaP study (in Japanese). Neurological Surgery 40:779–785
7. Celli P. Nofrone I, Palma L, Cantore G, Fortuna A (1994) Cerebral oligodendroglioma: prognostic factors and life history. Neurosurgery (Baltimore) 35:1018–1035

Metallothionein in Gliomas

Hisashi Nitta, Yutaka Hayashi, Yoshie Okada, Osamu Tachibana,
Masanao Mouri, Tetsumori Yamashima, and Junkoh Yamashita

Abstract. Metallothionein (MT) is a low molecular weight, intracytoplasmic protein
that has a high affinity for heavy metals. MT plays a role in the storage and metabolism
of essential trace elements and in detoxification of toxic heavy metals in normal
tissues. In systemic malignant tumors, MT is thought to be related to the cellular
mechanism of drug resistance to anticancer agents, especially platinum compounds.
We studied the expression of MT in 20 gliomas and 3 autopsied brains using immunohistochemical and reverse transcriptase-polymerase chain reaction (RT-PCR)
methods. In autopsied brains, MT expression was seen in astrocytes in the cerebral
gray matter and white matter and in the cerebellum. Neurons, ependyma, and oligodendrocytes did not show MT immunoreactivity. In gliomas, MT staining was seen in
both nucleus and cytoplasm of tumor cells. Expression of MT was most prominent in
glioblastomas and less intensive in low-grade gliomas. We concluded that intensity of
MT expression may correlate with histological grading of gliomas.

Key words. Metallothionein—Gliomas—Astrocytes—Chemotherapy

Introduction

Metallothionein (MT) is a low molecular weight, cytosolic protein found in various
eukaryotic cells [1]. MT is rich in cysteine (i.e., about one-third of all amino acids),
accounting for the high affinity of MT for heavy metals such as zinc, copper, mercury,
and cadmium. The highest concentrations of MT are in the liver, kidney, lung, and
skin [2,3]. In normal tissues, MT is of great importance in the metabolism of heavy
metals and detoxification of potentially toxic heavy metals [1].

cis-Platinum [cisplatin; *cis*-diamminedichloroplatinum, CDDP] has become the
one of the most popular anticancer agents in cancer therapy. CDDP has a platinum
atom as an active center [4]; MT can bind the platinum of CDDP and make it inactive.
This mechanism is assumed to be a cellular drug resistance to CDDP in various
tumors [5]. MT has also a radioprotective effect by its scavenging of free radicals [1].

In this study, we investigated the expression of MT in gliomas to examine whether
the intensity of MT expression can be correlated with the histological grading of
astrocytic tumors.

Department of Neurosurgery, Kanazawa University School of Medicine, Kanazawa 920, Japan

Materials and Methods

We used 20 postoperative specimens of gliomas (glioblastoma, 9; anaplastic astrocytoma, 3; low-grade astrocytoma, 2; oligodendroglioma or mixed glioma, 6) and 3 autopsied brains.

MT was detected using a labeled strepto-avidin biotin method with a monoclonal anti-MT antibody (DAKO-MT E9, DAKO corporation, Carpinteria, CA, USA) on formalin-fixed, paraffin-embedded sections. The expression of the MT-IA gene [6] was measured by reverse transcriptase-polymerase chain reaction (RT-PCR) (GeneAmp Thermostable rTth reverse transcriptase RNA PCR kit, Perkin-Elmer Cetus, Norwalk, CT, USA). Extracted RNA from the specimen was reverse transcribed and amplified by PCR for 40 cycles (1 min at 94°C, 1 min at 55°C, and 2 min at 70°C). The sequences of the up- and down stream primers for the MT-IA gene are as follows: upstream, 5′-TAAGGGATGCTAGGTTTCTG-3′; downstream, 5′-TTATGTCCTTA-ATCCCGAAA-3′.

Results

Immunohistochemistry of Metallothionen

Autopsied Brain

Pia mater and gray matter were stained with anti-MT antibody. Numerous astrocytes were visible throughout the gray matter except in the molecular layer. MT staining was prominent in astrocytes in both cerebral gray and white matter (Fig. la,b). No MT staining was seen in neurons, oligodendrocytes, or ependyma. Astrocytes in the granular layer of the cerebellum also showed positive MT staining.

Gliomas

There were few MT-positive cells in low-grade gliomas (Fig. 2). These MT-positive astrocytic cells were thought to be normal resident astrocytes in the tumor because of the configuration of cellular processes.

In anaplastic astrocytomas, MT-positive tumor cells were increased in number compared to those in low-grade gliomas (Fig. 3). In glioblastomas, many tumor cells were MT positive. MT staining was seen in both cytoplasm and nuclei (Fig. 4a). Tumor cells with plump cytoplasm also showed strong MT staining (Fig. 4b). The intensity of MT staining was correlated with the histological grading of the gliomas.

RT-PCR Analysis for the MT-IA Gene

MT expression was detectable in glioblastomas (Fig. 5, lane b), whereas meningiomas did not have a notable level of MT expression (Fig. 5, lane a).

Discussion

The biological functions of MT in pathological conditions are not clearly understood. The possible roles of MT in tumors are radioprotection and drug resistance [1,5]. MT-

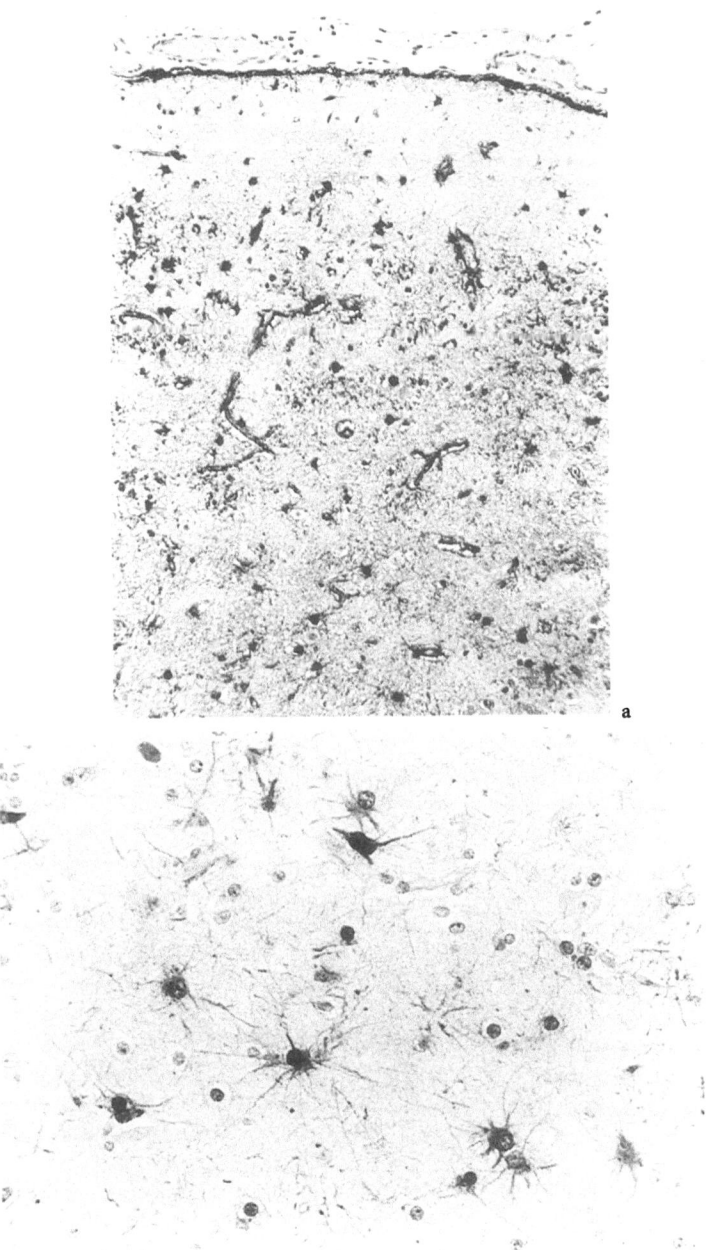

Fig. 1a,b. Immunohistochemistry with anti-MT (metallothionein). **a** Cerebral gray matter. Pia mater and astrocyotes are positive in MT staining; there is no MT staining in the molecular layer. ×80 **b** Higher magnification of **a**. MT-positive astrocytes are evident; oligodendrocytes and neurons are negative. ×160

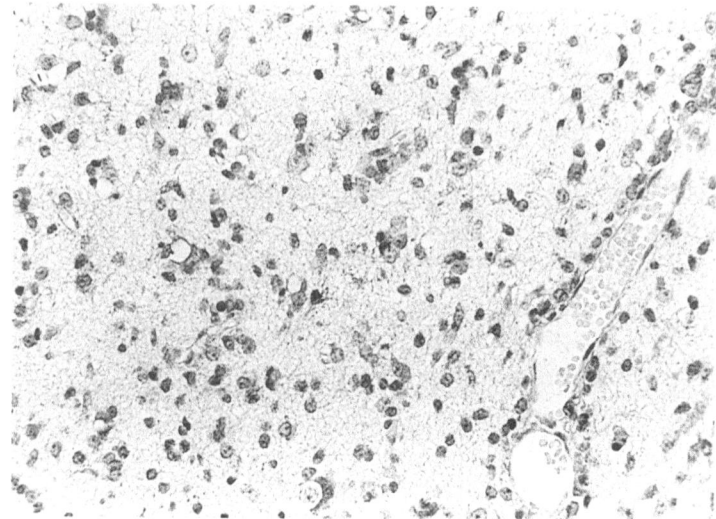

Fig. 2. Immunohistochemistry with anti-MT in a low-grade astrocytoma. Almost all tumor cells are MT negative; the few MT-positive cells are presumably normal astrocytes. ×80

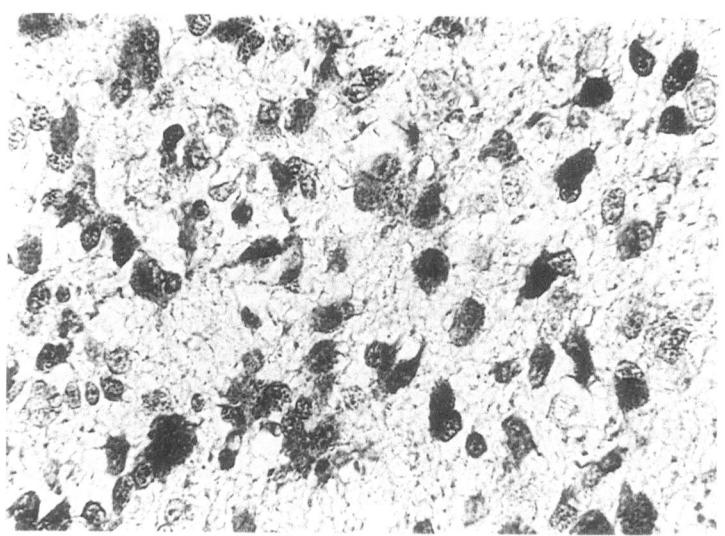

Fig. 3. Immunohistochemistry with anti-MT in an anaplastic astrocytoma. MT-positive tumor cells are more frequent than those of the low-grade astrocytoma shown in Fig. 2. ×160

positive cells show resistance to anticancer agents and radioresistance in vitro [7,8]. MT can easily bind heavy metals so that platinum compound (i.e., CDDP) is inactivated by MT in the cytoplasm. It has been reported that cells with abundant MT expression are less sensitive to other anticancer agents such as cyclophosphamide and doxorubicin as well [9].

In clinicopathological studies, it has been reported that systemic malignancy such as breast cancer exhibited intense MT expression and that its expression correlated

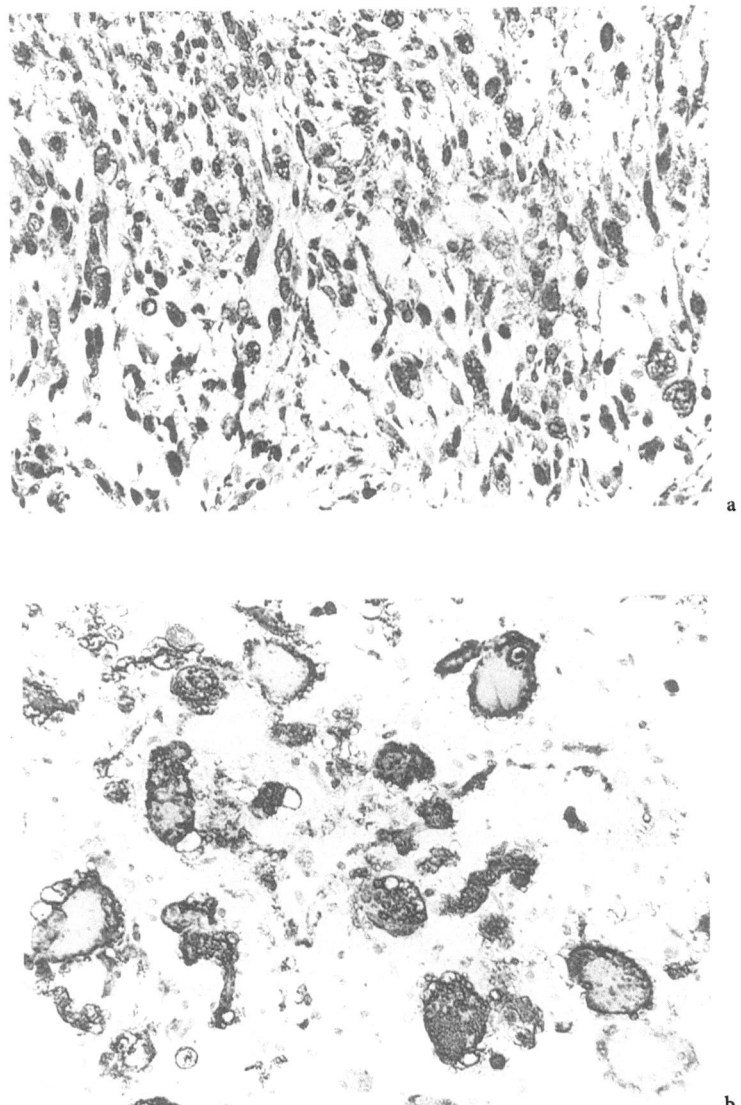

Fig. 4a,b. Immunohistochemistry with anti-MT in glioblastoma. **a** Numerous MT-positive tumor cells. ×80. **b** Giant tumor cells are also MT positive. ×160

with its prognosis. It is suggested that MT-positive glioma cells may have a chemo- and radioresistant character.

In experimental studies, various trials have been made to overcome MT-related drug resistance. A high zinc diet induces up-regulation of MT in normal tissue but not in tumor cells [10]. It enables an increase in drug intensity without increasing side effects. Proparglyglycine can provide downregulation of MT gene expression in tumor cells [5]. These observations indicate that tumor sensitivity to chemotherapy and radiotherapy may be modulated by these procedures.

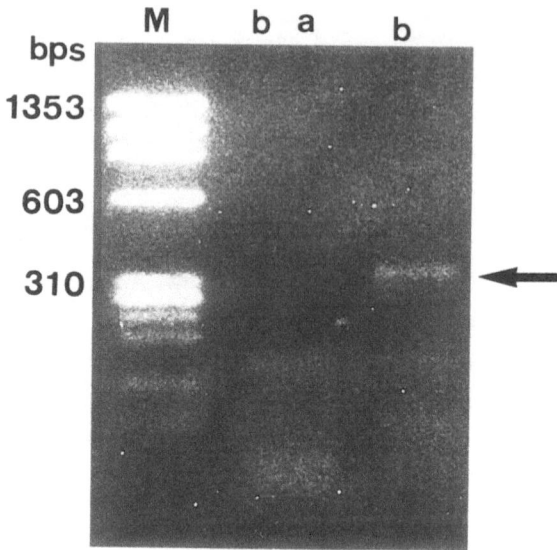

Fig. 5. Reverse transcriptase-polymerase chain reaction (RT-PCR) analysis of MT-IA gene. Ethidium bromide-stained gel shows an evident expression of MT-IA in glioblastoma (*arrow*) but not in meningioma. *Lane M*, marker; *lane a*, meningioma; *lane b*, glioblastoma; *bps*, base pairs

Because our study showed MT staining was correlated with the histological grading of gliomas, MT expression in gliomas may reflect one of the malignant behaviors of gliomas. In conclusion, an analysis of MT expression in gliomas may be useful as an adjunct to the histological grading of astrocytic tumors in diagnostic evaluation.

References

1. Dunn MA, Blalock TL, Cousins RJ (1987) Minireview: metallothionein (42525A). Proc Soc Exp Biol Med 185:107–119
2. Hamer DH (1986) Metallothionein. Annu Rev Biochem 55:913–951
3. Danielson KG, Ohi S, Huang PC (1982) Immunochemical detection of metallothionein in specific epithelial cells of rat organs. Proc Natl Acad Sci USA 79:2301–2304
4. Rosenberg B, Van Camp L, Trosko JE (1969) Platinum compounds: a new class of potent antitumor agents. Nature 222:385–386
5. Sato M, Kloth DM, Kadhim SA (1993) Modulation of both cisplatin nephrotoxicity and drug resistance in murine bladder tumor by controlling metallothionein synthesis. Cancer Res 53:1829–1832
6. Richards RI, Heguy A, Karin M (1984) Structural and functional analysis of the human metallothionein—IA gene: differential induction by metal ions and glucocorticoids. Cell 37:263–272
7. Bakka AB, Endresen L, Johnsen ABS (1981) Resistance against *cis*-dichlorodiammineplatinum in cultured cells with a high content of metallothionein. Toxicol Appl Pharmacol 61:215–226
8. Endresen L, Schjerven L, Rugstad HE (1984) Tumours from a cell strain with a high content of metallothionein show enhanced resistance against *cis*-dichlorodiammineplatinum. Acta Pharmacol Toxicol 55:183–187

9. Lazo JS, Basu A (1991) Metallothionein expression and transient resistance to electrophilic anti-neoplastic drugs. Semin Cancer Biol 2:266–271

10. Doz F, Berens ME, Deschepper CF (1992) Experimental basis for increasing the therapeutic index of *cis*-diamminedicarboxylato-cyclobutaneplatinum (II) in brain tumor therapy by a high-zinc diet. Cancer Chemother Pharmacol 29:219–226

Section 3. Meningioma

Histological Grading of Meningioma Based on MIB-1 Immunoreactivity

Junko Hirato[1], Yoichi Nakazato[1], and Masafumi Hirato[2]

Abstract. Atypical meningioma was added to the meningioma group in the revised World Health Organization classification, and thus meningioma was divided into three grades: histologically benign, atypical, and anaplastic. Several authors have defined the criteria of atypical meningioma, but there are still some practical problems in grading meningiomas histologically. We investigated the relationship between the histological features and proliferative ability assessed by immunoreactivity with MIB-1 monoclonal antibody and sought to apply this in grading of meningioma. In 73 meningioma specimens obtained from 49 cases, the following histopathological features and MIB-1 immunoreactivity were examined: mitotic index, prominent nucleoli, nuclear pleomorphism, small cells with high nuclear cytoplasmic ratios, hypercellularity, loss of architecture, brain invasion, and necrosis. Thirty-eight of 39 (97%) meningiomas with MIB-1 labeling index greater than 5.0 exhibited mitotic indices of more than 1. Necrosis, prominent nucleoli, loss of architecture, nuclear pleomorphism, hypercellularity, brain invasion, and small cells were observed in 92%, 64%, 62%, 56%, 56%, 21%, and 15% of these cases, respectively. Meningiomas with higher proliferative ability showed higher rates of presence of mitotic figures and necrosis. The mean MIB-1 labeling index of meningiomas with brain invasion was 19.80, and MIB-1 labeling indices correlated well with mitotic indices. Therefore, mitotic figures, necrosis, and brain invasion were more significant features for grading than other histological features. We propose a simplified diagnostic criteria: meningiomas exhibiting two or more of these three features are diagnosed as atypical meningioma. In addition, a MIB-1 labeling index of 5.0 in meningioma may be a border value between benign and atypical types.

Key words. Meningioma—MIB-1 antibody—Grading—Atypical—Proliferative ability

Introduction

Atypical meningioma was added to the meningioma group as Grade II in the revised World Health Organization (WHO) classification of brain neoplasms. This variant is defined as meningiomas that exhibit several of the following features: fre-

[1]Department of Pathology, [2]Department of Neurosurgery, Gunma University School of Medicine, Maebashi, Gunma, 371 Japan

quent mitoses, increased cellularity, small cells with high nuclear cytoplasmic ratios (N/C) and/or prominent nucleoli, uninterrupted patternless or sheetlike growth, and foci of spontaneous or geographic necrosis [1]. Meningiomas were then classified into three grades, excluding meningeal sarcoma. However, it is not always easy for pathologists to grade meningioma, even taking into account all these features.

Several authors have described diagnostic criteria for atypical and anaplastic meningiomas. Maier et al. [2] defined an atypical meningioma as one with focally increased cellularity and at least five mitotic figures per ten high-power fields (HPFs). This definition is concise, but the category of atypical meningioma established with this definition may be smaller than that of the WHO classification. Some investigators have estimated and graded the severity of histological signs of anaplasia as 0–3 [3,4]. The parameters included hypercellularity, nuclear pleomorphism, mitosis, necrosis, loss of architecture, and brain invasion, and meningioma was classified into four or three grades, depending on total scores. However, this method is too complicated to apply to grading of meningioma routinely. Scoring of some features is prone to subjectivity, and grading of identical cases may differ between pathologists. Furthermore, de la Monte et al. [5] reported that the presence of features such as large prominent nucleoli, tumor growth in sheets, individual cell, necrosis and nuclear pleomorphism may be used to predict the recurrence of meningiomas. The significance of each feature may be different in estimating the malignant potential of meningiomas.

On the other hand, Ki-67 immunoreactivity is a useful index for assessment of the proliferating activity of various tumors including meningiomas [6]. MIB-1 monoclonal antibody, which was raised against a recombinant peptide corresponding to the Ki-67 cDNA fragment, is applicable to paraffin-embedded tissue sections [7]. A study of the proliferative potential of brain tumors was also performed using this antibody [8].

In this study, we examined 73 meningiomas in terms of the relationship of the histopathological features and the proliferating activity as assessed by MIB-1 immunoreactivity, and investigated which histopathological features indicate higher proliferative ability of meningiomas. Then we sought to apply this method of assessment to a three-tiered meningioma grading system and proposed simplified diagnostic criteria for histological grading of meningiomas.

Materials and Methods

We examined 73 meningioma specimens obtained from 49 cases, which included cases exhibiting the histological signs of anaplasia published in the WHO classification or those showing recurrence once or several times. Histologically benign meningiomas were also included.

The specimens were fixed in 10% formalin and embedded in paraffin. The hydrolytic autoclaving method was employed for immunostaining with MIB-1 antibody (Immunotech, Marseille, France; 1:50). After deparaffinization, sections were treated in phosphate buffered saline at 121°C for 15 min and incubated in MIB-1 antibody overnight at 4°C. A Biotin-Streptavidin Immunostaining Kit (Nichirei, Tokyo, Japan) was used for staining; sections were then visualized with diaminobenzidine solution.

Microscopically, mitotic index and the presence of prominent nucleoli, nuclear pleomorphism, areas of small cells with high N/C (Fig. 1d), hypercellularity, loss of architecture, invasion of brain, and necrosis were examined. Mitotic index was defined as the average number of mitotic figures (Fig. 1a) in 10 HPFs after counting at least 20 serial HPFs. The presence or absence of other features, defined as follows, were noted. Prominent nucleoli meant large and eosinophilic nucleoli (Fig. 1b). The presence of irregularly shaped nuclei that were at least threefold as large as the nuclear size of common tumor cells was regarded as nuclear pleomorphism (Fig. 1c).

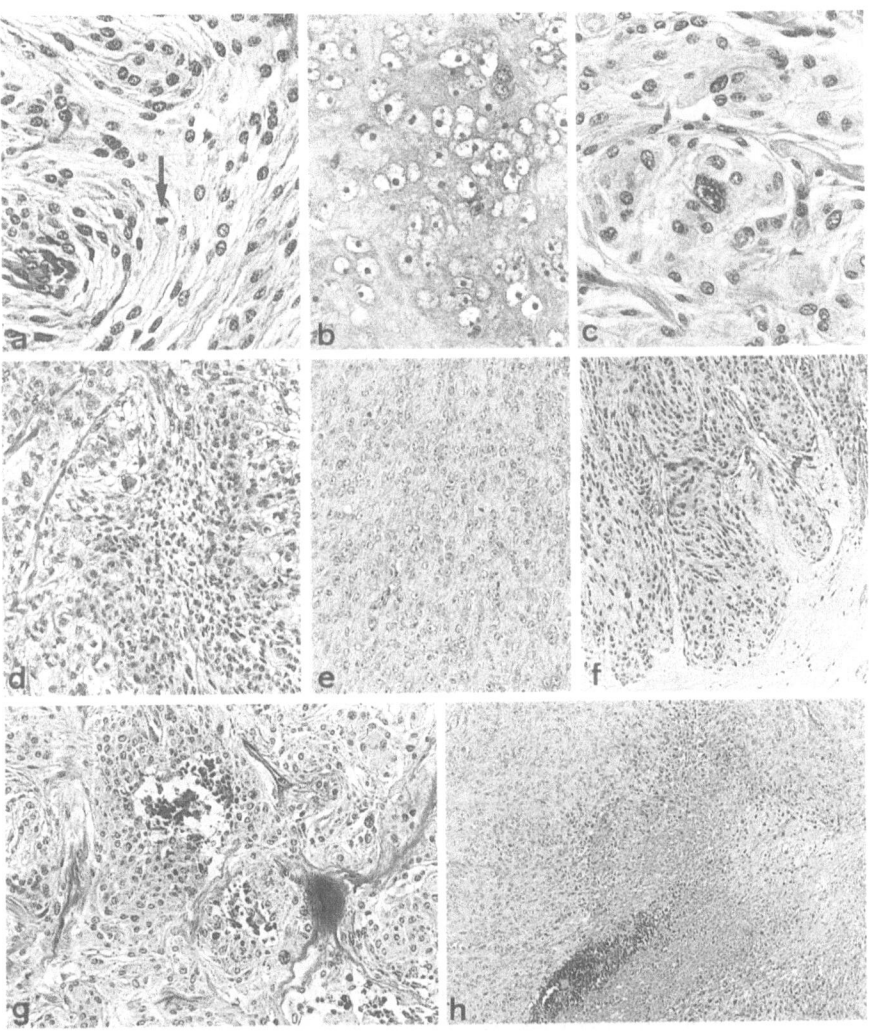

Fig. 1a–h. Histopathological features of meningioma. Hematoxylin and eosin staining. **a** A mitotic figure (*arrow*). ×250. **b** Prominent nucleoli. ×250. **c** Nuclear pleomorphism. ×250. **d** Small cell area with high nuclear cytoplasmic ratio (N/C). ×120. **e** Hypercellularity and loss of architecture. ×120. **f** Brain invasion. ×120. **g** Small foci of necrosis with karyorrhexis. ×120. **h** Conspicuous geographic necrosis. ×62

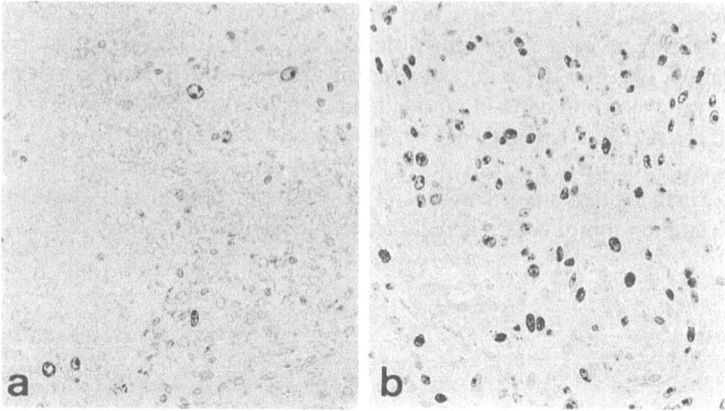

Fig. 2a,b. Anaplastic meningioma shows regional heterogeneity of MIB-1 immunoreactivity. MIB-1 immunostaining, ×170

Assessment of hypercellularity is more subjective than other features. When tumor cell nuclei were extensively piled up, we judged hypercellularity to be present (Fig. 1e). Loss of architecture meant that tumors showed growth in sheets in several microscopic fields at a magnification of ×200 (Fig. 1e). Brain invasion was judged positive when the tumor infiltrated to brain parenchyma in the form of tongues (Fig. 1f) or involved gliotic tissue. Necrosis was designated as both small foci of spontaneous necrosis (Fig. 1g) and extensive regions of geographic necrosis (Fig. 1h). MIB-1 antibody stained the nuclei of meningioma cells, and the staining pattern was diffuse or granular. Because the ratio of positive cells varied from region to region (Fig. 2a,b), the area with the greatest number of positive cells was selected and examined. The MIB-1 labeling index indicates the percentage of positive nuclei determined by counting 1000 nuclei in contiguous microscopic fields at a magnification of ×400 using a grid in the eyepiece.

Results

In our previous study [9], the mean Ki-67 (monoclonal antibody; Dako, Copenhagen, Denmark) labeling index of atypical meningioma according to the WHO classification was 4.82 in frozen sections, and the MIB-1 labeling index in paraffin sections was higher than the Ki-67 labeling index in frozen sections in identical tumors. On the basis of these findings, meningiomas with MIB-1 labeling indices of more than 5.0 were regarded as meningiomas with high proliferative ability. Of the 73 meningiomas examined in the current study, 39 belonged to this group. The histological features observed in meningiomas with high and low proliferative abilities are listed in Table 1. Thirty-eight (97%) of these meningiomas with high proliferative ability had mitotic indices equal to or more than 1, and the percentages with the presence of necrosis, prominent nucleoli, loss of architecture, nuclear pleomorphism, hypercellularity, brain invasion, and areas of small cells with high N/C were 92%, 64%, 62%, 56%, 56%, 21%, and 15%, respectively. In contrast, in the meningiomas with low proliferative activity, the incidence of each feature was low. The histological features of the meningioma group with the highest proliferative ability, of which labeling index was greater than 20.0, are given in Table 2. Mitosis and necrosis were observed in all the tumors. The mean mitotic index of the tumors was 23. The incidence of prominent nucleoli was increased in meningiomas with higher proliferative potential.

The mean MIB-1 labeling indices of meningiomas with or without each histological feature are listed in Table 3. The mean MIB-1 labeling index of meningiomas without brain invasion was not calculated, because the boundary zone was not always included in the tumor specimens and the absence of the feature thus was not definite. The mean MIB-1 labeling indices were significantly different between the tumors with and without mitosis or necrosis ($P < .0001$). Meningiomas with brain invasion showed a high mean MIB-1 labeling index, 19.8.

The area showing the highest MIB-1 immunoreactivity in each tumor corresponded to that showing the most mitotic figures on serial sections stained with hematoxylin and eosin. Linear regression analysis demonstrated that the MIB-1 labeling index was equivalent to $0.398 \times$ mitotic index $+6.963$: $r = .644$, $rs = .883$ (Fig. 3). A good correlation was found between the mitotic index and the MIB-1 labeling index. In contrast, there were only a few positive cells in the area of small cells with high

Table 1. Histopathological features of meningiomas with MIB-1 labeling indices more than 5.0.

Histological feature	MIB-1 LI > 5.0 ($n = 39$)		MIB-1 LI < 5.0 ($n = 34$)	
	n	%	n	%
Mitosis ($\geqq 1/10$ HPFs)	38	97	1	3
Necrosis	36	92	0	0
Prominent nucleoli	25	64	0	0
Loss of architecture	24	62	1	3
Nuclear plemorphism	22	56	1	3
Hypercellularity	22	56	0	0
Brain invasion	8	21	0	0
Small cells with high N/C	6	15	0	0

LI, labeling index; n, number; HPFs, high-power fields; N/C, nuclear cytoplasmic ratios.

Table 2. Histopathological features of meningiomas with MIB-1 LI greater than 20.0.

Histological feature	MIB-1 LI > 20	
	n	% ($n = 12$)
Mitosis ($\geqq 1/10$ HPFs)[a]	12	100
Necrosis	12	100
Prominent nucleoli	10	83
Loss of architecture	8	67
Nuclear pleomorphism	7	58
Hypercellularity	5	42
Brain invasion	4	33
Small cells with high N/C	1	8

[a] Mean mitotic number, 23/10 HPFs.

Table 3. Mean MIB-1 LI of meningiomas with or without various histological features.

Histological feature	Present (mean ± SD)	Absent (mean ± SD)
Mitosis (≧1/10 HPFs)	16.02 ± 7.94	1.93 ± 1.39*
Necrosis	16.72 ± 7.80	2.40 ± 2.31*
Prominent nucleoli	17.42 ± 8.00	5.06 ± 6.44*
Loss of architecture	16.92 ± 7.90	5.58 ± 7.22*
Nuclear pleomorphism	15.80 ± 8.01	6.54 ± 8.21*
Hypercellularity	15.48 ± 8.36	6.86 ± 8.31*
Brain invasion	19.80 ± 8.31	—
Small cells with high N/C	12.67 ± 8.68	9.18 ± 9.23

SD, standard deviation.
*, $P < .0001$.

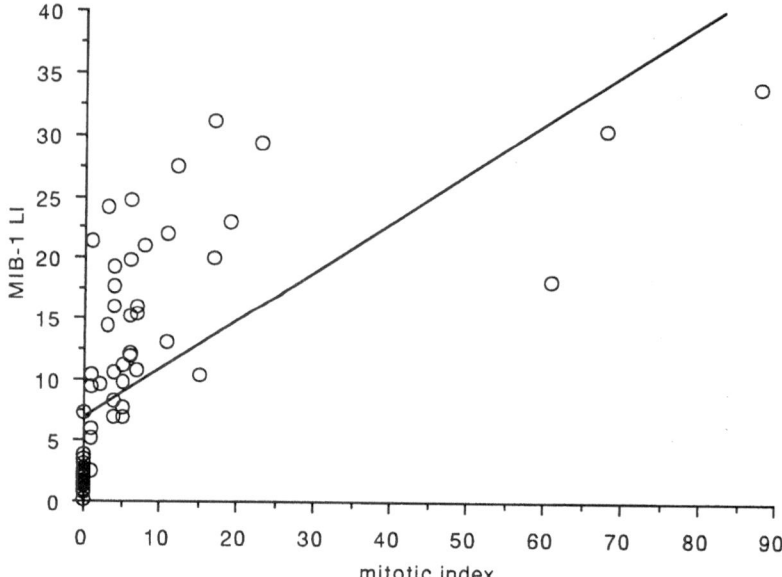

Fig. 3. Correlation between mitotic index (n/10 high-power fields) and MIB-1 labeling index (LI). Linear regression analysis showed good correlation: MIB-1 LI = 6.963 + 0.398 × mitotic index; $r = 0.644$, $rs = .883$, $P < .0001$

N/C. MIB-1-positive cells frequently showed relatively large nuclei with prominent nucleoli.

Discussion

Meningiomas with high proliferative potential were positive for mitotic figures and necrosis at high incidence. In addition, tumors infiltrating in the brain parenchyma exhibited markedly high proliferative activity. In grading of tumors, we generally evaluate cytological and histological anaplasia, proliferative activity, and invasive or metastatic ability. Atypical meningiomas are regarded as those with histological and cytological features that fall short of frank anaplasia [10]. Cellular anaplasia is judged from various features including irregularity of nuclear shape, increased chromatin, abnormal chromatin pattern, high N/C, pleomorphism, and prominent nucleoli; this grading is difficult to perform objectively. It seemed, with regard to the histological diagnosis of atypical meningiomas, that the assessment of proliferative ability may be the most important factor. Therefore, we considered that mitotic figures ($\geqq$1 per 10 HPFs), necrosis, and brain invasion were significant features for the diagnosis of atypical meningiomas. Simplifying the diagnostic criteria, meningiomas that have two or more of these three features may be diagnosed as atypical meningioma (Grade II). However, in practice the rarity of observation of brain invasion in histological preparations may decrease its value as a diagnostic criteria. Observation of mitotic figures and necrosis may be reliable features. Meningiomas without these three features are regarded as histologically benign meningiomas (grade I). If the specimens are small and only show either mitotic figures or necrosis, classification of atypical meningioma may depend on the other features including loss of architecture, prominent nucleoli, and hypercellularity.

There is a problem concerning the interpretation of necrosis. Recently, preoperative embolization has been frequently performed as a routine procedure to reduce bleeding. Several authors have reported, however, that necrosis occurred as a result of preoperative embolization [11,12]. It is necessary, therefore, for diagnosis to differentiate tumor necrosis from artificial necrosis evoked by embolization. Paulus et al. [11] described the following four features as histopathological changes caused by preoperative embolization: (1) a histological pattern composed of eosinophilic cytoplasm, small nuclei with condensed chromatin, and microcystic degeneration; (2) large necroses with indistinct borders; (3) presence of embolization material in large adjacent blood vessels; and (4) lack of additional histological criteria of malignancy. Empirically we considered that a small foci of necrosis with karyorrhexis and necrosis with fibrin deposits and replacement of collagen may not occur in 2 or 3 days after embolization. However, at present the morphological differences between these two types of necrosis are not sufficiently defined. The degree of interruption of blood flow and the period from embolization to surgical resection are considered to be responsible for the extent and morphology of necrosis. It is necessary to elucidate precisely the relationship between these factors and morphological changes.

In the WHO classification, anaplastic meningiomas are defined as those tumors exhibiting ominous histological features including obviously malignant cytology, a high mitotic index, and conspicuous necrosis [1]. We examined the histological features of tumors with MIB-1 labeling indices greater than 20.0 on the hypothesis that anaplastic meningiomas have markedly high proliferative ability. High mitotic index and necrosis were observed in all tumors. The average mitotic index was 23 per 10 HPFs. Necrotic areas were frequently large and geographic. Prominent nucleoli were found in 83% of these tumors. In addition, MIB-1-positive nuclei were frequently relatively large and had macronucleoli. Based on these data and published criteria, high mitotic index ($\geqq$10/10 HPFs), conspicuous necrosis, prominent nucleoli, loss of architecture, and brain invasion were taken to be discriminating features for the diagnosis of anaplastic meningioma. Meningiomas that satisfy the criteria of atypical meningioma and also exhibit three of these features can be regarded as anaplastic meningiomas (Grade III).

When we classified the primary meningiomas in the current study according to the presented criteria as shown in Fig. 4, they were graded as follows: 28 cases of histologically benign meningiomas, 16 cases of atypical types, and 5 cases of anaplastic types. Clinical outcomes of 19 cases of atypical and anaplastic meningiomas are shown in Table 4. In all except 2 patients, the tumor was resected totally. One case of atypical meningioma was subtotally resected and the tumor was again seen to be growing 23 months later. In another case, partial removal was performed, the tumor continued growing, and the patient died 26 months after surgery. These 2 cases were included in the recurrent group. Although interval time to recurrence in the anaplastic type was longer than that in cases of atypical meningioma, this may have been because the sizes of each group were small and follow-up time may have been insufficient.

After all tumor specimens were graded on the basis of current criteria, they were divided into 35 benign, 29 atypical, and 9 anaplastic meningiomas. The mean MIB-1 labeling indices in each type of meningioma in the current study are shown in Table 5. The MIB-1 labeling indices of atypical meningiomas ranged from 5.15 to 27.46. When a meningioma exhibits a MIB-1 labeling index more than 5.0, its histological features should be observed carefully, taking into account the possibility of an aggressive meningioma.

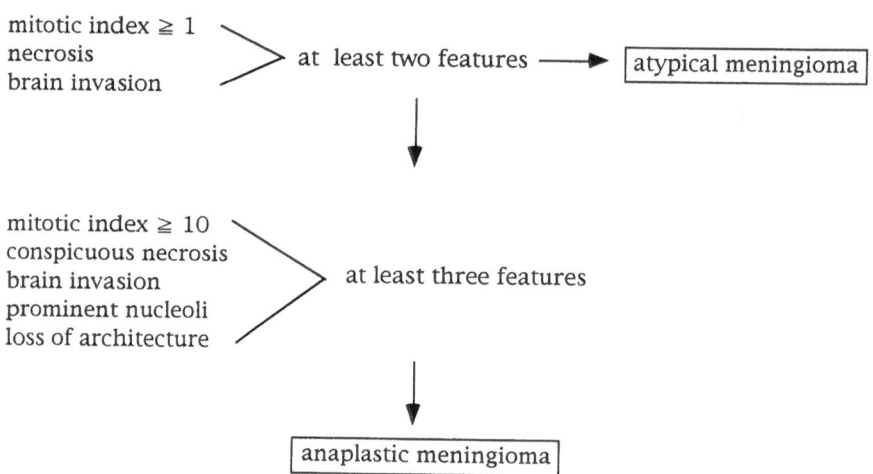

mitotic index ≥ 1
necrosis   > at least two features ──→ [atypical meningioma]
brain invasion

mitotic index ≥ 10
conspicuous necrosis
brain invasion   at least three features
prominent nucleoli
loss of architecture

[anaplastic meningioma]

Fig. 4. Diagnostic criteria of atypical and anaplastic meningioma

Table 4. Clinical outcomes of patients with atypical and anaplastic meningiomas.

	Atypical (n = 15)	Anaplastic (n = 4)
Recurrent	10	2
Interval time (mean)	5–48 mo (27 mo)	63, 97 mo (80 mo)
Dead	5	2
Nonrecurrent	5	2
Follow-up time	3–16 mo	8, 17 mo

Table 5. MIB-1 immunoreactivity in meningiomas.

Grade	Number of specimens	MIB-1 LI range	Mean ± SD
Benign (Grade I)	35	0.19–7.43	1.95 ±1.38
Atypical (Grade II)	29	5.15–27.46	14.13 ±6.22
Anaplastic (Grade III)	9	10.48–33.89	23.62 ±7.98

That histologically benign meningioma could recur is well known. Nine cases of meningioma of Grade I were recurrent in the present study. In five of these, total or subtotal removal had been performed. The average value ± SD of the MIB-1 labeling index of their primary tumors was 1.61 ± 1.11. In contrast, that of meningiomas which had not recurred for more than 5 years was 2.17 ± 1.56. There was no significant difference between proliferative potential of both groups. The MIB-1 labeling index was not predictable for the recurrence of histologically benign meningioma in this study. One meningioma of Grade I had an MIB-1 labeling index of 7.41. MIB-1 labeling index did not always correspond to histological grade, as has been reported previously [8,11]. Although the MIB-1 labeling index did not correlate infallibly with recurrence rate and histological grade, it may provide significant information for grading.

Conclusions

1. Mitotic figures, necrosis, and brain invasion in meningiomas show especially high correlations to their high proliferative ability as detected by MIB-1 immunostaining. These histological features contribute to the garding of meningiomas.
2. An MIB-1 labeling index of 5.0 may be a border value between common-type and atypical-type meningiomas.

Acknowledgments. We thank Ms. Machiko Yokota and Mr. Koji Isoda for their excellent technical assistance.

References

1. Kleihues P, Burger PC, Scheithauer BW (1993) Histological typing of tumours of the central nervous system, 2nd edn. Springer, Berlin, pp 36–37
2. Maier H, Ofner D, Hittmair A, Kitz K, Budka H (1992) Classic, atypical, and anaplastic meningioma; three histopathological subtypes of clinical relevance. J Neurosurg 77:616–623
3. Jääskeläinen J, Haltia M, Servo A (1986) Atypical and anaplastic meningiomas: radiology, surgery, radiotherapy, and outcome. Surg Neurol 25:233–242
4. Mahmood A, Caccamo DV, Tomecek FJ, Malik GM (1993) Atypical and malignant meningiomas: a clinicopathological review. Neurosurgery 33:955–963.
5. de la Monte SM, Flickinger J, Linggood RM (1986) Histopathologic features predicting recurrence of meningiomas following subtotal resection. Am J Surg Pathol 10:836–843

6. Roggendorf W, Schuster T, Peiffer J (1987) Proliferative potential of meningiomas determined with the monoclonal antibody Ki-67. Acta Neuropathol 73:361–364
7. Cattoretti G, Becker MHG, Key G, Duchrow M, Schlüter C, Galle J, Gerdes J (1992) Monoclonal antibodies against recombinant parts of the Ki-67 antigen (MIB-1 and MIB-3) detect proliferating cells in microwave-processed formalin-fixed paraffin sections. J Pathol 168:357–363
8. Karamitopoulou E, Perentes E, Diamantis I, Maraziotis T (1994) Ki-67 immunoreactivity in human central nervous system tumors: a study with MIB 1 monoclonal antibody on archival material. Acta Neuropathol 87:47–54
9. Hirato J, Nakazato Y, Satone A (1994) Application of proliferative ability using Ki-67 antibody and AgNORs method to brain tumor diagnosis (in Japanese). Neuropathol 14(suppl):315
10. Burger PC, Scheithauer BW (1994) Atypical and malignant meningiomas. In: Tumors of the central nervous system. Armed Forces Institute of Pathology, Washington, DC, pp 277–283
11. Paulus W, Meixensberger J, Hofmann E, Roggendorf W (1993) Effect of embolisation of meningioma on Ki-67 proliferation index. J Clin Pathol 46:876–877
12. Morimura T, Takeuchi J, Tani E (1994) Preoperative embolization of meningiomas: its efficacy and histopathological findings. Brain Tumor Pathol 11:123–129

Incidental Meningiomas in Autopsy Cases in Computed Tomography and Magnetic Resonance Imaging Era

Kazuhiko Sugiyama[1], Asao Hirano[1], Josefina F. Llena[1], Tohru Uozumi[2], Kaoru Kurisu[2], Kunyu Harada[2], Eiji Taniguchi[2], and Tohru Nishi[2]

Abstract. Between January 1980 and June 1994, autopsy was performed on 1979 cases at the Division of Neuropathology, Montefiore Medical Center. Intracranial meningioma was detected incidentally in 31 of these autopsies. These 31 cases were analyzed clinically and pathologically: the male-to-female ratio was about 1:2, and the average age at death was 76.8 years. A positive correlation was noted between tumor diameter and age. On histological study, the percentage of the psammomatous type of tumor was higher than that previously reported for clinical cases. When the proliferative activity was examined using antiproliferating cell nuclear antigen (anti-PCNA) antibody and silver-stained nucleolar organizer regions (Ag-NORs), the proliferative activity appeared lower in the psammomatous type than in any other histological type. These results suggest that clinical cases of meningioma incidentally detected in elderly persons have a low proliferative activity and persist in the individual for long periods of time.

Key words. Meningioma—Autopsy—Incidental tumor—Proliferating cell nuclear antigen—Nucleolar organizer region

Introduction

Meningioma is a tumor with an incidence rate of 2 per 100 000 population [1] that accounts for about 20% of all brain tumors [2,3]. Several reports [4–6] have concerned incidental meningiomas in autopsy cases. However, most of these reports were published before the introduction of computed tomography (CT) and magnetic resonance imaging (MRI). Very few reports have been published since then, and there has been no report in which findings were compared at the same facility before and after the introduction of CT and MRI. We analyzed, both clinically and pathologically, autopsy cases performed at the Montefiore Medical Center since the introduction of CT and MRI and compared these findings with these tumors from the same center reported soon after the introduction of CT [7]. In addition, the growth of the meningiomas was analyzed using a new technique.

[1] Division of Neuropathology, Department of Pathology, Montefiore Medical Center, The University Hospital for The Albert Einstein College of Medicine, Bronx, NY 10467, USA
[2] Department of Neurosurgery, Hiroshima University School of Medicine, Minami-ku, Hiroshima 734, Japan

Material and Methods

Specimens were obtained from 1979 autopsy cases examined at the Division of Neuropathology, Montefiore Medical Center, between January 1980 and June 1994. A diagnosis of incidental meningioma was made in cases in which all the following criteria were satisfied:

1. Intracranial meningioma was found incidentally in gross autopsy.
2. No medical records corresponded to meningioma.
3. No medical records indicated neurofibromatosis.

The age, sex, tumor site, tumor diameter, etc. were analyzed for each case. The tumor diameter was measured using Nakasu's method [7]. The tumor and the surrounding tissue were examined histologically [8]. Tumor growth was analyzed by examining percent positivity using immunohistochemical stains with MIB-1 [9] and antiproliferating cell nuclear antigen (PCNA) antibody [10], and nucleolar organizer regions (NORs) were scored using silver stain [11] in paraffin sections.

Results

Incidental meningioma that satisfied the listed criteria was detected in 31 cases; 29 cases had 1 lesion (single meningioma) and 2 cases had 2 lesions (multiple meningioma). In total, 33 lesions were detected. These 31 cases ranged from 46 to 98 years in age (mean, 76.8 years), including 11 men and 20 women with a male-to-female ratio about 1:2. The profiles of these 31 cases are shown in Table 1.

The tumors were located in the convexity in 18 cases, falx in 5 cases, parasagittal area in 5, sphenoidal ridge in 2, lateral ventricle in 1, olfactory groove in 1, and posterior fossa in 1. In 2 cases of multiple meningioma, all tumors were in the convexity. Figure 1 shows a case of meningothelial meningioma that developed in the choroid plexus of the inferior horn of the lateral ventricle; Fig. 2 shows the only case of meningioma accompanied by a microscopic daughter tumor. Tumor size in the 31 cases ranged from 3 to 30 mm in diameter (mean, 12.3 mm). According to the World Health Organization (WHO) classification [8], these tumors were histologically diag-

Table 1. Patient profiles[a].

Parameten	n
Sex	
Male	11
Female	20
Cause of death	
Neoplasm	10
Cardiovaseular disease	10
Aging	4
Infection	2
Diabetes mellitus	2
Other	3

[a] Patient ages ranged from 46 to 98 years (mean, 76.8).

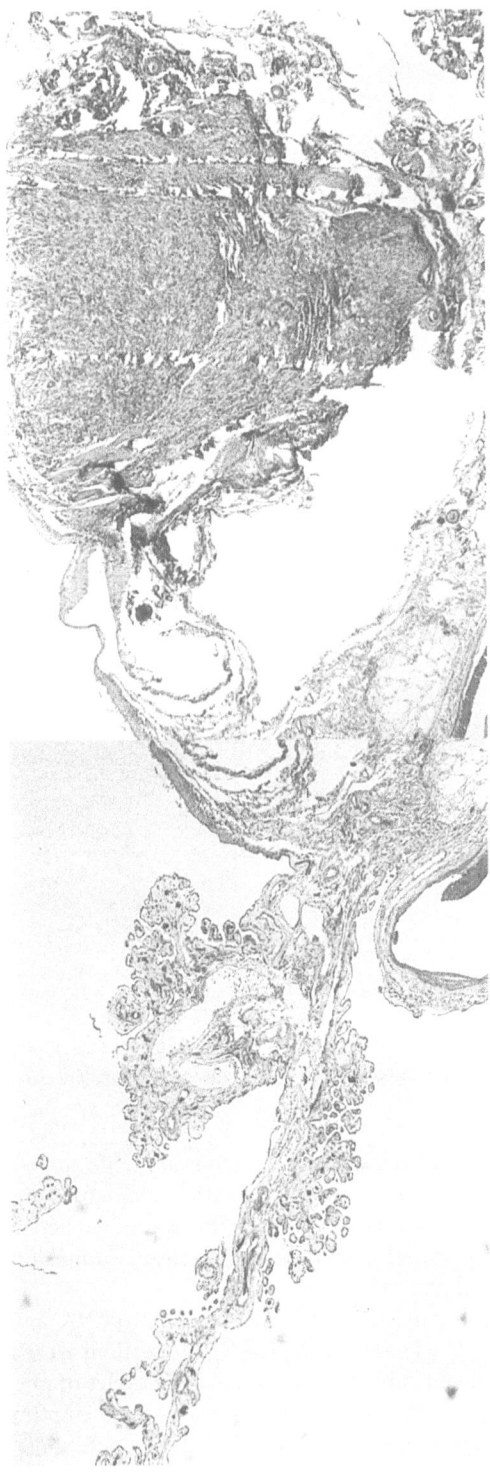

Fig. 1. Photomicrograph of meningothelial meningioma originating from the choroid plexus in the inferior horn of the lateral ventricle. Note hypertrophy of the mesenchyme around the tumor and disappearance of the epithelial cells. Hematoxylin and eosin (H&E), ×30

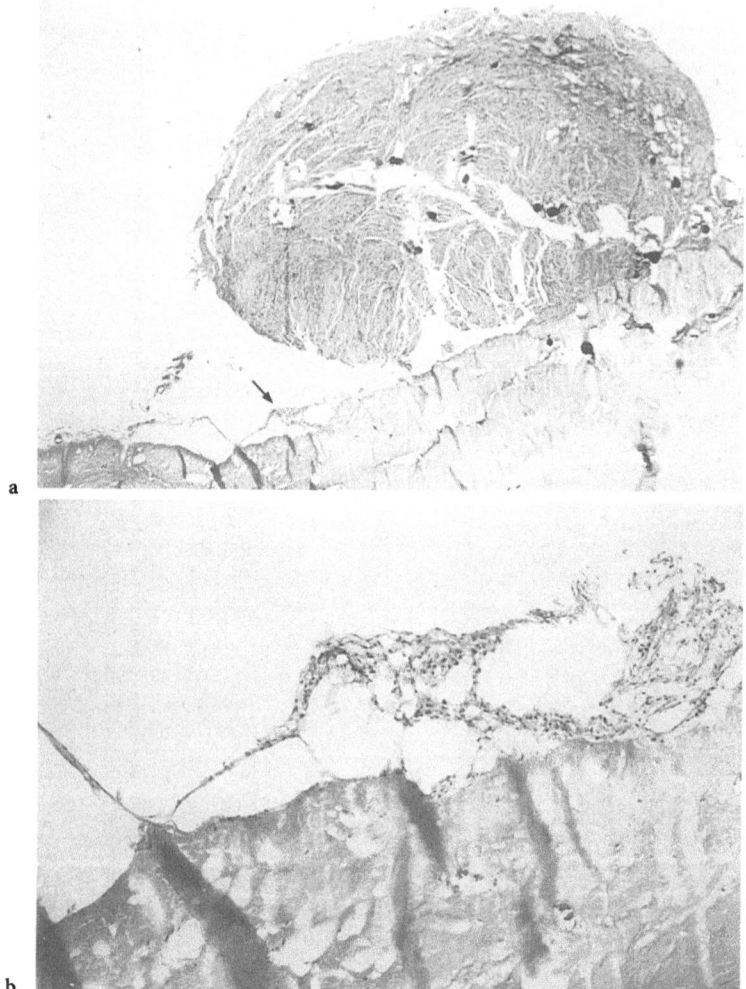

Fig. 2. a Photomicrograph of convexity meningioma with daughter tumor *(arrow)*. H&E, ×60. **b** Photomicrograph at high magnification of the daughter tumor. H&E, ×240

nosed as meningothelial in 14 cases, psammomatous in 12, fibrous in 5, transitional in 2, and angiomatous in 1. Figure 3 shows a case with angiomatous meningioma at the convexity (7 mm in diameter). A positive correlation was noted between tumor diameter and age of patient upon death, but there was no clear relationship between tumor diameter and histological type (Fig. 4).

Immunohistochemical staining with MIB-1 and anti-PCNA antibody was performed using the method of Linden et al. [12]. Tissue sections were placed in 0.01 M buffered citrate solution and subjected to 1, 3, 5, 7, or 9 cycles of microwave heating, each cycle lasting 3 min, to retrieve antigen and determine the optimal staining condition [13]. MIB antibody was negative under all these conditions, suggesting that antigenicity of the tissues is lost by the method of fixation used in this study (Fig. 5). The response to anti-PCNA antibody was greatest after 7 cycles of heating (Fig. 6).

Fig. 3. a Photomicrograph of angiomatous meningioma (7 mm in diameter). H&E, ×120. **b** Photomicrograph of
same case with silver impregnation for
reticulin. ×60

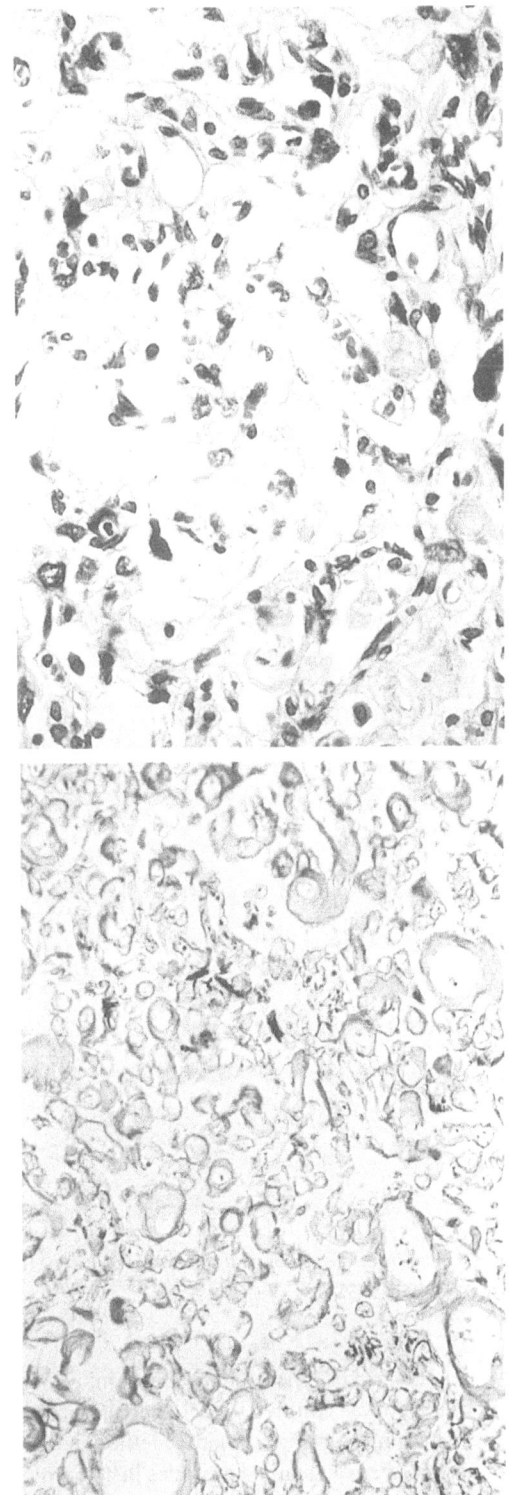

a

b

Size (mm)

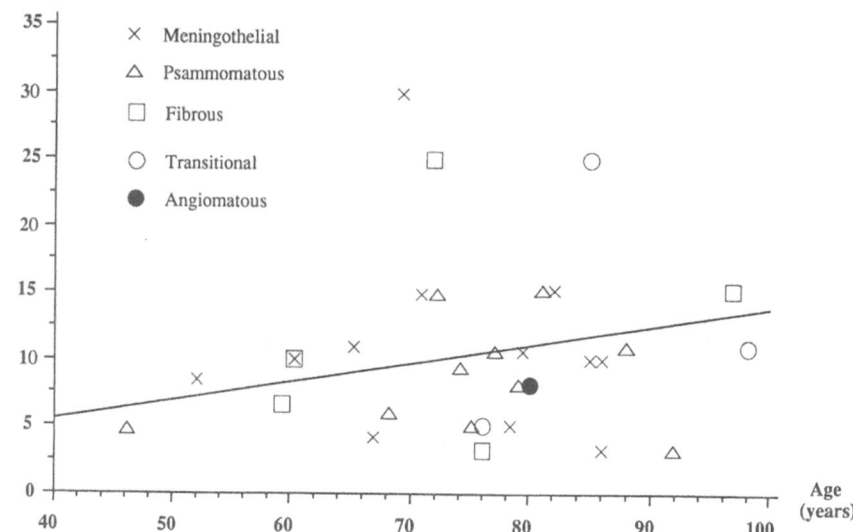

Fig. 4. Incidental meningioma: age (in years) plotted against tumor diameter (in millimeters). $Y = 0 + .14* X; R = .850$

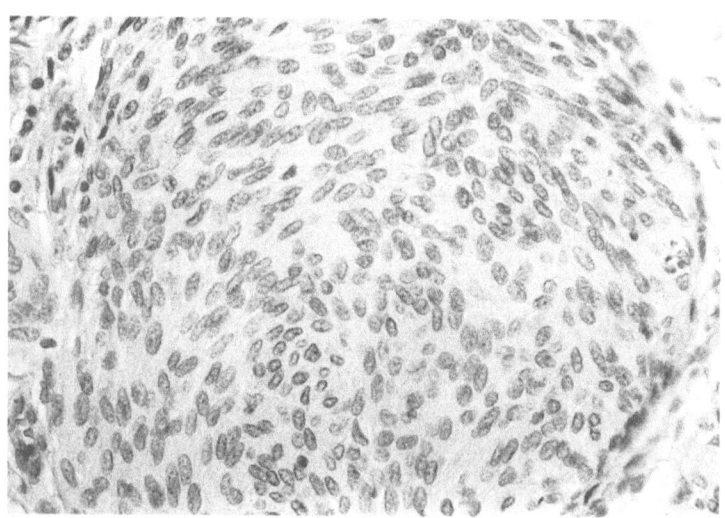

Fig. 5. Photomicrograph of no immunoreactivity for MIB-1. Immunostaining for MIB-1 with microwave treatment, ×120

Under the microscope (×400), the number of positive cells in 400 tumor cells from each section was counted to yield percent positivity (PP). NORs were examined using silver staining (Ag-NORs) by the method of Crocker et al. [14]. At ×1000, the number of positively silver-stained granules in 400 tumor cells from each section was counted to yield the Ag-NORs score (the average number of positively silver-stained granules

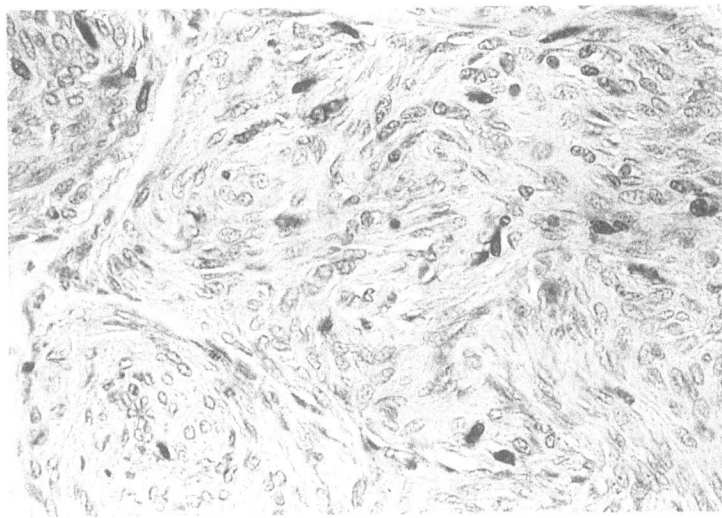

Fig. 6. Photomicrograph of sharp immunoreactivity for proliferating cell nuclear antigen (PCNA). Immunostaining for PCNA with microwave treatment, ×120

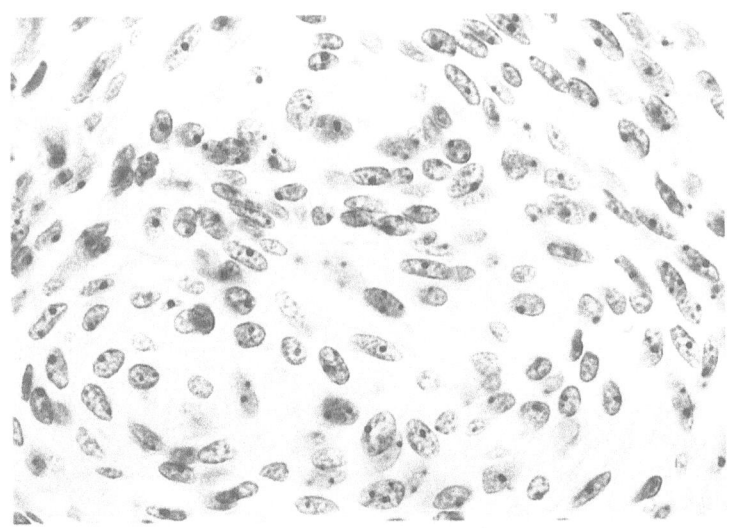

Fig. 7. Photomicrograph of nucleolar organizer region (NOR) staining. ×240

per cell) (Fig. 7). Table 2 summarizes the results from 15 cases; the PCNA PP ranged from 0.9% to 14.0% (mean, 5.0%) and the Ag-NORs score from 1.06 to 3.07 (mean, 1.89). Both parameters were significantly lower in the psammomatous type than in any other types ($P < .01$ for PCNA PP and $P < .05$ for Ag-NORs score, Mann–Whitney test). A positive correlation was noted between PCNA PP and the Ag-NORs score (Fig. 8).

Table 2. Incidental meningioma in autopsy cases.

Case	Age/Sex	Histological type	PCNA PP (%)	AgNOR counts
1	79/F	Me	2.4	2.00
2	78/F	Me	6.3	2.30
3	85/F	Me	6.2	2.58
4	67/F	Me	3.2	2.48
5	52/M	Me	5.1	1.24
6	86/M	Me	14.0	3.07
7	73/F	Ps	1.7	1.86
8	79/F	Ps	0.9	1.06
9	77/F	Ps	2.4	1.10
10	88/F	Ps	5.0	1.26
11	72/F	Ps	3.3	1.50
12	77/F	Ps	2.8	1.30
13	92/F	Fi	9.5	2.14
14	76/M	Tr	6.5	2.30
15	80/M	An	6.1	2.20

PCNA, Proliferating cell nuclear antigen; PP, percent positivity; AgNOR, silver-stained nucleolar organizer regions; Me, meningothelial; Ps, psammomatous; Fi, fibrous; An, angiomatous.

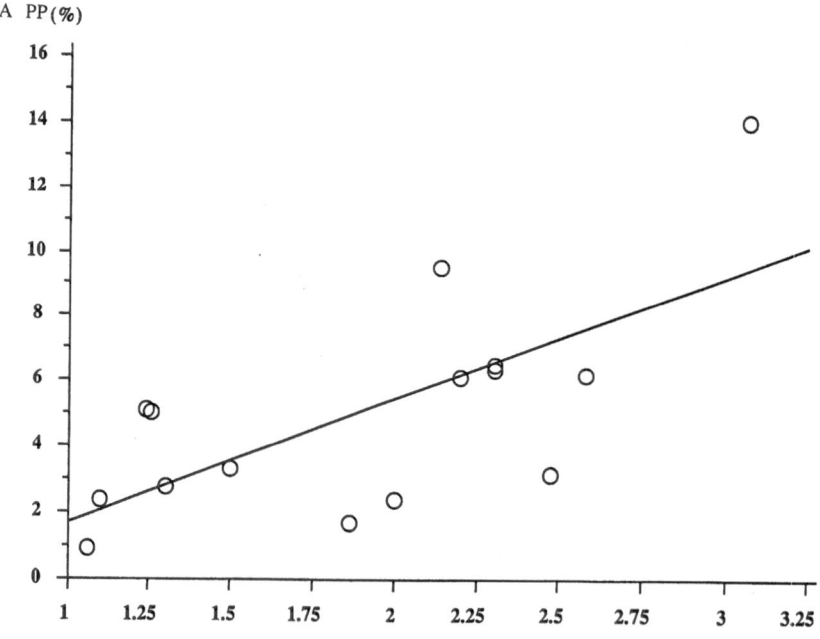

Fig. 8. Incidental meningioma in autopsy cases: percent positivity of proliferating cell nuclear antigen (PCNA PP) versus counts of silver-stained nucleolar organizer regions (AgNORs). $Y = -2.098 + 3.764^* X$; $R = .689$

Discussion

Meningioma develops in 2 of 100 000 persons [1] and accounts for about 20% of all brain tumors [2,3]. This tumor is often detected during autopsy because it develops from the arachnoid cup cell of the arachnoid granulation [15,16]. Several reports on incidental meningiomas in autopsy cases have appeared [4–6]. Most of these reports, however, were published before the introduction of CT and MRI, and very few reports have been published since then. Further, no investigators have compared features of this tumor before and after introduction of CT and MRI at the same facility. Nakasu et al. [7] reported on these tumors at the Montefiore Medical Center soon after the introduction of CT, having detected meningioma at an incidence of 2.3%. The meningioma detection rate in our study was 1.3% (31 of 1979 cases), lower than that reported by Nakasu et al. [7]. In addition, the multiple meningioma detection rate in the current study (6.5%) was lower than that reported by Nakasu et al. (8.2%) [7]. This decrease in the detection rates at this medical center seems to be related to the recent introduction and extensive use of CT and MRI.

The cases of meningioma found in our study are characterized by a lack of clinical symptoms and the considerably advanced age of the patients as compared to reported clinical cases [17,18]. In our study, a positive correlation was found between tumor diameter and the age of the patients, and the percentage of cases histologically diagnosed as psammomatous meningioma was higher than that of cases clinically diagnosed [11,19,20]. It was also found that the proliferative potential of psammomatous meningioma was lower than that of any other type. If these findings are combined with the knowledge that psammomatous meningioma has a lower recurrence rate and a better prognosis than any other histological type of meningioma [20], we may say that incidental meningioma detected in autopsy cases had a low proliferative activity and had remained for a long period. It is, therefore, necessary to review the conventional criteria that limit the use of surgery in elderly patients with incidental meningioma which has been increasingly detected following the introduction of MRI.

In the current study, small intraventricular meningioma (Fig. 1) and small angiomatous meningioma (Fig. 2) were also identified in pathological examination. Intraventricular meningioma is usually difficult to detect until it grows to be rather large [21], which is why small intraventricular meningiomas are rarely observed clinically. It is therefore very important to note the growth course of this tumor in our cases: tumor development in the choroid plexus, gradual replacement of the choroid plexus, and hypertrophy of mesenchyme. Although some investigators [22] have reported that angiomatous meningioma is a vessel-rich type of meningothelial meningioma, no meningothelial component was seen in this tumor on microscopy. It is likely that angiomatous meningioma was already present at the early stages of disease in this case, and that the growth of this tumor takes place while keeping a certain relation between tumor cells and tumor vessels. A microscopic daughter tumor was seen in 1 of the 31 cases examined. This finding is very important in consideration of the postoperative recurrence of this tumor [23], and may explain why about 10% of patients show recurrent tumor development even after treatment with Simpson's grade I surgery [24].

References

1. Rohringer M, Sutherland GR, Louw DF, Sims AF (1989) Incidence and clinicopathological features of meningiomas. J Neurosurg 71:665–672
2. Rachlin JR, Rosenblum ML (1989) Etiology and biology of meningiomas. In: Al-Mefty O (ed) Meningiomas. Raven, New York, pp 22–37
3. Committee of Brain Tumor Registry of Japan (1992) General features of brain tumors. Neurol Med Chir (Tokyo) 32:395

4. Nakasu S, Hirano A, Shimura T (1985) Incidental meningioma. Autopsy study. Neurol Med Chir (Tokyo) 25:928–932
5. Sayama I, Ito Z, Ohta H, Kobayashi H, Fukasawa H (1982) Incidental meningioma (in Japanese). Neurol Surg (Tokyo) 10:761–767
6. Wood MW, White RJ, Kernohan JW (1957) One hundred intracranial meningiomas found incidentally at necropsy. J Neuropathol Exp Neurol 16:337–340
7. Nakasu S, Hirano A, Shimura T, Llena JF (1987) Incidental meningiomas in autopsy study. Surg Neurol 27:319–322
8. Kleihues P, Burger PC, Scheithauer BW (1993) Histological typing of tumours of the central nervous system. Springer, Berlin, pp 33–37
9. Key G, Becker MHG, Duchrow W, Schluter C, Gerdes J (1992) New Ki-67 equivalent murine monoclonal antibodies (MIB-1) prepared against recombinant parts of the Ki-67 antigen. Anal Cell Pathol 4:181
10. Kim DK, Hoyt J, Bacci C, Keles GE, Mass M, Mayberg MR, Berger MS (1993) Detection of proliferating cell nuclear antigen in glioma and adjacent resection margin. Neurosurgery 33:619–626
11. Orita T, Kajiwara K, Nishizaki T, Ikeda N, Kamiryo T, Aoki H (1990) Nucleolar organizer regions in meningioma. Neurosurgery (Baltimore) 26:43–46
12. Linden MD, Torres FX, Kubus J, Zarbo RJ (1992) Clinical application of morphologic and immunocytochemical assessments of cell proliferation. Am J Clin Pathol 97:4–13
13. Shi S-R, Keu ME, Kalra KL (1991) Antigen retrieval in formalin-fixed, paraffin-embedded tissues: an enhancement method for immunohistochemical staining based on microwave oven heating of tissue sections. J Histochem Cytochem 39:741–748
14. Crocker J, Boldy DAR, Egan MJ: How should we count AgNORS? Proposal for standardized approach. J Pathol 158:185–188
15. Kepes JJ (1982) Meningiomas: biology, pathology and differential diagnosis. Masson, New York
16. O'Rahilly R, Miller F (1986) The meninges in human development. J Neuropathol Exp Neurol 45:588–608
17. Committee of Brain Tumor Registry of Japan (1992) General features of brain tumors. Neurol Med Chir (Tokyo) 32:401
18. Jaaskelainen J, Haltia M, Laasonnen E, Wahlstrom T, Valtonen S (1985) The growth rate of intracranial meningiomas and its relation to histology. An analysis of 43 patients. Surg Neurol 24:165–172
19. Mirimanoff RO, Dosoretz DE, Linggood RM, Ojemann RG, Martuza RL (1985) Meningioma: analysis of recurrence and prognosis following neurosurgical resection. J Neurosurg 62:18–24
20. Kunishio K, Ohmoto T, Furuta T, Matsumoto K, Nishimoto A (1994) Factors influencing recurrence rate of intracranial meningiomas after surgery. Neurol Med Chir (Tokyo) 34:81–84
21. Fornari M, Savoiardo M, Morello G, Solero C (1981) Meningiomas of the lateral ventricle. J Neurosurg 54:64–74
22. Russell SD, Rubinstein LJ (1989) Pathology of tumours of the central nervous system. Arnold, London, pp 473–479
23. Borovich B, Doron Y, Braun J, Guilburd JN, Zaaroor M, Goldsher D, Lemberger A, Gruszkiewicz J, Feinsod M (1986) Recurrence of intracranial meningiomas: the role played by regional multicentricity. Part 2: Clinical and radiological aspects. J Neurosurg 65:168–171
24. Simpson D (1957) Recurrence of intracranial meningiomas after surgical treatment. J Neurol Neurosurg Psychiatry 20:22–39

Clinicopathological Study of Malignant Meningiomas

Junichi Mizuno[1], Hiroshi Nakagawa[1], Kazuo Hara[2],
and Yoshio Hashizume[3]

Abstract. Although meningiomas are commonly benign brain tumors and curable by total surgical resection, malignant meningiomas with multiple recurrence have been long recognized. Of 68 primary intracranial meningiomas treated surgically at Aichi Medical University between 1985 and 1994, 6 cases were considered to be malignant in view of the clinical and pathological findings. These 6 cases were studied in terms of recurrence, radiological appearance, histological characteristics, and proliferation rate by monoclonal antibodies. Of this group of patients, 4 women and 2 men, 3 persons died eventually after multiple operations and 2 are alive with an episode of recurrence. These cases included 2 atypical, 1 papillary, 1 meningotheliomatous (invasive), and 1 hemangioblastic meningioma, and 1 hemangiopericytoma. On histological examination, hypervascularity and increased cellularity were noted in all cases. Radiological features were mushroom extension without calcification. Cell proliferation tended to increase at each recurrence. The authors would like to stress the combined evaluation of these histological and radiological characteristics and measurement of proliferation potential to predict the bizarre course of the patient.

Key words. Meningioma—Malignant—Recurrence—Monoclonal antibody—Hypervascularity

Introduction

There has been continuing debate on the clinicopathological characteristics of malignant meningiomas [1–3]. The World Health Organization (WHO) recently proposed a new classification of tumors of the central nervous system [4]. According to this classification on meningeal neoplasms, atypical, papillary, and anaplastic meningiomas are thought to be malignant. Various histopathological characteristics such as hypercellularity [1], mitotic activity [2], focal necrosis [5], hypervascularity [6], and pleomorphism [7] were termed malignancy. However, the aggressive behavior or recurrence of seemingly benign meningiomas without these findings cannot be well explained.

[1] Department of Neurological Surgery, [2] Department of Surgical Pathology, [3] Institute for Medical Science of Aging, Aichi Medical University, Aichi-gun, Aichi 480-11, Japan

Attempts were made to define nonbenign appearances from the radiological findings [8–10], but these definitions failed to grasp the exact behavior of the tumor at this moment. Therefore, the biological behavior of meningiomas often cannot be predicted from the histopathological or radiological findings alone. With the advent of monoclonal antibodies, including proliferating cell nuclear antigen (PCNA) and Ki-67 [11,12], the actual proliferative potential of human brain tumors has been calculated [13-15]. Determination of the proliferative rate using monoclonal antibodies in malignant meningiomas is of special value for recurrent tumors as positivity increases at each recurrence [11].

The purpose of this study was to investigate the prediction of malignant behavior of meningiomas by a "classic" clinicopathological method and a supplemental evaluation with monoclonal antibodies.

Patients and Methods

Sixty-eight patients with meningeal neoplasms proven neuropathologically underwent surgery at our institute from 1984 to 1993. Of these 68 meningiomas, 6 patients showing sinister histology are at the focus of this chapter. All cases were originally described as showing seemingly malignant features such as hypercellularity, high mitotic figures, focal necrosis, hypervascularity, nuclear pleomorphism, and brain invasion. A case of hemangiopericytoma of the meninges was included in this series, although a new WHO classification has excluded this neoplasm from the category of meningiomas. Location of the tumor, radiological appearance, Simpson's grading [16], recurrence, and histological features were reviewed. In addition, immunohistological labeling of proliferating cells with monoclonal antibodies including PCNA and Ki-67 (5 cases) were measured to evaluate the actual proliferation potential.

Results

The six patients, four women and two men, had a mean age of 49 years (range, 30 –68 years). Symptoms of the patients were essentially affected by the location of the tumor. All patients were available for follow-up study for a mean duration of 76 months (range, 3 – 10 years).

Location of Tumors

Tumor site was determined by computerized tomography (CT) or magnetic resonance imaging (MRI). In two cases, tumors were at the middle fossa; of the other four, there was one tumor each at the convexity, peritorcular, cavernous sinus, and petroclivus.

Clinical Course

A patient with a convexity meningioma was treated by total resection (Simpson's Grade I), but in the other five cases subtotal resection was done (between Simpson's Grade II and IV). Irradiation therapy was applied in four cases. No adjunctive chemotherapy was given.

Table 1. Clinical summary of malignant meningiomas.

Case no.	Age	Sex	Tumor location	Pathological diagnosis	Surgery (Simpson's grade)	Number of recurrences	Outcome
1	37	F	Convexity	Atypical	I	1	Alive
2	57	F	Middle fossa	Atypical	III	3	Dead
3	52	M	Middle fossa	Meningotheliomatous (invasive)	II	—	Alive
4	68	F	Peritorcular	Hemangiopericytoma	III	2	Alive
5	30	F	Cavernous sinus	Papillary	IV	2	Dead
6	48	M	Petroclivus	Hemangioblastic	IV	3	Dead

Table 2. Radiological summary of computed tomography (CT) and magnetic resonance imaging (MRI).

Case No.	Mushroom projection	Absence of calcification	Necrosis in the tumor	Transdural extension	Marked edema
1	+	+	−	−	−
2	+	+	−	+	I
3	+	+	+	−	−
4	+	+	+	+	−
5	+	+	+	−	−
6	+	+	+.	−	−

Five tumors showed recurrence or regrowth, and three patients died subsequently. The relationship between the location of the tumor, surgical resection, and recurrence is shown in Table 1.

CT and MRI Aspects

Calcification, commonly regarded as a sign of benign neoplasms, was absent in all cases. Hypodense or cystic areas within the tumor were seen in four cases. Two tumors exhibited transdural extension. Marked peritumoral edema was noted in only one case. Nodular irregularity of the tumor margins invading the adjacent brain, called mushrooming, was demonstrated in all cases (Table 2).

Histological Findings

Two cases were atypical and of the other cases there were one each of papillary type, meningotheliomatous type (invasive), hemangioblastic type, and a hemangiopericytoma. Of six cases, two showed histological change, one from meningotheliomatous to atypical type and the other from angiomatous to papillary type, at recurrence. Hypercellularity and hypervascularity were seen in all cases. Five cases revealed increased mitotic figures. Pleomorphism was evident in three and focal necrosis in two (Table 3).

Immunohistological Labeling of the Proliferating Cells

The relationship between positivity against PCNA and Ki-67 and recurrence is shown in Fig. 1. Although not statistically significant, positivity increased with recurrence.

Table 3. Pathological characteristics.

	Hypercellularity	Mitosis	Necrotic foci	Hypervascularity	Pleomorphism
1	++	+	−	++	++
2	++	+	+	++	+
3	+	+	−	+	−
4	++	−	−	++	+
5	++	+	+	++	+
6	+	+	−	++	−

++, positive (moderate to strong); +, positive (mild to moderate); −, negative.

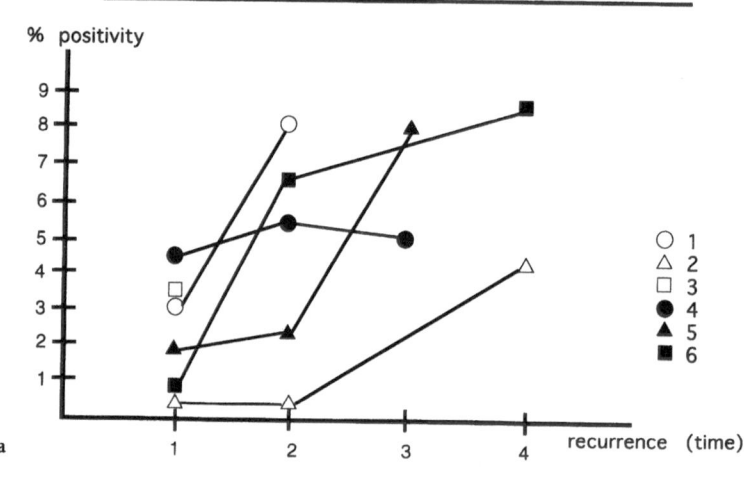

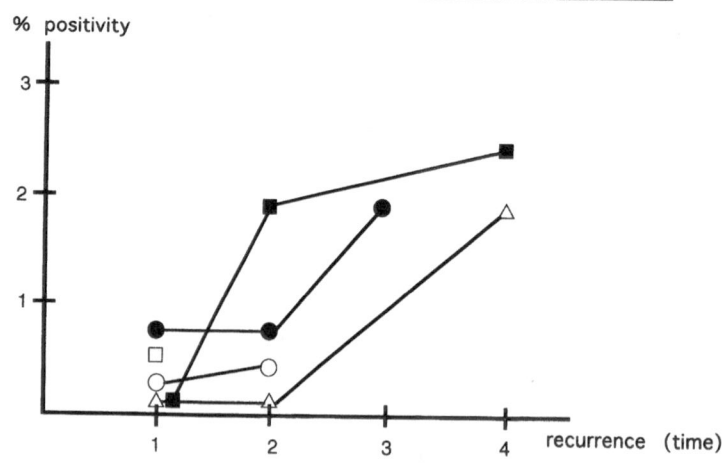

Fig. 1.a,b. Percent positivity of two monoclonal antibodies, proliferating cell nuclear antigen (PCNA) (**a**) and Ki-67 (**b**) in relation to recurrence. Positivity tends to increase with recurrence. Numbered symbols correspond to the six cases discussed in the text

Illustrative Cases

Case 1: Convexity Meningioma

This 37-year-old woman visited our hospital because of headache. MRI demonstrated a high-intensity mass of the right convexity (Fig. 2a). A total removal of the tumor was carried out (Simpson's grade I). Histological diagnosis was a meningotheliomatous meningioma (Fig. 2b). She was doing well as a housewife for 3 years and 9 months postoperatively. When she returned to us because of increasing head heaviness, MRI

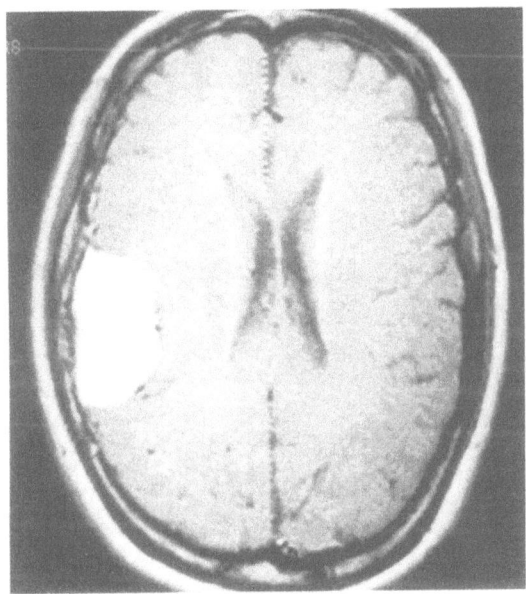

Fig. 2.a–d. Convexity meningioma. **a** A well-demarcated high-intensity area was noted in the right convexity on magnetic resonance imaging (MRI) with contrast enhancement. **b** Light photomicrograph shows typical pattern of whorl formation. Hematoxylin and eosin (H & E) stain, ×400. **c** A lobulated mass recurred at the same location. **d** Light photomicrograph reveals increased mitotic figures and pleomorphism with ample vascular networks. H & E, ×400

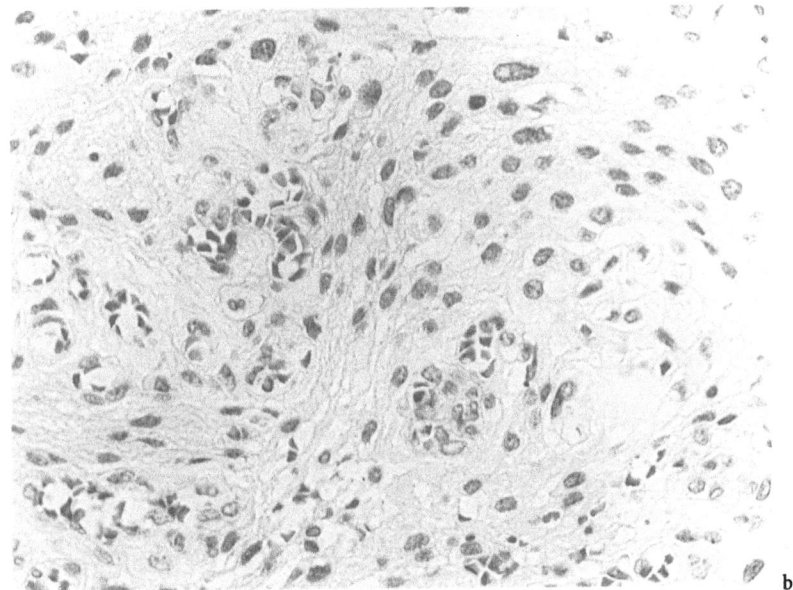

disclosed recurrence of the tumor at the same region (Fig. 2c). Complete resection of the tumor was attempted. Histologically her tumor was an atypical meningioma with increased pleomorphism, mitotic figures, and capillary networks (Fig. 2d). Positivity against PCNA and Ki-67 increased compared to that at the initial operation.

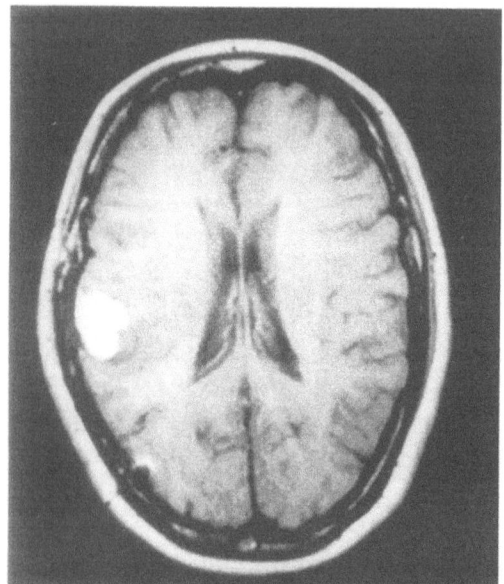

Fig. 2. *Continued*

c

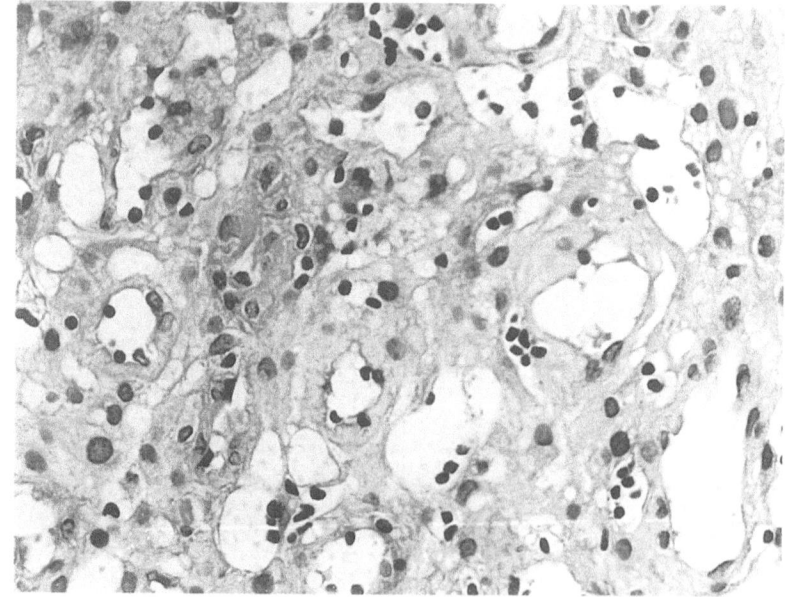

d

Case 2: Middle Fossa Meningioma

This 57-year-old housewife was admitted to our hospital because of a high-density mass in the right middle fossa extending into the posterior fossa on CT (Fig. 3a). A subtotal resection (Simpson's grade III) was performed. Histological diagnosis was atypical meningioma (Fig. 3b). She underwent surgical treatment four times during

Fig. 3.a–d. Middle fossa meningioma. **a** Computed tomography (CT) demonstrates an uniformly enhanced high-density mass in the right middle fossa with extension into the posterior fossa. **b** Light photomicrograph shows increased pleomorphism, signifying atypical meningioma. H & E, ×400. **c** Mushroom enlargement of the tumor projects into the adjacent brain with extracranial extension. **d** Election micrograph shows irregularity of nucleus; no desmosome or interdigitation was seen. ×20 000

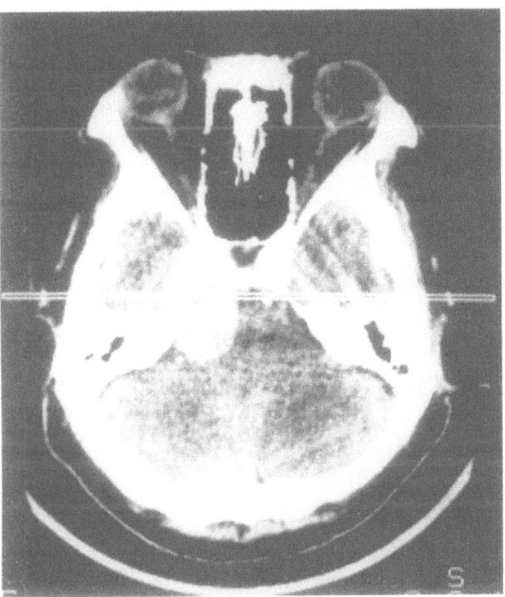

a

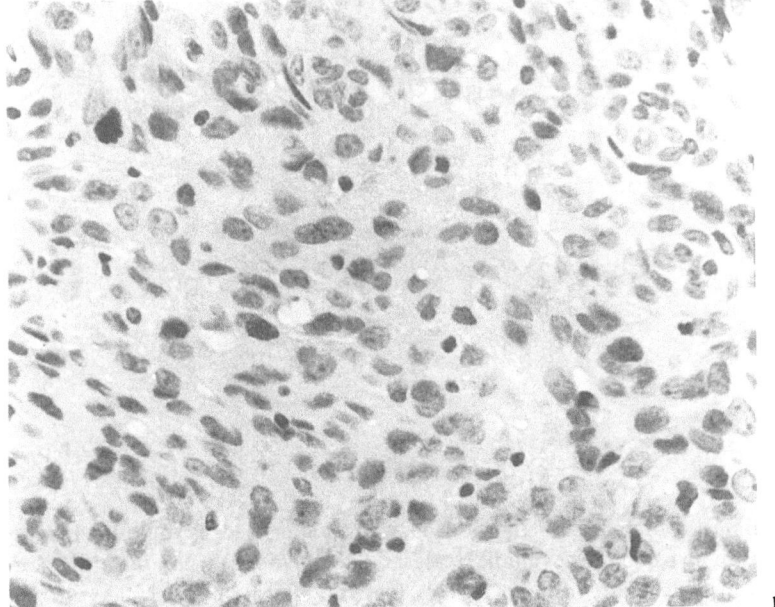

b

Fig. 3. *Continued*

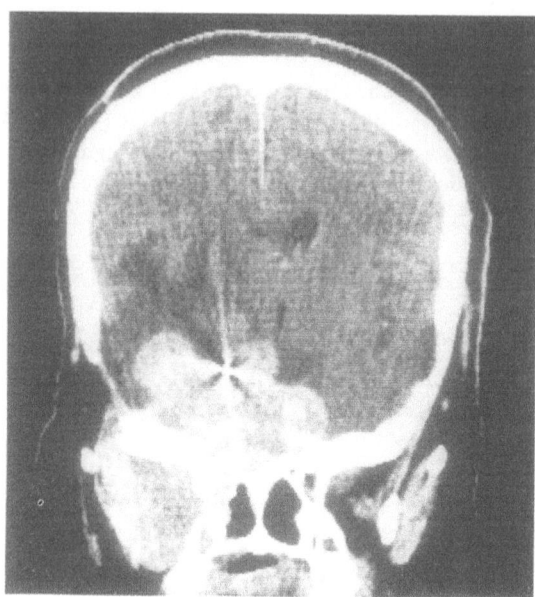

c

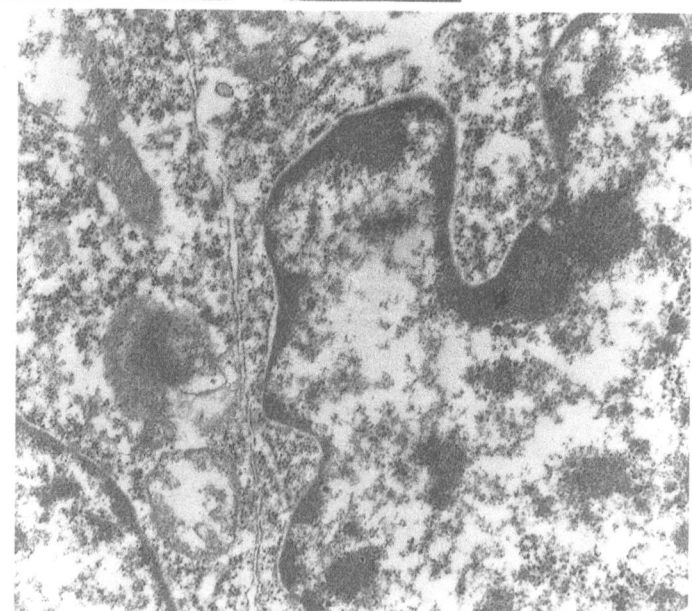

d

her clinical course. Eventually she died, 4 years later, because of brainstem dysfunction from invasion by the tumor. Her last CT revealed mushrooming projection of the tumor into the adjacent brain (Fig. 3c). Electron microscopy views lacked the typical morphological features of meningiomas (Fig. 3d).

Discussion

Meningiomas have been classified according to their grade of malignancy [17,18]. It seems to be unrealistic to establish criteria of malignant meningiomas by any single clinical behavior, radiological appearance, or classic histological feature.

On CT and MR imagings, there are unique appearances that discriminate atypical or malignant meningiomas from classic meningiomas, for instance, indistinct margins toward the adjacent brain, heterogeneous enhancement, and mushroom enlarging [8–10]. Of the six cases in this series all cases showed mushroom enlargement without calcification. Heterogeneously irregular enhancement was positive in four cases, and two cases showed extension along the dura.

We wish to put special emphasis on mushroom enlargement without calcification, reflecting a specific derangement of growth by malignant meningiomas. Heterogeneous enhancement may not be as important a radiological sign as malignancy, because low-density areas often appear in benign meningiomas [10,19].

The process of malignant transformation of benign meningiomas has not been well explained, nor has prediction of recurrence after complete resection of the tumor been well established, although there are several reports [20,21]. In our series, there was a similar case of histological changes from meningotheliomatous type to atypical type 3 years and 9 months after a total removal. This case showed increased pleomorphism and hypervascularity at recurrence. Skullerud et al. [1] regarded high cellularity as indicative of recurrence, Jellinger et al. [2] preferred high cellularity and increased mitotic rate, Christensen et al. [5] necrosis, de la Monte et al. [6] hypervascularity, and Cho et al. [7], pleomorphism.

Hypervascularity and hypercellularity were noticed in all cases of our series. Increased mitotic figures were noticed in five cases and pleomorphism in three. Although much larger series on this critical issue should be accumulated, we would like to emphasize that the ample capillary networks in packed tumor cells are an important histological feature for recurrence and malignant transformation of meningiomas.

A useful method of monitoring the growth rate of a meningioma would be to measure cell kinetics by an immunohistological method using the monoclonal antibodies PCNA and Ki-67 [22,23]. Several investigators have reported the prognostic utility of proliferation markers in malignant meningiomas in determining malignancy of the tumor [24–26]. The authors analyzed recurrence of malignant meningiomas using those monoclonal antibodies and found that positivity to antibodies tended to increase with each recurrence despite various levels of positive reaction at the initial operation. Roggendorf et al. [11] reported Ki-67 labeling indices correlated well with the rate of tumor recurrence. The issue of biologically meaningful atypia as well as the malignancy of menigiomas has been widely discussed. The monoclonal antibody method would provide supplemental information about the active proliferating rate of brain tumors.

Conclusion

The line of demarcation between benign and malignant meningiomas is still equivocal. There is no single reliable guideline to predict a bizarre course of patients with nonbenign meningiomas. Although there are only a few cases in our series, densely packed tumor cells with abundant capillary networks and mushroom enlargement are considered to be malignant signs. Observation of proliferative potential using PCNA and Ki-67 was useful for follow-up.

References

1. Skullerud K, Loken AC (1974) The prognosis in meningiomas. Acta Neuropathol 29:337–344
2. Jellinger K, Slowik F (1975) Histological subtypes and prognostic problems in meningiomas. J Neurol 208:279–298
3. Thomas HG, Dolman CL, Berry K (1981) Malignant meningiomas: clinical and pathological features. J Neurosurg 55:929–934
4. Kepes JJ (1990) Review of the WHO's new proposed classification of brain tumors. In: Proceedings of the Xlth International Congress of Neuropathology, Kyoto, Japan, pp 87–97
5. Christensen D, Laursen H, Klinken L (1983) Prediction of recurrence in meningiomas after surgical treatment. Acta Neuropathol 61:130–134
6. de la Monte SM, Flickinger J, Linggood R (1986) Histopathologic features predicting recurrence of meningiomas following subtotal resection. Am J Surg Pathol 10:836–843
7. Cho KG, Hoshino T, Nagashima T, et al (1986) Prediction of tumor doubling time in recurrent meningiomas. J Neurosurg 65:790–794
8. Dietemann JL, Heldt N, Burquet JL, et al (1982) CT findings in malignant meningiomas. Neuroradiology 23:207–209.
9. New PFJ, Hesselink JR, O'Carroll CP, et al (1982) Malignant meningiomas: CT and histological criteria, including a new CT sign. AJNR 3:267–276
10. Vassilouthis J, Anbrose J (1979) Computerized tomography scanning appearances of intracranial meningiomas. J Neurosurg 50:320–327
11. Roggendorf W, Schuster T, Peiffer F (1987) Proliferative potential of meningiomas determined with the monoclonal antibody Ki-67. Acta Neuropathol 73:361–364
12. Hall PA, Levison DA, Woods AL, et al (1990) Proliferating cell nuclear antigen (PCNA) immunolocalization in paraffin sections: an index of cell proliferation with evidence of deregulated expression in some neoplasms. J Pathol 162:285–294
13. Burger PC, Shibata T, Kleihues P (1986) The use of the monoclonal antibody Ki-67 in the identification of proliferating cells. Am J Surg Pathol 10:611–617
14. Louis DN, Edgerton S, Thor AD, et al (1991) Proliferating cell nuclear antigen and Ki-67 immunohistochemistry in brain tumors. A comparative study. Acta Neuropathol 81:675–679
15. Plate KH, Rueschoff J, Behnke, et al (1990) Proliferative potential of human brain tumors as assessed by nucleolar organizer regions (Ag NORs) Ki67-immunoreactivity. Acta Neurochir (Wien) 104:103–109
16. Simpson D (1957) The recurrence of intracranial meningiomas after surgical treatment. J Neurol Neurosurg Psychiatry 20:22–39
17. Turner OA, Craig WM, Kernohan JW (1942) Malignant meningiomas. A clinical and pathologic study. Surgery 11:81–100
18. Zulch KJ, Mennel HD (1975) The question of malignancy in meningiomas (abstract). Acta Neurochir 31:275–276
19. Russell EJ, Ajax EG, Kricheff II et al (1980) Atypical computed tomographic features of intracranial meningiomas. Radiology 135:673–682
20. Pasquier B, Gasnier F, Pasquier D (1986) Papillary meningioma: clinicopathologic study of seven cases and review of the literature. Cancer 58:299–305
21. Yamazaki Y, Kawano N, Suwa T, et al (1994) Recurrent meningioma with malignant transformation: a case which changed from meningothelial type to papillary type (in Japanese). No Shinkei Geka 22:285–289

22. Allegranza A, Girlando S, Arrigoni GL et al (1991) Proliferating cell nuclear antigen expression in central nervous system neoplasms. Virchows Arch A Pathol Anat 419:417–423
23. Shibata T, Burger PC, Kleihues P (1988) Cell kinetics of human meningiomas and neurinomas in Ki-67 PAP stain (in Japanese). No Shinkei Geka 16:939–944
24. Hoshino T, Nagashima T, Murovic JA, et al (1986) Proliferative potential of human meningiomas of brain. Cancer 58:1466–1472
25. Orita T, Kajiwara K, Nishizaki T, et al (1990) Nuclear organizer regions in meningioma. Neurosurgery 26:43–46
26. Scarpelli M, Montironi R, Sisti S, et al (1989) Quantitative evaluation of recurrent meningiomas. Pathol Res Pract 185:746–751

Part II
Dynamic Aspects of the Biology of Brain Tumor Cells

Section 1. Cell Motility

Expression of L1CAM in Brain Tumors: Immunohistochemical Study Using Anti-L1CAM Antibodies

Shuichi Izumoto, Norio Arita, Takanori Ohnishi, Shoju Hiraga, Takuyu Taki, and Toru Hayakawa

Abstract. We investigated expression of L1CAM, a neural cell adhesion molecule, in brain tumors using three different antibodies. All six olfactory neuroblastomas, three primitive neuroectodermal tumors, two central neurocytomas, and three gangliogliomas showed positive immunoreactivity. One of six medulloblastomas also showed positive staining, but six glioblastomas and five oligodendrogliomas did not stain. Tumor cells were immunoreactive to the antibodies that recognized the fibronectin type III domain or intracellular domain of L1CAM, but vascular endothelial cells alone were immunoreactive to the antibody recognizing the immunoglobulin C2 domain. L1CAM is a useful immunohistochemical marker of embryonic or neuronal tumors in the central nervous system but not of astrocytic or oligodendroglial tumors.

Key words. Cell adhesion molecule—L1CAM—Brain tumor—Immunohistochemistry

Introduction

Adhesion molecules play important roles in cell interaction during development, maintenance, and regeneration of the nervous system, each of them having distinct functions involving different cells at different stages. Neural cell adhesion molecule L1 (L1CAM) is one of the adhesion molecules that belongs to an immunoglobulin superfamily [1,2] and is involved not only in neuron–neuron adhesion but also in neurite fasciculation, outgrowth of neurites, neurite outgrowth on Schwann cells, and neuron cell migration [3–7]. L1CAM consists of six immunoglobulin C_2-like domains, five fibronectin type III-like domains, a transmembrane segment, and a relatively small cytoplasmic region [1]. Expression of L1CAM is developmentally regulated and has been demonstrated to exist only on neurons in the central nervous system [8]. The present study was undertaken to investigate whether neuronal tumors as well as non-neuronal tumors in the central nervous system express L1CAM protein.

Department of Neurosurgery, Osaka University Medical School, Suita, Osaka 565, Japan

Materials and Methods

Materials

Thirty-one surgical specimens of neuroepithelial tumors were studied: 11 neuronal tumors (6 olfactory neuroblastomas, 2 central neurocytomas, 3 gangliogliomas), 9 embryonic tumors (6 medulloblastomas, 3 primitive neuroectodermal tumors [PNETs]), 6 glioblastomas, and 5 oligodendrogliomas.

Methods

Tumor specimens were fixed with paraformaldehyde and embedded in paraffin. Sections of the tumors 6 μm thick were cut and mounted on slides that had been coated with 3′-aminopropyltriethoxysilan. The sections were incubated with three different rabbit anti-rat L1CAM antibodies (generous gifts from Dr. Asou, Keio University [9]), which recognize the immunoglobulin C_2 domain of L1CAM (antibody Ig-C_2), fibronectin type III domain (antibody FN), and intracellular domain (antibody IC), respectively. The sections were stained by the avidin–biotin complex peroxidase method as described previously [10] using Vectastain ABC kit (Vector Lab., Inc., Burlingame, CA). Briefly, they were deparaffinized and rehydrated through graded ethanols. The endogenous peroxidase activity was blocked with hydrogen peroxide (0.3% in methanol for 20 min). The sections were washed with $0.01 M$ phosphate buffered saline (PBS, pH 7.4) containing 0.1% Triton X-100. They were then incubated with normal goat serum diluted 1:70. After washing, the sections were incubated with one of the primary anti-L1CAM antibodies diluted 1:200 for 18 h at 4 °C and then with biotinylated second antibody of rabbit anti-rat IgG for 1 h at room temperature; this was followed by incubation with avidin DH–biotinylated horseradish peroxidase H complex for 1 h at room temperature. After each incubation, the sections were washed with $0.01 M$ PBS (pH 7.4) and 0.1% Triton X-100. Sections were then incubated with 3, 3′-diaminobenzidinehydrogen peroxidase substrate. The slides were counterstained in hematoxylin and mounted with EUKITT. The intensity of staining was graded as intensely positive, positive, or negative.

Results

The results of immunostaining are summarized in Table 1. Three (9.7%) of 31 tumors stained with antibody Ig-C_2, 15 (48%) with antibody FN, and 6 (19%) with antibody IC. All olfactory neuroblastomas were positive. One of these, with widespread dural invasion, strongly stained with antibody FN (Fig. 1A–C). All three PNETs stained positively with antibody FN. The intensity of positive staining varied from one tumor to another (Fig. 2). One medulloblastoma was focally immunoreactive to antibody FN, but most medulloblastoma cells lacked immunoreactivity. Diffuse but weak positive staining was observed in two central neurocytomas. In three gangliogliomas, immunoreactive cells were focally seen, but none of these were large ganglionic cells. Neither oligodendrogliomas or glioblastomas were immunoreactive. With antibody FN or antibody IC, tumor cells stained positively. With antibody Ig-C_2, however, vascular endothelial cells in two olfactory neurobla-

Table 1. Results of immunohistochemical study with L1CAM antibodies.

	n	Antibodies		
		FN-III	Ig-C2	IC
Olfactory neuroblastoma	6	6 (2)	2	6
Central neurocytoma	2	2	0	0
Ganglioglioma	3	3	0	0
PNET	3	3 (1)	0	0
Medulloblastoma	6	1	1	0
Glioblastoma multiforme	6	0	0	0
Oligodendroglioma	5	0	0	0
Total:	31	15 (3)	3	6

FN, Ig-C_2, and IC represent antibodies recognizing the fibronectin type III domain, immunoglobulin C_2 domain, and intracellular domain of L1CAM molecule, respectively. PNET, primitive neuroectodermal tumor.
Numbers in parentheses indicate number of tumors showing intense positive staining.

stomas and one medulloblastoma were imunoreactive, while tumor cells were poorly reactive.

Discussion

Cell adhesion molecules (CAMs) are involved in several morphogenetic events and are regulated to fulfill changing demands during cell development. Among neural cell adhesion molecules expressed in the central nervous system, the amount of L1CAM varies with age, showing a peak value in early postnatal life [8]. In rat brain, expression of L1CAM on neurons increased from embryonic day 17 and decreased postnatally.

Our immunohistochemical study demonstrated that embryonic and neuronal tumors expressed L1CAM but glial tumors did not. L1CAM may be an immunohistochemical marker for neuronal or embryonic tumors.

We have no clear explanation for the fact that the immunostaining results with three antibodies were different. Tumor cells stained positively with antibodies FN and IC, while vascular endothelial cells in olfactory neuroblastoma and medulloblastoma stained with antibody Ig-C_2. One possible explanation is that endothelial cells of these tumors have some molecules that are cross-reactive to L1CAM, which is recognized by antibody Ig-C_2. Positive staining with antibody Ig-C_2, however, was limited to the sections in which tumor cells stained with antibodies FN or IC. This fact suggests another possibility: that the L1CAM identified on the endothelial cells was its soluble form, which was produced by tumor cells and migrated to endothelial cells. Indeed, L1CAM was reported to exist as not only a phosphorylated insoluble form of 200-kDa polypeptides on the cell surface but also as a soluble form of 170-, 140-, and 80-kDa polypeptides.

We found that an olfactory neuroblastoma showing widespread dural invasion had diffuse and intense positive staining with antibody FN. L1CAM has been reported to

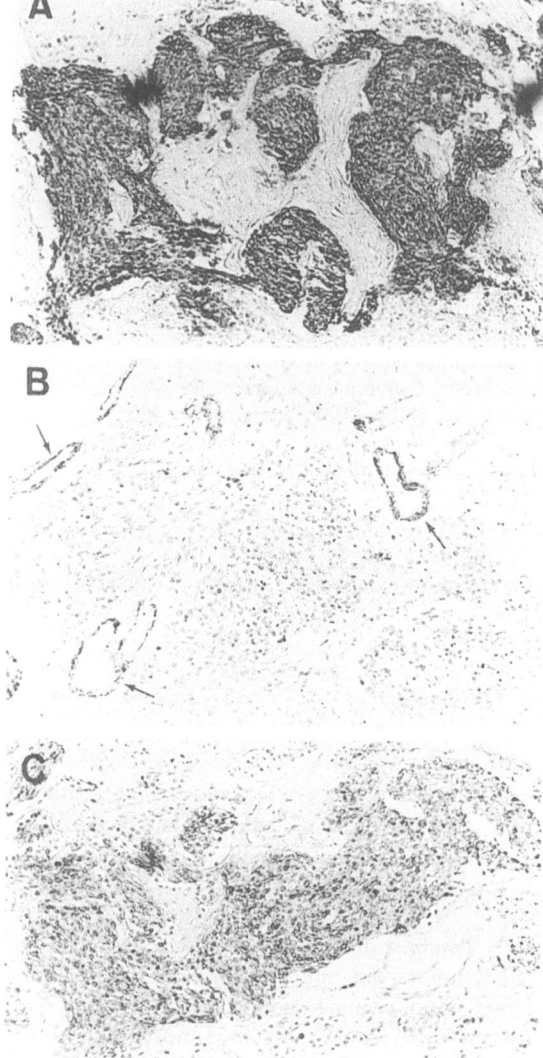

Fig. 1A–C. Olfactory neuroblastoma with prominent dural invasion. **A** Tumor cells diffusely and intensely stained with antibody FN. ×100. **B** Vascular endothelial cells were immunoreactive to antibody Ig-C₂, but tumor cells (*arrows*) were not. ×100. **C** Tumor cells diffusely stained with antibody IC. ×100

be involved in neural migration of cerebellar granular cells in the pre- and postnatal period in rats. L1CAM might be involved in the process of cell invasion into the dura mater in olfactory neuroblastomas.

Glioblastomas and oligodendrogliomas did not stain with L1CAM antibodies in this study. We have, however, detected L1CAM mRNA expressed by cultured glioma cells with reverse transcriptase-polymerase chain reaction (RT-PCR). The biological function of L1CAM as detected on tumor cells is currently unknown and should be elucidated.

Acknowledgments. We are grateful to Dr. H. Asou (Keio University, Tokyo) for generous gifts of anti-L1CAM antibodies.

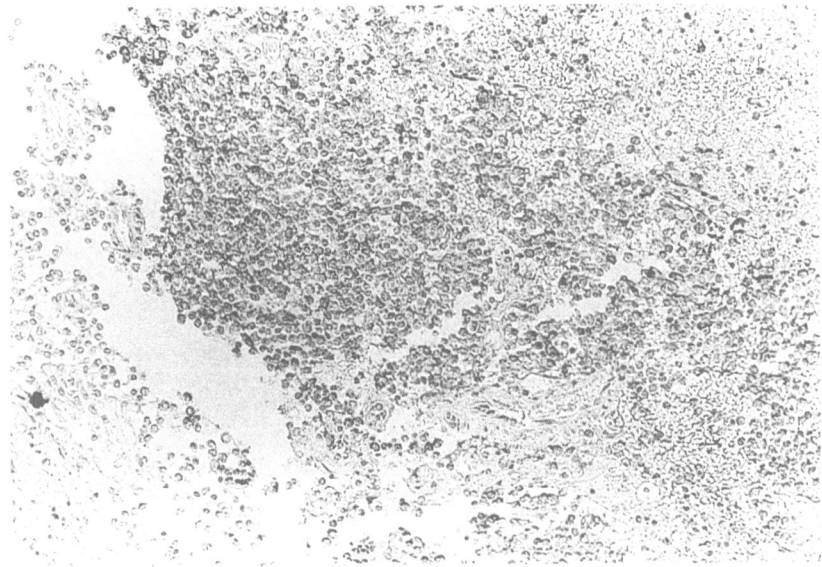

Fig. 2. Primitive neuroectodermal tumor (PNET) shows focal intense staining with antibody FN. ×100

References

1. Moos M, Tacke R, Scherer H, Teplow D, Fruh K, Schachner M (1988) Neural adhesion molecule L1 as a member of the immunoglobulin superfamily with binding domains similar to fibronectin. Nature 334:701–703
2. Sonderegger P, Rathjen FG (1992) Regulation of axonal growth in the vertebrate nervous system by interactions between glycoproteins belonging to two subgroups of the immunoglobulin superfamily. J Cell Biol 119:1387–1394
3. Lemmon V, Farr KL, Lagenaur C (1989) L1-mediated axon outgrowth occurs via a homophilic binding mechanism. Neuron 2:1597–1603
4. Kadmon G, Kowitz A, Altevogt P, Schachner M (1990) The neural cell adhesion molecule N-CAM enhances L1-dependent cell-cell interactions. J Cell Biol 110:193–208
5. Asou H, Miura M, Kobayashi M, Uyemura K, Itoh K (1992) Cell adhesion molecule L1 guides cell migration in primary reaggregation cultures of mouse cerebellar cells. Neurosci Lett 144:221–224
6. Miura M, Asou H, Kobayashi M, Uyemura K (1992) Functional expression of a full-length cDNA coding for rat neural cell adhesion molecule L1 mediates homophilic intercellular adhesion and migration of cerebellar neurons. J Biol Chem 267:10752–10758
7. Appel F, Holm J, Conscience JF. Schachner M (1993) Several extracellular domains of the neural cell adhesion molecule L1 are involved in neurite outgrowth and cell body adhesion. J Neurosci 13:4764–4755
8. Linnemann D, Edvardsen K, Bock E (1988) Developmental study of the cell adhesion molecule L1. Dev Neurosci 10:34–42
9. Asou H, Miura M, Kobayashi M, Uyemura K (1992) The cell adhesion molecule L1 has a specific role in neural cell migration. NeuroReport 3:481–484
10. Hsu SM, Raine L, Fanger H (1981) Use of avidin-biotin peroxidase complex (ABC) in immunoperoxidase techniques. A comparison between ABC and unlabelled antibody (PAP) procedures. J Histochem Cytochem 29:577–580

Expression and Biological Functions of L1 Cell Adhesion Molecule in Malignant Glioma Cells

Takanori Ohnishi, Shuichi Izumoto, Norio Arita, Shoju Hiraga, Takuyu Taki, and Toru Hayakawa

Abstract. Human and rat glioma cells were screened for their expression of the L1 cell adhesion molecule (L1 CAM) gene and protein by reverse transcriptase-polymerase chain reaction (RT-PCR) and immunodot analysis, respectively. All glioma cells tested expressed the L1 gene in various degrees. They also produced L1 molecules to a certain extent, while normal rat glia did not produce L1. The amount of expression of the L1 gene was related to the cell morphology and cell–cell aggregation patterns in a monolayer cell culture. That is, the more glioma cells expressed the L1 gene, the less polarity they had in cell shape and the more compactly they aggregated when growing in the early phase of cell culture. The glioma cells strongly migrated not only to a synthetic L1 polypeptide but also to L1- or L1cs-transfected fibroblast cells. These results suggest that L1 expressed in glioma cells may play an important role in the migration of the glioma cells through homophilic or heterophilic cell adhesion, thus participating in tumor invasion, particularly along the nerve fibers.

Key words. L1—Cell adhesion molecule—Glioma—Invasion—Cell migration

Introduction

Malignant gliomas are characterized by their high invasiveness into surrounding normal brain tissues, particularly along the nerve fibers including corupus callosum. Such translocation of tumor cells might be mediated by adhesion and motility of individual cells to extracellular matrices and host cells [1]. We have demonstrated that glioma-derived motility factor (GMF) promotes the migration of glioma cells in an autocrine fashion [2,3]. The propensity of glioma cells to infiltrate along the nerve fibers, however, cannot be explained by the function of the GMF alone. Several adhesion molecules in the central nervous system have been reported that can regulate neural cell adhesion and motility [4,5]. Among them, L1, one of the cell adhesion molecules belonging to the immunoglobulin superfamily, has been shown to have the strongest migration activity for neural cells [6]. L1 is, so far, believed to be involved in neuron–neuron homophilic adhesion by a calcium-independent mechanism [7,8]. Although an L1 involvement in cell adhesion other than neuron–neuron adhesion is

Department of Neurosurgery, Osaka University Medical School, Suita, Osaka 565, Japan

more controversial, recent studies have shown that antibodies to L1 readily inhibit neuron–glial adhesion in both the mouse and the chicken [7,9]. In addition, it has been shown that L1 may also engage in a heterotypic binding mechanism with the axon-associated cell adhesion molecule axonin-1 [10]. Other ligands for L1 have been postulated but have not been identified [11]. There have been no reports on gene expression of L1 in gliomas or the biological functions of L1 in glioma cells. In this study, we have demonstrated a novel expression of the L1 gene and production of L1 molecules in human and rat malignant glioma cells. Furthermore, we have investigated the migratory activity of L1 in glioma cells to clarify the biological functions of L1 in the process of tumor invasion.

Materials and Methods

Cells and Cell Culture

Human glioma cell lines, T98G and U373MG, and rat glioma cell lines, C6 and 9L, were maintained as previously described [2,12]. Nine different human glioma cells (h-1, h-2, h-3, h-4, h-5, h-6, h-7, h-8, and h-9) obtained from patients with glioblastoma were cultured and grown in Dulbecco's modified Eagle's medium with 10% fetal bovine serum (FBS). Normal rat glia was obtained from the brain of day 18 fetuses of a pregnant Wistar rat as previously described [3]. A neuroblastoma cell line, GOTO (from the Japanese Cancer Research Resources Bank), was maintained in medium containing 45% RPMI1640, 45% minimal essential medium, and 10% FBS.

Reverse Transcriptase Polymerase Chain Reaction

Total RNA(2μg), extracted from each cell line using Isogen (Nippon Gene, Toyama, Japan), was incubated at 42°C for 20min in 20μl of a reaction mixture containing 2.5pmol of random hexamer, 1U of RNase inhibitor (RNasin), 2.5U of M-MLV reverse transcriptase (RT), 20nmol of each dNTPs, 4ml of 5 × RT buffer (0.25M Tris-HCl (pH 8.3), 0.37M KCl, 15mM MgCl$_2$, and 200pmol of DTT. The solution was then heated at 99°C for 5min and cooled at 5°C for 5min. The cDNA solution thus prepared (20μl) was combined with 55.4μl of sterile water containing 25pmol of each of the two primers (p21, CGCAGCAAGGGCGGCAAATA; p22, TGGCCCCTGAGCTGTCATTG), 140nmol of MgCl$_2$, 3.5mmol of KCL, and 2.5U of Taq polymerase. This solution was subjected to 35 cycles of amplification (each cycle being composed of denaturation at 94°C for 1min, annealing at 55°C for 1min, and extension at 72°C for 2min). The solution was then subjected to electrophoresis on 2% agarose gel and stained with ethidium bromide.

Immunodot Analysis

Whole cell lysates were obtained from 10^7 of each cell type using a lysis buffer containing 1% (vol/vol) NP-40, 1mM phenylmethanesulfonyl fluoride (PMSF), 0.15M NaCl, and 1mM EDTA in 10mM Tris-HCl (pH 7.4) buffer. The lysates whose protein was adjusted to the same concentration (1mg/ml) among each cell line were serially diluted, and 100μl of each sample was spotted onto Immobilon-P membranes

(Millipore). The dot was blocked with Block-Ace (Dainippon Pharmaceutical, Osaka, Japan), incubated for 1 h with a rabbit anti-L1 polyclonal antibody (gift from Dr. H. Asou), washed in Tris-HCl buffered saline (TBS) containing 0.1% Tween, and then incubated with a biotinylated goat anti-rabbit IgG antibody (Vector, Burlingame, CA, USA) for 1 h. After incubation with avidin–biotin-conjugated horseradish peroxidase (Vector) for 30 min, the immunoreactive products were visualized with diaminobenzidine in 0.01% H_2O_2 in 0.05 M TBS.

Cell Migration Assay

Assays were carried out by using two different forms of L1 as stimulants: synthetic polypeptides that include a part of the fibronectin domain of the L1 molecule, and human fibroblast cells in which the L1 gene is transfected and the L1 molecule is normally expressed (gift from Dr. H. Asou). Forty-eight-well microchemotaxis chambers (NeuroProbe, Cabin John, MD, USA) were used for the fomer stimulant, and chemotactic cells (Kurabo) were used for the latter. Both contained 8-μm-pore-size polycarbonate membranes as a filter. Details of the assay method have been previously described [2,3]. All experiments were performed in triplicate.

Results

Expression of L1 Gene

All glioma cell lines tested expressed the L1 gene in various degrees, although the amounts of L1 in glioma cells were less than one-half of that in the positive control, GOTO cells (Fig. 1). T98G, h-7, and h-9 glioma cells in which the L1 gene was expressed in relatively high amounts showed a morphology of polygonal epithelium-like cells and had a tendency to grow in close contact each other from the early phase of cell culture (Fig. 2A). On the other hand, h-5, h-6, and h-8 glioma cells in which the L1

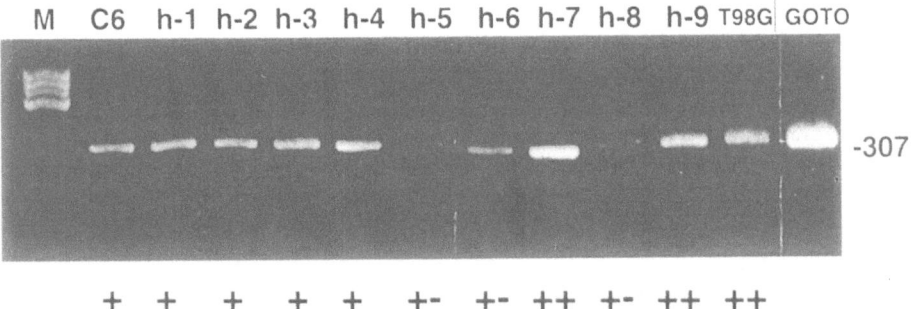

Fig. 1. L1 cell adhesion molecule (CAM) gene expression determined by reverse transcriptase-polymerase chain reaction (RT-PCR). A definitive band of 307 bp (L1 cDNA by RT-PCR) was detected in all glioma cell lines and a neuroblastoma cell line, GOTO, which served as a positive control. Among samples of glioma cell lines, T98G, h-7, and h-9 showed a relatively high-intensity band (pluses + +); h-5, h-6, and h-8 cells had a weak band (+ −); the remaining cell lines showed medium intensity (+)

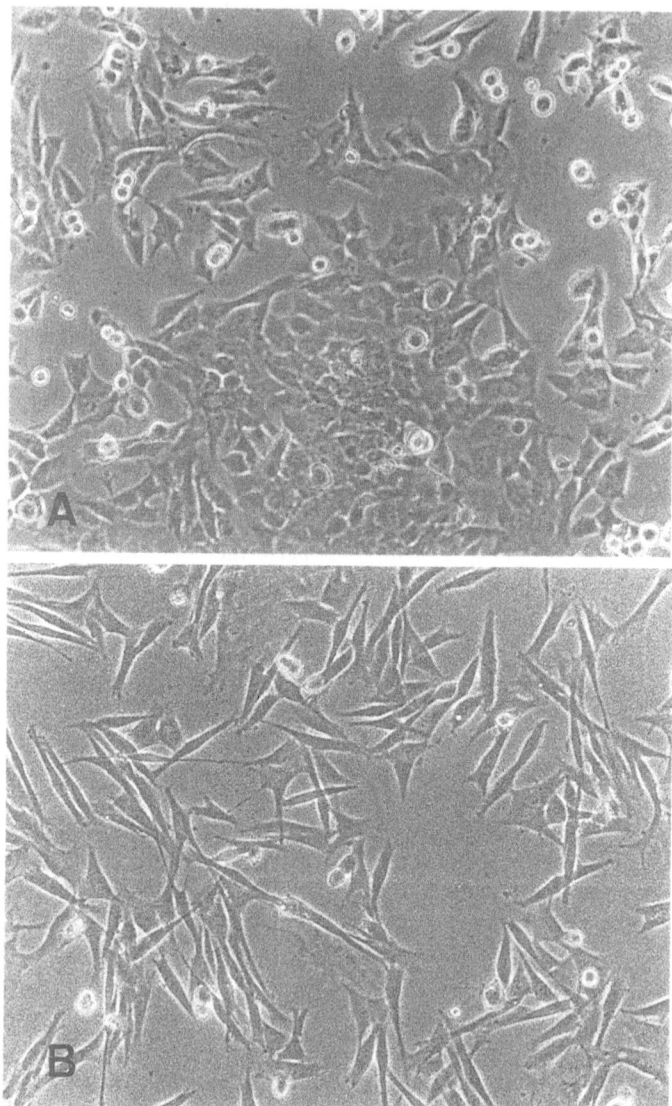

Fig. 2. Phase-contrast micrographs show two typical glioma cells with different morphology. **A** T98G cells are round with less polarity and with a tendency to growth aggregation during the early phase of cell culture. **B** h-8 human glioma are spindle-shaped cells that grow sparsely with less contact among the cells

gene was expressed in much smaller amounts had a spindle-shaped cell morphology and was distibuted sparsely in cell culture (Fig. 2B). The correlation between the amount of L1 gene expression and cell morphology in culture is summarized in Fig. 3. The more that glioma cells expressed L1 gene, the more compactly the cells aggregated when growing and the less polarity in cell shape was shown by the cells.

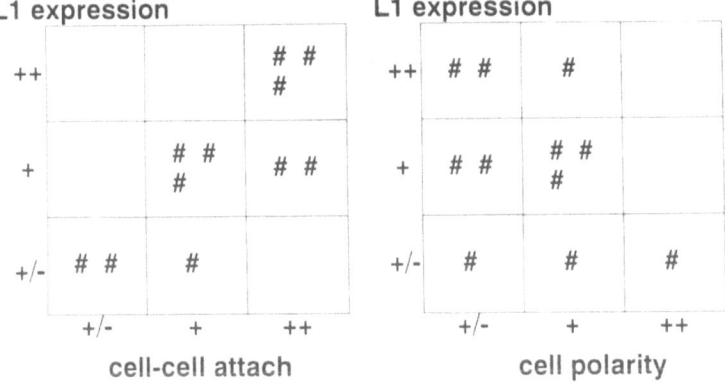

Fig. 3. Correlation between amount of L1 gene expression and human glioma cell morphology in a monolayer culture. A positive correlation was observed between the amounts of L1 and the intensity of cell–cell attachment; a negative correlation was seen between the amount of L1 and cell polarity. Each cell is denoted by the symbol #

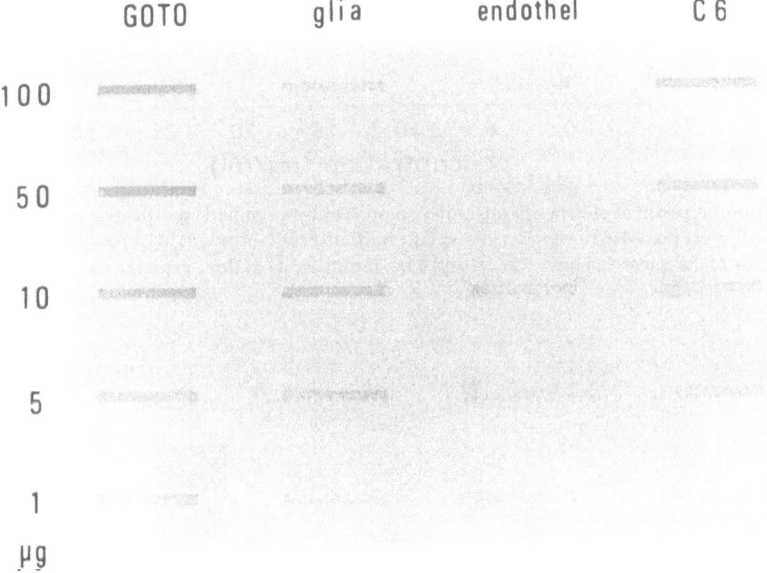

Fig. 4. Immunodot analysis of L1 in cultured cells. The cell lysates from each cell line were serially diluted and spotted on Immobilon-P transfer membranes under negative pressure. The numbers on the *left side* show amounts of total protein in each sample applied to the membrane. GOTO cells are the positive control; endothel is a negative control. C6 glioma cells expressed the L1 molecule one-fifth to one-tenth as much as did GOTO cells

Production of L1 Molecules

Immunodot analyses disclosed that glioma cells produced L1 molecules to a certain extent. C6 glioma cells produced the L1 molecule about one-fifth to one-tenth as much as GOTO cells (Fig. 4). Neither normal rat glias nor endothelial cells (which served as a negative control) produced L1 in a detectable amount in our assay.

Migratory Responses of Glioma Cells to L1

Glioma cells strongly migrated to L1 polypeptides in solution in a dose-dependent manner (Fig. 5). The glioma cells also showed a high migratory response to both L1 and L1cs (a short-type isoform of L1) gene-transfected fibroblast cells. Although there

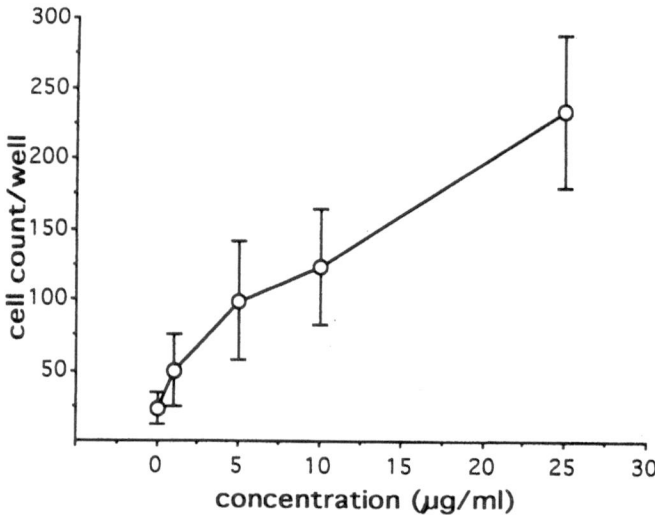

Fig. 5. Dose response of glioma cell migration stimulated by a synthetic polypeptide of L1. The C6 glioma cells were placed in the upper wells and the indicated concentrations of L1 polypeptides in the lower wells of the microchambers. *Circles* and *bars*, means ± SD of three experiments

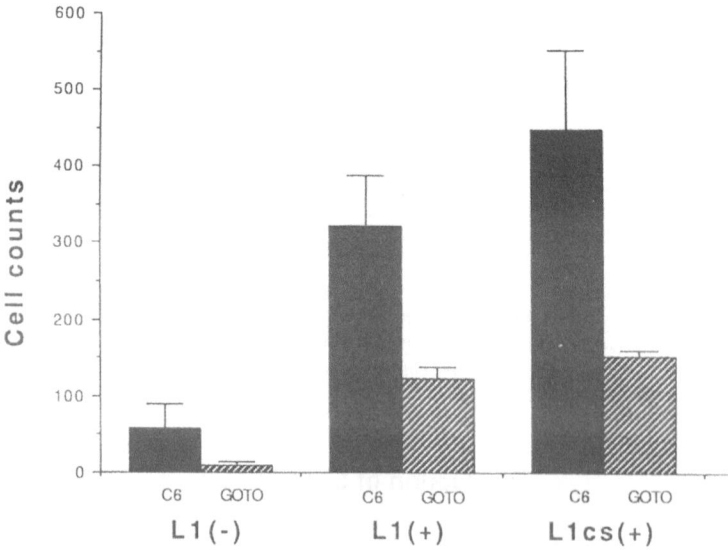

Fig. 6. Migratory responses of C6 glioma cells and neuroblastoma GOTO cells to the L1-[*L1 (+)*] and L1cs-[*L1cs (+)*] transfected fibroblast cells. *L1(−)*, fibroblast cells without the L1 gene as a control; *blocks* and *bars*, means + SD of three experiments

was no difference in the migration of GOTO cells between L1-and L1cs-transfected fibroblasts as stimulant cells, glioma cells migrated more strongly to the solution containing L1cs cells than that containing L1 cells. Fibroblast cells without L1 gene as control had only a little migratory glioma cell activity (Fig. 6).

Discussion

Cell adhesion has been implicated not only in several morphogenic processes during development but also in multistep processes of invasion and metastasis in malignant tumors. In the central nervous system, several cell adhesion molecules have been characterized, including N-cadherin, the neural cell adhesion molecule (NCAM), and the myelin-associated glycoprotein [13–15]. L1, one of these cell–cell adhesion molecules, is a transmembrane glycoprotein of approximately 200 kDa belonging to the calcium-independent immunoglobulin superfamilies (IgCAMs) [16]. The expression and distribution of L1 is highly restricted both spatially and temporally compared to NCAM, and the appearance of L1 is closely correlated with neuronal maturation, migration, and neurite extension [17,18].

Although it has been reported that neuroblastomas and hematopoietic tumors express L1 molecules [19,20], the expression of L1 gene in malignant gliomas has not been investigated. In the this study, we have shown that all malignant glioma cells tested express L1 gene and produce the molecule in a different degree among cell lines. It is well known that malignant tumors characteristically reproduce structural elements resembling those found during embryonic development [21]. In cultures of immature astrocytes, transforming growth factors-β_1 (TGF-β_1) and -β_2 (TGF-β_2) increased expression of L1, leading to a glia-mediated, L1-specific increase in neurite outgrowth of dorsal root ganglion neurons on the astrocyte substrate [22]. In addition, osteogenic protein-1 (OP-1), a member of the TGF-β superfamily, has been shown to markedly induce L1 expression in neuroblastoma $\times$ glioma hybrid cells by acting on a transcriptional mechanism of gene regulation [23].

In malignant gliomas, upregulation of L1 gene might occur by molecular mechanisms similar to those seen in immature astrocytes and neural cells because the prominent expressions of TGF-β_1 and TGF-β_2 mRNA have been identified in these glial tumors [24]. The biological functions of L1 expressed on glioma cells remain unknown. The present observation, that glioma cells with a high expression of L1 showed polygonal and epithelium-like cell morphology and had a tendency to aggregate in the early phase of cell culture, may indicate that L1 molecules play a role in cell–cell adhesion even in glioma cells. Although it is in dispute whether L1 molecules are involved in cell adhesion other than homophilic neuronal adhesion, discrepancies in the previous experiments are most likely caused by the cell cultures used in the studies. It is possible that expression of L1 or the L1 ligand in such cells may be regulated and thereby may be present under some culture conditions and absent under others.

It has been postulated that the binding sites on L1 for neuron–glia adhesion are different from those for neuron–neuron adhesion [9]. Our analyses of the L1 gene in glioma cells disclosed that L1 expressed in all glioma cells was a short-type isoform of L1 (L1cs) in which 12 bases encoding a part of the cytoplasmic domain of L1 molecules are deleted (data not shown). Thus, L1-mediated interactions of glioma cells with glioma cells and glioma cells with other cells can occur through the L1cs isoform on glioma cells.

In addtion to intercellular adhesion, L1 has been shown to play a role in cell motility such as the migration of cerebellar granule cells during early postnatal development [5,25]. Miura et al. [26] have demonstrated that fibroblast cells in which a full-length cDNA of L1 was transfected strongly promoted the migration of rat cerebellar neural cells in coculture of these cells. The current results, showing that glioma cells strongly migrated to a synthetic polypeptide of L1 which contained a region of fibronectin type III-related repeats (FNIII) of L1, indicate that the FNIII domain of L1 molecules may have an essential role in the activity of glioma cell migration. This hypothesis may be supported by the findings not only that anti-L1 antibodies recognize immunoglobulin domains but also that the FNIII domains of L1 inhibit the L1-promoted migration of glioma cells (unpublished data). In this study, L1cs-transfected fibroblast cells promoted glioma cell migration much more strongly than did L1-tranfected cells. Because the migration assay consisted of a two-chamber system separated via a medium solution, the cells placed in the upper chamber might respond to soluble forms of L1 rather than the intact L1 bound to the cell membrane in the lower chamber. Thus, the cells having L1cs may release more soluble forms of L1 outside the cells than those having L1. However, GOTO cells expressing L1 migrated to both the L1- and L1cs-transfected fibroblasts to a similar extent.

The dissimilarity in migratory responses between C6 glioma cells and GOTO cells may be thought to result from the differences of L1 molecules that are expressed in these cells. This suggests that the L1cs isoform characteristically expressed on glioma cells may regulate the adhesive and migratory properties of the tumor cells in a way different from that in which the L1 is expressed on neuronal cells. It may be postulated that malignant glioma cells release a soluble form of L1 which can stimulate glioma cell motility. Then, the cells migrate to the glioma-derived L1 molecules that have bound to L1 which is constitutively expressed on neuronal fibers, thus resulting in spreading and infiltration of glioma cells from the original sites to the normal brain around the tumor. Because the cytoplasmic domain of L1 has several sites to be phosphorylated by protein kinase C and other kinases [27], L1cs-directed augmentation of glioma cell migration may actually occur by an alteration of signal transduction.

Approaches at the molecular level to clarify the mechanism of invasive growth of malignant gliomas are just beginning. Although further studies including in vivo experiments are needed to directly demonstrate the role of L1 CAM in glioma invasion, this study implies that malignant glioma cells do not spread at random within the central nervous system but can migrate via cell adhesion molecules such as the L1 that is expressed on both glioma and neuronal cells.

Acknowledgments. We thank Dr. H. Asou for his kind gift of the anti-L1 antibody, L1 polypeptides, and L1-transfected fibroblast cells.

References

1. Nicolson GL (1988) Organ specificity of tumor metastasis: role of preferential adhesion, invasion and growth of malignant cells at specific secondary sites. Cancer Metastasis Rev 7:143–188

2. Ohnishi T, Arita N, Hayakawa T, Izumoto S, Taki T, Yamamoto H (1990) Motility factor produced by malignant glioma cells: role in tumor invasion. J Neurosurg 73:881–888

3. Ohnishi T, Arita N, Hayakawa T, Kawahara K, Kato K, Kakinuma A (1993) Purification of motility factor (GMF) from human malignant glioma cells and its biological significance in tumor invasion. Biochem Biophys Res Commun 193:518–525

4. Keilhauer G, Faissner A, Schachner M (1985) Differential inhibition of neurone–neurone, neurone–astrocyte and astrocyte–astrocyte adhesion by L1, L2 and NCAM antibodies. Nature 316:728–730

5. Lindner J, Rathjen FG, Schachner M (1983) L1 mono- and polyclonal antibodies modify cell migration in early postnatal mouse cerebellum. Nature 305:427–430

6. Asou H, Miura M, Kobayashi M, Uyemura K, Itoh K (1992) Cell adhesion molecule L1 guides cell migration in primary reaggregation cultures of mouse cerebellar cells. Neurosci Lett 144:221–224

7. Grumet M, Hoffman S, Edelman GM (1984) Two antigenically related neuronal cell adhesion molecules of different specificities mediate neuron–neuron and neuron–glia adhesion. 81:267–271

8. Rathjen FG, Schachner M (1984) Immunocytological and biochemical characterization of a new neuronal cell surface component (L1 antigen) which is involved in cell adhesion. EMBO J 3:1–10

9. Grumet M, Edelman GM (1988) Neuron–glia cell adhesion molecule interacts with neurons and astroglia via different binding mechanisms. J Cell Biol 106:487–503

10. Kuhn TB, Stoeckli TE, Condrau MA, Rathjen GJ, Sonderegar P (1991) Neurite outgrowth on immobilized axonin-1 is mediated by a heterophilic interaction with L1 (G4). J Cell Biol 115:1113–1126

11. Werz W, Schachner M (1988) Adhesion of neural cells to extracellular matrix constituents: involvement of glycosaminoglycans and cell adhesion molecules. Brain Res 471:225–234

12. Izumoto S, Arita N, Hayakawa T, Ohnishi T, Taki T, Yamamoto H, Ushio Y (1990) Effect of MX2, a new morpholino anthracycline, against experimental brain tumors. Anticancer Res 10:735–740

13. Noble M, Albrechtsen M, Moller C, Lyles J, Bock E, Goridis C, Watanabe M, Rutishauser U (1985) Glial cells express N-CAM/D2-CAM-like polypeptides in vitro. Nature 316:725–728

14. Takeichi M (1988) The cadherins: cell-cell adhesion molecules controlling animal morphogenesis. Development (Camb) 102:639–655

15. Poltorak M, Sadoul R, Keilhauer G, Landa C, Fahrig T, Schachner M (1987) Myelin-associated glycoprotein, a member of the L2/HNK-1 family of neural cell adhesion molecules, is involved in neuron–oligodendrocyte and oligodendrocyte–oligodendrocyte interaction. J Cell Biol 105:1893–1899

16. Moos M, Tacke R, Scherer H, Teplow D, Fruh K, Schachner M (1988) Neural adhesion molecule L1 as a member of the immunoglobulin superfamily with binding do mains similar to fibronectin. Nature 334:701–703

17. Daniloff JK, Chuong CM, Levi G, Edelman GM (1986) Differential distribution of cell adhesion molecules during histogenesis of the chick nervous system. J Neurosci 6:739–758

18. Thiery J-P, Delouvee A, Grumet M, Edelman GM (1985) Initial appearance and regional distribution of the neuron–glia cell adhesion molecule in the chick embryo. J Cell Biol 100:442–456

19. Figarella-Branger DF, Durbec PL, Rougon GN (1990) Differential spectrum of expression of neural cell adhesion molecule isoforms and L1 adhesion molecules on human neuroectodermal tumors. Cancer Res 50:6364–6370

20. Kowiz A, Kadmon G, Verschueren H, Remels L, Baetselier PD, Hubbe M, Schachner M, Schirrmacher V, Altevogt P (1993) Expression of L1 cell adhesion molecule is associated with lymphoma growth and metastasis. Clin Exp Metastasis 11:419–429

21. Kennedy PGE (1982) Neural cell markers and their applications to neurology. J Neuroimmunol 2:35–53

22. Saad B, Constam DB, Ortmann R, Moos M, Fontana A, Schachner M (1991) Astrocyte-derived TGF-β2 and NGF differentially regulate neural recognition molecule expression by cultured astrocytes. J Cell Biol 115:473–484

23. Perides G, Hu G, Rueger DC, Charness ME (1993) Osteogenic protein-1 regulates L1 and neural cell adhesion molecule gene expression in neural cells. J Biol Chem 268:25197–25205
24. Scneider J, Hofman FM, Apuzzo MLJ, Hinton DR (1992) Cytokines and immunoregulatory molecules in malignant glial neoplasms. J Neurosurg 77:265–273
25. Hoffman S, Friedlander DR, Chuong C-M, Grumet M, Edelman GM (1986) Differential contributions of Ng-CAM and N-CAM to cell adhesion in different neural regions. J Cell Biol 103:145–158
26. Miura M, Asou H, Kobayashi M, Uyemura K (1992) Functional expression of a full-length cDNA coding for rat neural cell adhesion molecule L1 mediates homophilic intercellular adhesion and migration of cerebellar neurons. J Biol Chem 267:10752–10758
27. Sadoul R, Kirchhoff F, Schachner M (1989) A protein kinase activity is associated with and specifically phosphorylates the neural cell adhesion molecule L1. J Neurochem 53:1471–1478

The Role of Urokinase-Type Plasminogen Activator in the Invasion and Proliferation of Malignant Brain Tumors

Shingo Takano[1], Yoshihiko Yoshii[1], Tadao Nose[1], Barry Landau[2], and Steven Brem[2]

Abstract. Matrix-degrading enzymes, particularly urokinase-type plasminogen activator (u-PA) and its endogenous inhibitor, plasminogen activator inhibitor-1 (PAI-1), are hypothesized to mediate tumor cell invasion. To study the link between these enzymes and the invasive phenotype of gliomas, we examined (1) the enzyme levels in a series of human brain tumors, and (2) enzyme levels and the invasiveness of four glioblastoma cell lines (U118, U138, U373, A172). The enzyme levels were measured by their activity (zymography), concentration of antigen (enzyme-linked immunosorbent assay, ELISA), and mRNA expression (Northern blot analysis). The u-PA and PAI-1 levels were significantly higher in glioblastomas and metastatic brain tumors than in astrocytoma, meningioma, and neurinoma. The invasiveness of glioblastoma cells, determined by Matrigel chemoinvasion assay, was highly correlated with the ratio of u-PA/PAI-1 expression. The growth rate of glioblastoma cells also correlated with the u-PA/PAI-1 expression ratio. These findings demonstrate that the ratio of u-PA to PAI-1 modulates glioblastoma invasiveness and proliferation.

Key words. Glioblastoma—Invasiveness—Plasminogen activator—Plasminogen activator inhibitor

Introduction

Human glioblastoma is characterized by local invasive spread into the surrounding brain [1]. The microscopic spread of neoplastic cells into the brain adjacent to the tumor is the principal reason for the local recurrence of glioblastomas that renders all forms of current therapy, including surgery, irradiation, or chemotherapy, ultimately futile [2].

Proteolytic degradation of the extracellular matrix, mediated in particular by urokinase-type plasminogen activator (u-PA), controlled by endogenous inhibitors, plasminogen activator inhibitor (PAI), is an essential first step in the tumor cell invasion [3]. We tested the hypothesis that the upregulation of the proteolytic enzymes u-PA and PAI-1 in malignant brain tumors and the expression of these

[1] Department of Neurosurgery, Tsukuba University School of Medicine, Tsukuba, Ibaraki 305, Japan
[2] Department of Neurosurgery, Northwestern University School of Medicine, Chicago, Illinois 60611, USA

enzymes would predict the degree of invasiveness among heterogeneous glioblastoma cell lines. We report that the proteolytic balance of uPA/PAI-1 showed a striking correlation to the invasive phenotype.

Materials and Methods

Tissue Preparation

Brain tumor samples (glioblastoma 15, astrocytoma 8, metastatic brain 18, meningioma 4, neurinoma 4) and normal brain (4 cases) were collected at the time of surgery, snap-frozen in isopentane, and stored at $-70°C$. Samples were then thawed and weighed. Tissue fragments were homogenized with a motor-driven pestle for 3 min in 1 ml of extraction buffer per 50 mg of tissue weight (0.075 M potassium acetate, 0.3 M NaCl, 0.1 M L-arginine. 10 mM ethylenediaminetetraacetate (EDTA), 0.25% Triton X-100 (Rohmand Haas, Philadelphia, PA, USA), pH 4.2) [4]. The homogenates were centrifuged at 12 000 g for 10 min at 4°C and the supernatants were aliquoted. Protein concentrations were determined using the Bio-Rad protein determination reagent (Bio-Rad, Richmond, CA, USA) using bovine serum albumin as the standard [5].

Cell Culture

Human glioblastoma cells (U118 MG, U138 MG, U373 MG, and A172) (American Type Culture Collection) were grown in Dulbecco's modified Eagle's medium (DMEM) with 10% fetal calf serum (FCS). For plasminogen activator determination and chemoattractant of chemoinvasion assays, glioma cells were grown in 6-well culture dishes. When the cell layer reached 90% confluence, the medium was discarded and the cultures were washed and incubated in 2 ml of serum-free DMEM for 24 h. The conditioned medium was collected, centrifuged, and stored at $-70°C$. The cells were extracted with 500 µl of extraction buffer. The extracts were sonicated, centrifuged at 12000 g for 10 min at 4°C, aliquoted, and stored at $-70°C$. Protein concentrations were determined.

Plasminogen Activator Determination

Zymographic analysis was carried out as previously described [6]. The cell extract and the conditioned medium adjusted to protein concentration were electrophoresed on a 10% polyacrylamide gel. The gels were transferred onto plasminogen (200 µg) containing casein-agarose gel. The zymograms were incubated overnight at 4°C, then at 37°C, and photographed as the lytic bands appeared. The activity was quantitated by an imaging densitometer (Bio-Rad Model GS-670). Quantification of antigen was performed using commercially available ELISA kits (Biopool, Umea, Sweden).

RNA Extraction and Northern Blot Analysis

Total cytoplasmic RNA from glioma cells was prepared by the acid guanidinum thiocyanate-phenol-chloroform extraction method [7]. Ten micrograms of each total

RNA were size fractionated through 1% w/v agarose gels containing 2.0 M formaldehyde. RNA was transferred to Duralose UV membranes (Stratagene, La Jolla, CA, USA) by capillary transfer in 10× standard saline citrate (SSC) and ultraviolet-cross-linked with 120000 µJ/cm^2 using an ultraviolet Stratalinker 2400 (Stratagene). After prehybridization, the membranes were hybridized with ^{32}P-labeled cDNA probes in 50% formamide, 5× saline-sodium phosphate-EDTA, 0.1% sodium dodecyl sulfate (SDS), 5× Denhardt's solution, and 100 µg/ml salmon sperm DNA overnight at 42°C. Hybridized filters were washed in 0.1× SSC/0.5% SDS at 50°C for 30 min before autoradiography at −70°C using XAR-5 (Kodak, Rochester, NY, USA) film with intensifying screens. Signals were quantitated using an imaging densitometer. The probes used were 2 133-bp BamHI-HindIII fragment of the pEUK-C1 for PAI-1 [8], 1.5-kb PstI-PstI fragment of the pHUK-8 for u-PA (American Type Culture Collection), and 2100-bp XhoI-XhoI fragment of the pHFβA-1 for β-actin (American Type Culture Collection).

Chemoinvasion Assay

The chemoinvasion assay was performed as reported previously [9] using a BioCoat Matrigel Invasion Chamber (Becton Dickinson, Bedford, MA, USA). Cells (1 × 10^4) were suspended in a final volume of 200 µl of DMEM with 0.1% bovine serum albumin. A 200-µl sample of the glioma cell suspension was then placed in the upper compartment of the Boyden chambers and 500 µl of serum-free glioblastoma cell conditioned medium was placed in the lower chamber as a chemoattractant. Assembled chambers were incubated for 24 h. At the end of the incubation period, the filters were removed and fixed in methanol. Cells on the upper filter surface were carefully removed by rubbing with a cotton swab. The filters were stained with hematoxylin and mounted on glass slides. The number of cells on the lower surface was quantitated by computer-assisted image analysis (Quantimet 570, Leica, Deerfield, IL, USA). Using 10× magnification, the size of the measured area was 0.24 mm^2. The total number of cells withins nine fields at the center of the filter was measured.

Cell Proliferation Assay

Cell proliferation assays were performed using the CellTiter 96TM Aqueous Non-Radioactive Proliferation Assay (Promega, Madison, WI, USA) as previously described [6]. Glioma cells, 5 × 10^4/ml in DMEM with 10% FCS, were plated in 96-well plates (Becton Dickinson, Lincoln Park, NJ, USA) at 5000 cells/well. On day 1 and day 3 of incubation, 20 µl of tetrazolium compound and phenazine methosulfate solution was added to each well and incubated for 2 h at 37°C. The optical density at 490 nm was read on an engyral-linked immunosorbent assay (ELISA) plate reader (Bio-Tek, Winooski, VT, USA). Cell proliferation was calculated by the ratio of optical density at 490 nm on day 3 compared to day 1.

Statistical Analysis

Results are expressed as mean ± SD. Statistically significant differences between means were determined utilizing a one-way analysis of variance and the Tukey test. Differences were considered significant at P values less than .05.

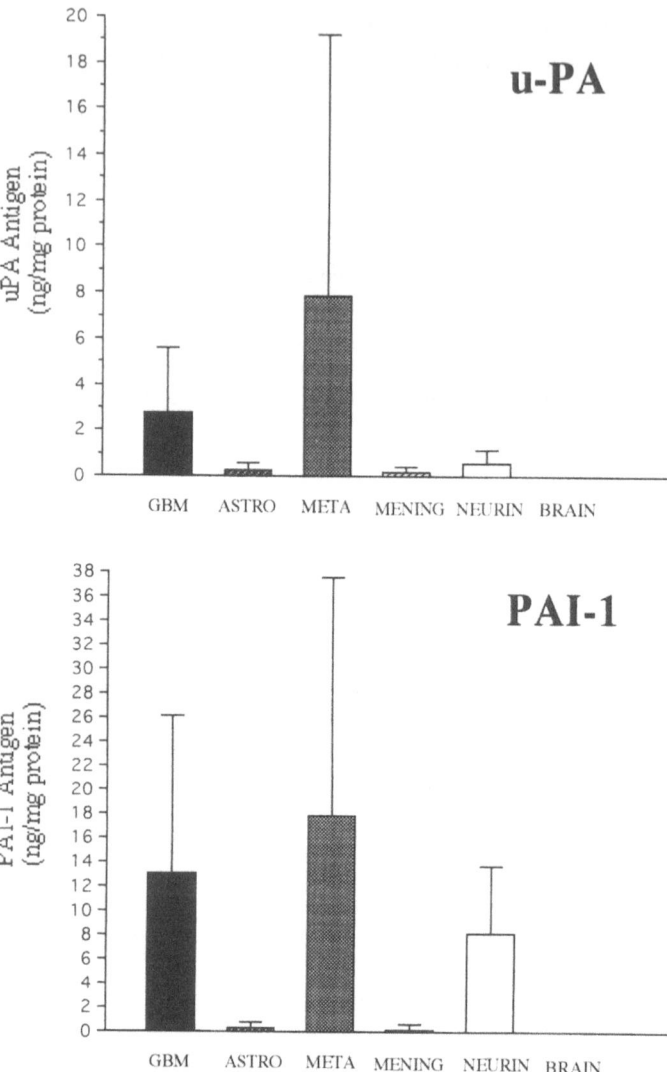

Fig. 1. Tissue urokinase-type plasminogen activator (u-PA, *top*) and plasminogen activator inhibitor-1 (PAI-1, *bottom*) antigen concentrations determined by enzyme-linked immunosorbent assay (ELISA) in tissue extracts of 53 surgical specimens. u-PA antigen concentrations in glioblastomas (*GBM*) and metastatic brain tumors (*META*) are significantly higher than those of astrocytomas (*ASTRO*), meningiomas (*MENING*), neurinomas (*NEURIN*), and normal brains (*BRAIN*). PAI-1 antigen concentrations in glioblastomas and metastatic brain tumors are significantly higher than those of astrocytomas, meningiomas, and normal brains. Values are the mean ± SD of each group

Results

The u-PA and PAI-1 antigen levels were undetectable in normal brains and significantly higher in glioblastomas and metastatic brain tumors compared to astrocytomas, meningiomas, and neurinomas (Fig. 1).

The four cell lines showed a heterogeneous spectrum of cell proliferation and invasiveness (Table 1). The four cell lines showed a heterogeneous spectrum of u-PA and PAI-1 activity, antigen, and mRNA (Table 2, Fig. 2). The proliferation of glioblastoma cells was significantly correlated with ratio of u-PA/PAI-1 expression in conditioned medium as determined by ELISA ($r = .952$, $P < .05$) and Northern blot analysis ($r = .951$, $P < .05$). The glioblastoma invasiveness was significantly correlated with the ratio of uPA/PAI-1 expression determined by ELISA of glioma-conditioned medium ($r = .992$, $P < .01$) and Northern blot analysis (Fig. 3). Moreover, there was a strong correlation between glioblastoma invasiveness and u-PA activity determined by zymography of the glioblastoma-conditioned medium ($r = .995$, $P < .01$).

Discussion

This study clearly demonstrated that (1) malignant brain tumors (glioblastoma and metastatic brain tumor) possessed higher concentrations of u-PA as well as PAI-1 compared to less malignant glioma (astrocytoma) and benign brain tumors (meningioma and neurinoma), and (2) glioblastoma invasiveness and proliferation highly correlated with enhanced production of u-PA.

The finding that glioblastoma cellular proliferation correlates with u-PA production of glioma cells suggests a mitogenic role for u-PA [10] separate from he matrix-degrading function of the enzyme, possibly using the growth factor-like domains of the u-PA molecule [11]. We demonstrated that glioma invasiveness highly correlated with enhanced u-PA production using three different determinations: (1) mRNA

Table 1. Invasiveness and proliferation of glioblastoma cell lines.

Malignant phenotype	U118	U138	U373	A172
Proliferation[a]	1.83 ± 0.04	1.75 ± 0.15	2.25 ± 0.16	1.54 ± 0.18
Invasiveness (cell number)	190.3 ± 14.1	85.1 ± 34.8	685.8 ± 68.0	21.0 ± 12.9

[a] Ratio of OD490 of day 3/day 1.

Table 2. u-PA and PAI-1 profiles of glioblastoma cell lines.

Matrix-degrading enzyme		U118	U138	U373	A172
ELISA (ng/ml/10^5 cells)	u-PA				
	Extract	0.98	0[a]	0.16	0.06
	Medium	0.33	0[a]	0.48	0[a]
	PAI-1				
	Extract	1.1	3.5	1.5	24.2
	Medium	13.1	65.7	3.8	32.7
Zymogram[b]	u-PA				
	Extract	7.5	0.63	13.76	5.96
	Medium	3.71	1.01	10.61	0.68
mRNA[b]	u-PA	64.5	3.5	41.3	1.3
	PAI-1				
	3.0 kb	72.2	65.2	6.7	40.3
	2.0 kb	71.4	78.9	10.1	18.7

u-PA, urokinase-type plasminogen activator; PAI-1, plasminogen activator inhibitor-1.
[a] Not detectable by ELISA (enzyme-linked immunosorbent assay).
[b] Zymogram value and mRNA value (adjusted by β-actin signal) from densitometry.

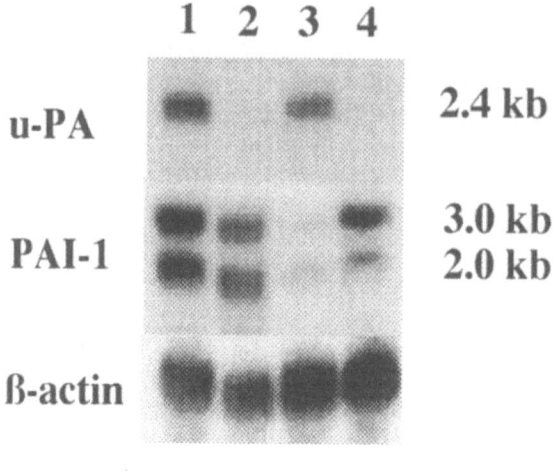

Fig. 2. Northern blot analysis of glioblastoma cells. Lane 1, U118; lane 2, U138; lane 3, U373; lane 4, A172

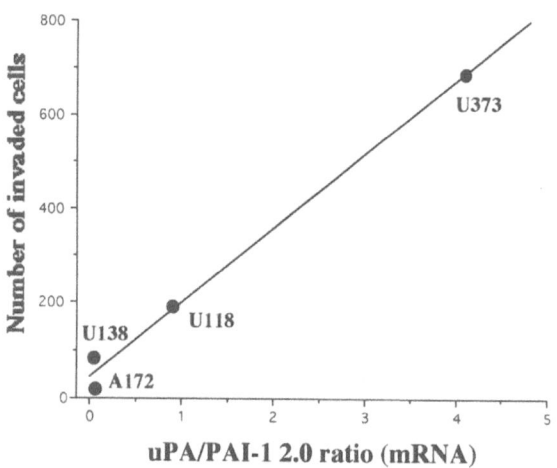

Fig. 3. Correlation between glioblastoma invasiveness and u-PA/PAI-1 expression ratio in Northern analysis ($r = .996$, $P < .01$)

expression by Northern analysis, (2) secreted protein activity by zymography, and (3) secreted protein antigen levels by ELISA. We have chosen to use the ratio of u-PA to PAI-1 mRNA and proteins as a reflection of the net proteolytic of the cells [12]. The results obtained with correlation of invasion and enhanced u-PA production indicate that u-PA could be required for the glioblastoma cells to invade basement membrane structures. In glioblastoma tissues, we have demonstrated elevation of PAI-1 as well as u-PA. In tissues, the source of PAI-1 may be proliferative endothelial cells, and PAI-1 could protect against excess proteolysis with elevated u-PA [13].

In summary, malignant brain tumors possessed high concentrations of u-PA and PAI-1, and the balance in favor of excess u-PA associated with less PAI-1 was critical for glioma cell invasion. These results provide a therapeutic target to inhibit the invasive phenotype of gliomas using protease inhibitors.

Acknowledgments. The authors thank David Ivancic, Elaine Verrusio, and Marguerite Wotozcek-Obadia for their expert technical assistance.

References

1. Daumas-Duport C, Scheithauer BW, Kelly PJ (1987) A histologic and cytologic method for spatial definition of gliomas. Mayo Clinic Proc 62:435–449
2. Kornblith PL (1985) Malignant gliomas. In: Long DM (ed) Current therapy in neurological surgery. Mosby, Toronto, pp 25–27
3. Mignatti P, Rifkin DB (1993) Biology and biochemistry of proteinases in tumor invasion. Physiol Rev 73:161–195
4. Camiolo SM, Siuta MR, Madeja JM (1982) Improved medium for extraction of plasminogen activator from tissue. Prep Biochem 12:297–305
5. Bradford MM (1976) A rapid and sensitive method for quantitation of microgram quantities of protein utilizing the principle of protein dye binding. Anal Biochem 72:248–254
6. Takano S, Gately S, Neville ME, Herblin WF, Gross JL, Engelhard H, Perricone M, Eidsvoog K, Brem S (1994) Suramin, an anticancer and angiosuppressive agent, inhibits endothelial cell binding of basic fibroblast growth factor, migration, proliferation, and induction of urokinase-type plasminogen activator. Cancer Res 54:2654–2660
7. Chomczynski P, Sacchi N (1987) Single-step method of RNA isolation by acid guanidium thiocyanate-phenol-chloroform extraction. Anal Biochem 162:156–159
8. Pannekoek H, Veerman H, Lambers H, Diergaarde P, Verweil PCL, van Zonnerveld AJ, Mourik JA (1986) Endothelial plasminogen activator inhibitor (PAI): a new member of the serpin gene family. EMBO J 5:2539–2544
9. Albini A, Melchiori A, Santi L, Liotta LA, Brown PD, Steler-Stevenson WG (1991) Tumor cell invasion inhibited by TIMP-2. J Natl Cancer Inst 83:775–779
10. De Petro G, Copeta A, Barlati S (1994) Urokinase-type and tissue-type plasminogen activators as growth factors of human fibroblasts. Exp Cell Res 213:286–294
11. Saksela O, Rifkin DB (1988) Cell-associated plasminogen activation: regulation and physiological functions. Annu Rev Cell Biol 4:93–126
12. Pepper MS, Belin D, Montesano R, Orci L, Vassalli JD (1990) Transforming growth factor-beta 1 modulates basic fibroblast growth factor-induced proteolytic and angiogenic properties of endothelial cells in vitro. J Cell Biol 111:743–755
13. Grondahl-Hansen J, Christensen IJ, Rosenquist C, Brunner N, Mouridsen HT, Dano K, Blichert-Toft M (1993) High levels of urokinase-type plasminogen activator and its inhibitor PAI-1 in cytosolic extracts of breast carcinomas are associated with poor prognosis. Cancer Res 53:2513–2521

Section 2. Cell Kinetics

Stemline Study Based on the Nuclear Characterization and Image Cytometry in Resected Brain Tumors

Yoshihiko Yoshii, Atsushi Saito, Koji Tsuboi, Shingo Takano,
Yoji Komatsu, Hideo Tsurushima, and Tadao Nose

Abstract. We examined nuclear morphometry and DNA content in SG2M phase tumor cells by using image analysis in relation to time to tumor progression (TTP) in 73 brain tumor patients from whom clinical follow-up was obtained. The patients with hypertetraploid tumors in G2M ploidy had a shorter TTP than those of patients with tetraploid tumors in G2M ploidy. Nuclei size in SG2M phase cells was larger and nuclear shape in SG2M phase cells much more deformed than those in the G0G1 phase cells in all tumors studied. Tumors with hyperT in G2M ploidy indicated highly malignant and proliferative stem cells with DNA content above 4C in the SG2M phase cells. Tumors with T in G2M ploidy indicated malignancy by the number of SG2M fractions, and those tumor cells showed stemlines with DNA content of 4C in the SG2M phase cells. Our results indicated that heterogeneity is composed of many stem cell lines differing densitometrically and morphometrically in gliomatous and nongliomatous brain tumors. This classification in G2M ploidy may suggest the degree of heterogeneity or stemlines in the resected tumors and may also help to select the therapeutic modality for these brain tumors.

Key words. Human brain tumors—G2M ploidy—Image analysis—Time to tumor progression—Stem cell line

Introduction

Nuclear DNA content has been widely studied in human brain tumors by flow cytometry (FCM) and has served as a useful prognostic factor in a variety of neoplasms [1–9]. On the other hand, the S-phase fraction is a major factor in determining the proliferative potential of cell populations [10–21].

Automated image cytometry (ICM) of DNA content has been used increasingly in cytopathology and histopathology to detect aneuploid cell populations within neoplastic lesions [7–9,16,20–32]. The advantage of this technique is direct visualization of the tumor sample. Malignant cells can be preferentially selected for analysis. These cytometric DNA analyses provide good prognostic information as well as the FCM study.

The experimental and clinical evidence suggest that malignant neoplasms are not homogenous in their cell composition but are composed of heterogenous cell types.

Department of Neurological Surgery, University of Tsukuba, Tsukuba, Ibaraki 305, Japan

127

The degree of heterogeneity in the tumor tissue plays an important role in treatment. Some authors have already suggested that this factor contributes to variable response to tumor chemotherapy [33,34] as well as to variations in cell-surface markers [35], tumor antigens [33,36], and growth rates [37,38]. The evidence for heterogeneity of malignant brain tumors has so far only been suggested by their pathological appearance. There have been some cytometric studies of heterogeneity in the tumor tissue [21,22,39–43]. Our previous work by image analysis suggested that there were different stem cells in the aneuploid tumor cells in brain tumors [20]. Image analysis is available to investigate stemlines in tumor cells cytometrically or morphometrically.

In this study, the following factors were investigated in human brain tumors: histological grade, DNA content, SG2M phase fraction, G2M ploidy pattern, and stemlines. The time to tumor progression (TTP) of the patients was estimated as well. The purpose of this work, as described here, was to see whether the heterogeneity observed in tumor growth characteristics represented the different stemlines in a single tumor and if alteration of the DNA content would also be associated with the morphological change of each nucleus in those stemlines.

Materials and Methods

Clinical Data and Histopathological Diagnosis

The 73 patients underwent surgery at Tuskuba University Hospital between 1985 and 1993. The 20 patients with glioblastoma multiforme (GM) and the 17 with anaplastic glioma (AG) were routinely treated with surgery and postoperative radiotherapy (RT) of 60–65 Gy combined with adjuvant chemotherapy such as ACNU (1-(4-amino-2-methyl pyrimine-5-yl)-methyl-3-(2-chloroethyl)-3-nitrosourea hydrochloride) alone or ACNU combining interferon-beta (IFN-β) or PAV (provarbezine, ACNU, and vincristine). The 11 patients with low-grade glioma (LGG) and the 5 with malignant meningioma were also routinely treated with surgery and postoperative RT. Brain metastases (BMs) were present in 21 patients. Those with a single BM were treated by surgery, and postoperative RT was added depending on control of the primary cancer or the existence of metastases in other organs. Those patients with multiple BMs were treated by surgery to improve their performance state and to lower the increased intracranial pressure. Time to tumor progression (TTP) was correlated with DNA ploidy and proliferation index.

Cytological Samples and Cell Image Analysis

Samples obtained from surgical resections were fixed in formalin and embedded in paraffin. Sections were cut serially from one block to be 4 μm thick. Some slides were routinely stained with periodic acid–Schiff (PAS), Kluver-Barrera, reticulin silver impregnation, Azan-Mallory, Bodian, phosphotungstic acid hematoxylin (PTAH), hematoxylin and eosin (H&E), and Feulgen stains. For Feulgen staining, the slide was brought to room temperature and rinsed in distilled water.

Cell image analysis was performed using a TAS plus microscope image processor (Leitz, Wetzlar, Germany) with a 100× magnification lens (numerical aperture, 1.32). The nuclear integrated optical density (IOD) was estimated on the densitometric levels on each pixel. The nuclear DNA content was calculated from the sum of the optical density (OD) values of each pixel of the nucleus. The IOD was measured using a wavelength of 545 nm [23,29,30]. The nuclei of 100 well-preserved cells with neighboring nuclei were selected by eye and measured with image analysis (Fig. 1). The programming software for the TAS plus was supplied by Drs. Becker and Mikel (Armed Forces Institute of Pathology, Washington, DC, USA). The IOD values of 10–20 lymphocytes from the same specimen were used to calculate the mean value of the control diploid cell population.

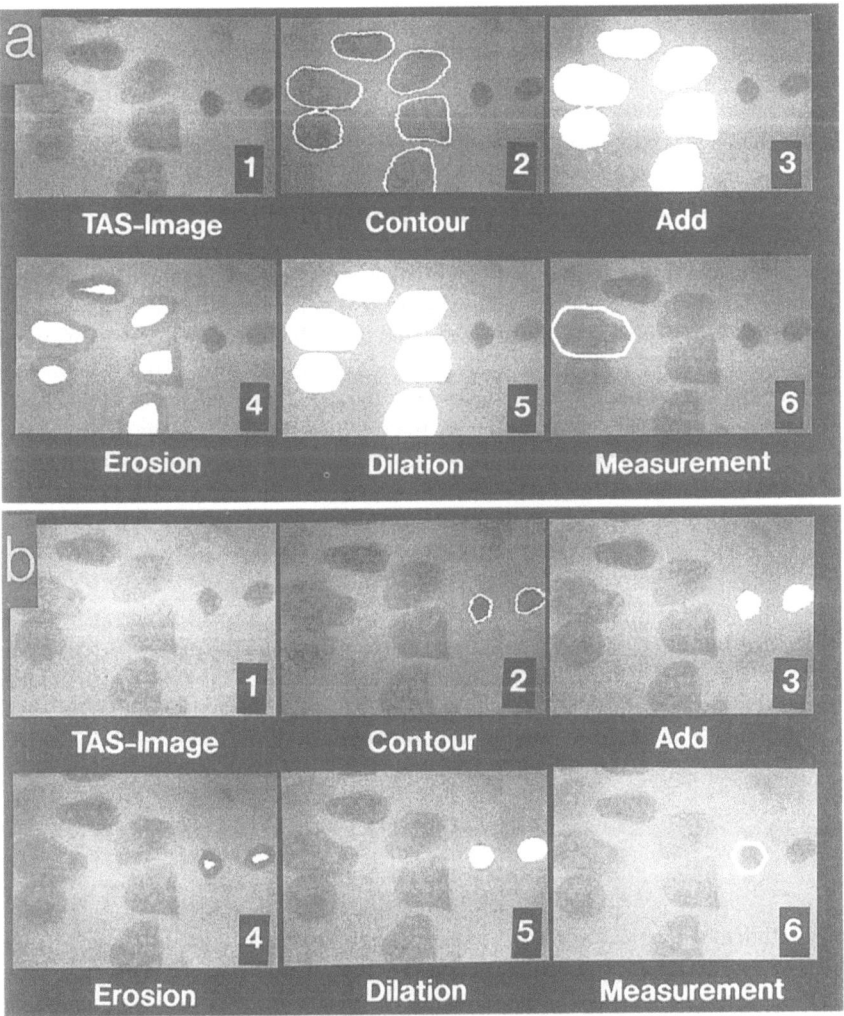

Fig. 1a,b. Morphometric DNA analysis by means of monitor images of a TAS micrograph of metastatic brain tumor cells and lymphocytes. Images of nuclei were displayed at magnification of ×3200 on a monitor via a television camera mounted on the vertical phototube of an optical microscope. Measurement is shown in order of the number. Measurements were performed by drawing the contour of each nucleus using a light pen. Those outlines were corrected in relationship to their true shape by erosion and dilation methods. The nuclear integrated optical density was estimated on the densitometric level in the final limit of those nuclei, and the morphological measurements were performed on their final outline. **a** An example of measurement of tumor cell nuclei. **b** An example of measurement of lymphocytes as an internal control in the same sample

Nuclear Morphology

The morphometric nuclear parameters included form factor (FF), number of nuclei, and nuclear area (μm^2). FF was calculated as $4\pi \times area /(perimeter)^2$. An FF of 1.0 means that the nucleus is round, while an FF of 0.01 indicated an irregular shape. The nuclear size was estimated from the number of pixels occupied by a nucleus.

DNA Index

The absolute IOD value of each tumor was normalized using the value obtained from lymphocytes within the same tissue. The DNA index (DI) of each tumor nuclei was determined by dividing the tumor IOD by the mean IOD of the diploid lymphocyte nuclei. The DI was expressed by arbitrary units.

Determination of G0G1 and SG2M Phase Cells

The crude histogram of the DIs of 100 tumor cells was prepared using arbitrary units. The mean G0G1 DIs were calculated by the crude G0G1 phase cells with a nucleus less than 2.0 DIs. The diploid cells were considered to be those cells with a nucleus in the range of mean $\pm$ (1 SD + 0.1) G0G1 DIs. The SG2M phase cells were defined as the value (1 SD + 0.1) above the mean diploid DIs [20]. All DIs in the nuclei of those cells were averaged, and the mean values were the calculated G2M DIs. The percentage of tumor cells with SG2M DI was calculated in each patient. This percentage of SG2M phase cells (%SG2M) corresponds to the proliferation index (PI) of the tumor.

Determination of G2M Ploidy in Image Cytometry

A previous study of brain tumors [20] established a mean diploid DI of 1.2 $\pm$ 0.32 in G0G1 phase tumor cells. We used this number to determine the ploidy pattern of the tumor in this series (Fig. 2). Theoretically, the estimated G2M DIs of 4C could be calculated as twice the mean G0G1 DIs of 2C. The G2M ploidy pattern in each patient was estimated and classified into three ploidy patterns in relation to the estimated G2M DIs; hypotetraploid (hypoT), tetraploid (T), and hypertetraploidy (hyperT) (Fig. 3).

Statistical Analysis

Paired student's t test (two-tailed) was used for the comparison of the mean $\pm$ SD of the mean of the factors studied. Correlation and variation analysis were also applied.

Results

DNA Index and Histology

Table 1 illustrates the distribution of the mean DIs in the five histopathological group of all studied patients. The mean DIs of the patients with brain metastasis were

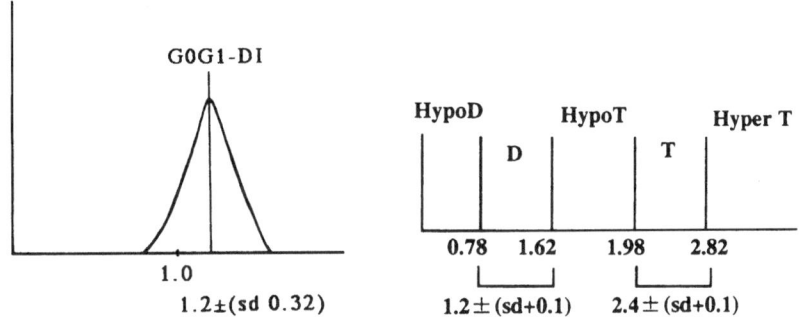

Fig. 2. Determination of ploidy pattern from image cytometry using a TAS plus. Because there were relatively large SD for G0G1 DNA index (DI), the range of the diploid DIs was decided by the mean G0G1 DI within 1 SD to +0.1, and that of tetraploid DIs was by twice the mean G0G1 DIs within 1 SD to +0.1

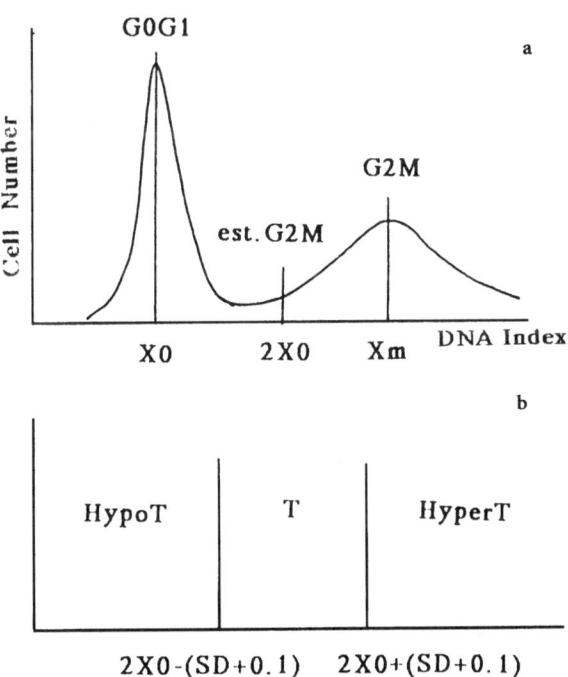

Fig. 3a,b. Determination of ploidy represented by the mean DIs in all G2M phase cells. **a** The estimated G2MDIs (2 Xo) were obtained by multiplying the mean G0G1 DI (Xo). The calculated G2M DIs (Xm) were obtained by averaging the DIs of all cells with DIs more than 2 SD above the mean G0G1 DIs. **b** The range of the tetraploid DIs in G2M ploidy was based on 2 Xo ± (1 SD + 0.1) and indicated those averages are within estimated G2M DIs. Hypotetraploid in G2M ploidy pattern indicates that the mean SG2M DIs are less than 1 SD and 0.1 point below the estimated G2M DIs. Hypertetraploid in G2M ploidy pattern indicates that the mean SG2M DIs are more than 1 SD and 0.1 point above the estimated G2M DIs

Table 1. Relationship between mean DNA index (DI) and pathology.

Pathology	Number of cases	DNA Index	
		Mean	SD
Glioblastoma multiforme	20	1.93*	0.57
Anaplastic glioma	17	2.07*	0.92
Low-grade glioma	11	1.20*	0.40
Brain metastasis	21	1.63*	0.67
Malignant meningioma	5	1.25*	0.55

*, $P < .001$.

Table 2. Relationship between mean SG2M DNA index, %SG2M, and pathology.

Pathology	Number of cases	SG2M DNA Index		%SG2M	
		Mean	SD	Mean	SD
Glioblastoma multiforme	20	3.16*	0.52	33.8*	16.1
Anaplastic glioma	17	3.11*	0.77	38*	24.2
Low-grade glioma	11	2.27*	0.39	11.6*	11.3
Brain metastasis	21	2.82**	0.67	23.1**	15.6
Malignant meningioma	5	2.25**	0.79	17**	11.4

%SG2M, percentage of SG2M phase fraction.
*, $P < .001$; **, $P < .05$.

significantly greater than those of patients with malignant meningioma. The mean DIs of patients with LGG were significantly different from those of patients with GM and AG.

SG2M DNA Index and %SG2M

Table 2 shows the relationship between the mean SG2M DIs, %SG2M, and histopathology in the five groups of 73 patients. The mean SG2M DIs of patients with brain metastasis were significantly greater than those of patients with malignant meningioma. The mean SG2M DIs of patients with GM and AG were significantly higher than those of patients with LGG. The %SG2M was significantly higher for GM, AG, and brain metastasis than for LGG.

The mean SG2M DIs fitted to an exponential curve when plotted against the mean DIs ($P < .001$) (Fig. 4a), and mean %SG2M values also significantly fitted to a linear curve when plotted against the mean DIs ($P < .001$) (Fig. 4b).

G2M Ploidy, %SG2M, and TTP

The patients with hyperT tumors had a shorter mean TTP than those with T tumors ($P < .01$) (Table 3). There was no significant correlation in TTP between the patients with hypoT and T, or between the patients with hyperT and hypoT, although the four patients with hypoT had a tendency for a longer TTP. In the patients with tetraploid gliomas in G2M ploidy, patients with high-grade glioma had a shorter mean TTP and a higher mean %SG2M than those with low-grade glioma (Fig. 5a). In patients with high-grade glioma, although the patients with hyperT glioma had a shorter mean TTP

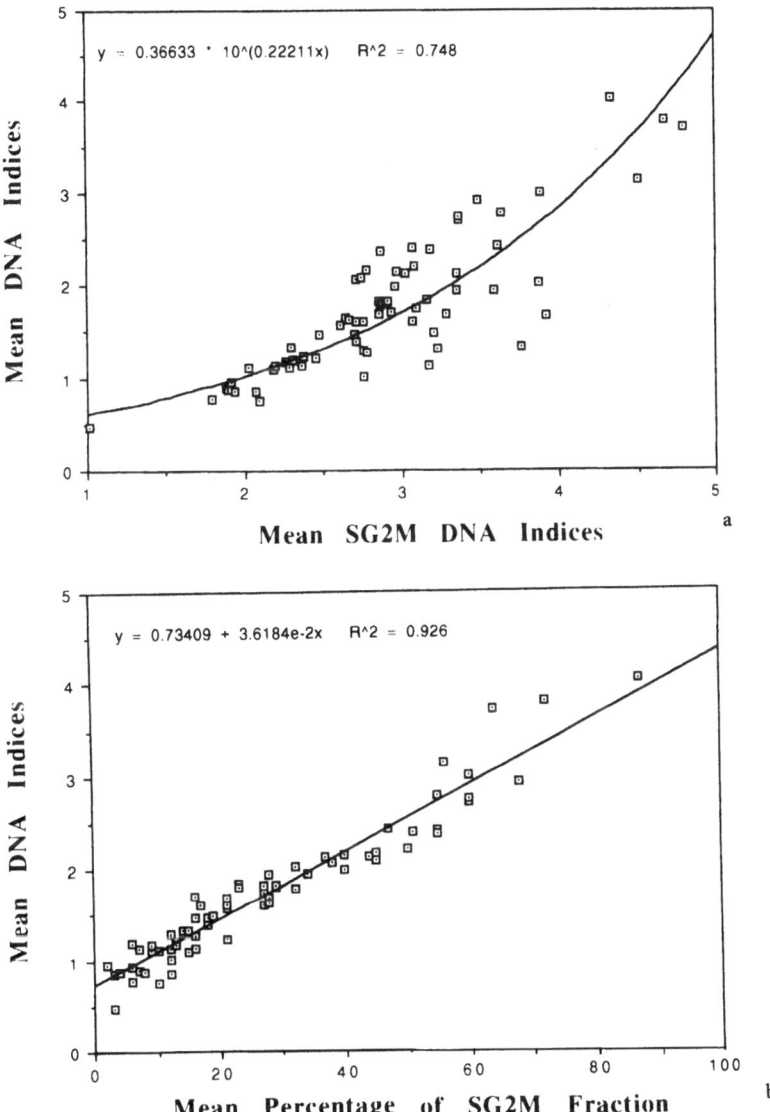

Fig. 4a,b. Relationship between mean DNA index (DI), SG2M-DI, and percentage of SG2M fraction (%SG2M). The mean SG2M DIs (a) and %SG2M (b) values fitted significantly to each curve when plotted against the mean DI ($P < .001$)

than patients with T glioma, the %SG2M values showed significant difference between the patients with T and hyperT gliomas (Fig. 5b).

Morphometry in G0G1 and SG2M Phase Nuclei

In all patients with brain tumors who were studied, the mean area of nuclei in SG2M phase cells was significantly larger than in G0G1 phase cells (Table 4). In patients with

Table 3. Relationship between G2M ploidy, pathology, and time to tumor progression (TTP).

G2M Ploidy	Pathology	TTP (mean ± SD) (mo)
Hypo T (4)	GM (1), AG (2), Meta (1)	25.3 ± 30.2
T (42)	GM (9), AG (8), LGG (11), Meta (9), Maling. M (5)	18.9 ± 20.5*
Hyper T (27)	GM (10), AG (7), Meta (10)	9.2 ± 11.8*

T, tetraploidy; TTP, time to tumor progression; GM, glioblastoma multiforme; AG, anaplastic glioma; LGG, low-grade glioma; Meta, brain metastasis; Malig. M, malignant meningioma.
*, $P < .01$.
Number of cases are in parentheses.

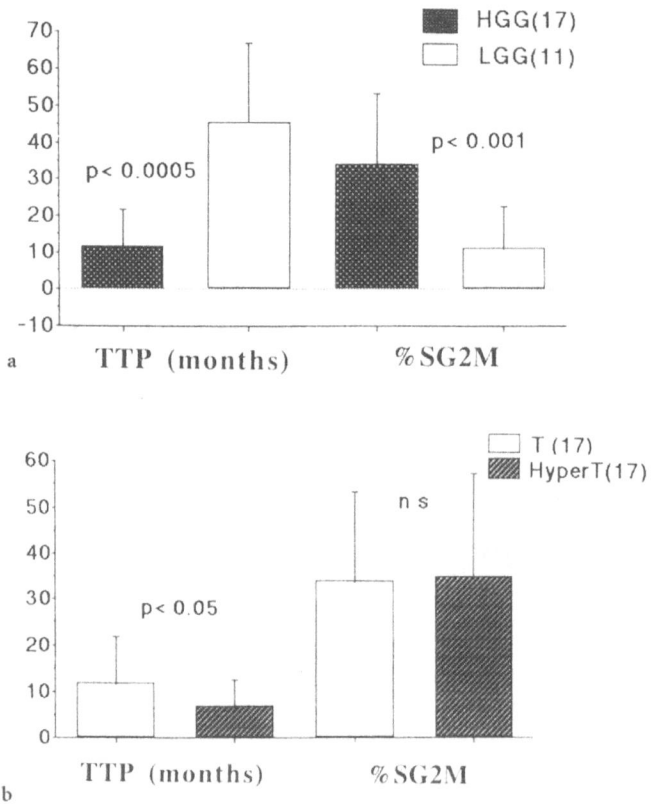

a

b

Fig. 5a,b. Relationship among time to tumor progression (TTP), %SG2M, and G2M ploidy in the patients with glioma. **a** The patients with tetraploid HGG in G2M ploidy had a shorter TTP and a larger %SG2M than those of the patients with LGG. **b** Although the patients with hyperT HGG in G2M ploidy had a shorter TTP than those of the patients with T HGG, the %SG2M values had no significant difference between the patients with T and hyperT HGG in G2M ploidy. *TTP*, time to tumor progression; *%SG2M*, percentage of the SG2M phase fractions; *HGG*, high-grade glioma; *LGG*, low-grade glioma; *ns*, not significant; *T*, tetraploidy; *hyper T*, hypertetraploidy. Parentheses enclose number of cases studied

Table 4. Relationship between nuclear area and cell cycle phased nuclei in 73 patients with brain tumors.

Pathology	Number of cases	Nuclear area (mean ± SD μm^2)	
		G0G1 nuclei	SG2M nuclei
Brain metastasis	21	44.3 ± 10.3*	70.5 ± 23.9*
Malignant meningioma	5	41.7 ± 2.8**	58.1 ± 8.5**
Glioblastoma multiforme	20	33.0 ± 8.8*	59.2 ± 16.9*
Anaplastic glioma	17	33.1 ± 9.7*	52.4 ± 21.2*
Low-grade glioma	11	29.9 ± 4.5*	47.7 ± 11.0*

Note the area is larger in SG2M phase nuclei than in G0G1 phase nuclei in all tumors.
*, $P < .001$; **, $P < .05$.

Table 5. Relationship between form factor (FF) and cell cycle phased nuclei in 73 patients with brain tumors.

Pathology	Number of cases	Form factor (mean ± SD)	
		G0G1 nuclei	SG2M nuclei
Brain metastasis	21	0.90 ± 0.03*	0.88 ± 0.04*
Malignant meningioma	5	0.9 ± 0.04**	0.9 ± 0.04**
Glioblastoma multiforme	20	0.85 ± 0.04*	0.82 ± 0.07*
Anaplastic glioma	17	0.86 ± 0.05*	0.83 ± 0.07*
Low-grade glioma	11	0.89 ± 0.04**	0.87 ± 0.06**

Note shape of nuclei is more irregular in SG2M phase than in G0G1 phase in brain metastasis, glioblastoma multiforme, and malignant glioma.
*, $P < .05$; **, not significant.

Table 6. Relationship between nuclear area and form factor (FF) of different tumors in hypotetraploidy in G2M ploidy.

Pathology	Number of cases	Nuclear area (mean ± SD μm^2)	Form factor (mean ± SD)
Glioblastoma multiforme	1	75.2	0.84
Anaplastic glioma	2	35.0 ± 5.9	0.94 ± 0.04
Brain metastasis	1	35.7	0.89

brain metastasis, GM, and AG, the mean FFs of nuclei in SG2M phase cells were significantly lower than those in G0G1 phase cells (Table 5).

G2M Ploidy Pattern and Morphometry

Among the patients with each G2M ploidy pattern (Tables 6–8), the group with nongliomatous tumors showed a significantly larger nuclear area than the group with gliomatous tumors.

In patients with brain metastasis in particular, the nuclear area in hyperT in G2M ploidy was significantly larger than in T in G2M ploidy (Fig. 6a). However, in the FFs of those nuclei there was no significant difference between hyperT and T tumor cells in G2M ploidy patterns (Fig. 6b).

The morphological changes in the nuclei of hyperT and T tumor cells in G2M ploidy may not correlate with the DNA content in those nuclei.

Table 7. Relationship between nuclear area and form factor (FF) of different tumors in tetraploidy in G2M ploidy.

Pathology	Number of cases	Nuclear area (mean ± SD μm²)	Form factor (mean ± SD)
Glioblastoma multiforme	9	56.2 ± 17.2	0.84 ± 0.05
Anaplastic glioma	8	48.9 ± 14.9*	0.84 ± 0.06
Low-grade glioma	11	47.7 ± 11.0**	0.87 ± 0.06
Brain metastasis	9	61.3 ± 16.2*	0.89 ± 0.04
Malignant meningioma	5	58.1 ± 8.5**	0.89 ± 0.05

*, $P < .05$; **, $P < .0005$.

Table 8. Relationship between nuclear area and form factor (FF) of different tumors in hypertetraploidy in G2M ploidy.

Pathology	Number of cases	Nuclear area (mean ± SD μm²)	Form factor (mean ± SD)
Glioblastoma multiforme	10	60.3 ± 17.3*	0.80 ± 0.08
Anaplastic glioma	7	61.3 ± 26.9	0.80 ± 0.06
Brain metastasis	10	84.1 ± 24.1*	0.87 ± 0.04

*, $P < .05$.

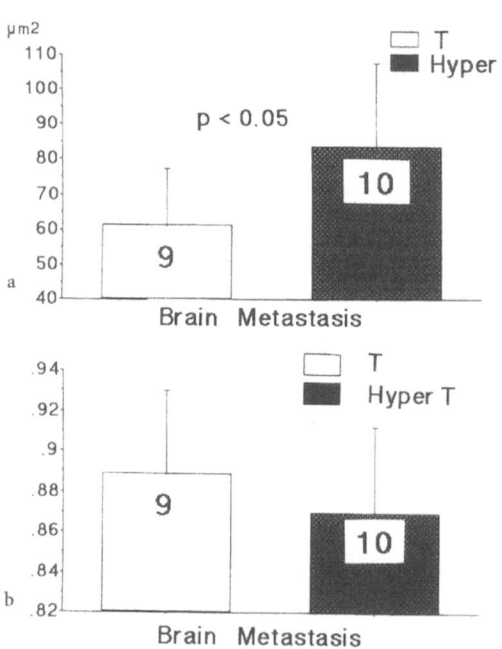

Fig. 6a,b. Relationship between nuclear morphometry in the SG2M phase cells with T and hyperT in G2M ploidy in patients with brain metastasis. **a** The nuclear area in those cells with hyperT was significantly larger than those with T. **b** The nuclear form factor (FF) in those cells with hyperT showed no significant difference from those with T. Numbers are number of cases

Discussion

Our previous analysis of DNA ploidy showed that there was a positive correlation between diploidy and long TTP in benign brain tumors, but that there was no consistent correlation between aneuploidy, such as hyperT, hypoD, hypoT, and T, and TTT in malignant brain tumors [20].

Our results showed that mean DIs were mainly affected by mean SG2M DIs. A distribution of SG2M cells appeared in the same sample, and a higher number of SG2M DIs and a higher percentage of SG2M tumor cells occurred in malignant brain tumors than in benign tumors. Those results are similar to other reports [1–9,11–17,21,39–41,44–47]. This in turn suggests investigating the DNA content and nuclear morphology in SG2M phase cells as a main prognostic factor in malignant brain tumors. We analyzed the difference between the estimated SG2M DIs and the crude mean SG2M DIs to evaluate, by this method, whether a stemline in which the diploid (2C) tumors consisted of a first major peak have a G2M tetraploid (4C) whose cells consisted of a second major peak.

We found that the population of patients who survived longer included those with hypoT tumors in G2M ploidy. In contrast, we found that patients with hyperT tumors in G2M ploidy survived for a shorter time both with and without high SG2M fractions than those of hypoT and T. The patients with T tumors in G2M ploidy without a high SG2M fraction survived relatively longer than those of hyperT and T with high SG2M fraction. We believe that our classification in the G2M ploidy pattern is useful for the prognostic evaluation in patients with brain tumors.

It was interesting, in SG2M phase cells, that the nuclear area was larger and the form factor showed greater deformity than those in G0G1 phase cells in GM, AG, and brain metastasis. We can understand this result to reflect the high cellular metabolism of SG2M phase cells. A large variability of nuclear volumes was considered to be a quantitative expression of aneuploidy [28].

In a stemline study in brain tumors, Kawamoto et al. [41] reported multimodal aneuploidy in the classification of ploidy pattern and that the tumor tissue with such ploidy was composed of two types (stemlines) of tumor cell.

In our studies, the stem cells with hyperT glioma in G2M ploidy have a highly abnormal DNA content except for the proliferative potential of the S-fraction. In contrast, stem cells with T glioma in G2M ploidy have a DNA content with two peaks of 2C and 4C. Furthermore, stem cells with hypoT glioma in G2M ploidy have a DNA content between 2C and 4C in the SG2M phase cells. However, in the glioma group the morphological nuclear change had no significant correlation with hyperT and T tumor cells in the G2M ploidy patterns. Stem cells with hyperT glioma in G2M ploidy mainly had an abnormal DNA content rather than variable nuclear morphology.

In patients with brain metastasis, the nuclear area of hyperT tumor cells in G2M ploidy was significantly larger than those of T tumor cells in G2M ploidy. Stem cells of hyperT metastatic tumors in G2M ploidy not only have a densitometrically abnormal DNA content but also a morphologically abnormal nuclear character.

Thus, our results indicate that heterogeneity is composed of many stem cell lines differing both densitometrically and morphometrically in gliomatous and nongliomatous brain tumors. Our results indicated in particular that the increase of DNA content in SG2M phase cells in human glioma was not associated with the increase of those nuclear areas and the deformity of those nuclear shapes. In human brain tumors, analysis of the heterogeneity in the tumor cells appears to contribute to the improvement of the therapeutic method applied to the tumors [33,34]. Our studies indicated that analysis of tumor heterogeneity should also be investigated from two standpoints: the densitometric DNA content and the morphological nuclear character.

Conclusion

Tumors with hyperT in G2M ploidy indicated highly malignant and proliferative stem cells with DNA content above 4C in the SG2M phase cells. Tumors with T in G2M ploidy indicated malignancy by the number of the SG2M fraction, and those tumor cells showed the stem lines with DNA content of 4C in the SG2M phase cells. In contrast, tumors with hypoT in G2M ploidy indicated less malignant and proliferative stem cells, with DNA content between 2C and 4C in the SG2M phase cells. However, in human gliomas the chromosomal heterogeneity did not always correlate with the morphological heterogeneity. Our classification in G2M ploidy may suggest the degree of heterogeneity or stemlines in the resected tumors, and may contribute to selecting the therapeutic modality for brain tumors.

Further investigation of the heterogenous nature of brain tumors using image analysis is needed to understand tumor biology and to improve treatment of this disease.

Acknowledgments. The authors thank Drs. RL Becker and UV Mikel, Division of Quantitative Pathology, Departmant of Cellular Pathology, Armed Forces Institute of Pathology, Washington, DC, USA, for their technical support.

References

1. Frederiksen P, Raske-Nelson E, Bichel P (1978) Flow cytometry in tumors of the brain. Acta Neuropathol 41:179–183
2. Hoshino T, Nomura K, Wilson CB, et al (1978) The distribution of nuclear DNA from human brain-tumor cells: flow cytometric studies. J Neurosurg 49:13–21
3. Kawamoto K, Herz F, Wolley RC, et al (1979) Flow cytometric analysis of DNA distribution in human brain tumors. Acta Neuropathol 46:39–44
4. Lehmann J, Krug H (1980) Flow-through fluorocytophotometry of different brain tumors. Acta Neuropathol 49:123–132
5. Mork SJ, Laerum OD (1980) Modal DNA content of human intracranial neoplasms studied by flow cytometry. J Neurosurg 53:198–204
6. Nishizaki T, Orita T, Furutani Y, et al (1989) Flow cytometric DNA analysis and immunohistochemical measurement of Ki-67 and BUdR labeling indices in human brain tumors. J Neurosurg 70:379–384
7. Salmon I, Kiss R, Dewitte O, et al (1992) Histopathologic grading and DNA ploidy in relation to survival among 206 adult astrocytic tumor patients. Cancer 70:538–546
8. Salmon I, Kiss R, Levivier M, et al (1993) Characterization of nuclear DNA content, proliferation index, and nuclear size in a series of 181 meningiomas, including benign primary, recurrent, and malignant tumors. Am J Surg Pathol 17:239–247
9. Salmon I, Levivier M, Camby I, et al (1993) Assessment of nuclear size, nuclear DNA content and proliferation index in stereotaxic biopsies from brain tumors, Neuropathol Appl Neurobiol 19:507–518
10. Broggi G, Franzini A, Costa A, Melcarne A, Allegranza A (1985) Cell kinetics of neuroepithelial tumors in serial stereotactic biopsies. A new combined approach. Appl Neurophysiol 48:472–476
11. DeReuck J, Sieben G, DeCoster W, et al (1980) Cytophotometric DNA determination in human oligodendroglial tumors. Histopathology 4:225–232
12. Hoshino T, Wilson CB (1979) Cell kinetic analyses of human malignant brain tumors (gliomas). Cancer 44:956–962
13. Hoshino T, Townsend JJ, Muradea I, et al (1980) An autoradiographic study of human gliomas: growth kinetics of anaplastic astrocytoma and glioblastoma multiforme. Brain 103:967–984

14. Hoshino T, Nagashima T, Murovic JA, et al (1986) In situ cell kinetics studies on human neuroectodermal tumors with bromodeoxyuridine labeling. J Neurosurg 64:453–459

15. Nagashima T, DeArmond SJ, Murovic J, et al (1985) Immunocytochemical demonstration of S-phase cells by antibromodeoxyuridine monoclonal antibody in human brain tumor tissues. Acta Neuropathol 67:155–159

16. Saito A, Yoshii Y, Nose T (1994) Image analysis of nuclear DNA content and morphometrical characteristics of the tumor cells in human astrocytomas. Brain Tumor Pathol 11

17. Yoshii Y, Maki Y, Tsuboi K, et al (1986) Estimation of growth fraction with bromodexyuridine in human central nervous system tumors. J Neurosurg 65:659–693

18. Yoshii Y, Narushiama K, Tsuboi K, et al (1988) Tumor cord and growth in human brain tumors based on mathematical morphology. J Neurol Oncol 6:119–128

19. Yoshii Y, Sugiyama K (1988) Intercapillary distance in the proliferating area of human glioma. Cancer Res 48:2938–2941

20. Yoshii Y, Saito A, Tsuboi K, et al (1994) Nuclear characterization and G2M ploidy in human brain tumors using semiautomated image analysis. Brain Tumor Pathol

21. Zaprianov Z, Christov K (1988) Histological grading, DNA content, cell proliferation and survival of patients with astroglial tumors. Cytometry 9:380–386

22. Banner BF, Branczio L, Bahnson RR, et al (1990) DNA analysis of multiple synchronous renal cell carcinomas. Cancer 66:2180–2185

23. Becker RL, Mikel UV (1990) Interrelation of formalin fixation, chromatin compactness and DNA values as measured by flow and image cytometry. Anal Quant Cytol Histol 12:333–341

24. Cope C, Rowe D, Delbridge L, et al (1991) Comparison of image analysis and flow cytometric determination of cellular DNA content. J Clin Pathol 44:147–151

25. Davenport RD, Mckeever PE (1987) Ploidy of endothelium in high-grade astrocytomas. Anal Quant Cytol Histol 9:25–29

26. Martin H, Voss K (1982) Automated image analysis of glioblastomas and other gliomas. Acta Neuropathol 58:9–16

27. Martin H, Voss K (1982) Computerized classification of gliomas by automated microscope pictur analysis (AMPA). Acta Neuropathol 58:261–268

28. Martin H, Voss K, Hufnagl P, et al (1984) Automated image analysis of glimas: an objective and reproducible method for tumor grading. Acta Neuropathol 63:160–169

29. Mikel UV, Becker RL (1991) A comparative study of quanititative stains for DNA in image cytometry. Anal Quant Cytol Histol 13:253–259

30. Mikel UV, Fishbein WN, Bahr GF (1985) Some practical considerations in quantitative absorbance microspectro-photometry; preparation techniques in DNA cytophotometry. Anal Quant Cytol Histol 7:107–118

31. Schad LR, Schmitt HP, Oberwittler C, et al (1987) Numerical grading of astrocytoma. Med Inform 12:11–22

32. Ullen H, Falkmer UG, Collins VP, et al (1991) Methodologic aspects of nuclear DNA assessment of gliomas with astrocytic and/or oligodendrocytic differentiation. Correlation of image and flow cytometric studies on paraffin-embedded specimens. Anal Quant Cytol Histol 13:168–176

33. Calabresi P, Dexter DL, Heppner GH (1979) Clinical and pharmacological implications of cancer cell differentiation and hetergeneity. Biochem Pharmacol 28:1933–1941

34. Heppner GH, Dexter DL, DeNucci T, et al (1978) Heterogeneity in drug sensitivity among tumor cell subpopulations of single mammary tumor. Cancer Res 38:3758–3763

35. Raz A, McLellan WL, Hart IR, et al (1980) Cell surface properties of B16 melanoma variants with differing metastatic potential. Cancer Res 40:1645–1651

36. Miller FR, Heppner GH (1979) Immunologic heterogeneity of tumor cell subpopulations from a single mouse mamnary tumor. J Natl Cancer Inst 63:1457–1463

37. Dexter DL, Kowalski HM, Blazar BA, et al (1978) Heterogeneity of tumor cells from a single mouse mammary tumor. Cancer Res 38:3174–3181

38. Gray JM, Pierce GB (1964) Relationship between growth rate and differentiation of melanoma in vivo. J Natl Cancer Inst 32:1201–1211

39. Appley AJ, Fitzgibbons PL, Chandrasoma PT, et al (1990) Multiparameter flow cytometric analysis of neoplasms of the central nervous system: correlation of nuclear antigen p105 and DNA content with clinical behavior. Neurosurgery 27:83–96

40. Giangaspero F, Chieco P, Lisignoli G, et al (1987) Comparison of cytologic composition with microfluorometric DNA analysis the glioblastoma multiforme and anaplastic astrocytoma. Cancer 60:59–65

41. Kawamoto K, Sakai N, Numa Y, et al (1991) Significance of flow cytometric measurement of DNA index in gliomas. Brain Tumor Pathol 8:177–181

42. Shapiro JR, Yung WKA, Shapiro WR (1981) Isolation, karyotype, and clonal growth of heterogeneous subpopulation of human malignant gliomas. Cancer Res 41:2349–2359

43. Coons SW, Johnson PC (1993) Regional heterogeneity in the DNA content of human gliomas. Cancer 72:3052–3060

44. Ahyai A, Spaar FW (1987) DNA and prognosis of meningiomas: a comparative cytological and fluorescence-cytophotometrical study of 71 tumors. Acta Neurochir 87:119–128

45. Ironside JW, Battersby RDE, Lawry J, et al (1987) DNA in meningioma tissues and explant cell cultures: a flow cytometric study with clinicopathological correlates. J Neurosurg 66:588–594

46. May PL, Broome JC, Lawry J, et al (1989) The prediction of recurrence in meningiomas. A flow cytometric study of paraffin-embedded archival meterial. J Neurosurg 71:347–351

47. Sparr FW, Ahyai A, Blech M (1987) DNA fluorescence cytometry and prognosis (grading) of meningiomas. A study of 104 surgically removed tumors. Neurosurg Rev 10:35–39

Efficiency of Glioma Score in Glioma Patients Using Proliferating Potential with MIB-1 Monoclonal Antibody

Tatsuhiro Maeda, Kazuhiko Saruta, Satoyuki Ito, Hiroki Sawa, and Isamu Saito

Abstract. We have proposed a "glioma score" that includes malignancy as determined histologically, the patient's age, and the MIB-1 proliferating cell index (PCI) as the prognostic indicator for patients with malignant gliomas. Each part of the glioma score (GS), is assigned points from 1 to 4 based on histological malignancy, patient's age, and value of MIB-1 PCI, respectively. The total score then sums the points of each group. The MIB-1 PCIs for glioma patients were correlated with tumor grade. Cases with a GS of 10 points or more showed a shorter time to progression (TTP) of less than 2 years. The incidence of cases with a TTP of less than 2 years is significantly higher for a GS of 10 points or more and less than 10 as analyzed by contingency table analysis ($P = .02$). Kaplan–Meier proportional survival curves were generated for cases with GS of 10 or over and less than 10. Patients whose GS was more than 10 had a tendency toward a shorter TTP than those patients whose GS was less than 10 but no significant survival advantage was demonstrated between them. Therefore, the proposal of a glioma score may provide important information for therapeutic intervention and prognosis of patients with gliomas.

Key words. MIB-1 proliferating cell index—Proliferative potential—Malignant gliomas—Prognosis

Introduction

Malignant gliomas constitute about 40% of central nervous system neoplasms. They directly invade and grow in brain tissue and rarely metastasize. Because they invade normal brain tissue, complete removal of the tumor could be devastating, so subtotal resection is frequently the procedure of choice. Therapy for most malignant gliomas therefore consists of surgery followed by radiation therapy and chemotherapy. Recurrence is almost always at the local site.

The most important prognostic factors for malignant gliomas are age, performance status, and histological malignancy. In general, younger patients have a better prognosis than older patients, and the more intact and functional patients survive longer than those with poor status regardless of other factors.

Department of Neurosurgery, Kyorin University School of Medicine, Shinkawa Mitaka, Tokyo 181, Japan

Unfortunately, histopathological features do not always correlate well with the biological behavior of the tumor or with the survival of the patients. For example, cellularity increases and nuclei become more irregular in size and shape with grade of malignancy. Necrosis and hemorrhage occur in the highest grade tumors such as glioblastoma multiforme. However, glioblastoma multiforme often fails to show mitoses, whereas some slow-growing oligodendrogliomas present many mitoses. Moreover, survival within each patient group that includes low-grade astrocytoma, highly anaplastic astrocytoma, and glioblastoma multiforme is still highly variable.

One possible prognostic factor is proliferative potential. A monoclonal antibody has been developed that can identify 5-bromo,2-deoxyuridine (BUdR); it is an analog of thymidine and like [³H]thymidine it is incorporated into the nuclear DNA of cells during DNA synthesis [1–3]. The BUdR labeling index (LI) appears to reflect the proliferative potential more accurately than the histopathological grading and should therefore be considered a more important factor in determining the prognosis of the patient with glioma [2]. However, it did not perform well as a prognostic indicator for glioblastoma multiforme. Thus, improved prognostic criteria are still needed.

The monoclonal antibody MIB-1 is a newly designed proliferation marker that recognizes the Ki-67 antigen even in formalin-fixed, paraffin-embedded tissues [4,5]. The MIB-1 antibody reacts with the nuclear matrix of cells presented in G_1, G_2, S, and M phases. The value of MIB-1 for the assessment of cell proliferating activity has been widely documented in various human tumors, including brain tumors, to be as good as BUdR-LI [6].

The aim of this study was to test the applicability of MIB-1 antibody as a prognostic marker in malignant gliomas. We also proposed a "glioma score," including histological malignancy, patient's age, and MIB-1 proliferating cell index (PCI) as the prognostic indicator for patients with malignant gliomas. Another objective of this study was to evaluate the prognostic significance of the glioma score for patients with malignant gliomas and to compare this score with patient survival.

Clinical Materials and Methods

Thirty-seven patients with human gliomas who underwent surgery between 1990 and 1994 in the Department of Neurosurgery, Kyorin University School of Medicine, entered this study. There were 11 cases of low-grade astrocytoma (WHO grade II), 16 of highly anaplastic astrocytoma (WHO grade III), and 10 of glioblastoma multiforme (WHO grade IV). The patients were aged from 1 to 76 years (mean, 47 years). Juvenile pilocytic astrocytomas were excluded from this analysis.

Surgical specimens were fixed in 70% ethanol and embedded in paraffin wax; the 5-μm-thick sections were routinely stained with hematoxylin and eosin. Immunohistochemical reactions were carried out using the streptavidin/peroxydase method (Dako Strept ABComplex/HRP Duet mouse/rabbit kit, Dako, Santa Barbara, CA, USA) and MIB-1 mouse mAb (Dianova, Hamburg, Germany), which recognizes an epitome on the Ki-67 antigen.

Sections were deparaffinized in xylene and dehydrated through graded ethanol to water. The slides were placed in glass jars filled with $10\,mM$ citrate buffer and processed 20 min in an autoclave oven at 800 W. The slides were allowed to cool in the jars at room temperature for 20 min and then incubated sequentially with the monoclonal MIB-1 antibody (Immunotech S.A., Marseille, France) at 1:50 for 45 min, with biotinylated link antibody for 30 min, and then streptavidin labeled with peroxidase for 30 min (LSAB code 681, Dacopatts, Copenhagen, Denmark). A light hematoxylin counterstain was used. The method is described in detail in the manufacturer's instructions included with the antibody. Negative control staining was obtained by substituting MIB-1 with a nonnuclear antibody.

Evaluation of MIB-1 Proliferative Cell Index

The ratio of positive cell nuclei to the total number of tumor cell nuclei as the PCI was calculated in several homogenous, highly labeled microscopic fields. At least 1000 cells per case were counted. Positive and negative control slides were incubated with each stained batch. Vascular endothelial cells and hematopoietic cells were not counted.

Glioma Score

We proposed that the glioma score consist of the factors that relate to prognosis of the patients such as histological diagnosis, patient age, and MIB-1 proliferating index in Table 1. Each part is given points from 1 to 4 based on histological malignancy, the patient's age, and the value of MIB-1 PCI. The glioma score was then totaled to show the score including the points of each group.

Statistical Analysis

Patients were arbitrarily divided into two groups: those whose tumors had PCIs of less than 3% and those with tumors with PCIs of 3% or more, and also into those whose tumors had a GS of less than 10 points and those with a GS of 10 or more. The time to progression (TTP) in these groups was estimated nonparametrically from incomplete observations by the method of Kaplan and Meier.

Results

The clinical data and MIB-1 PCI for 37 patients including 11 grade II, 16 grade III, and 10 grade IV tumors are analyzed. The median PCI for anaplastic astrocytomas grade III and glioblastoma multiformes were 7.2% and 11.8%, respectively, while low-grade astrocytomas (grade II) demonstrated a median PCI of 1%. These MIB-1 PCI for each grade of tumor were significantly different by simple regression

Table 1. Glioma score components.

Score	Grade[a]	Patient age (years)	MIB-1 PCI (%)
1	I	<20	<1.0
2	II	20–40	$1 \leq PCI < 5$
3	III	41–60	$5 \leq PCI < 10$
4	IV	>61	≥ 10

PCI, proliferating cell index.
[a] Grade of histological malignancy, using WHO grading.

Table 2. Relationship between glioma score (GS) and time to proliferation (TTP).

TTP	GS ≥ 10	GS ≤ 9
Less than 2 years	12 cases (86%)	9 cases (39%)
More than 2 years	2 cases (14%)	14 cases (61%)

$P = .02$.

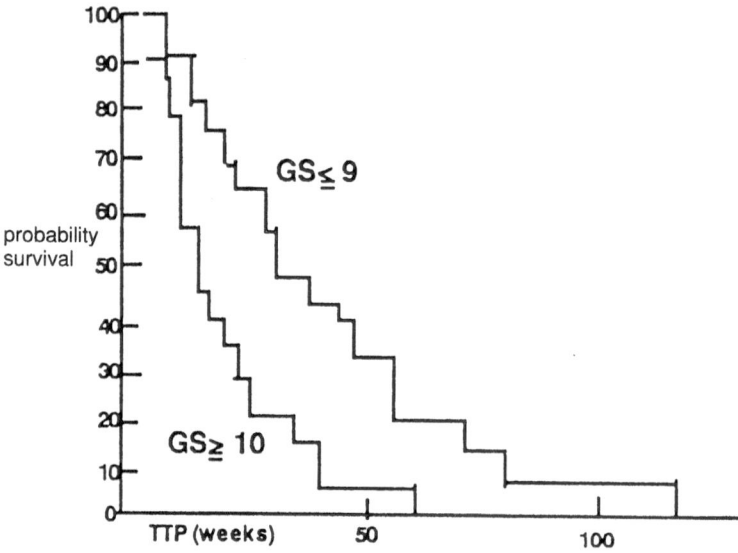

Fig. 1. Kaplan–Meier survival curves for glioma patients show the relationship of glioma score (GS) to time to progression (TTP). Patients whose GS was 10 or over tended to have a shorter TTP than the cases whose GS was less than 10, but the difference was not significant ($P > .05$)

analysis. Therefore, the MIB-1 PCIs for glioma patients were correlated with tumor grade.

The cases with a GS of 10 points or more showed a shorter TTP of less than 2 years (Table 2). The prevalence of cases with a TTP of less than 2 years is significantly different between GS of 10 or more and less than 10 points as analyzed by contingency table analysis ($P = .02$). Kaplan–Meier proportional survival curves were generated for these cases with GS of 10 points and over or less than 10 points. No significant survival advantage was demonstrated between these two groups of patients. However, there was a tendency for cases whose GS was 10 or over to show a shorter TTP than cases whose GS was under 10. (Fig. 1).

Illustrative Cases

Case 1

A 74-year-old man presented with left motor weakness and headache. Postcontrast computed tomography (CT) showed an irregular enhancing mass with cystic formation in the right frontal region. He had undergone craniectomy and partical removal of the tumor, which was histologially diagnosed as glioblastoma multiforme. The adjuvant therapy included radiation therapy followed by ACNU as chemotherapy. The MIB-1 PCI of this tumor specimen was 7.9%; the glioma score in this case totaled 11 points, consisting of 4 points for grading, 4 for age, and 3 for MIB-1 PCI. The TTP was only 5 months, and this patient survived only 6 months.

Case 2

A 28-year-old woman presented with headache. Postcontrast CT showed an irregular and heterogenous enhancing mass in the corpus callosum. Partial removal of tumor was performed; its diagnosis was glioblastoma multiforme. The adjuvant therapy included radiation therapy, chemotherapy, and immunotherapy. The MIB-1 PCI was 2.9%, and the glioma score, totaling 8 points, consisted of 4 points for grading, 2 for age, and 2 for MIB-1 PCI. The TTP was 26 months, and the patient died after surviving for 45 months.

Case 3

A 40-year-old man presented with generalized convulsion. Postcontrast CT demonstrated a low-density area without an enhancing region in right parietal lobe. An operation was performed and the tumor removed subtotally. The diagnosis was anaplastic astrocytoma grade III. The adjuvant therapy included radiation therapy and chemotherapy. The TTP was 45 months, and no recurrence of the tumor is evident. The glioma score totaled 6 points: 3 points for grading, 2 for age, and 1 for MIB-1 PCI.

Discussion

Hoshino et al. [7–9] established that cell kinetic studies by BUdR LI can be applied to elucidate the complex proliferation kinetics of human brain tumors in situ and to better understand their malignant behavior. Recently, however, it has not been easy to acquire the drug for BUdR; BUdR labeling studies can only be applied with some restrictions because tetragenic and mutagenic effects could be induced by administration of BUdR, although the doses required for in vivo labeling studies of BUdR are samll [10–12]. Moreover, it is necessary that the patients take the drugs to evaluate BUdR labeling studies. Thus, the proliferative activity of malignant glioma should be evaluated by tests other than BUdR.

The monoclonal antibody MIB-1 detects the nuclear Ki-67 antigen that is present in all active parts of the cell cycle including G_1, S, G_2, and mitosis, but is absent in G_0 [5]. Immunostaining with MIB-1 provides a reliable means of evaluating the growth fraction of the glioma cell populations. Of the various immunohistochemical proliferation markers used in histology and histopathology, the MIB-1 antibody against the Ki-67 antigen probably has the greatest relevance for the study of tumor cells. Because MIB-1 is able to detect the Ki-67 antigen in formalin-fixed, paraffin-embedded sections following microwave heating of the specimen, immunohistochemistry opens a larger time window than BUdR and proliferating cell nuclear antigen techniques. Moreover, recent studies demonstrated that MIB-1 has been used to estimate the growth fraction in different groups of solid tumors including non-Hodgkin lymphomas [13,14], carcinomas [15–18], and a wide range of intracranial tumors [19–23], and the percentage of MIB-1-positive cell nuclei was found to reflect the histological grade of malignancy.

In our study, the difference between MIB-1 value and histological malignancy was significant. According to Karamitopoulou et al. [4], on the other hand, glioblastomas and anaplastic astrocytomas exhibited statistically significant higher mean Ki-67 LI values than their benign counterparts, while no significant difference was found between anaplastic astrocytoma and glioblastomas [4]. Their findings clearly indicated that MIB-1 values generally correlated well with the histological features and grading. Several studies on the proliferative potential of gliomas using either the Ki-67 index or BUdR LI have strongly suggested that the percentage of Ki-67 or BUdR immunopositive cells correlates closely with the histological features and grading of anaplasia [24–28]. Shibuya et al. [29] suggested that cell proliferating activity in brain tumors as determined by Ki-67 index is closely related to the BUdR LI. Hoshino et al. [30] suggested that the higher BUdR LI indicate a faster rate of tumor growth and shorter time to recurrence, especially in low-grade gliomas, and that the relationship between the proliferative potential and prognosis appears to be more accurately evaluated using BUdR LI than by histopathological diagnosis alone. The factors influencing patient prognosis could not be evaluated by the proliferative potential in the individual tumors alone. In this study, we propose a glioma score that will indicate glioma prognosis more accurately than the evaluation of proliferative potential by the immunohistochemical findings alone. One of the other important prognostic factors for malignant gliomas is patient age; in general, younger patients do better than older patients. Therefore, the glioma score contains factors of histological malignancy, patient age, and MIB-1 PCI, which are the important factors of prognosis in glioma patients.

In our results, the cases with a glioma score of 10 points or over showed a shorter time to progression, i.e., less than 2 years. Thus, the prevalence of cases with time to progression of less than 2 years is significantly higher among those with a glioma score of 10 and over.

Kaplan–Meier survival curves for patients with malignant gliomas relating time to progression with the glioma score showed there was a tendency toward a higher incidence of a short time to progression with a glioma score of 10 points or more although the difference was not significant. The MIB-1 proliferating index and BUdR LI are the only methods for predicting the proliferative potential of tumors. Monoclonal antibodies to proliferating cell nuclear antigen or cyclin [31], thymididylate syntheses [32], deoxyribonucleic acid polymerase-alpha [33], and nuclear organizing region [34,35] are also potentially useful for cell kinetic studies. So far, the MIB-1 PCI and BUdR-LI have provided more reliable results than studies with other monoclonal antibodies currently available. These cell kinetic analyses will be of great theoretical and practical importance for understanding the biological and clinical behavior of individual gliomas. The proliferating potential is not the only factor influencing patient prognosis; histological features and patient age are also important to evaluate the prognosis. In this study, we propose a glioma score including some known prognostic factors influencing patient survival with malignant gliomas. The glioma score may also provide more important information for therapeutic intervention and prognosis of patients with gliomas. Nevertheless, efforts to obtain more accurate prognostic information whether by this glioma score or other elements, are of great theoretical and practical importance.

Acknowledgments. The authors thank Hideko Sato for immunohistochemical assistance.

References

1. Hoshino T, Nagashima T, Cho KG, Davis RL, Donegan J, Slusarz M, Wilson CB (1989) Variability in the proliferative potential of human gliomas. J Neurooncol 7:137–143
2. Hoshino T, Prados M, Wilson CB, Cho KG, Lee KS, Davis RL (1989) Prognostic implications of the bromodeoxyuridine labeling index of human gliomas. J Neurosurg 71:335–341
3. Germano IM, Ito M, Cho KG, Hoshino T, Davis RL, Wilson CB (1989) Correlation of histopathological features and proliferative potential of gliomas. J Neurosurg 70:701–706
4. Karamitopoulou E, Perentes E, Diamantes I, Maraziotis T (1994) Ki-67 immunoreactivity in human central nervous system; a study with MIB-1 monoclonal antibody on archival material. Acta Neuropathol 87:47–54
5. Gattoretti G, Becker MHG, Key G, Duvchrow M, Schluter C, Galle J, Gerdes J (1992) Monoclonal antibodies recombinant parts of the Ki-67 antigen (MIB-1 and MIB-3) detect proliferating cells in microwave-processed formalin paraffin sections. J Pathol 168:357–363
6. Nielsen AL, Nyhorm HCJ, Engel P (1994) Expression of MIB-1 (paraffin Ki-67) and AgNOR morphology in endometrial adenocarcinomas of endometrioid type. Int J Gynecol Pathol 13:(1):37–44
7. Hoshino T, Ahn D, Prados MD, Lamborn K, Wilson CB (1993) Prognostic significance of the proliferative potential of intracranial gliomas measured by bromodeoxyuridine labeling. Int J Cancer 53:550–555
8. Hoshino T, Nagashima T, Cho KG, Murovic JA, Hodes JE, Wilson CB, Edwards MS, Pitts LH (1986) S-Phase fraction of human brain tumors in situ measured by uptake of bromodeoxyuridine. 38:369–374
9. Hoshino T, Nagashima T, Murovic JA, Wilson CB, Edwards MS, Gutin FH, Davis RL, DeArmond SJ (1986) In situ cell kinetic studies on human neuroectodermal tumors with bromodeoxyuridine labeling. J Neurosurg 64:453–459
10. Goz B (1978) Effects of incorporation of 5-halogenated deoxyuridines into the DNA of eukaryotic cells. Pharmacol Rev 29:249–272
11. Heartlein MW, O'Neill JP, Pal BC, Preston RJ (1982) The induction of specific locus mutations and sister-chromatid exchanges by 5-bromo- and 5-chlorodeoxyuridine. Mutat Res 92:441–446
12. San Sebastian J, O'Neill JP, Pal BC, Preston RJ (1980) The induction of chromosome aberrations, sister chromatid exchanges, and specific locus mutations in Chinese hamster ovary cells by 5-bromodeoxyuridine. Cytogenet Cell Genet 28:47–54
13. Gerdes J, Dallenbach F, Lennert K, Lemke H, Stein H (1984) Growth fraction in malignant non-Hodgkin's lymphomas (NHL) as determined in situ with the monoclonal antibody Ki-67. Hematol Oncol 2:365–371
14. Hall PA, Richards MA, Gregory WN, d'Ardenne AJ, Lister TA, Stanfield AG (1988) The prognostic value of Ki-67 immunostaining in non-Hodgkin's lymphoma. J Pathol 154:223–235
15. Gerdes J, Lelle RJ, Pickartz H, Heidenreich W, Schwarting R, Kurtsiefer L, Stauch G, Stein H (1986) Growth fractions in breast cancers determined in situ with monoclonal antibody Ki-67. J Clin Pathol 39:977–980
16. McGurrin JF, Doria MI, Dauson PJ, Karison T, Stein HO, Franklin WA (1987) Assessment of tumor cell kinetics by immunohistochemistry in carcinoma of breast. Cancer 59:1744–1750
17. Shepherd NA, Richman PI, England J (1988) Ki-67-derived proliferative activity in colorectal adenocarcinoma with prognostic correlations. J Pathol 155:213–219
18. Yonemura Y, Kimura H, Ooyama S, Kamata T, Yamaguchi A, Matsumoto H, Ninomiya I, Miyazaki I (1991) Immunocytochemical staining of proliferating cells in endoscopically biopsied tissues of gastric carcinomas with monoclonal antibody Ki-67. Oncology 48:162–165

19. Burger PC, Shibata T, Kleihues P (1986) The use of monoclonal antibody Ki-67 in the identification of proliferating cells; application to surgical pathology. Am J Surg Pathol 10:611–617

20. Giangaspero F, Dogllioni C, Rivano MT, Pileri S, Gerdes J, Stein H (1987) Growth fraction of human brain tumors defined by the monoclonal antibody Ki-67. Acta Neuropathol (Berl) 74:179–182

21. Morimura T, Kitz K, Budka H (1989) In situ analysis of cell kinetics in human brain tumors. A comparative immunocytochemical study of S-phase cells by the new in vitro bromodeoxyuridine-labeling technique and proliferating pool cells by monoclonal antibody Ki-67. Acta Neuropathol 77:276–282

22. Schroder R, Bien K, Kott R, Meyers I, Vossing R (1991) The relationship between Ki-67 labeling and mitotic index in glioblastoma and meningiomas: demonstration of the viability of the intermitotic cycle time. Acta Neuropathol 82:389–394

23. Zuber P, Hamou MF, de Tribolet N (1988) Identification of proliferating cells in human gliomas using the monoclonal antibody Ki-67. Neurosurgery (Baltimore) 22:364–368

24. Nagashima T, DeArmond SJ, Murovic J, Hoshino T (1985) Immunohistochemical demonstration of S-phase cells by anti-bromodeoxyuridine monoclonal antibody in human brain tumor tissues. Acta Neuropathol (Berl) 67:155–159

25. Nishizaki T, Orita T, Saiki M, Furutani Y, Aoki I (1988) Cell kinetic studies of human brain tumors by in vitro labeling using anti-BUdR monoclonal antibody. J Neurosurg 69:371–374

26. Patosouris E, Stocker U, Kallmeyer V, Keiditsch E, Mehraein P, Stavrou D (1988) Relationship between the Ki-67 positive cells, growth rate and histological type of human intracranial tumors. Anticancer Res 8:537–544

27. Raghavan R, Steart PV, Weller RO (1990) Cell proliferation patterns in the diagnosis of astrocytomas, anaplastic astrocytomas and glioblastoma multiforme: Ki-67 study. Neuropathol Appl Neurobiol 16:123–133

28. Yoshii Y, Maki Y, Tsuboi K, Tsumoto Y, Nakagawa K, Hoshino T (1986) Estimation of growth fraction with bromodeoxyuridine in human central nervous system tumors. J Neurosurg 65:659–663

29. Shibuya M, Ito S, Miwa T, Davis RL, Wilson CB, Hoshino T (1993) Proliferating potential of brain tumors. Analyses with Ki-67 and anti-DNA polymerase alpha monoclonal antibodies, bromodeoxyuridine labeling and nuclear organizer region antigen counts. Cancer 71:199–206

30. Hoshino T, Rodoriquez LA, Cho KG, Lee KS, Wilson CB, Edwards MS, Levin VA, Davis RL (1988) Prognostic implication of the proliferating potential of low grade astrocytomas. J Neurosurg 69:839–842

31. Tabuchi K, Honda C, Nakane P (1987) Demonstration of proliferating cell nuclear antigen (PCNA/cyclin) in glioma cells. Neurol Med Chir (Tokyo) 27:1–5

32. Shibui S, Hoshino T, Iwasaki K, Nomura K, Jastreboff MM (1989) Cell cycle phase dependent emergence of thymidylate syntheses studied by monoclonal antibody (M-TS-4). Cell Tissue Kinet 22:259–268

33. Mushima N, Miwa T, Suzuoki T, Hayashi K, Masaki S, Kaneda T (1988) Detection of proliferating cells in dysplasia, carcinoma in situ, and invasive carcinoma of the uterine cervix by monoclonal antibody against DNA polymerase alpha. Cancer 61:1182–1186

34. Gerdes J, Schwab U, Lemme H, Stein H (1983) Production of a mouse monoclonal antibody reactive with a human nuclear antigen associated with cell proliferation. Int J Cancer 31:13–20

35. Kajiwara K, Nishizaki T, Orita T, Nakayama H, Aoki H, Ito H (1990) Silver colloid staining technique for analysis of glioma malignancy. J Neurosurg 73:113–117

Part III
Molecular Neuro-Oncology and
Its Impact on the Clinical Management of
Brain Tumors

Part III
Molecular Neuro-Oncology and
the Clinical Mind to Research on
Brain Tumors

Section 1. Molecular Biology and Genetics

Molecular Analysis of Phosphorylated Tyrosine-Binding Proteins in the Transduction of Proliferation and Differentiation Signals

Kazuo Nagashima[1], Shinya Tanaka[1], Satoshi Ota[1], Hideki Hasegawa[1], and Michiyuki Matsuda[2]

Abstract. The human CRK protein consists of an SH2 region that binds to phosphotyrosine-containing peptides and an SH3 region which associates with cellular factors to modulate transformation. The microinjection of CRK protein induced neurite formation in PC12, a rat pheochromocytoma cell line. This activity was abolished by mutation of the CRK protein at either SH2 or SH3, and was suppressed by monoclonal antibodies against CRK SH2 or p21^{ras}. This set of observations suggests that both the SH2 and the SH3 domains of human CRK protein are required for neuronal differentiation of PC12 cells, and that they function upstream of Ras. In addition, from the search for proteins that bind to the SH3 domain of CRK and activate Ras, we identified a new guanine nucleotide-releasing protein which was designated C3G. The nucleotide sequence of the 4.1-kb C3G cDNA contains a 3.2-kb open reading frame that encodes a 121-kDa protein. The mRNAs of both the C3G and the CRK proteins are expressed ubiquitously in adult and fetal human tissues. The overall results of this investigation suggest that the complex of CRK and C3G may transduce signals from tyrosine kinases to Ras in a number of different tissues.

Key words. Tyrosine phosphorylation—SH2 and SH3—Far Western blot—CRK and C3G—Ras

Introduction

Recent investigations have demonstrated a close relationship between the development, differentiation, and proliferation of brain tumors and oncogenes [1,2]. Oncogenes are usually activated by point mutation, amplification, rearrangement, or translocation, with gene amplification being the most frequent cause of activation in gliomas [3]. The activated oncogenes thus far identified in brain tumors are listed in Table 1 [2]. They include epidermal growth factor (EGF) receptor, c-erbB-2, platelet-derived growth factor (PDGF) receptors, PDGFs, *ros*1, *ras*, *src*, *raf*, *gli*, *fos*, and *myc*. The products of many of these oncogenes have enhanced tyrosine kinase activity (Table 1). Because cell-transforming activity has been related to activated tyrosine kinases [4], the study of signal propagation pathways from activated tyrosines to the

[1] Department of Pathology, Hokkaido University School of Medicine, Kita-ku, Sapporo 060, Japan
[2] Department of Pathology, National Institute of Health, Shinjuku-ku, Tokyo 162, Japan

Table 1. Oncogenes in brain tumors.[a]

Oncogene	MW (×10³)	Domain	Chromosome	Function	Brain tumors
src	60	Tyrosine kinase	20q11.2-q13	Development	Glioblastoma
H-*ras*	21	GTPase	11p15.5	Signaling	Glioblastoma
c-*myc*	64, 67	DNA binding	8q24	Embryogenesis	Medulloblastoma
N-*myc*	60, 63	DNA binding	2p23-24		Astrocytoma
EGFR (erbB-1)	170	Tyrosine kinase	7p13-12	EGFR	Glioblastoma
c-*erbB-2/neu*	185	Tyrosine kinase	17q21	EGFR homolog	Astrocytoma Glioblastoma
PDGFRα	180	Tyrosine kinase	4q11-q12	PDGF binding	Glioma
PDGFRβ	180	Tyrosine kinase	5q31-q32	PDGF binding	Glioma
PDGF-A	16	—	7pter-p21	PDGFR ligand	Glioma
PDGF-B (sis)	14	—	22q12.3-q12.1	PDGFR ligand	Glioma
*ros*1	259	Tyrosine kinase	6q22	Differentiation	Glioblastoma
raf/mil	74	Serine-threonine kinase	3p25	Serine-threonine kinase	Glioblastoma
gli	118	Zinc finger	12q13	Transcription	Glioblastoma
fos	62	Zinc finger	14q21-q31	Proliferation	Pituitary adenoma

EGF, epidermal growth factor; R, receptor; PDGF, platelet-derived growth factor.
[a] Modified from Tabuchi [2].

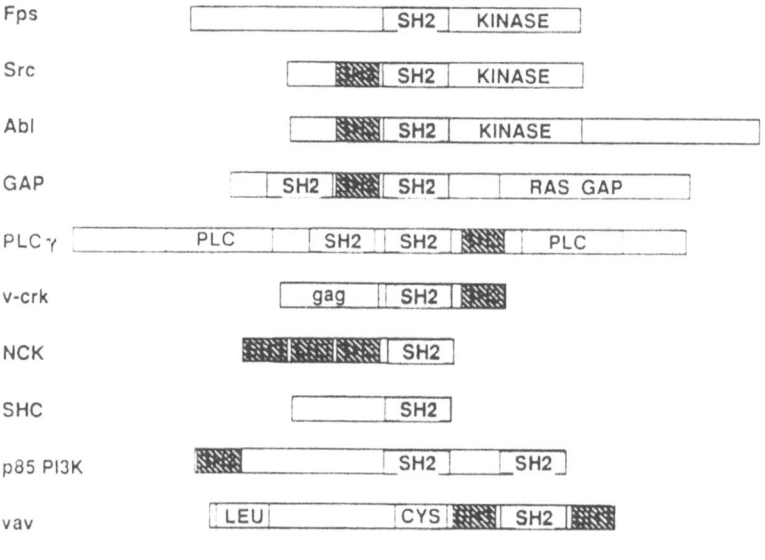

Fig. 1. The oncogenes *fps*, *src*, and *abl* contain a tyrosine kinase domain and an SH2 or SH3 domain. GTPase activating protein (*GAP*) and phospholipase Cγ (*PLC*γ) have enzymatic domains. By contrast, v-CRK, NCK, and SHC consist mostly of SH2 and SH3 domains and are therefore called adaptor molecules

nucleus and the cell cycle can provide important data toward understanding the mechanisms involved in transformation and differentiation.

Several cytoplasmic signaling proteins have two distinct Src homology (SH) regions essential for binding to phosphotyrosine-containing proteins. The SH2 domain recognizes such proteins and regulates protein–protein interactions, and the SH3 domain modulates further signal transduction [5,6]. The SH2- and SH3-containing proteins are divided into two categories: those with catalytic domains and those consisting mostly of SH2 and SH3 domains (Fig. 1). The v-CRK protein, originally identified as the oncoprotein of a chicken retrovirus, is an example of an adaptor molecule that consists mostly of SH2 and SH3 domains [7].

In this chapter we present the results of examining the functions of the SH2 and SH3 domains of the human CRK protein using cultures of PC12 cells. This cell line, derived from a rat pheochromocytoma, has been extensively employed to study signal transduction by growth factors [8]. We further provide the details pertaining to the isolation and characterization of the cDNA that encodes a specific CRK SH3-binding protein.

Materials and Methods

In our cell culture technique, PC12 cells were grown at 37°C in a humidified atmosphere of 5% CO_2 in air; 35-mm culture dishes precoated with 10 μg/ml of poly-D-lysine and Dulbecco's modified Eagle's minimum essential medium supplemented with 10% heat-inactivated fetal bovine serum and 5% horse serum were used throughout.

An anti-CRK (SH2) mouse monoclonal antibody (mAb), AD2, was produced as previously described [9]. This mAb blocks the binding of SH2 to phosphotyrosine-containing proteins. We also used the commercial anti-p21^{ras} rat mAb Y13-259 [10] and a mouse mAb to glutathione S-transferase (GST), provided by Dr. Yoichi Tachibana.

Two alternatively spliced cDNAs of the CRK gene, CRK-I and CRK-II, were used [11]. pGEX-CRK-I and pGEX-CRK-II, derived from pGEX2T [12] and containing the CRK-I and CRK-II coding regions downstream of the GST gene, were used to generate fusion proteins. The expression plasmids for mutant CRK proteins were constructed by a combination of restriction enzyme cleavage, fragment preparation, and ligation, together with site-directed mutagenesis [13]. All mutated proteins were expressed as GST fusion proteins.

Microinjection was carried out with an automated injection system (Zeiss, Jena, Germany), by means of which PC12 cells were injected with 0.5 pl of a given protein solution following the previously described protocol [14]. The cells were fixed 24 h after microinjection and probed with the anti-GST mAb. GST-positive cells were considered as successfully injected, and PC12 cells whose extended neurites were longer than the diameter of the cell body were counted as differentiated cells.

Cells were fixed for 15 min at 37°C with 4% paraformaldehyde in (PBS) phosphate buffered saline, permeabilized with 0.2% Triton X-100 (Nacalai Tesque, Kyoto, Japan) in PBS, probed with mAbs, and incubated with fluorescein isothiocynate-(FITC) conjugated anti-mouse IgG. The cells thus treated were examined by fluorescence-activated or confocal microscopy (Bio-Rad, Hercules, CA, USA).

Probes used for Far Western blotting were peptides containing the SH3 domain of the CRK-I expressed in *Escherichia coli* as fusion proteins of GST and purified on a glutathione-Sepharose 4B column (Pharmacia, Uppsala, Sweden).

A λgt11 cDNA expression library constructed from mRNA of human spleen cells was obtained from Clontech (Palo Alto, CA, USA). Recombinant clones expressing SH3-binding proteins were identified by Far Western blotting using GST-CRK-SH3 and anti-GST mAb [13].

A temperature-sensitive *cdc25* mutant of the yeast *Saccharomyces cerevisiae* was used for genetic manipulations. The yeast shuttle vector pKT10 was ligated with the 3'-region of the C3G gene to generate pKC3GPv (nt 1982–3393) and pKC3GHc (nt 2452–3393). The expression vectors pKT10 and YRp7 were used as negative controls, and pL25/SP, which is a YRp7 derivative containing the wild-type CDC25 gene, as a positive control

Filters blotted with mRNAs from adult and fetal human tissues (Clontech) were incubated at 42°C with ^{32}P-labeled probes. The bound probes were analyzed with the FUJIX radioanalytic imaging system (Fuji, Tokyo, Japan).

Results

When the CRK-I protein, expressed in *E. coli* as a GST fusion protein, was microinjected into PC12 cells induction of neurite outgrowth was evident within 16h. Verification that these cells did indeed contain the CRK-I protein was obtained by immunocytochemical examination with the anti-GST mAb. These tests revealed that all cells with neurite outgrowth were positively stained (Fig. 2). The microinjection

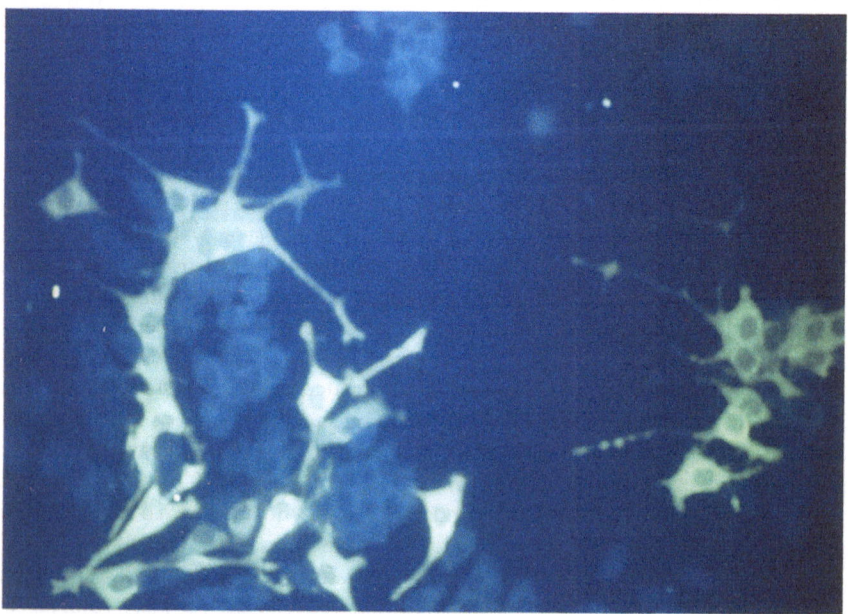

Fig. 2. Immunostaining of PC12 cells microinjected with the CRK-I protein expressed as a glutathione S-transferase (GST) fusion protein. The cells showing neurite outgrowth were positively stained by the anti-GST monoclonal antibody (mAb), thus demonstrating that CRK-I promotes neuronal differentiation of PC12 cells. Note that round cells lacking neurite outgrowth were not stained by the mAb to GST fluorescein isothiocynate (FITC) technique, ×400

experiments were repeated 17 times, and the data obtained showed that an average of 51% ± 15% of cells injected with CRK-I had undergone neuronal differentiation.

To define the region required for the CRK-mediated neuronal differentiation, we microinjected PC12 cells with a series of mutated CRK proteins (Fig. 3). We found that the CRK-II protein, a product of alternative splicing that has an extra SH3 at the carboxyl terminus of CRK-I, also induced neurite outgrowth. By contrast, a deletion or a point mutation in SH2 [SH3(N), SH3(C), PST, V38], which abolished binding to phosphotyrosine-containing proteins, prevented these proteins from inducing neurite outgrowth in PC12 cells. Moreover, deletions or three of five amino acid substitutions in SH3(N) [SH2, KPN, SAL, BGL, K150, TQ, L169] impaired the ability of

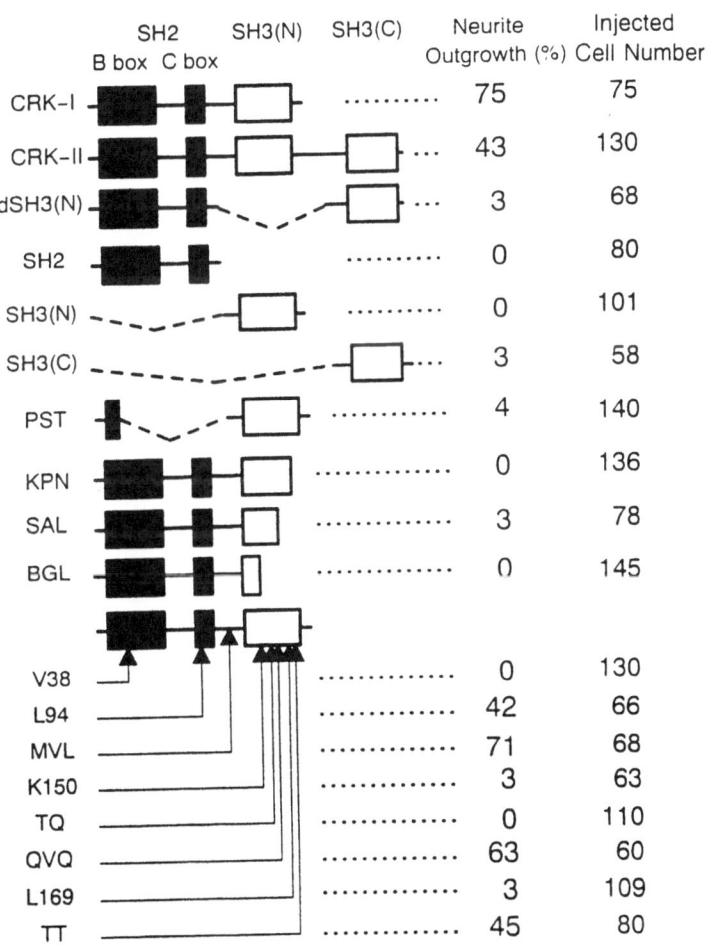

Fig. 3. Schematic structure of the CRK proteins and their respective efficacy in inducing neuronal differentiation of PC12 cells [13]. The *filled boxes* represent the B and C boxes of SH2; the *open boxes* represent the amino terminal [SH3(N)] and the carboxyl terminal [SH3(C)] portions of SH3. CRK-I and CRK-II are wild types. SH3(N), SH3(C), and PST are deletion forms. KPN, SAL, and BGL are partial deletions of SH3. V38 to TT have amino acid substitutions in SH2 or SH3. The percentage of successfully injected cells with neurite outgrowths and the total number of injected cells are indicated for each protein

CRK-I to induce neuronal differentiation. These results documented that both SH2 and SH3(N) are required for neurite outgrowth. On the other hand, L94, MVL, QVQ, and TT were efficient inducers of neurite outgrowth, suggesting that the amino acids substituted in these mutant proteins were not directly involved in CRK-induced neuronal differentiation.

To obtain the cDNA of the CRK SH3-binding proteins, Far Western blotting was performed using bacterially expressed SH3 peptides fused with GST in combination with the anti-GST mAb. We screened 1.5×10^6 plaque-forming units (pfu) from a human spleen λgt11 library and identified four positive plaques. We selected two clones that contained overlapping fragments and isolated and sequenced the full-length cDNA. The nucleotide sequence obtained consisted of 4070 bp and contained a 3231-bp open reading frame encoding 1077 amino acids (Fig. 4A). As the protein had a region homologous to a guanine nucleotide-releasing protein (GNRP) for Ras, we designated this protein as C3G, for CRK SH3-binding GNRP. The predicted molecular mass of C3G is 121 kDa.

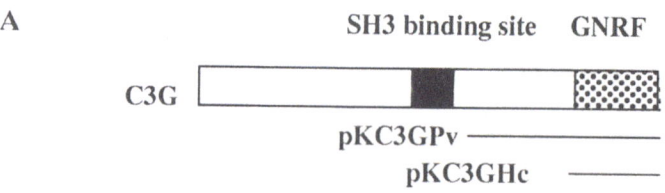

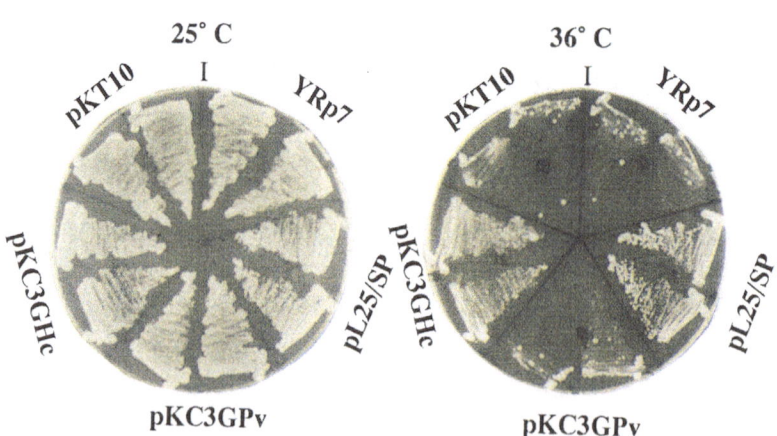

Fig. 4. **A** Structure of C3G and schematic representation of the C3G expression vectors used in the experiments. The *black box* represents the SH3 binding site; the *dotted box* is the guanine nucleotide-releasing factor (*GNRF*) function domain. **B** Temperature-dependent growth of the *cdc25* *Saccharomyces cervisiae* strain was examined after transformation with the plasmids indicated in A. Transformants of pKT10 and YRp7 grew at 25°C but failed to grow at 36°C. pL25/SP, a plasmid containing the wild-type CDC25 gene, was used as positive control, and its transformants grew at 36°C. The pKC3GHc (the truncated form of C3G) transformants grew at 36°C, thus demonstrating the substitution of the CDC25 (GNRF) function in yeast [23]

To assess the function of C3G, we examined whether the 3' region of C3G can complement the loss of CDC25, a Ras-GNRP of *S. cerevisiae*. The KMY172-5A strain of *S. cerevisiae*, which contains temperature-sensitive *cdc25*, was transformed with expression vectors containing either pKC3GHc or pKC3GPv. The pKC3GHc transformant grew at 36°C, as did cells transformed by pL25/SP, a YRp7-derived plasmid that contained the wild-type CDC25 gene (Fig. 4B). By contrast, cells transformed by pKC3GPv or by expression vectors YRp7 and pKT10 could not grow at 36°C. These results demonstrate that the C3G gene can complement the loss of CDC25 function in *S. cervisiae*, and that appropriate truncation of the C3G gene may be necessary for this activity.

By Northern blotting for which C3G cDNA served as probe, we detected a transcript of approximately 7.5 kb in all human tissues examined. Adult skeletal muscles, placentae, fetal brain, and heart contained large amounts of C3G mRNA, whereas livers of adults and fetuses contained lesser amounts. The distribution of the C3G mRNA was very similar to that of the 4.8-kb CRK mRNA.

Discussion

The CRK protein belongs to a new class of proteins that play an important role in signal transduction from tyrosine kinases. These proteins, CRK, and GRB2/ASH/Sem-5 consist mostly of SH2 and SH3 domains [15–17]. Of these, human GRB2 promotes cell growth with overexpression of the H-Ras protein [16], while antisense RNA of mouse ASH inhibits cell replication [17]. Our results demonstrate that the CRK protein also transduces signals by activating p21^{ras}, thus documenting that this group of proteins have the common property of activating proteins of the Ras family, considered as switch devices for signal transduction.

There is consensus that in vitro binding of SH2 to phosphotyrosine-containing proteins reflects an essential in vivo function [18]. Thus, the microinjection of neutralizing anti-CRK (SH2) mAb has provided direct evidence that the SH2-mediated protein–protein interaction is an indispensable in vivo function of SH2. Because mutations in the SH3 domain of CRK abolished the signal for neurite formation through activation of p21^{ras}, it is conceivable that this protein domain may bind cytoplasmic proteins so as to transmit the signal to activated Ras.

Moreover, by screening an expression library with the SH3 peptides of CRK, we did isolate the cDNA of the protein designated C3G, which represents an additional member of the GNRPs. It should be indicated in this context that CDC25 [19] and SCD25 [20] of yeast, CDC25^{Mm} of rats, mice, and humans [21], and SOS of *Drosophila* [22] have been proven to be Ras GNRFs. Since the amino acid sequence of the C3G protein is strikingly similar to those of Ras GNRPs and because this protein complements the loss of CDC25 function in yeast, it is conceivable that C3G could be a GNRF for Ras protein [23].

Conclusions

CRK protein belongs to the adaptor-type Src homology (SH), SH2- and SH3-containing molecules that transduce signals from tyrosine kinases. A novel Ras guanine nucleotide-releasing protein, C3G, was identified as a CRK SH3-binding protein. The possibility that the complex of CRK and C3G may transduce signals from tyrosine kinases to Ras is postulated.

References

1. Batra SK, Ahmed Rasheed BK, Bigner SH, Bigner DD (1994) Biology of disease. Oncogenes and anti-oncogenes in human central nervous system tumors. Lab Invest 71:621–637
2. Tabuchi K (1994) Cytogenetic diagnosis and gene therapy of brain tumor: its current status and future prospect (in Japanese). Jpn J Cancer Clin 40:1031–1042
3. Hurtt MR, Moossy J, Donovan-Peluso M, Locker L (1992) Amplification of epidermal growth factor receptor gene in gliomas: histopathology and prognosis. J Neuropathol & Exp Neurol 51:84–90
4. Yamazaki H, Fukui Y, Ueyama Y, Tamaoki N, Kawamoto T, Taniguchi S, Shibuya M (1988) Amplification of the structurally and functionally altered epidermal growth factor receptor gene (c-erbB) in human brain tumors. Mol Cell Biol 8:1816–1820
5. Pawson T, Gish GD (1992) SH2 and SH3 domains: from structure to function. Cell 71:359–362
6. Mayer BJ, Baltimore D (1993) Signaling through SH2 and SH3 domains. Trends Cell Biol 3:8–13
7. Pawson T (1988) Non-catalytic domains of cytoplasmic protein-tyrosine kinases; regulatory elements in signal transduction. Oncogene Res 3:491–495
8. Greene LA, Tischler AS (1976) Establishment of a nonadrenergic clonal line of rat adrenal pheochromocytoma cells which respond to nerve growth factor. Proc Natl Acad Sci USA 73:2424–2428
9. Matsuda M, Nagata S, Tanaka S, Nagashima K, Kurata T (1993) Structural requirement of the CRK SH2 region for the binding to phosphotyrosine-containing proteins; evidence by the reactivity to monoclonal antibodies. J Biol Chem 268:4441–4446
10. Smith MR, DeGudicibus SJ, Stacey DW (1986) Requirement for c-ras proteins during viral oncogene transformation. Nature 320:540–543
11. Matsuda M, Tanaka S, Nagata S, Kojima A, Kurata T, Shibuya M (1992) Two species of human CRK cDNA encode proteins with distinct biological activites. Mol Cell Biol 12:3482–3489
12. Smith DB, Johnson KS (1988) Single-step purification of polypeptides expressed in *Escherichia coli* as fusions with glutathione S-transferase. Gene 67:31–40
13. Tanaka S, Hattori S, Kurata T, Nagashima K, Fukui Y, Nakamura S, Matsuda M (1993) Both the SH2 and SH3 domains of human CRK protein are required for neuronal differentiation of PC12 cells. Mol Cell Biol 13:4409–4415
14. Ansorge W, Pepperkok R (1988) Performance of an automated system for capillary microinjection into living cells. J Biochem Biophys Methods 16:283–292
15. Clark SG, Stern MJ, Horvitz HR (1992) *C. elegans* cell-signaling gene *sem*-5 encodes a protein with SH2 and SH3 domains. Nature 356:340–344
16. Lowenstein EJ, Daly RJ, Batzer AG, Li W, Margolis B, Lammers R, Ullrich A, Skolnik EY, Barsagi D, Schlessinger J (1992) The SH2 and SH3 domain-containing protein GRB2 links receptor tyrosine kinases to Ras signaling. Cell 70:431–442
17. Matsuoka K, Shibata M, Yamakawa A, Takenawa T (1992) Cloning of ASH, a ubiquitous protein composed of one Src homology region (SH)-2 and 2 SH3 domains, from human and rat cDNA libraries. Proc Natl Acad Sci USA 89:9015–9019
18. Koch CA, Anderson D, Moran MF, Ellis C, Pawson T (1991) SH2 and SH3 domains: elements that control interactions of cytoplasmic signaling proteins. Science 252:668–674
19. Jones S, Vignais ML, Broach JR (1991) The CDC25 protein of *Saccharomyces cerevisiae* promotes exchange of guanine nucleotides bound to *ras*. Mol Cell Biol 11:2641–2646
20. Crechet J-B, Poullet P, Mistou M-Y, Parmeggiani A, Camonis J, Boy-Marcotte E, Damak F, Jacquet M (1990) Enhancement of the GDP-GTP exchange of RAS proteins by the carboxyl-terminal domain of SCD25. Science 248:866–868
21. Feig LA (1993) The many roads that lead to Ras. Science 260:767–768

22. Bonfini L, Karlovick CA, Dasgupta C, Banerjee U (1993) The *son of sevenless* gene product: a putative activator of Ras. Science 255:603–606
23. Tanaka S, Morishita T, Hashimoto Y, Hattori S, Nakamura S, Shibuya M, Matsuoka K, Takenawa T, Kurata T, Nagashima K, Matsuda M (1994) C3G, a guanine nucleotide-releasing protein expressed ubiquitously, binds to the Src homology 3 domains of CRK and GRB2/ASH proteins. Proc Natl Acad Sci USA 91:3443–3447

Gene Alterations in Glial Tumors

C. David James

Abstract. The occurrence and stepwise accumulation of mutations are thought to both cause and chronicle the malignant progression of cancer. Evidence in support of this interpretation of tumor evolution has come from numerous investigations demonstrating that increasing tumor histopathological malignancy is associated with increasing numbers of detectable mutations. One group of tumors for which this relationship is evident are the gliomas, among which frequent losses of genetic information from chromosomes 17p, 9p, and 10, and amplification of the epidermal growth factor receptor gene, have been noted. It is now clear that these and additional alterations accumulate as gliomas become more malignant. Specific gene targets have been identified for some of the glioma-associated chromosomal alterations, including the genes that encode the p53 (17p) and p16 (9p) proteins. The identification of these mutations provides a starting point from which to investigate growth-regulatory pathways whose perturbations underlie glial tumor development. It is anticipated that information obtained from such investigations will contribute important concepts for the development of directed, effective, and rational therapies for the treatment of a cancer that is currently fatal in nearly all instances.

Key words. Oncogenes—Tumor suppressor genes—Amplification—Deletion—Malignancy

Introduction

Less than 7 years ago, our knowledge of glioma genetics was for the most part limited to information detailing the numerous karyotypic abnormalities that are apparent in cell cultures from these tumors. During the latter portion of the past decade, several groups of investigators determined that abnormal ploidy of chromosomes 7 and 10, as well as structural alterations of several chromosomes, particularly 9p and 19p, were common to these tumors [1–3]. The information gathered from these studies, especially with respect to chromosomal deletions, has provided a springboard from which to launch molecular genetic investigations directed at the localization and identification of genes whose alterations are known to be critical for tumor development.

Department of Neurosurgery, Emory University School of Medicine, 1327 Clifton Rd., N.E., Atlanta, GA 30322, USA

From such investigations it now seems reasonably certain that several specific gene alterations occur during the evolution of malignancy in glioma. Various models have been advanced to explain the multistep nature of glial tumor genetics [4–7], the underlying conceptual basis for which was established in a report by Nowell [8] (Fig. 1).

Explained in the context of Nowell's model, the sequence of events involved in the malignant progression of a tumor is initiated by a mutation (T_1) in an affected cell that confers a growth advantage and promotes the cell's clonal expansion. Subsequent to this mutation, cells of the initial variant clone acquire additional growth-advantageous alterations (T_2–T_6) that give rise to more aggressive (malignant) subclones. Evidence in support of this model stems from the results of studies in which like tumors (e.g., gliomas) of varying histological malignancy have been examined for cumulative genetic alterations. Such studies have revealed a correlation between increasing tumor alterations and increasing malignancy in several types of cancer [9–11].

The perspective offered by this model has been helpful in interpreting data from the molecular genetic analysis of the most common of central nervous system neoplasms, the gliomas. For the purpose of this review, the molecular genetic events associated with the malignant progression of such tumors will be considered as involving either the inactivation of gene products that normally suppress cell growth (tumor suppressor genes, TSGs) or the activation of gene products that promote cell growth (oncogenes).

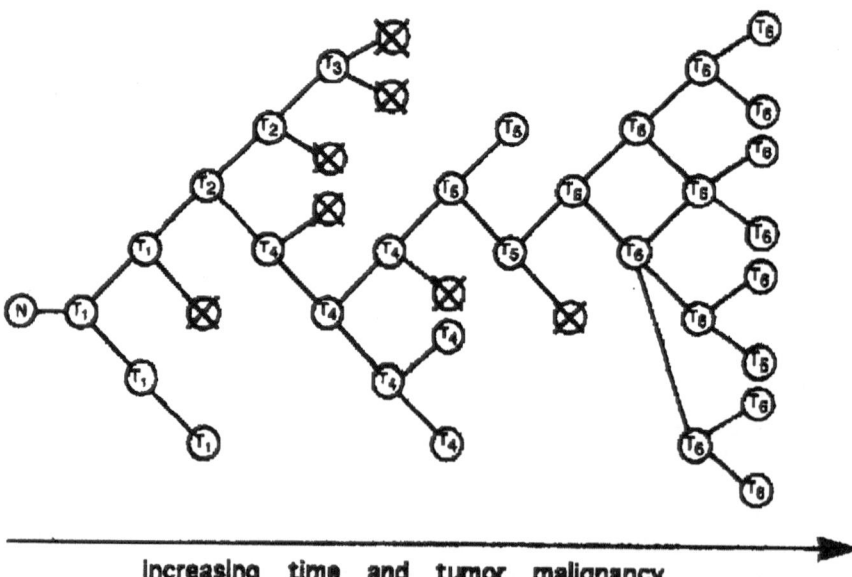

Increasing time and tumor malignancy

Fig. 1. Cellular model for tumor progression. The composition and malignancy of a solid tumor depends on the time elapsed since occurrence of the initiating mutation and the cumulative growth advantage conferred by various combinations of mutations. Lethal mutations are indicated by cells that have been *crossed out*. (From [8], with permission)

Localization and Accumulation of TSG Alterations in Glial Tumors

The localization or identification of genes whose products have a negative growth-regulatory function has been accomplished through two approaches, both of which rely on restriction fragment length polymorphisms (RELPs). One of these approaches involves the localization of TSGs through the linkage analysis of families with hereditary tumor syndromes [12]. In such families, the segregation pattern of parental alleles is followed in a kindred, and the linkage (chromosomal proximity) of a marker with a cancer-predisposing TSG is established by the consistent cosegregation of an allele with the disease phenotype. In the case of gliomas, few families have been identified as having a glial tumor syndrome, and to date there are no reports involving their study by linkage analysis. There are, however, several syndromes in which there is an elevated incidence of glioma, and consequently glial tumors are considered as part of their constellation of disease manifestation. Such syndromes include neurofibromatosis type 1, type 2, and Li-Fraumeni. For these, the application of linkage analysis has been of fundamental importance to the identifcation of corresponding TSGs [13–15].

The other application of RFLPs toward the localization of TSGs is referred to as deletion mapping. A chromosomal deletion map is obtained through the application of loss of heterozygosity (LOH) analysis in which restriction fragment patterns are compared in a patient's normal DNA (obtained from peripheral white blood cells) and tumor DNAs. Loss of a restriction fragment length allele in a tumor DNA sample is indicative of a TSG that has been inactivated through deletion [12]. By applying a battery of mapped probes (markers) from a chromosome of interest, one can limit the chromosome location of a TSG by determining the smallest common region of deletion among a panel of similar tumors (Fig. 2). This type of analysis has been applied extensively to gliomas and has revealed several associations between detectable alterations and tumor histopathology.

Perhaps the most striking of these has been the loss of genetic information from chromosome 10 and its association with glioblastoma; such a loss has consistently been shown in 50%–90% of glioblastomas examined in several independent studies [9,16–19]. LOH on chromosome 10 occurs much less frequently in glial tumors of

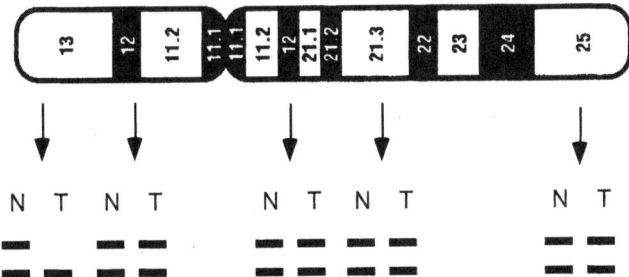

Fig. 2. Hypothetical results associated with the deletion mapping analysis for markers (chromosomal locations indicated by *arrows*) on chromosome 17. In this example, the tumor DNA loss of heterozygosity demonstrated by the marker in 17p13 in combination with maintenance of tumor DNA heterozygosity by all other markers suggests the existence of a tumor suppressor gene distal (p-terminus direction) to the marker in 17p12. *N*, normal DNA; *T*, tumor DNA

intermediate (anaplastic) malignancy, and no losses of heterozygosity on chromosome 10 have been reported in low malignancy grade gliomas. In the context of Nowell's model (see Fig. 1), the loss of genetic information from chromosome 10 appears to be a late event in the malignant progression of glioma.

LOH analysis of chromosome 9 has revealed the frequent loss of one (hemizygous deletion) or both (homozygous deletion) copies of markers localized to the region 9p21–22 [20,21]. Significantly, hemizygous deletions are most frequently seen in the anaplastic tumors whereas homozygous deletions have been primarily observed in the glioblastomas. Such data suggest the occurrence of discrete 9p deletion events in association with glial tumor attainment of intermediate and high-grade malignancy.

As opposed to the consistent occurrence of chromosome 10 LOH in glioblastomas, losses of genetic information from chromosomes 17p, 19q, and 22q occur at similar frequencies in all malignancy grades of glioma, suggesting these alterations may be early events in glial tumorigenesis. Interestingly, each of these alterations displays a preferential association with gliomas of specific cellular differentiation: 17p loss with astrocytomas [22–24], 19q loss with tumors of oligodendroglial composition [25–27], and 22q loss with tumors showing ependymal differentiation [25,28]. Although these observations suggest differences between the primary TSG inactivation events that occur in different types of glioma, it is interesting to note that the more malignant forms of oligodendroglioma and astrocytoma show frequent loss of genetic information from 9p and chromosome 10. Taken together, such data suggest distinct early genetic events of glial tumorigenesis with respect to tumor cellular differentiation, and that the pathways of glioma genetic evolution converge during tumor progression.

Current Status Regarding TSG Identifications

The molecular genetic studies conducted thus far indicate that a minimum of five tumor suppressor gene inactivation events are of significance to the development of glial tumors. The LOH on chromosome 10 is perhaps the most important of these because of its specific association with and frequency of loss in tumors of highest histopathological malignancy. Data from a few studies indicate the existence of a TSG on the distal portion of the chromosome's long arm [19,29]. Currently, its location is not well resolved, and there are data suggesting the existence of additional TSGs residing in distinct regions of this chromosome [16,30]. No candidate genes have yet to be advanced as potential targets of these deletions.

As noted, allelic deletions on chromosome 19q are frequent in tumors with oligodendroglial composition, and such deletions occur at similar frequencies in oligodendrogliomas of low and intermediate malignancy grade [27]. Loss of genetic information from 19q has also been demonstrated in a significant proportion of oligoastrocytomas, anaplastic astrocytomas, and glioblastomas. Although deletion mapping has been useful toward limiting the location of the implied TSG, no candidate genes have been advanced as targets of associated LOH.

The locus targeted for LOH on chromosome 22 in gliomas, especially ependymomas, may involve the gene whose alteration predisposes to NF2 [31]. Although this possibility has yet to be addressed in detail, a recent study in which the inactivation of both NF2 genes was shown in a sporadic (non-NF2) ependymoma supports this hypothesis [32].

In contrast to the analysis of LOH on chromosomes 10 and 19, which have localized but thus far failed to identify respective target genes, deletion mapping of chromosomes 9p and 17p has met with considerable success. For 9p, alterations that result in loss of genetic information have been reported in many cancers. The first indication as to which genes were involved in these alterations was provided by the analysis of leukemias [33,34] in which homozygous deletions of the class I interferon (IFN) gene cluster were demonstrated. Homozygous deletions of the 9p-localized IFNs have subsequently been shown in bladder cancer [35], small cell lung carcinoma [36], and melanoma [37] as well as glioma [20,38]. However, as efforts were directed at determining whether the IFN loci defined the critical region of 9p deletion, it became apparent that not all deletions included the IFN genes and that a common region of loss residing centromere-proximal to the IFN gene cluster was shared by various neoplasms [39,40]. Approximately 6 months before this conference, two groups simultaneously published the localization of a candidate tumor suppressor gene, *p16*, to the common region of deletion [41,42]. High frequencies of *p16* gene homozygous deletion in various types of tumor cell lines suggests that inactivation of *p16* function is important to the development of many forms of cancer.

The most extensively studied of the LOH events in glial tumors are the chromosome 17p deletions; such loss is most commonly seen in tumors of astrocytic differentiation. The majority of 17p deletions are thought to be targeted at the *p53* gene [43–45]. As is the case with chromosome 9p, 17p alterations have been reported in numerous cancers, and astrocytomas were initially investigated for *p53* mutations [46] on the basis of a correlation first determined in colorectal tumors: p53 mutations are frequently associated with loss of heterozygosity of sequences from the distal portion of 17p where the *p53* gene is located. Loss of genetic information from 17p and p53 mutations have been reported in all malignancy grades of astrocytoma and as such are thought to represent an early event in astrocytoma development [45]. In addition to mutation frequency, other evidence that favors the involvement of *p53* mutations in CNS neoplasia stems from the demonstration of glioblastoma cell growth suppression by introduction and expression of an exogenous wild-type (normal) *p53* gene [47]. With regard to familial cancer, predisposition to tumor development in Li-Fraumeni sydrome has been shown to be associated with inherited *p53* mutations [15].

Oncogene Activation in Gliomas

Amplification of the epidermal growth factor receptor (EGFR) gene represents the most common oncogene activation in gliomas and has been reported by several investigatory groups [48–51]. The frequency of amplification cited among glial tumors of highest histopathological malignancy has consistently been 40%–50% of examined cases. The frequency of EGFR amplification in glial tumors of intermediate or anaplastic malignancy is less clearly known, partly because fewer such tumors have been analyzed. In total, frequencies between 10% and 30% have been reported. Few instances of EGFR amplification have been reported in low-grade glial tumors. Therefore, the amplification of EGFR is associated with increasing glial tumor malignancy.

Recent analysis of amplified EGFR genes in malignant gliomas has revealed additional factors associated with this genetic alteration. At least two regions of the EGFR gene have been shown to undergo alteration in glioblastomas with gene amplification

[52–54]. One type of alteration is particularly frequent, occurring in as many as half the tumors with EGFR gene amplification [52,53]. We recently determined that the protein encoded by this altered EGFR gene is a constitutively activated tyrosine kinase that promotes cell proliferation [55], and others have shown that its expression enhances glioblastoma cell tumorigenicity [56]. It is currently unclear whether this mutant receptor participates in signal transduction in a manner similar to that of activated wild-type receptor, or whether it acts to promote cell proliferation through novel intracellular molecular interactions.

By demonstration of the presence of double-minute (DM) particles in glioma cell cultures, cytogenetic analysis provided the first evidence supporting the possibility of frequent gene amplification in glial tumors. EGFR amplification is usually, but not always, associated with the presence of tumor DMs [57]. It has been determined that the cyclin-dependent kinase (CDK4) or MDM2 genes are amplified in nearly 15% of malignant gliomas [58]; the relationship between their amplification and presence of tumor DM particles is currently unknown. The functions of cdk4 and mdm2 proteins are discussed in the next section.

Interrelationships Between Gene Alterations and Growth-Regulatory Pathways

The models that have been useful for describing the occurrence and accumulation of gene alterations in gliomas unfortunately offer little information concerning the molecular mechanisms of glial tumorigenesis. In fact, it appeared until recently that the identification of glioma gene alterations was merely producing a detailed catalog of seemingly disparate events. This has changed, however, as it is becoming increasingly apparent that alternative genetic mechanisms exist for the disruption of a few, key regulatory systems which govern the growth rate of cells.

p16-cdk4-pRb-Cyclin D System

The p16 protein, for which the gene on chromosome 9p is frequently deleted, is thought to exert a negative type of control over cell proliferation through its binding to cyclin-dependent kinase (cdk) 4 and preventing its forming an active complex with cyclin D proteins [59] (Fig. 3). It has been proposed that sufficiently high concentrations of cyclin D–cdk4 complex could result in the functional inactivation of retinoblastoma protein (pRb, a substrate of activated cdk4) [60], and thereby promote transit through the G_1 phase of the cell cycle [59]. Consequently, the relative abundance of D-type cyclins and p16 could regulate the cumulative intracellular activity of cdk4 kinase and therefore determine whether a cell is in a quiescent or proliferative state. The information that has emerged regarding interactions between p16, pRb, cyclin D, and cdk4 provides many opportunities to investigate tumor cell mechanisms that disrupt the growth-regulatory system constituted by these proteins. For instance, a relationship has been described between the expression of pRb and cyclin D1 in tumors [61] and tumor cell lines [61,62], which indicates that pRb cell growth inhibition can be abrogated either through loss of RB gene expression or by increased expression of the cyclin D1 gene.

We have shown that CDK4 amplification occurs as an alternative mechanism to *p16* gene homozygous deletion in glial tumors and cell lines [63]. These reports [61–63]

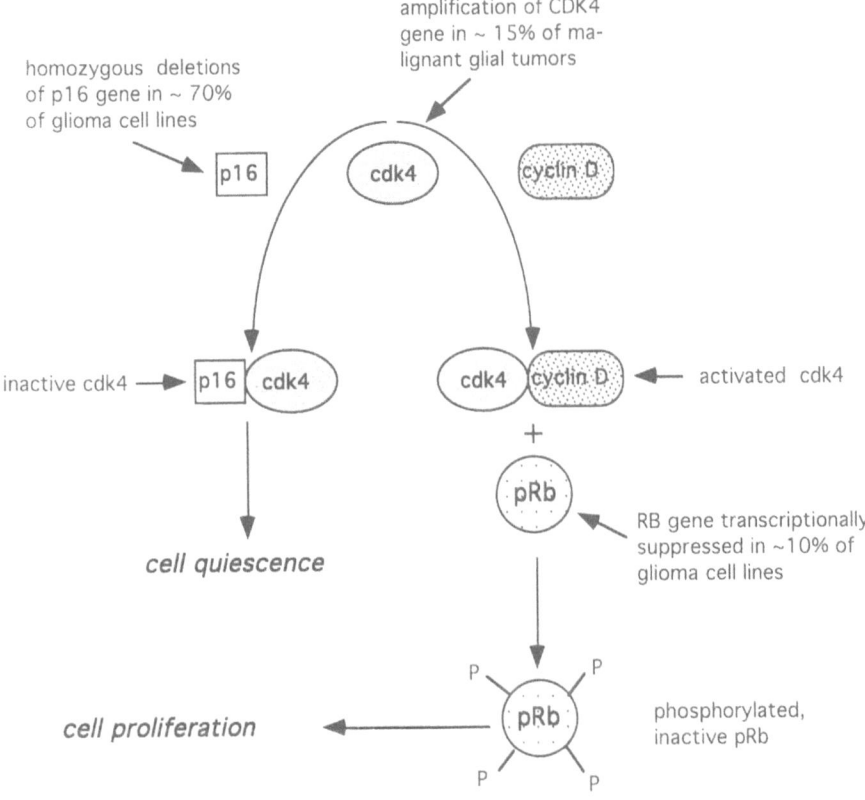

Fig. 3. Model of control of cell proliferation through regulation of cdk4 activity

are among a rapidly growing body of literature that suggests that pRb inactivation is essential to tumor development and that such inactivation can occur through a variety of mechanisms. For gliomas, RB gene deletions and alterations have been shown in only a few tumors [64], and RB transcriptional suppression has been shown in some malignant glioma cell lines [65]. Abrogation of pRb function in gliomas does not, however, appear to generally involve mechanisms that completely suppress pRb synthesis. The combined frequency of *p16* gene homozygous deletion and CDK4 amplification in these tumors suggest, however, that pRb functional inactivation is important to the development of most gliomas.

p53-MDM2-p12-Cyclin-cdk System

Since the association between inactivating mutations of *p53* and tumor development was initially established, the publication of *p53*-related investigations has increased rapidly [66]. The frequency and content of these reports suggest that the *p53* growth-regulatory system is complex and that our understanding of its molecular interactions and function is far from mature. For instance, a molecular-based rationale has only recently been advanced to account for the manner in which *p53* regulates cell proliferation. Data from independent investigatory groups [67,68] now suggest *p53* as a

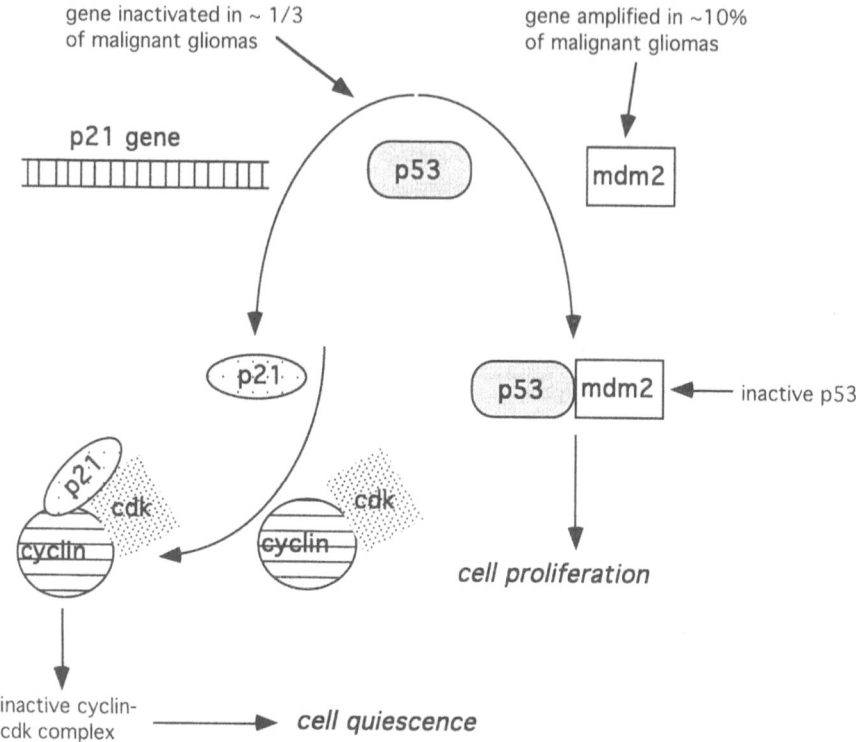

gene inactivated in ~ 1/3
of malignant gliomas

gene amplified in ~10%
of malignant gliomas

p21 gene

p53

mdm2

p21

p53 mdm2 ←——— inactive p53

p21

cdk

cdk

cyclin

cyclin

cell proliferation

inactive cyclin-
cdk complex ——————→ *cell quiescence*

Fig. 4. Model of control of cell proliferation through regulation of p53 activity

positive transcriptional regulator of a gene encoding a protein, p21, that binds to and inhibits the activity of cyclin–cyclin-dependent kinase complexes (Fig. 4).

Of equal importance to the effects of *p53* function is the regulation of its function. One form of *p53* regulation has been determined through studies of tumors that show that a gene encoding a p53-binding protein, mdm2, is sometimes amplified in sarcomas [69] as well as malignant gliomas [58].

The binding of mdm2 functionally inactivates *p53* [70,71], and we [72] as well as others [69] have shown that gene amplification-associated overexpression of mdm2 occurs in tumors and cell lines as an alternative mechanism to *p53* mutations for abrogating its growth suppressive effects. Regulation of *p53* function through phosphorylation has also been indicated [73,74]. As is the case with pRb, therefore, *p53* functional inactivation can also occur through numerous mechanisms, including mutation and interaction with other proteins.

Conclusions

The molecular genetic characterization of glial tumorigenesis has already identified specific TSGs and oncogenes whose corresponding protein function in normal and neoplastic tissue can be examined in detail. For three of the mutations described here, p53, p16, and EGFR, it is apparent that alteration of each results in increased intracellular kinase activity that stimulates cell cycling. Although it is encouraging to identify a common theme associated with different mutations, in this case deregulated protein phosphorylation, it is nonetheless entirely unlikely that all or even a majority of the genes have been identified whose alteration are associated with glial tumor development. Consequently, it may be unreasonable to suppose that a sufficient amount of information can be gathered from existing reports from which to develop rational therapies for the treatment of glioma. However, it is becoming increasingly apparent that the gene alterations which are being identified are directed toward disrupting a few key pathways that maintain control over cell proliferation. As additional glioma-associated gene alterations are identified and subsequent functional studies performed, it is anticipated that an integrated schema will evolve that describes relationships between the genetic events involved in the development of glioma. The understanding of such events is anticipated to lead to the effective treatment of these tumors.

References

1. Rey JA, Bello MJ, de Campos JM, Kusak ME, Ramos C, Benitez J (1987) Chromosomal patterns in human malignant astrocytomas. Cancer Genet Cytogenet 29:201–221
2. Bigner SH, Mark J, Burger PC, Mahaley MS Jr, Bullard DE, Muhlbaier LH, Bigner DD (1988) Specific chromosomal abnormalities in malignant human gliomas. Cancer Res 48:405–411
3. Jenkins RB, Kimmel DW, Moertel CA, Schultz CG, Scheithauer BW, Kelly PJ, Dewald GW (1989) A cytogenetic study of 53 human gliomas. Cancer Genet Cytogenet 39:253–279
4. Steck PA, Saya H (1991) Pathways of oncogenesis in primary brain tumors. Curr Opin Oncol 3:476–484
5. Collins VP, James CD (1993) Gene and chromosomal alterations associated with the development of human gliomas. FASEB J 7:926–930
6. Wong AJ, Zoltick PW, Moscatello DK (1994) The molecular biology and molecular genetics of astrocytic neoplasms. Semin Oncol 21:139–148
7. Lang FF, Miller DC, Koslow M, Newcomb EW (1994) Pathways leading to glioblastoma multiforme: a molecular analysis of genetic alterations in 65 astrocytic tumors. J Neurosurg 81:426–436
8. Nowell P (1976) The clonal evolution of tumor cell populations. Science 194:23–28
9. James CD, Carlbom E, Dumanski J, Hansen M, Nordenskjold M, Collins VP, Cavenee WK (1988) Clonal genomic alterations in glioma malignancy stages. Cancer Res 48:5546–5551
10. Vogelstein B, Fearon ER, Kern SE, Hamilton SR, Preisinger AC, Nakamura Y, White R (1989) Allelotype of colorectal carcinoma. Science 244:207–211
11. Sato T, Tanigami A, Yamakawa K, Akiyama F, Kasumi F, Sakamoto G, Nakamura Y (1990) Allelotype of breast cancer: cumulative allele losses promote tumor progression in primary breast cancer. Cancer Res 50:7184–7189
12. Cavenee WK, Dryja TP, Phillips RA, Benedict WF, Godbout R, Gallie BL, Murphree AL, Strong LC, White RL (1983) Expression of recessive alleles by chromosomal mechanisms in retinoblastoma. Nature 305:779–784
13. Rouleau GA, Wertelecki W, Haines JL, Hobbs WJ, Trofatter JA, Seizinger BR, Martuza RL, Superneau DW, Conneally PM, Gusella JF (1987) Genetic linkage of bilateral acoustic neurofibromatosis to a DNA marker on chromosome 22. Nature 329:246–248
14. Seizinger BR, Rouleau GA, Ozelius LJ, Lane AH, Faryniarz AG, Chao MV, Huson S, Korf BR, Parry DM, Pericak-Vance MA, et al (1987) Genetic linkage of von Recklinghausen neurofibromatosis to the nerve growth factor receptor gene. Cell 49:589–594
15. Malkin D, Li FP, Strong LC, Fraumeni JF, Nelson CE, Kim DH, Kassel J, Gryka MA, Bischoff FZ, Tainsky MA, et al (1990) Germ line p53 mutations in a familial syndrome of breast cancer, sarcomas, and other neoplasms. Science 250:1233–1238

16. Fujimoto M, Fults DW, Thomas GA, Nakamura Y, Heilbrun MP, White R, Stroy JL, Naylor SL, Kagan-Hallet KS, Sheridan PJ (1989) Loss of heterozygosity on chromosome 10 in human glioblastoma multiforme. Genomics 4:210–214

17. Watanabe K, Nagai M, Wakai S, Arai T, Dawashima K (1990) Loss of constitutional heterozygosity on chromosome 10 in human glioblastoma. Acta Neuropathol 80:251–254

18. Venter DJ, Thomas DG (1991) Multiple sequential abnormalities in the evolution of human gliomas. Br J Cancer 63:753–757

19. Rasheed ABK, Fuller GN, Friedman AH, Bigner DD, Bigner SH (1992) Loss of heterozygosity for chromosome 10 loci in human gliomas. Genes Chromosomes & Cancer 5:75–82

20. James CD, He J, Carlbom E, Nordenskjold M, Cavenee WK, Collins VP (1991) Chromosome 9 deletion mapping reveals interferon alpha and interferon beta-1 gene deletions in primary glial tumors. Cancer Res 51:1684–1688

21. Ichimura K, Schmidt EE, Yamaguchi N, James CD, Collins VP (1994) A common region of homozygous deletion in malignant human gliomas lies between the IFN-α/ω gene cluster and the D9S171 locus. Cancer Res 54:3127–3130

22. James CD, Carlbom E, Nordenskjold M, Collins VP, Cavenee WK (1989) Mitotic recombination of chromosome 17 in astrocytomas. Proc Natl Acad Sci USA 86:2858–2862

23. El-Azouzi M, Chung RY, Farmer GE, Martuza RL, Black PM, Rouleau GA, Hettlich C, Hedley-Whyte ET, Zervas NT, Panagopoulos K, Nakamura Y, Gusella JF, Seizinger BR (1989) Loss of distinct regions of the short arm of chromosome 17 associated with tumorigenesis of human astrocytomas. Proc Natl Acad Sci USA 86:7186–7190

24. Fults D, Tippets RH, Thomas GA, Nakamura Y, White R (1989) Loss of heterozygosity for loci on chromosome 17p in human malignant astrocytoma. Cancer Res 49:6572–6577

25. Ransom DT, Ritland SR, Kimmel DW, Moertel CA, Dahl RJ, Scheithauer BW, Kelly PJ, Jenkins RB (1992) Cytogenetic and loss of heterozygosity studies in ependymomas, pilocytic astrocytomas, and oligodendrogliomas. Genes Chromosomes & Cancer 5:348–356

26. Von Deimling A, Louis DN, von Ammon K, Petersen I, Wiestler OD, Seizinger B (1992) Evidence for a tumor suppressor gene on chromosome 19q associated with human astrocytomas, oligodendrogliomas, and mixed gliomas. Cancer Res 52:4277–4279

27. Reifenberger J, Reifenberger G, Liu L, James CD, Wechsler W, Collins VP (1994) Molecular genetic analysis of oligodendroglial tumors shows preferential allelic losses on chromosome arms 19q and 1p. Am J Pathol 145:1175–1190

28. James CD, He J, Carlbom E, Mikkelsen T, Ridderheim P-A, Cavenee WK, Collins VP (1990) Loss of genetic information in central nervous system tumors common to children and young adults. Genes Chromosomes & Cancer 2:94–102

29. Fults D, Pedone C (1993) Deletion mapping of the long arm of chromosome 10 in glioblastoma multiforme. Genes Chromosomes & Cancer 7:173–177

30. Karlbom AE, James CD, Boethius J, Cavenee WK, Collins VP, Nordenskjold M, Larsson C (1993) Loss heterozygosity in malignant gliomas involves at least three distinct regions on chromosome 10. Hum Genet 92:169–174

31. Trofatter JA, MacCollin MM, Rutter JL, Murrell JR, Duyao MP, Parry DM, Eldridge R, Kley N, Menon AG, Pulaski K, Hasse VH, Ambrose CM, Munroe D, Bove C, Hains JL, Martuza RL, MacDonald ME, Seizinger BR, Short MP, Buckler AJ, Gusella JF (1993) A novel moesin-ezrin-, radixin-like gene is a candidate for the neurofibromatosis 2 tumor suppressor. Cell 72:791–800

32. Rubio MP, Correa KM, Ramesh V, MacCollin MM, Jacoby LB, von Deimling A, Gusella JF, Louis DN (1994) Analysis of the neurofibromatosis 2 gene in human ependymomas and astrocytomas. Cancer Res 54:45–47

33. Diaz MO, Ziemin S, Le Beau MM, Pitha P, Smith SD, Chilcote RR, Rowley JD (1988) Homozygous deletion of the alpha- and beta 1-interferon genes in human leukemia and derived cell lines. Proc Natl Acad Sci USA 85:5259–5263

34. Diaz MO, Rubin CM, Harden A, Ziemin S, Larson RA, Le-Beau MM, Rowley JD (1990) Deletions of interferon genes in acute lymphoblastic leukemia. N Engl J Med 322:77–82

35. Cairns P, Tokino K, Eby Y, Sidransky D (1994) Homozygous deletions of 9p21 in primary human bladder tumors detected by comparative multiplex polymerase chain reaction. Cancer Res 54:1422–1424

36. Olopade OI, Buchhagen DL, Malik K, Sherman J, Nobori T, Bader S, Nau MM, Gazbar AF, Minna JD, Diaz MO (1993) Homozygous loss of the interferon genes defines the critical region on 9p that is deleted in lung cancers. Cancer Res 53:2410–2415

37. Holland EA, Beaton SC, Edwards BG, Kefford RF, Mann GJ (1994) Loss of heterozygosity and homozygous deletions on 9p21–22 in melanoma. Oncogene 9:1361–1365

38. James CD, He J, Collins VP, Allalunis-Turner MJ, Day RS (1993) Localization of chromosome 9p homozygous deletions in glioma cell lines with markers constituting a continuous linkage group. Cancer Res 53:3674–3676

39. Olopade OI, Bohlander SK, Pomykala H, Maltepe E, Van Melle E, Le Beau MM, Diaz MO (1992) Mapping the shortest region of overlap of deletions of the short arm of chromosome 9 associated with human neoplasia. Genomics 14:437–443

40. Einhorn S, Heyman M (1993) Chromosome 9 short arm deletions in malignant diseases. Leuk & Lymphoma 11:191–196

41. Kamb A, Gruis NA, Weaver-Feldhaus J, Liu Q, Harshman K, Tavtigian SV, Stockert E, Day RS III, Johnson BE, Skolnick MH (1994) A cell cycle regulator potentially involved in genesis of many tumor types. Science 264:436–440

42. Nobori T, Miura K, Wu DJ, Lois A, Takabayashi K, Carson DA (1994) Deletions of the cyclin-dependent kinase-4 inhibitor gene in multiple human cancers. Nature 368:753–756

43. Fults D, Brockmeyer D, Tullous MW, Pedone CA, Cawthon RM (1992) p53 mutation and loss of heterozygosity on chromosomes 17 and 10 during human astrocytoma progression. Cancer Res 52:674–679

44. Frankel RH, Bayona W, Koslow M, Newcomb EW (1992) p53 mutations in human malignant gliomas: comparison of loss of heterozygosity with mutation frequency. Cancer Res 52:1427–1433

45. von-Deimling A, Eibl RH, Ohgaki H, Louis DN, von-Ammon K, Petersen I, Kleihues P, Chung RY, Wiestler OD, Seizinger BR (1992) p53 mutations are associated with 17p allelic loss in grade II and grade III astrocytoma. Cancer Res 52:2987–2990

46. Nigro JM, Baker SJ, Preisinger AC, Jessup JM, Hostetter R, Cleary K, Bigner SH, Davidson N, Baylin S, Davilee P, Vogelstein B (1989) Mutations in the p53 gene occur in diverse human tumor types. Nature 342:705–708

47. Mercer WE, Shields MT, Amin M, Sauve GJ, Appella E, Romano JW, Ullrich SJ (1990) Negative growth regulation in a glioblastoma tumor cell line that conditionally expresses human wild-type p53. Proc Natl Acad Sci USA 87:6166–6170

48. Libermann TA, Nusbaum HR, Razon N, Kris R, Lax I, Soreq H, Whittle N, Waterfield MD, Ullrich A, Schlessinger J (1985) Amplification, enhanced expression and possible rearrangement of EGF receptor in primary human brain tumors of glial origin. Nature 313:144–147

49. Wong AJ, Bigner SH, Bigner D, Kinzler KW, Hamilton SR, Vogelstein B (1987) Increased expression of the epidermal growth factor receptor gene in malignant gliomas is invariably associated with gene amplification. Proc Natl Acad Sci USA 84:6899–6903

50. Ekstrand AJ, James CD, Cavenee WK, Seliger B, Pettersson RF, Collins VP (1991) Genes for the epidermal growth factor receptor, transforming growth factor alpha, and epidermal growth factor and their expression in human gliomas in vivo. Cancer Res 51:2164–2172

51. Hurtt MR, Moosy J, Donovan PM, Locker J (1992) Amplification of epidermal growth factor receptor gene in gliomas: histopathology and prognosis. J Neuropathol Exp Neurol 51:84–90

52. Sugawa N, Ekstrand AJ, James CD, Collins VP (1990) Identical splicing of aberrant epidermal growth factor receptor transcripts from amplified rearranged genes in human glioblastomas. Proc Natl Acad Sci 87:8602–8606

53. Ekstrand AJ, Sugawa N, James CD, Collins VP (1992) Amplified and rearranged EGFR genes in human glioblastomas reveal deletions of sequences coding for portions of the amino-and/or carboxyl-terminal tails. Proc Natl Acad Sci USA 89:4309–4313

54. Wong AJ, Ruppert JM, Bigner SH, Grzeschik CH, Humphrey PA, Bigner DS, Vogelstein B (1992) Structural alterations of the epidermal growth factor receptor gene in human gliomas. Proc Natl Acad Sci USA 89:2965–2969

55. Ekstrand AJ, Longo N, Hamid ML, Olson JJ, Collins VP, James CD (1994) Functional characterization of an EGF receptor with a truncated extracellular domain expressed in glioblastomas with EGFR gene amplification. Oncogene 9:2313–2320

56. Nishikawa R, Ji XD, Harmon RC, Lazar CS, Gill GN, Cavenee WK, Huang HJ (1994) A mutant epidermal growth factor receptor common in human glioma confers enhanced tumorigenicity. Proc Natl Acad Sci USA 91:7727–7731

57. Bigner SH, Wong AJ, Mark J, Muhlbaier LH, Kinzler KW, Vogelstein B, Bigner DD (1987) Relationship between gene amplification and chromosomal deviations in malignant human gliomas. Cancer Genet Cytogenet 29:165–170

58. Reifenberger G, Reifenberger J, Ichimura K, Meltzer PS, Collins VP (1994) Amplification of multiple genes from chromosomal region 12q13–14 in human malignant gliomas; preliminary mapping of the amplicon shows preferential involvement of CDK4, SAS, and MDM2. Cancer Res 54:4299–4303

59. Serrano M, Hannon GJ, Beach D (1993) A new regulatory motif in cell-cycle control causing specific inhibition of cyclin D/CDK4. Nature 366:704–707

60. Kato J-Y, Matsushime H, Hiebert SW, Ewen ME, Sherr CJ (1993) Direct binding of cyclin D to the retinoblastoma gene product (pRb) and pRb phosphorylation by the cyclin D-dependent kinase, CDK4. Genes Dev 7:331–342

61. Jiang W, Zhang YJ, Kahn SM, Hollstein MC, Santella RM, Lu SH, Harris CC, Montesano R, Weinstein IB (1993) Altered expression of the cyclin D1 and retinoblastoma genes in human esophageal cancer. Proc Natl Acad Sci USA 90:9026–9030

62. Muller H, Lukas J, Schneider A, Warthoe P, Bartek J, Eilers M, Strauss M (1994) Cyclin D1 expression is regulated by the retinoblastoma protein. Proc Natl Acad Sci USA 91:2945–2949

63. He J, Allen JR, Collins VP, Godbout R, Allalunis-Turner MJ, Day RS III, James CD (1994) CDK4 amplification is an alternative mechanism to p16 gene homozygous deleletion in glioma cell lines. Cancer Res 54:5804–5807

64. Venter DJ, Bevan KL, Ludwig RL, Riley TE, Jat PS, Thomas DG, Noble MD (1991) Retinoblastoma gene deletions in human glioblastomas. Oncogene 6:445–448

65. Godbout R, Miyakoshi J, Dobler KD, Andison R, Matsuo K, Allalunis-Turner MJ, Takebe H, Day RS III (1992) Lack of expression of tumor-suporessor genes in human malignant glioma cell lines. Oncogene 7:1879–1884

66. Marx, J (1993) Learning how to suppress cancer. Science 261:1385–1387

67. Harper JW, Adami GR, Wei N, Keyomarsi K, Elledge SJ (1993) The p21 Cdk-interacting protein Cip1 is a potent inhibitor of G1 cyclin-dependent kinases. Cell 75:805–816

68. el-Deiry WS, Tokino T, Velculescu VE, Levy DB, Parsons R, Trent JM, Lin D, Mercer WE, Kinzler KW, Vogelstein B (1993) WAF1, a potential mediator of p53 tumor suppression. Cell 75:817–825

69. Leach FS, Tokino T, Meltzer P, Burrell M, Oliner JD, Smith S, Hill DE, Sidransky D, Kinzler KW, Vogelstein B (1993) p53 mutation and MDM2 amplification in human soft tissue sarcomas. Cancer Res 53:2231–2234

70. Oliner JD, Pietenpol JA, Thiagalingam S, Gyuris J, Kinzler KW, Vogelstein B (1993) Oncoprotein MDM2 conceals the activation domain of tumour suppressor p53. Nature 362:857–860

71. Momand J, Zambetti GP, Olson DC, George D, Levine AJ (1992) The mdm-2 oncogene product forms a complex with the p53 protein and inhibits p53-mediated transactivation. Cell 69:1237–1245

72. He J, Reifenberger G, Lu L, Collins VP, James CD (1994) Analysis of glioma cell lines for amplification and overexpression of MDM2. Genes Chromosomes & Cancer 11:91–96

73. Sturzbecher HW, Maimets T, Chumakov P, Brain R, Addison C, Simanis V, Rudge K, Philip R, Grimaldi M, Court W, et al (1990) p53 Interacts with p34cdc2 in mammalian cells: implications for cell cycle control and oncogenesis. Oncogene 5:795–781

74. Bischoff JR, Friedman PN, Marshak DR, Prives C, Beach D (1990) Human p53 is phosphorylated by p60-cdc2 and cyclin B-cdc2. Proc Natl Acad Sci USA 87:4766–4770

A Model for the Molecular Pathogenesis of Astrocytic Gliomas

Otmar D. Wiestler and Andreas von Deimling

Abstract. Astrocytic gliomas are the most common human cerebral neoplasms. The WHO classification of brain tumors recognizes four malignancy grades based on histopathological parameters. Recently, there has been remarkable progress in studies on the molecular pathogenesis of these tumors. In this chapter, we summarize data from an ongoing study that has been initiated to molecularly characterize human astrocytomas. The data from 150 human astrocytic gliomas are compiled. These gliomas were assessed for characteristic genomic alterations, i.e., loss of portions of chromosomes 10, 17p, 17q, and 19q, and point mutations of the *p53* tumor suppressor gene and for amplification of the epidermal growth factor (EGF) receptor (*EGFR*) gene. Our findings support the hypothesis that distinct genetic pathways result in the formation of astrocytomas of different malignancy grades and that glioblastoma multiforme can be subdivided into at least two genetic subsets. It is to be expected that molecular genetic studies will have a major impact on both diagnostic and clinical neurooncology.

Key words. Astrocytomas — Molecular genetics — Oncogenes — Tumor suppressor genes — Loss of heterozygosity — Molecular classification

Introduction

Astrocytic tumors are the most common, primary human central nervous system tumors. Histopathological parameters have been employed to distinguish four grades of malignancy: pilocytic astrocytoma (WHO grade I), astrocytoma (WHO grade II), anaplastic astrocytoma (WHO grade III), and glioblastoma multiforme (WHO grade IV) [1]. Although classical histopathological methods have not been able to characterize pathogenic factors contributing to the formation of astrocytic gliomas, recent molecular genetic studies have uncovered several genetic alterations that appear to play a role in the pathogenesis of astrocytic neoplasms. In this chapter, we summarize the findings of an ongoing molecular genetic study on human astrocytomas. A preliminary model for the molecular pathogenesis of these neoplasms is introduced.

Department of Neuropathology, University of Bonn Medical Center, D-53105 Bonn, Germany

As in most human cancers, two families of genes appear to be involved in the formation of gliomas: oncogenes and tumor suppressor genes. A major property of activated oncogenes is their potential to actively drive and deregulate the growth of susceptible cells. Activation of one allele will suffice to induce this growth-stimulating action. The products of tumor suppressor genes, on the other hand, are characterized by their potential to inhibit cell growth. Such genes can only be inactivated through loss or functional inhibition of both alleles. Genetically, oncogenes act as dominant genetic elements whereas tumor suppressor genes act in a recessive fashion. Over the years, many genes with properties of oncogenes or tumor suppressor genes have been identified in the eukaryotic genome and their number continues to increase. From studies in many laboratories, there is evidence for an involvement of both oncogenes and tumor suppressor genes in the formation of human gliomas.

One oncogene that has received considerable attention in neurooncology is the epidermal growth factor receptor (*EGFR*) oncogene. It encodes a transmembrane tyrosine kinase receptor protein with the capacity to bind epidermal growth factor (EGF), transforming growth factor-α, and several other growth-stimulating peptides. Amplification and subsequent overexpression of this gene are detectable in 30%–40% of glioblastomas (Fig. 1). The frequent activation of the *EGFR* gene has already prompted attempts to interfere with the EGFR pathway by subjecting glioblastoma patients to treatment with an antibody to the receptor protein. However, these therapeutic efforts have not been successful. Attempts to correlate amplification of the *EGFR* gene with histopathological parameters and patient survival have produced conflicting results [2,3]. Recently, the *mdm-2*, *CDK4*, and *SAS* genes have been identified as components of an amplicon on chromosome 12 in a subpopulation of glioblastomas. These oncogenes appear to be involved in an advanced stage of astrocytoma progression. They are not usually affected in low-grade gliomas or nonastrocytic neural tumors.

On the other hand, there is ample evidence for a role of tumor suppressor genes in the formation of human gliomas. The most commonly affected tumor suppressor gene in astrocytic gliomas is the *p53* gene. Several studies have reported a 30%–50% incidence of mutations in the *p53* tumor suppressor gene in both low- and high-grade astrocytomas (see following). This indicates that *p53* plays a role during an early stage of astrocytoma formation. However, a detailed model for its molecular functions has not yet emerged, and genes interacting with or substituting for *p53* are still largely unknown. Recent reports have demonstrated homozygous deletions of an interesting region on chromosome 9p in malignant gliomas [4]. This chromosomal area harbors the p16 and p15 cell cycle regulatory genes, both of which may substitute for p53 alterations as they are involved in the same cell cycle pathway as the p53 protein [5].

In contrast to astrocytomas, nonastrocytic gliomas including oligodendrogliomas and ependymomas and other tumors of the brain such as meningiomas, schwannomas, central neurocytomas, or primitive neuroectodermal tumors do not exhibit significant incidences of *p53* mutations [6]. We conclude from this observation that the *p53* gene exerts a surprising tropism for astrocytic cells in the central nervous system.

In many instances of tumor suppressor gene inactivation, one allele carries a point mutation while the other is destroyed by a major structural alteration such as chromosomal deletion, inversion, or translocation. This second type of genetic change can be identified using polymorphic DNA markers for the affected chromosomal locus. Such

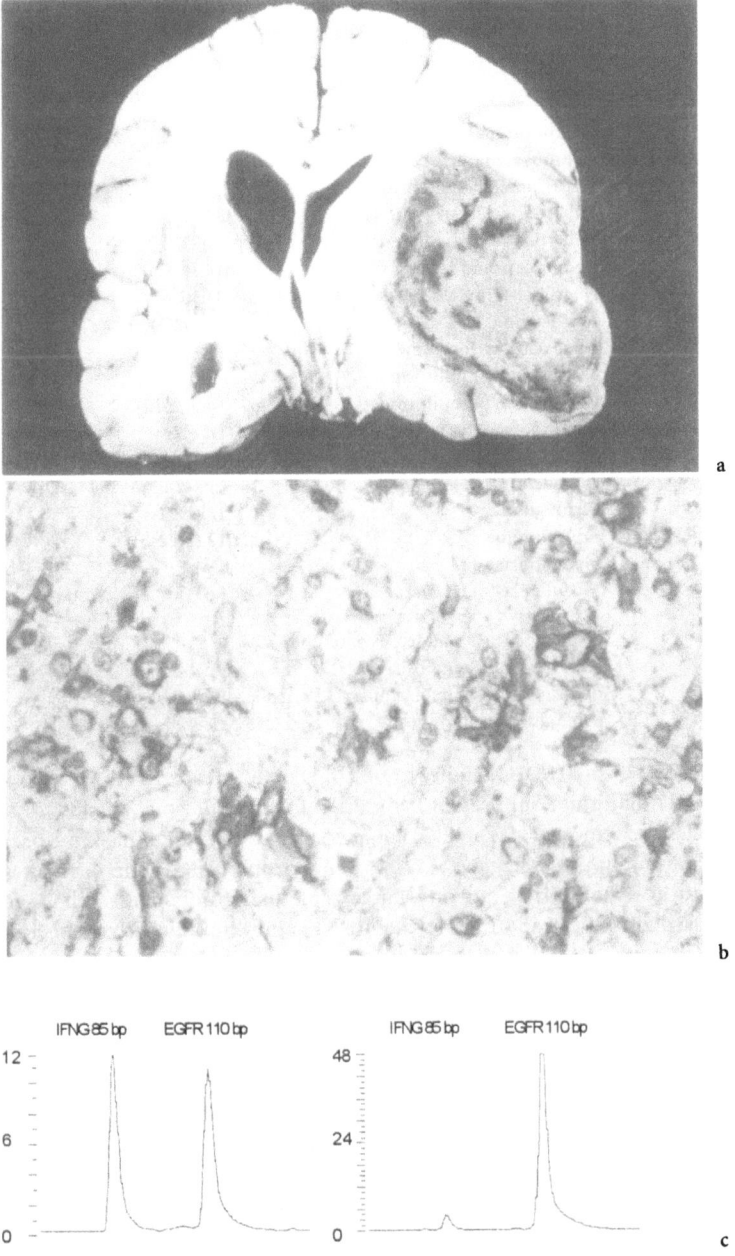

Fig. 1a–c. Neuropathological and molecular features of glioblastoma multiforme. **a** Macroscopic section through the brain of a patient with a large glioblastoma in the right temporal lobe. **b** Immunoreactivity for the epidermal growth factor (EGF) receptor oncogene product in a glioblastoma. **c** Differential polymerase chain reaction (PCR) analysis for the detection of EGF receptor gene amplification. A fragment of the interferon γ gene (IFN-γ), which is located on the same human chromosome, was coamplified as control gene. The *right panel* shows a glioblastoma with striking amplification of the EGF receptor (*EGFR*) oncogene. The reactions in the *left panel* were carried out with DNA from a glioblastoma that does not exhibit amplification of this oncogene

Table 1. Chromosomal localization of putative and identified tumor suppressor genes involved in the formation of central nervous system neoplasms.

Tumor entity	Chromosome (gene)
Neurofibromatosis type 1	17q11.2 (NF1)
Neurofibromatosis type 2	22q12 (NF2)
von Hippel–Lindau disease	3p25 (VHL)
Tuberous sclerosis (type 1)	9q33–34
Tuberous sclerosis (type 2)	16p13 (TSC-2)
Retinoblastoma	13q14 (RB1)
Neuroblastoma	1p36
Astrocytoma	17p13 (p53)
Anaplastic astrocytoma	19q13.2–13.3
Glioblastoma multiforme	10
Glioblastoma multiforme	9p21 (p16, p15)
Pilocytic astrocytoma	17q11.2 (NF1?)
Oligodendroglioma	1p36
Oligodendroglioma	19q13.2–13.3
Meningioma	22q12 (NF2)
Schwannoma	22q12 (NF2)
Medulloblastoma	17pter
Medulloblastoma	9p31

Cloned genes are added in parentheses.
NF, neurofibromatosis; VHL, von Hippel–Lindau disease; RB, retinoblastoma; TSC, tuberous sclerosis; p16, inhibitor of cyclin-dependent kinase type 4.

loss of heterozygosity (LOH) studies are a convenient means to analyze the involvement of potential tumor suppressor genes in human neoplasms. The loss of chromosomal alleles, as demonstrated by LOH analysis, is thought to unmask the presence of mutant tumor suppressor genes. With polymorphic DNA microsatellites, these studies can now be carried out on a large scale using polymerase chain reaction- (PCR-) based amplification of microsatellite loci and nonradioactive detection of the PCR fragments [7]. A major prerequisite is the availability of blood DNA samples as a DNA reference from each tumor patient. LOH studies in human brain tumors have uncovered various candidate loci on chromosomes 9p, 10, 17p, 17q, and 19q, some of which are listed in Table 1.

The involvement of already identified cloned genes (*EGFR*, *p53*) and putative tumor suppressor genes raises the question whether astrocytic gliomas can be characterized and molecularly classified on the basis of molecular genetic alterations. We here present the compiled data of an ongoing study based on the analysis of a large series of human astrocytic gliomas: pilocytic astrocytomas, WHO grade I; astrocytomas, WHO grade II; anaplastic astrocytomas, WHO grade III; and glioblastoma multiforme, WHO grade IV. All tumors were examined for structural genetic alterations in the most frequently affected regions on chromosomes 10, 17, and 19q and in the *EGFR* gene.

Pilocytic Astrocytoma, WHO Grade I

Pilocytic astrocytomas are astrocytic brain tumors of low malignancy that occur predominantly in childhood and adolescence. Typical sites for this tumor are the cerebellar hemispheres and midline structures of the central nervous system such as the hypothalamus, brainstem, and optic nerves. Pilocytic astrocytomas usually follow a benign course and may be cured by surgical resection. These tumors occur both sporadically and in association with neurofibromatosis type 1 (NF1, von Recklinghausen's neurofibromatosis). One-third of all patients with pilocytic astrocytomas of the optic nerve (optic glioma) have NF1 [8], and 1%–5% of all patients with NF1 develop optic glioma [9]. The histopathological features of pilocytic astrocytomas are identical in the sporadic and NF1-associated forms. They include elongated piloid cells, a coarse glial fibrillary matrix, microcysts, Rosenthal fibers, and granular bodies. These features readily distinguish pilocytic astrocytomas from adult supratentorial astrocytomas, which are often clinically and histologically malignant tumors.

In our series of 20 pilocytic astrocytomas, 4 (20%) showed LOH on chromosome 17 [10]. Three of these tumors had allelic losses confined to the long arm, and one had lost the entire chromosome. Analysis with multiple probes mapped on chromosome 17q defined a commonly affected region extending from the centromere to 17q21. These allelic losses suggest the involvement of a tumor suppressor gene on the long arm of chromosome 17, located between the centromere and 17q21, in the pathogenesis of pilocytic astrocytoma. Allelic loss on chromosome 17q was not associated with any of the special histopathological features of pilocytic astrocytoma such as Rosenthal fibers, protein droplets, or microcystic change, and was observed in both supratentorial and infratentorial pilocytic astrocytomas. Only 1 of the tumors with LOH 17q was from a documented NF1 patient.

The long arm of chromosome 17 harbors several genes that are involved in tumorigenesis. Among these genes, the *NF1* tumor suppressor gene is a particularly interesting candidate because patients afflicted with NF1 are prone to developing pilocytic astrocytomas [9]. The *NF1* gene exhibits 6TPase activating protein (6AP) activity, interacts with *ras* proto-oncogenes, and may be involved in the control of cell growth [11–13]. Alterations in the *NF1* gene in patients with NF1 and in tumors from patients with NF1 have been detected in only a few cases [14–18]. However, large regions of the gene have not been studied in detail. The patient with NF1 demonstrated LOH on 17q that included the NF1 locus, but the remaining copy of the *NF1* gene has not yet been examined. Studies to analyze the *NF1* gene in sporadic and NF1-related pilocytic astrocytomas are currently in progress. A detailed molecular analysis has been hampered considerably by the large size of both the *NF1* gene and *NF1* gene transcripts. This will require single-strand conformation polymorphism (SSCP) screening of cDNA fragments from tumors and normal cells.

LOH on the short arm of chromosome 17 has been noted frequently in adult astrocytomas [19–21]. However, only 1 of the 20 pilocytic astrocytomas in this study displayed LOH on 17p, and a search for mutant p53 in these tumors by SSCP analysis failed to uncover mutations in exons 5–8 of the *p53* gene. On the other hand, allelic losses on the long arm of chromosome 17, while found in 20% of the pilocytic astrocytomas, were not detected in our series of adult WHO grade II and III astrocytomas. Furthermore, allelic losses on chromosomes 10 and 19q and amplification of the *EGFR* gene, which are frequently encountered in adult astrocytomas, have not been observed in pilocytic astrocytomas. These molecular genetic findings support the clinicopathological separation of pilocytic astrocytomas from adult astrocytomas.

Astrocytoma, WHO Grade II

Astrocytomas of WHO grade II typically arise in middle-aged patients and are preferentially located in the cerebral hemispheres. These tumors are histopathologically benign but display a significant infiltration potential. Fibrillary, protoplasmic, and gemistocytic variants can be distinguished microscopically [1]. Survival periods of 5 years or longer may be achieved. However, WHO grade II astrocytomas frequently progress to anaplastic variants within several years. The most commonly observed genetic alteration in these tumors is LOH 17p, which occurs in approximately half of all WHO grade II and grade III astrocytomas. The affected chromosomal region includes the *p53* tumor suppressor gene. Mutations in the conserved domains of the *p53* gene, which span exons 5 to 8, have been identified in numerous human malignancies such as carcinomas of the breast, lung, and colon [22–24]. These mutations are often associated with a corresponding loss of the second copy of chromosome 17 [22,25], thus meeting the classical paradigm of recessive tumor suppressor gene inactivation [26].

Because LOH on chromosome 17p is frequently detectable in lower grade astrocytomas, we explored the possibility that *p53* mutations may occur in WHO grade II and III astrocytomas. We analyzed 19 astrocytomas (WHO grade II) and 26 anaplastic astrocytomas (26 WHO grade III) for mutations in the conserved regions of the *p53* gene by SSCP analysis and direct DNA sequencing. In addition, we evaluated all tumors for LOH of chromosome 17p by Southern blot restriction fragment length polymorphism (RFLP) analysis to assess the relationship of *p53* mutations to allelic losses on chromosome 17p. Both LOH 17p and *p53* mutations were detected in approximately 50% of astrocytomas of WHO grade II and grade III, and there was a striking association of these two changes. These results show that loss of chromosome 17p is more common in lower grade astrocytomas than had been previously suggested [19,27,28]. In addition, the percentage of LOH 17p does not appear to differ between WHO grade II and grade III astrocytoma, thus indicating that loss of chromosome 17p may be involved in an early stage of astrocytoma formation. All cases with *p53* mutations had LOH of 17p, while only four tumors exhibited LOH 17p without detectable *p53* mutations. These data reveal that *p53* mutations are not restricted to glioblastoma multiforme, but are found in lower grade astrocytic tumors as well. In addition, they demonstrate an association between *p53* mutations and LOH of 17p, which suggests that the genetic locus on chromosome 17p affected in the tumors is the *p53* gene. An interesting problem not yet resolved concerns the nature of alternative tumor-associated genes that substitute for *p53* mutations in those astrocytomas without detectable lesions on chromosome 17p.

LOH 10, LOH 17q, LOH 19q, and *EGFR* gene amplification were not present at a significant incidence in astrocytoma WHO grade II.

Anaplastic Astrocytoma, WHO Grade III; and Malignant Progression of Astrocytic Gliomas

Low-grade astrocytomas in adult patients bear a significant risk of progression to a more malignant astrocytoma variant, that is, anaplastic astrocytoma (WHO grade III) or glioblastoma multiforme. This development occurs in more than 50% of initially low-grade astrocytomas and represents a major prognostic factor for these patients.

Histopathological signs of anaplastic change include increased cellularity, nuclear and cellular pleomorphism, and elevated mitotic activity. A detailed neuropathological analysis of biopsy specimens has not revealed morphological parameters that would reliably predict the individual course and risk for malignant progression of low-grade astrocytomas. However, molecular genetic studies may promise significant progress for this serious problem in clinical neurooncology.

To identify genes or genetic loci associated with the development of malignancy in astrocytic gliomas, we have analyzed a series of 19 astrocytomas (WHO grade II) and 27 anaplastic astrocytomas (WHO grade III) for LOH 17p, *p53* mutations, LOH 9p, and LOH 19q. The p53 and chromosome 9p loci were selected as they had previously been considered as progression-related genetic loci [29–31]. We were not able to establish a significant association with anaplastic astrocytoma for either candidates. LOH 17p and *p53* mutations were observed at high incidence in both low-grade and anaplastic astrocytomas. However, there was no significant difference between the two groups suggesting that the *p53* gene is likely to play a role at an early stage of astrocytoma formation. LOH 9p was present at low frequency in both astrocytoma variants. This locus can now be reexamined in detail as the cell cycle-associated p16 and p15 genes have recently been identified as candidate genes affected in this chromosomal region.

An intriguing novel mode of inactivation of these genes involves homozygous deletion of both alleles. Experiments to specifically analyze homozygous deletions of the chromosome 9p21 target region in WHO grade II and grade III astrocytomas are in progress. Our study has uncovered an interesting novel candidate for a progression-associated genetic locus in astrocytomas. This locus resides on the long arm of chromosome 19; 50% of the anaplastic astrocytomas exhibited LOH 19q while only 3 of 17 astrocytomas of WHO grade II showed allelic loss in this region [32]. This may indeed indicate that the chromosomal arm 19q contains a putative tumor suppressor involved in the malignant progression of astrocytic gliomas. Current and future studies will focus on an analysis of the chromosome 19q candidate locus in other brain tumors, on a molecular characterization and detailed mapping of the affected region on chromosome 19q13.3–13.4, and on the clinical follow-up of patients enrolled in this molecular genetic analysis [33].

In contrast to glioblastoma multiforme, LOH 10 and EGFR gene amplification were not detected at a significant incidence in anaplastic astrocytoma, WHO grade III. These loci appear to play a role in advanced stages of malignancy in glioblastoma multiforme.

Glioblastoma Multiforme, WHO Grade IV

Glioblastomas are the most frequent and most malignant astrocytic gliomas (Fig. 1). They predominantly occur in older patients. Histopathological hallmarks of this highly malignant glioma are tumor necrosis and glomeruloid vascular endothelial proliferation. The majority of these tumors develop *de novo*, that is, without a history of a previous astrocytic glioma (primary glioblastoma multiforme). However, glioblastoma multiforme may also arise in patients with a previously diagnosed lower grade astrocytoma (secondary glioblastoma multiforme). In this latter group of patients, alterations in tumor-associated genes are likely to mediate the process of malignant progression to glioblastoma multiforme. Although the histopathological appearance of glioblastoma multiforme is extremely heterogeneous, it has not been possible to differentiate by light microscopy tumors that arise from previous astrocytomas from those that develop *de novo* [34]. Neither immunohistochemical nor ultrastructural analyses have provided evidence for subdividing glioblastoma multiforme into clinically or biologically distinct entities.

Young age of the patient at the time of diagnosis and high Karnovsky performance status score are favorable prognostic parameters in glioblastoma multiforme [34]. In addition, glioblastoma multiforme patients with a history of a previous lower grade tumor (secondary glioblastoma multiforme) appear to have a better prognosis than those whose tumors arose in a clinically de novo manner [35]. These observations thus hint at the possibility of subdividing glioblastoma multiforme with an alternative approach, and suggest that younger patients with a clinical history or histological evidence of a previous lower grade tumor (i.e., patients with secondary glioblastoma multiforme) may represent a more favorable subgroup of glioblastoma multiforme.

Several LOH studies in malignant astrocytomas have demonstrated specific defects, most frequently involving chromosomes 9p, 10, 17p, 19q, and 22 [19–21,27,36–39]. Allelic losses of chromosome 10 are predominantly observed in glioblastoma multiforme whereas chromosome 17p deletions appear to be associated with both lower grade diffuse astrocytomas and glioblastoma multiforme. While LOH studies have not been able to differentiate glioblastomas into molecular variants, they have suggested that molecular genetic data may provide information on the origin of glioblastoma multiforme, i.e., whether glioblastoma multiforme arises through dedifferentiation from lower grade tumors or develops *de novo* [36]. We have investigated the incidence of LOH of chromosomes 10p, 10q, 17p, and 19q and amplification of the *EGFR* gene in a large series of glioblastomas to determine whether these tumors can be subtyped on a genetic basis. Our findings show that LOH on chromosome 17p and *EGFR* gene amplification do not usually occur together in glioblastoma multiforme ($P = .01$). This allows the separation of glioblastoma multiforme into at least two distinct genetic subsets (Fig. 2). Loss of chromosome 10, however, was present in all patients with *EGFR* gene amplification and in many patients with loss of chromosome 17p and was, therefore, not useful for subdividing glioblastoma multiforme. From these data we propose a model of at least two molecular pathways resulting in distinct variants of glioblastoma multiforme [40].

The genetic pathway to glioblastoma multiforme type 1 is associated with loss of genetic material on the short arm of chromosome 17. Because LOH on chromosome 17p and mutations of the corresponding *p53* gene both occur as commonly in WHO grade II and III astrocytomas as in glioblastoma multiforme, LOH 17p and *p53* mutations most likely represent early steps in astrocytoma formation [20,21]. Those glioblastomas exhibiting allelic loss on chromosome 17p may, therefore, arise through progression from lower grade astrocytic lesions. In some cases, the precursor lesion could be a microscopic focus that is not clinically symptomatic. Progression to glioblastoma multiforme may involve further genetic alterations, such as loss of chromosome 10.

The genetic pathway to glioblastoma multiforme type 2 involves both *EGFR* gene amplification and loss of chromosome 10. We have shown that amplification of the *EGFR* gene is closely associated with loss of chromosome 10, and have suggested that loss of a tumor suppressor gene on chromosome 10 precedes *EGFR* gene amplification

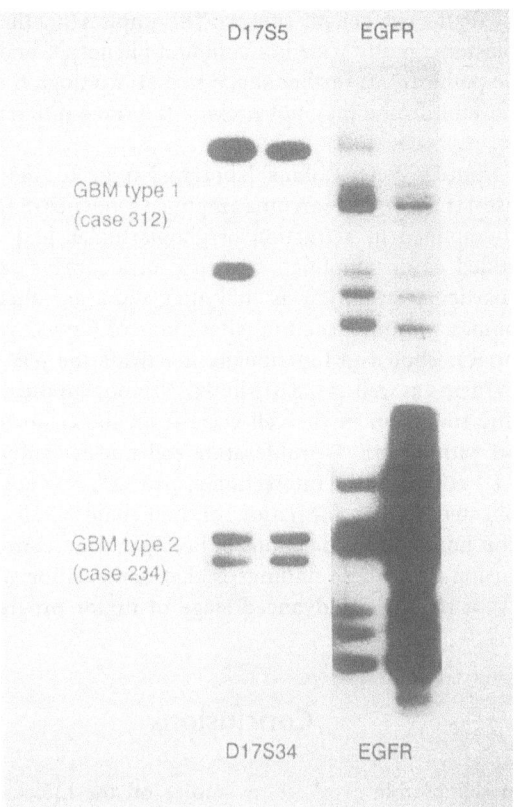

Fig. 2. Molecular genetic differentiation of glioblastoma (*GBM*) type 1 and type 2. Representative Southern blots demonstrate the characteristic molecular genetic features of glioblastoma multiforme type 1 and type 2. Loss of heterozygosity on the short arm of chromosome 17 at D17S5 without EGF receptor (*EGFR*) gene amplification in glioblastoma multiforme type 1 (*upper panels*); maintenance of heterozygosity at D17S34 with amplification of the EGFR gene in glioblastoma multiforme type 2 (*lower panels*). In each panel, the left lane represents constitutional DNA, and the right lane, tumor DNA

[41]. These tumors can also exhibit LOH on other chromosomes, such as 19q [42]. It is tempting to speculate that this glioblastoma variant arises *de novo*, without a preceding lower grade astrocytoma. None of the patients in our study with *EGFR* gene amplification had a history of an earlier lower grade astrocytoma.

Patients with glioblastoma multiforme type 1 had a mean age of 40.5 years, whereas patients with glioblastoma multiforme type 2 had a mean age of 56.3 years. The observation that glioblastoma multiforme type 1 occurs in significantly younger patients than glioblastoma multiforme type 2 ($P = .001$) lends further support to the genetic subclassification of glioblastoma multiforme. These data may also indicate that the age-based difference in prognosis reflects the predominance of glioblastoma multiforme type 1 in younger patients. In addition, it is likely that those glioblastoma patients with a previous history of lower grade glioma who do better clinically [35] are also in the glioblastoma multiforme type 1 group.

Despite the identification of putatively distinct genetic subsets of glioblastoma multiforme, histological evaluation failed to reveal any association of specific histological features with the two genetic subsets. This implies that the histological heterogeneity of glioblastoma multiforme is a common phenotype and may not reflect the different genetic pathways. It further suggests that histological attempts of separating glioblastoma multiforme may not provide the same differential information as genetic analyses.

Recent work from Dr. Peter Collins' laboratory indicates that the *mdm-2*, cyclin-dependent kinase 4 (*CDK4*), and sarcoma amplified sequence (*SAS*) genes on chromosome 12 are coamplified in a fraction of glioblastomas [43]. *mdm-2*, which was originally identified as an amplified sequence in a murine sarcoma, and *CDK-4* have received particular attention as they may represent alternative tumorigenic pathways in gliomas without structural alterations of the *p53* gene. The product of the *mdm-2* gene was shown to functionally inactivate the p53 protein by complex formation. These genes as well as the p16 and p15 tumor suppressors on chromosome 9p21 regulate the transition in the cell cycle from the G_1 to the S phase through their interaction with a CDK-4–proliferating cell nuclear antigen–cyclin D (CDK-4/PCNA/cyclin D) complex [5]. Interestingly, p16 (MTS-1) and p15 (MTS-2) have also been implicated in the formation of malignant gliomas as these tumors frequently exhibit homozygous deletions of both genes on chromosome 9p21 [4]. A potential conclusion from these findings is that deregulation of the G_1/S cell cycle checkpoint plays a role at an advanced stage of tumor progression in malignant gliomas.

Conclusions

There has been remarkable progress in studies on the molecular pathogenesis of astrocytic gliomas. Distinct molecular pathways that lead to the formation of pilocytic astrocytomas, to WHO grade II and III astrocytomas in adult patients, and to the common, *de novo* glioblastoma multiforme are beginning to emerge. A current and preliminary model for these pathways is outlined in Fig. 3. This model differentiates at least three molecular pathways for astrocytic gliomas. The key lesion in diffusely infiltrating astrocytomas of WHO grade II are mutations of the *p53* gene on the short arm of chromosome 17. Malignant progression to the anaplastic astrocytoma involves a putative tumor suppressor on chromosome 19q and, potentially, the *p16* and *p15* cell cycle regulatory genes on chromosome 9p. Secondary glioblastomas in younger individuals represent the end stage of this progression cascade. They additionally exhibit a high incidence of allelic losses on chromosome 10, indicating the presence of a pathogenetically relevant glioblastoma-associated tumor suppressor on this human chromosome.

According to our model, glioblastomas may be divided into at least two subsets. One molecular variant is characterized by allelic losses on the short arm of chromosome 17, which presumably affect the *p53* gene, and by the absence of *EGFR* gene amplification. This type of glioblastoma multiforme occurs primarily in younger patients (glioblastoma multiforme type 1) and may arise through progression from low-grade astrocytomas. The other subset is characterized by *EGFR* gene amplification without loss of chromosome 17p and occurs primarily in older patients (glioblastoma multiforme type 2). As glioblastoma multiforme at a younger age is usually associated with a better clinical outcome, this molecular distinction of two glioblastoma variants may well be of prognostic significance.

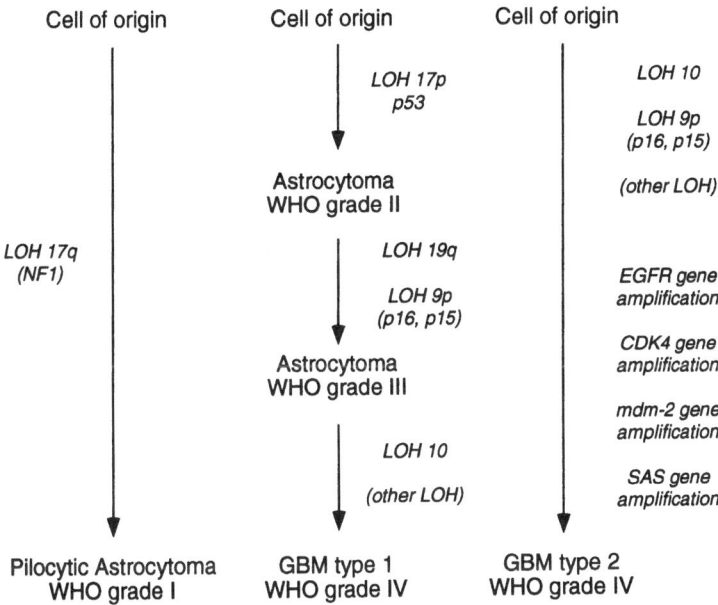

Fig. 3. Hypothetical model for the molecular pathogenesis of human astrocytomas. Three distinct molecular genetic pathways lead to pilocytic astrocytoma WHO grade I (*left column*); astrocytoma WHO grade II and WHO grade III, and glioblastoma multiforme type 1 (*middle column*); and glioblastoma multiforme type 2 (*right column*). LOH, loss of heterozygosity

The pilocytic astrocytoma (WHO grade I) with clearly distinct clinical and neuropathological features can also be differentiated on a molecular genetic basis. A characteristic molecular genetic alteration in pilocytic astrocytomas is LOH on chromosome 17q, a feature not seen in WHO grade II and grade III astrocytoma and only rarely observed in glioblastoma multiforme. This emphasizes an independent pathway in the formation of these tumors that may involve the NF1 tumor suppressor gene.

It is clear that this current model for the molecular pathogenesis of astrocytic gliomas is in a preliminary stage and will require considerable additional effort to be further refined. Future studies will focus on (a) the identification of novel tumor-associated genes and gene loci, (b) the characterization of patterns of complementary genetic changes, (c) a molecular differentiation of morphologically homogeneous tumor entities, and (d) the use of molecular genetic parameters as novel diagnostic and prognostic criteria. It is to be expected that these studies will have a major impact on both diagnostic and clinical neurooncology.

Acknowledgments. We gratefully acknowledge our colleagues who have contributed to these studies, in particular D.N. Louis, K. v. Ammon, P. Kleihues, H. Ohgaki, I. Petersen, J. Schramm, B.R. Seizinger, M.G. Yasargil, and many enthusiastic students and young coworkers in Bonn. Our research is supported by grants from the DFG (Sonderforschungsbereich 400), and by a center grant from the University of Bonn Medical Center and the State of Nordrhein-Westfalen.

References

1. Kleihues P, Burger PC, Scheithauer BW (1994) Histological typing of tumors of the central nervous system, 2nd edn, WHO international classification of tumors. Springer, Berlin Heidelberg New York
2. Bigner SH, Burger PC, Wong AJ, Werner MH, Hamilton SR, Muhlbaier LH, Vogelstein B, Bigner DD (1988) Gene amplification in malignant human gliomas: clinical and histopathologic aspects. J Neuropathol & Exp Neurol 47:191-205
3. Hurtt MR, Moossy J, Donovan-Peluso M, Locker J (1992) Amplification of epidermal growth factor receptor gene in gliomas: histopathology and prognosis. J Neuropathol & Exp Neurol 51:84-90
4. Jen J, Harper JW, Bigner SH, Bigner DD, Papadopoulos N, Markowitz S, Willson JKV, Kinzler KW, Vogelstein B (1994) Detection of p16 and p15 genes in brain tumors. Cancer Res 54:6353-6358
5. Hunter T, Pines J (1994) Cyclins and cancer: cyclin D and CDK inhibitors come of age. Cell 79:573-582
6. Ohgaki H, Eibl RH, Schwab M, Reichel M, Mariani L, Gehring M, Petersen I, Höll T, Wiestler OD, Kleihues P (1993) Mutations of the p53 tumor suppressor gene in neoplasms of the human nervous system. Mol Carcinog 8:74-80
7. von Deimling A, Bender B, Louis DN, Wiestler OD (1993) A rapid and nonradioactive PCR-based assay for the detection of allelic loss in human tumors. Neuropathol Appl Neurobiol 19:524-529
8. Garner A, Klinworth GK (1982) Tumors of the orbit, optic nerve and lacrimal sack. Dekker, New York
9. Lewis RA, Gerson LP, Axelson KA, Riccardi VM, Whitford RP (1984) Von Recklinghausen neurofibromatosis. II. Incidence of optic gliomata. Ophthalmology 91:929
10. von Deimling A, Louis DN, Menon AG, von Ammon K, Petersen I, Ellison D, Wiestler OD, Seizinger BR (1993) Deletions on the long arm of chromosome 17 in pilocytic astrocytoma. Acta Neuropathol 86:81-85
11. Xu G, O'Connell P, Viskochil D, Cawthon R, Robertson M, Culver M, Dunn D, Stevens J, Gesteland R, White R, Weiss R (1990) The neurofibromatosis type 1 gene encodes a protein related to GAP. Cell 62:599-608
12. Han J-W, McCormick F, Macara IG (1991) Regulation of ras-GAP and the neurofibromatosis 1 gene product by eicosanoids. Science 252:576-579
13. DeClue JE, Papageorge AG, Fletcher JA, Diehl SR, Ratner N, Vass WC, Lowy DR (1992) Abnormal regulation of mammalian p21ras contributes to malignant tumor growth in von Recklinghausen (type 1) neurofibromatosis. Cell 69:265-273
14. Cawthon RM, Weiss R, Xu G, Viskochil D, Culver M, Stevens J, Robertson M, Dunn D, Gesteland R, O'Connell P, White R (1990) A major segment of the neurofibromatosis type 1 gene: cDNA sequence, genomic structure, and point mutations. Cell 62:193-201
15. Viskochil D, Buchberg AM, Xu G, Cawthon RM, Stevens J, Wolff RK, Culver M, Carey JC, Copeland NG, Jenkins NA, White R, O'Connell P (1990) Deletions and a translocation interrupt a cloned gene at the neurofibromatosis type 1 locus. Cell 62:187-192
16. Wallace MR, Marchuk DA, Andersen LB, Letcher R, Odeh HM, Saulino AM, Fountain JW, Brereton A, Nicholson J, Mitchell AL, Brownstein BH, Collins FS (1990) Type 1 neurofibromatosis gene: identification of a large transcript disrupted in three NF1 patients. Science 249:181-186
17. Stark M, Assunm G, Krone W (1991) A small deletion and an adjacent base exchange in a potential stem-loop region of the neurofibromatosis 1 gene. Hum Genet 87:685-687
18. Li Y, Bollag G, Clark R, Stevens J, Conroy L, Fults D, Ward K, Friedman E, Samowitz W, Robertson M, Bradley P, Cawthon R (1992) Somatic mutations in the neurofibromatosis 1 gene in human tumors. Cell 69:275-281
19. Fults D, Tippets RH, Thomas GA, Nakamura Y, White R (1989) Loss of heterozygosity for loci on chromosome 17p in human malignant astrocytoma. Cancer Res 49:6572-6577
20. James CD, Carlbom E, Nordenskjold M, Collins VP, Cavenee WK (1989) Mitotic recombination of chromosome 17 in astrocytomas. Proc Natl Acad Sci USA 86:2858-2862

21. von Deimling A, Eibl RH, Ohgaki H, Louis DN, von Ammon K, Petersen I, Kleihues P, Chung RY, Wiestler OD, Seizinger BR (1992) p53 mutations are associated with 17p allelic loss in grade II and grade III astrocytoma. Cancer Res 52:2987–2990

22. Nigro JM, Baker SJ, Preisinger AC, Jessup JM, Hostetter R, Cleary K, Bigner SH, Davidson N, Baylin S, Devilee P, Glover T, Collins FC, Weston A, Modali R, Harris CC, Vogelstein B (1989) Mutations in the p53 gene occur in diverse tumor types. Nature 342:705–708

23. Takahashi T, D'Amico D, Chiba I, Buchhagen DL, Minna JD (1990) Identification of intronic point mutations as an alternative mechanism for p53 inactivation in lung cancer. J Clin Invest 86:363–369

24. Hollstein M, Sidransky D, Vogelstein B, Harris CC (1991) p53 mutations in human cancers. Science 253:49–53

25. Baker SJ, Preisinger AC, Jessup JM, Paraskeva C, Markowitz S, Wilson JKV, Hamilton SR, Vogelstein B (1990) p53 mutations occur in combination with 17p allele deletions as late events in colorectal tumorigenesis. Cancer Res 50:7717–7722

26. Knudson AG (1993) Antioncogenes and human cancer. Proc Natl Acad Sci USA 90:10914–10921

27. El-Azouzi M, Chung RY, Farmer GE, Martuza RL, Black PM, Rouleau GA, Hettlich C, Hedley-Whyte ET, Zervas NT, Panagopoulos K, Nakamura Y, Gusella J, Seizinger BR (1989) Loss of distinct regions on the short arm of chromosome 17 associated with tumorigenesis of human astrocytomas. Proc Natl Acad Sci USA 86:7186–7190

28. Venter DJ, Thomas DGT (1991) Multiple sequential molecular abnormalities in the evolution of human gliomas. Br J Cancer 63:753–757

29. James CD, He J, Carlbom E, Nordenskjold M, Cavenee WK, Collins VP (1991) Chromosome 9 deletion mapping reveals interferon α and interferon β-1 gene deletions in human glial tumors. Cancer Res 51:1684–1688

30. Olopade OI, Jenkins RB, Ransom DT, Malik K, Pomykala H, Nobori T, Cowan JM, Rowley JD, Diaz MO (1992) Molecular analysis of deletions of the short arm of chromosome 9 in human gliomas. Cancer Res 52:2523–2529

31. Sidransky D, Mikkelsen T, Schwechheimer K, Rosenblum ML, Cavenee W, Vogelstein B (1992) Clonal expansion of p53 mutant cells is associated with brain tumour progression. Nature 355:846–847

32. von Deimling A, Bender B, Jahnke R, Waha A, Albrecht S, Wellenreuther R, Fassbender F, Nagel J, Kraus J, Menon AG, Louis DN, Lenartz D, Schramm J, Wiestler OD (1994) Loci associated with malignant progression in astrocytomas: a candidate on chromosome 19q. Cancer Res 54:1–5

33. von Deimling A, Nagel J, Bender B, Lenartz D, Schramm J, Louis DN, Wiestler OD (1994) Deletion mapping of a putative tumor suppressor gene on chromosome 19q associated with human gliomas. Int J Cancer 57:676–680

34. Burger PC, Green SB (1987) Patient age, histologic features, and length of survival in patients with glioblastoma multiforme. Cancer 59:1617–1625

35. Winger MJ, Macdonald DR, Cairncross JG (1989) Supratentorial anaplastic gliomas in adults. J Neurosurg 71:487–493

36. James CD, Carlblom E, Dumanski JP, Hansen M, Nordenskjold M, Collins VP, Cavenee WK (1988) Clonal genomic alterations in glioma malignancy stages. Cancer Res 48:5546–5551

37. Fujimoto M, Fults DW, Thomas GA, Nakamura Y, Heilbrun MP, White R, Story JL, Naylor SL, Kagan-Hallet KS, Sheridan PJ (1989) Loss of heterozygosity on chromosome 10 in human glioblastoma. Genomics 4:210–214

38. Fults D, Pedone CA, Thomas GA, White R (1990) Allelotype of human malignant astrocytoma. Cancer Res 50:5784–5789

39. Watanabe K, Nagai M, Arai T, Kawashima K (1990) Loss of constitutional heterozygosity in chromosome 10 in human glioblastoma. Acta Neuropathol 80:251–254

40. von Deimling A, von Ammon K, Schoenfeld D, Wiestler OD, Seizinger BR, Louis DN (1993) Subsets of glioblastoma multiforme defined by molecular genetic analysis. Brain Pathol 3:19–26

41. von Deimling A, Louis DN, von Ammon K, Petersen I, Hoell T, Chung RY, Martuza R, Schoenfeld D, Yasargil MG, Wiestler OD, Seizinger BR (1992) Association of epidermal

growth factor receptor gene amplification with loss of chromosome 10 in human glioblastoma multiforme. J Neurosurg 77:295–301

42. von Deimling A, Louis DN, von Ammon K, Petersen I, Wiestler OD, Seizinger BR (1992) Evidence for a tumor suppressor gene on chromosome 19q associated with human astrocytomas, oligodendrogliomas and mixed gliomas. Cancer Res 52:4277–4279

43. Reifenberger G, Reifenberger J, Ichimura K, Meltzer PS, Collins VP (1994) Amplification of multiple genes from chromosomal region 12q13-14 in human malignant gliomas: preliminary mapping of the amplicons shows preferential involvement of CDK4, SAS, and MDM2. Cancer Res 54:4299–4303

Molecular Genetics of Oligodendroglial Tumors

G. Reifenberger[1], J. Reifenberger[1], L. Liu[2], C.D. James[3], W. Wechsler[1], and V.P. Collins[2]

Abstract. This review discusses molecular genetic alterations associated with the development and progression of oligodendroglial tumors of the central nervous system. The current data suggest that early events in the oncogenesis of oligodendroglial tumors are distinct from those associated with astrocytomas and ependymomas and characteristically involve the loss of genetic information from chromosome arms 19q and 1p. The target genes of these deletions are not identified yet. However, the chromosomal position of the suspected oligodendroglioma-associated tumor suppressor gene on 19q has already been narrowed down to an area of about 5 megabases at 19q13.2–19q13.3. In contrast to astroglial neoplasms, allelic loss on 17p or mutations of the *TP53* tumor suppressor gene appear to be rare in oligodendroglial neoplasms. However, similarities between molecular genetic alterations in astroglial and oligodendroglial tumors are indicated by allelic losses on 9p and 10 and amplification of the epidermal growth factor receptor gene in anaplastic tumors, suggesting the utilization of common pathways in the progression of glial tumors.

Key words. Oligodendroglioma—Molecular genetics—Oncogenes—Tumor suppressor genes—Loss of heterozygosity

Introduction

The oligodendrocyte was first described as a distinct glial cell type in the central nervous system by the Scottish pathologist W.F. Robertson in 1900 [1]. Robertson believed these cells to be of mesodermal origin and therefore named them "mesoglia." This term was abandoned by the later studies of del Rio-Hortega [2], Penfield [3], and Bailey and Hiller [4], which firmly established to oligodendrocyte as a cytological entity and clearly demonstrated the morphological differences distinguishing it from astrocytes and microglia. In addition, these classical studies already suggested that

[1] Department of Neuropathology, Heinrich-Heine-University, 40225 Düsseldorf, Germany
[2] Ludwig Institute for Cancer Research, Stockholm Branch, and Institute for Oncology and Pathology, Division of Tumor Pathology, Karolinska Hospital, S-17176 Stockholm, Sweden
[3] Laboratory of Molecular Neuro-Oncology, Department of Neurosurgery, Emory University, Atlanta, GA 30322, USA

oligodendrocytes are of neuroectodermal origin and play a role in the formation and maintenance of myelin in the central nervous system.

The first description of an oligodendroglioma was published by Bailey and Cushing in 1926 [5], and 3 years later the classical work of Bailey and Bucy on "Oligodendrogliomas of the brain" appeared [6]. These authors provided the first comprehensive description of the clinical and pathological characteristics of this tumor type. They noted that oligodendrogliomas are relatively slow growing tumors that are frequently calcified and preferentially occur in the cerebral hemispheres of adults. Using silver impregnation techniques they could already demonstrate that, in addition to the neoplastic oligodendrocytes, other glial cells such as astrocytes and, more frequently, transitional cells between oligodendrocytes and astrocytes may be present in these tumors, and thus the concept of mixed oligoastrocytomas was outlined. Since the publication of this landmark paper, a large number of studies have confirmed and extended the original findings of Bailey and Bucy and described in detail the clinical, neuroradiological, and neuropathological characteristics of oligodendrogliomas (for review, see [7–9]).

Before discussing recent results on the molecular genetics of oligodendroglial tumors we briefly review some general characteristics of oligodendroglial tumors and particularly focus on the morphological criteria forming the basis for their histopathological classification. This appears to us of great importance for a reasonable discussion of correlations between morphological features and biological behavior on the one hand and molecular genetic alterations on the other hand. We classify our tumors according to the WHO classification of tumors of the central nervous system [10], and we strongly argue for the general use of this classification as the morphological baseline to facilitate comparison of scientific results from different laboratories around the world.

Clinical and Neuropathological Characteristics of Oligodendroglial Tumors

The frequency of oligodendroglial tumors is estimated to be between 5% and 18% of all gliomas [7,8]. The peak incidence lies in the fifth and sixth decades of life [11]. Men appear to be slightly more frequently affected than women, with ratios ranging from 3:2 [11] to 2:1 [12]. With respect to the localization of oligodendrogliomas, the vast majority occur in the cerebral hemispheres with preference for the frontal and temporal lobes [7,8,13]. More rarely, oligodendrogliomas may originate in the brainstem, cerebellum, or spinal cord.

The WHO classification of tumors of the central nervous system [10] lists two subtypes in the group of oligodendroglial tumors, namely the oligodendrogliomas of WHO grade II and the anaplastic (malignant) oligodendrogliomas of WHO grade III. By definition, both are composed predominantly of neoplastic oligodendrocytes. Macroscopically, oligodendroglial tumors typically appear as solid greyish-pink masses growing in the cerebral cortex and subcortical white matter. Infiltration of the leptomeninges is common as is central cystic degeneration and calcification, usually accentuated in the peripheral parts of the tumor. Histologically, WHO grade II oligodendrogliomas are moderately cellular neoplasms characterized by uniformity of cellular and nuclear size and shape. The tumor cells typically have round hyperchromatic nuclei, an artifactually swollen clear cytoplasm, and a well-defined plasma membrane. This characteristic "fried-egg" or "honeycomb" appearence, although representing a fixation artifact, is a very distinctive diagnostic feature of oligodendrogliomas. Other histological hallmarks include focal calcifications and a typical capillary vascularization pattern often referred to as "chicken-wired." In addition, oligodendrogliomas tend to infiltrate the cerebral cortex where they form so-called secondary structures such as perinuclear satellitosis, perivascular accumulation, and subpial aggregations.

In contrast to the well-differentiated oligodendrogliomas, anaplastic oligodendrogliomas (WHO grade III) are characterized by signs of increased anaplasia such as high cellularity, nuclear polymorphism, increased mitotic activity, vascular proliferations, and foci of necrosis [10]. In some anaplastic oligodendrogliomas, polymorphic multinucleated giant cells may be numerous ("polymorphous variant") [7]. With regard to grading and prognosis of oligodendroglial tumors, Burger et al. [14] reported necrosis and increased mitotic activity as the most significant criteria. According to Smith et al. [15], necrosis and pleomorphism were the best indicators for anaplasia while microcysts appeared to be related to a better prognosis. Similar results were reported by Mørk et al. [16], who found necrosis, cell density, and microcysts the most important prognostic parameters in oligodendroglial tumors.

The classification of mixed oligoastrocytomas may be difficult with regard to the distinction from "pure" oligodendroglial or astroglial tumors. According to the WHO classification [10], an oligoastrocytoma is "a tumor with a conspicious mixture of neoplastic oligodendrocytes and astrocytes, either diffusely intermingled or separated into distinct areas." For those tumors in which the two components are geographically distinct, there is general agreement that the classification of such lesions as oligoastrocytoma is appropriate. However, the situation becomes controversial for cases with a diffuse admixture of oligodendroglial and astrocytic elements because astroglial tumor cells may be present in oligodendrogliomas, as already noted by Bailey and Bucy [6], and particularly "anaplastic oligodendrogliomas often contain a significant admixture of neoplastic astrocytes" [10]. As a guideline, Mørk et al. [16] distinguished oligoastrocytomas from oligodendrogliomas by the presence of at least 25% neoplastic astrocytes. While this figure may be of some help, in many cases it is difficult to determine an exact percentage because of the considerable morphological overlap of neoplastic glial cells and the variable degree to which the whole tumor has been sampled. Thus, in practice we use the definition of the WHO classification and only diagnose an oligoastrocytoma in cases with unequivocal and substantial astrocytic and oligodendroglial components.

Immunohistochemically, oligodendrogliomas are consistently positive for the carbohydrate epitope recognized by the monoclonal antibody anti-Leu-7 (CD57) and for S100 protein [17–19]. Immunoreactivity for γ-enolase (the so-called neuron-specific enolase) is also frequently found [20]. However, immunoreactivity for these antigens is not specific for oligodendrogliomas and is also found in many other types of neuroectodermal tumors [19,21]. Immunoreactivity for glial fibrillary acidic protein (GFAP) in oligodendrogliomas can be present not only in intermingled reactive or neoplastic astrocytes but also in transitional cell forms, for example, the so-called mini-gemistocytes, as well as in typical oligodendroglial tumor cells [18,19,22]. According to Russell and Rubinstein [8], about 50% of the "pure" oligodendrogliomas contain GFAP-immunopositive neoplastic oligodendrocytes.

Thus, immunohistochemistry for GFAP cannot be regarded as a reliable marker for the discrimination between astroglial and oligodendroglial tumor cells.

A number of differentiation antigens specifically expressed by normal oligo-dendrocytes in vivo or in vitro have been identified. These include myelin proteins such as myelin basic protein (MBP), proteolipid protein (PLP), or myelin-associated glycoprotein (MAG), galactolipids like galactocerebroside (GC) or galactosulphatide, certain gangliosides as well as several enzymes such as carbonic anhydrase C, 2'-3'-cyclic nucleotide-3'-phosphatase (CNP), glycerol-3-phosphate dehydrogenase, and lactate dehydrogenase (LDH). However, none of these antigens has gained significance as a diagnostically useful marker for oligodendrogliomas. Either they are no longer expressed by neoplastic oligodendrocytes, as MBP [18,20], or they are expressed in only a minority of cases, as MAG [18], or their expression is not restricted to oligodendroglial tumor cells, for example, carbonic anhydrase C [23]. Whether galactocerebroside is a diagnostically useful marker for oligodendroglial tumors [24] remains to be corroborated.

The primary treatment of oligodendroglial tumors consists of surgical resection, frequently followed by radiation therapy either as part of the initial therapy or at relapse. These therapeutic approaches are usually not curative, as indicated by the reported 10-year survival rates that vary between 10% and 38% [11,13,25]. Thus, the prognosis for oligodendroglioma patients is still relatively poor and very difficult to predict in individual case. Recent studies, however, have suggested that postoperative chemotherapy may significantly prolong survival of patients with anaplastic oligodendroglial tumors and mixed gliomas [26,27].

Cytogenetics and Molecular Genetics of Oligodendroglial Tumors

Until recently, only little was known about the molecular genetic etiology of oligodendroglial tumors because most of the published studies concerning genetic alterations in glial tumors have focused on the more common astrocytomas and glioblastomas. For such tumors, characteristic chromosomal deletions as well as amplification of certain cellular oncogenes have been identified (for review see [28–30]). In addition, mutations in certain tumor suppressor genes, including the TP53 gene on 17p [31–33] and the RB1 gene on 13q [34], as well as homozygous deletions of the MTS1 gene on 9p21 [35–38], have been described in astrocytic tumors. In contrast, knowledge about the gene and chromosomal alterations in oligodendroglial tumors is relatively scarce. However, several groups have recently addressed this topic in greater detail [39–44], and our chapter reviews the current knowledge concerning the cytogenetic and molecular genetic alterations associated with the development and progression of oligodendroglial tumors.

Allelic Losses on the Long Arm of Chromosome 19

Several studies employing restriction fragment length polymorphism (RFLP) analysis have indicated that allelic deletions on 19q occur at high frequency in oligo-dendroglial tumors [39–41,43–44]. According to our own data [43], loss of alleles from chromosome 19q is the most frequent alteration in these tumors and may be detected in more than 80% of cases (Fig. 1). In contrast to the findings of von Deimling et al. [40,41] and Kraus et al. [44], who both described approximately equal frequencies of allelic loss on 19q in oligodendrogliomas and mixed oligoastrocytomas, our results

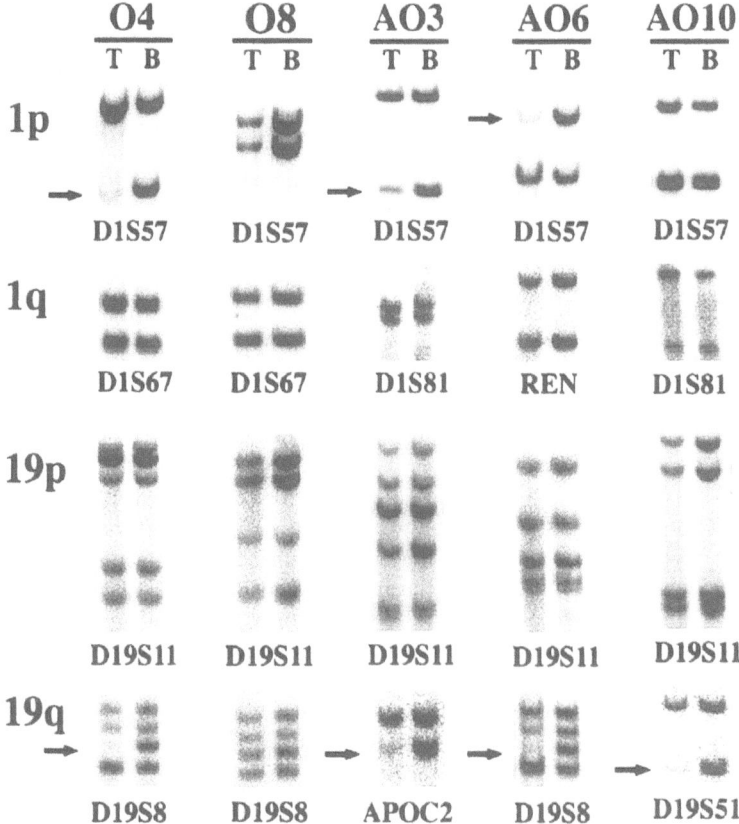

Fig. 1. Examples of loss of heterozygosity (LOH) on chromosomes 1 and 19 in oligodendroglial tumors and mixed gliomas. Case numbers appear at *top* of figure (*O*, oligodendroglioma; *AO*, anaplastic oligodendroglioma; *T*, tumor DNA; *B*, blood DNA; for details see Reifenberger et al. [43]). For each case and chromosome arm, the hybridization result obtained for one selected locus is shown. *Arrows* indicate constitutional alleles absent in corresponding tumor DNAs. The tumors O4, AO3, and AO6 demonstrate LOH on 1p and 19q. Case O8 shows no allelic loss on 1 and 19. The only detectable abnormality in this tumor was an allelic deletion on 11p (not shown). Tumor AO10 has lost alleles on 19q but not on chromosome 1. Densitometric analysis demonstrated simple loss of alleles for all affected loci shown

indicate that the incidence in the latter group may be lower, i.e., in about 30% of cases [43]. In either case, the available data suggest that mixed oligoastrocytomas have clonal genomic alterations. Kraus et al. [44] found the same alterations, i.e., loss of alleles on 19q and 1p, in differentially analyzed oligodendroglial and astroglial tumor parts of three mixed gliomas. These authors suggested a common origin of oligodendrogliomas and oligoastrocytomas. Our data, however, show more heterogeneous alterations in oligoastrocytomas that either resemble those associated with oligodendroglial tumors (allelic losses on 19q and 1p) or those typically seen in astrocytic tumors (allelic losses on 17p) [43].

In most oligodendrogliomas and mixed gliomas with loss of heterozygosity (LOH) on 19q, the losses involve all informative loci on this chromosomal arm, suggesting that most of or even the entire q-arm had been deleted. However, individual cases may demonstrate partial or interstitial losses. This phenomenon allowed us to assign a commonly deleted region to the area distal to the *CYP2a* gene and proximal to the *D19S22* locus, that is, bands 19q13.2 to 19q13.4 [43]. Rubio et al. [45] identified nine gliomas with partial deletions on 19q and were thereby able to further narrow down the chromosomal location of the suspected tumor suppressor gene to an approximately 8-cM/5-megabase region at 19q13.2–19q13.3 between the loci *APOC2* and *HRC*. This region does not include the *D19S8* locus at 19q13.2, which Ransom et al. [39] had described as homozygously deleted in one oligo-dendroglioma.

Alterations of 19q seem not to be restricted to oligodendroglial tumors as cytogenetic studies of glioblastomas have demonstrated structural abnormalities of 19q in a significant percentage of cases [46,47]. According to Bigner et al. [46], a clustering of breakpoints occurred at 19q13 in glioblastomas, a finding that fits very well to the commonly deleted region in gliomas as determined by LOH analyses [43,45]. In addition, allelic loss on 19q has been demonstrated in about 40% of anaplastic astrocytomas, 25% of glioblastomas, but less than 20% of WHO grade II astrocytomas [40,41,44,48]. Therefore, it has been suggested that 19q also contains a tumor suppressor gene involved in the progression of astrocytic tumors [48].

Taken in combination, these findings indicate that the inactivation of one or more tumor suppressor gene(s) on the q-arm of chromosome 19 is of importance in the majority of oligodendroglial tumors as well as in a considerable fraction of mixed gliomas, anaplastic astrocytomas, and glioblastomas. At present, the identification of the target gene(s) is complicated by the relatively large region of interest covering approximately 5 megabases at 19q13.2 to 19q13.3. The development of additional markers in this region and the examination of more oligodendroglial tumors will likely lead to the identification of cases with small interstitial deletions, thereby permitting a narrowing of the chromosomal localization of the suspected tumor suppressor gene(s). This would allow the use of positional cloning methods for gene identification and cloning. In addition, a candidate gene approach seems to be reason-able because a number of potential tumor suppressor genes have already been mapped to this region. These include such interesting genes as *ERCC1*, *ERCC2*, and the gene for DNA-ligase 1 (*LIG1*), which all code for enzymes involved in DNA excision and repair, the interleukin 11 (*IL11*) gene, and several genes coding for zinc-finger proteins [49,50]. The *XRCC1* gene, another DNA excision and repair gene at 19q13.2, has already been excluded as a candidate because it maps centromeric to the commonly deleted region in gliomas [45]. With regard to the *ERCC1* and *ERCC2* genes, Southern hybridization revealed that both genes frequently showed loss of one allele, and no gross rearrangement of the remaining alleles were seen [43]. Northern blot hybridizations also showed no loss of mRNA expression or aberrant transcripts in oligodendrogliomas. It remains to be shown whether more subtle changes such as point mutations are present in these two or any of the other candidate genes within the deleted region.

Allelic Losses on the Short Arm of Chromosome 1

Allelotyping of oligodendroglial tumors has demonstrated that the second most fre-quent genetic alteration in these neoplasms is the loss of alleles on the short arm of chromosome 1 [43–44] (see Fig. 1). According to our data, LOH on 1p occurs in about 67% (14/21) of the oligodendroglial tumors and 19% (3/16) of the oligoastrocytomas

[43]. These findings are in line with the results of two other recent studies. Bello et al. [42] found LOH on 1p in 6 of 6 oligodendrogliomas, 5 of 6 anaplastic oligodendrogliomas, and 2 of 3 oligoastrocytomas, while the incidences in the series of Kraus et al. [44] were 33% (3/9) in oligodendrogliomas, 50% (3/6) in anaplastic oligodendrogliomas, 50% (6/12) in oligoastrocytomas, and 46% (6/13) in anaplastic oligoastrocytomas. Earlier RFLP studies on small numbers of oligodendrogliomas had reported LOH on 1p in 3 oligodendrogliomas [39,51]. Taking these data together, it is evident that allelic deletions on 1p are frequent in oligodendroglial tumors as well as in mixed gliomas and appear to occur in all WHO malignancy grades. A striking coincidence of LOH on 1p with allelic deletions on 19q (Fig. 1) was noted in our series [43] as well as in the cases of Kraus et al. [44]. This finding may suggest a synergistic effect of both alterations with regard to the provision of a selective growth advantage to the affected oligodendroglial cells.

The frequent LOH on 1p in oligodendroglial tumors determined by molecular genetic methods was anticipated by several cytogenetic studies that had reported karyotypic abnormalities of this chromosome, especially translocations involving the p-arm [39,47,52,53]. Structural and numerical aberrations of chromosome 1 as well as LOH for loci on 1p are not specific to oligodendrogliomas and have been demonstrated in a variety of other tumor types including neuroblastoma [54], malignant melanoma [55], medulloblastoma [56], male germ cell tumors [57], meningioma [58–60], and certain epithelial tumors [61–64]. With regard to nonoligodendroglial gliomas, several cytogenetic studies have demonstrated that alterations of 1p are present in a significant fraction of glioblastomas [46,47,65,66]. These data were recently supplemented by molecular cytogenetic studies employing comparative genomic hybridization that reported loss of genetic information from 1p in more than 40% of the glioblastomas [67]. In contrast, previous LOH studies did not report loss of alleles on chromosome 1 as a particularly frequent event in glioblastomas [51,66,68]. These studies had analyzed only few loci on chromosome 1 and might therefore have underestimated the frequency of LOH on this chromosome. However, two more recent RFLP studies analyzed multiple loci and also found a relatively low incidence of LOH on 1p in astrocytomas and glioblastomas [42,44]. Together these two studies found losses on 1p in only 5 of 98 low- and high-grade astrocytomas (5%) and 8 of 90 glioblastomas (9%) [42,44]. Thus, it appears that alterations of 1p seem to be less frequent in astrocytic than in oligodendroglial tumors.

With regard to the exact chromosomal localization of the oligodendroglioma-associated tumor suppressor gene on 1p, we identified only one case with a partial deletion of 1p indicating a position distal to the NGFB locus on 1p13 [43]. Most oligodendrogliomas had LOH at all informative loci on 1p, a result also observed by Bello et al. [42]. However, these authors found one oligodendroglioma with a terminal retention of heterozygosity at the D1Z2 locus (1p36.3) and a glioblastoma with an interstitial deletion between D1S57 and D1Z2 (1p32–1p36.3).

In summary, current data suggest that 1p contains at least one tumor suppressor gene whose inactivation, in addition to the one suspected on 19q, is of significance in the development of oligodendroglial tumors. Whether this putative tumor suppressor gene on 1p is the same as the one affected in neuroblastomas or other types of tumors remains to be determined. Recent studies on breast carcinomas and male germ cell tumors indicate that more than one tumor suppressor gene may be located on this chromosome arm [57,69]. Future studies should aim at narrowing down the exact chromosomal position of the oligodendroglioma-associated tumor suppressor gene on 1p by analyzing a larger number of cases with multiple markers. This will hopefully lead to the identification of cases with small interstitial deletions that would eventually facilitate the positional cloning of this gene or genes.

Allelic Losses on 17p and *TP53* Mutations

Allelic deletions on 17p are present in about 35% of astrocytic tumors of all malignancy grades [70–72] and are frequently associated with mutation of the remaining *TP53* tumor suppressor gene allele [31–33]. According to our results the frequency of allelic deletions on 17p is much lower in oligodendroglial tumors (<10%), whereas the incidence in mixed gliomas (31%) was nearly the same as observed for astrocytomas [43]. It is noteworthy that in the mixed gliomas LOH on 17p only occurred in cases without LOH on 19q and 1p [43].

A study by Oghaki et al. [73] found mutations of the *TP53* gene in 2 of 17 oligodendrogliomas (12%). Rasheed et al. [74] detected LOH on 17p and mutation of *TP53* in 1 of 11 (9%) oligodendrogliomas. In our series, sequencing of the *TP53* transcripts from exon 2 to 10 revealed no mutation in 9 tumors (3 anaplastic oligodendrogliomas, 3 oligoastrocytomas, and 3 anaplastic oligoastrocytomas), including 7 cases with LOH on 17p encompassing the *TP53* gene. Thus, in contrast to the situation in astrocytic tumors, allelic deletions on 17p in oligodendroglial tumors and mixed gliomas seem not to be closely associated with *TP53* mutations. This finding suggests that a second tumor suppressor gene may reside on 17p, a hypothesis supported by studies on breast cancers [75], medulloblastomas [76,77], and astrocytomas [78] that identified tumors either showing a lack of association between 17p deletions and *TP53* mutations or 17p deletions distal to the *TP53* locus. In addition, the recent experimental study has provided functional evidence for a second tumor suppressor gene on 17p [79]. Thus, a second tumor suppressor gene on 17p could be of importance in a fraction of oligodendrogliomas and mixed gliomas. In contrast to astrocytic tumors, genomic alterations of the *TP53* gene seem to be of minor significance in oligodendroglial tumors.

Genetic Alterations Associated with the Progression of Oligodendroglial Tumors

The data discussed so far indicate that the primary genetic alterations in oligodendroglial tumors differ from those associated with the development of astrocytomas. However, when it comes to alterations related to the progression from low-grade (WHO grade II) to high-grade (WHO grade III and IV) lesions, gliomas appear to utilize common pathways. This statement is based on our finding that anaplastic oligodendrogliomas and anaplastic mixed gliomas frequently show additional LOH on 9p and 10 (Fig. 2) [43]. Both are genetic alterations that have already been associated with the progression of astrocytic tumors (for review see [28,30]). Previous cytogenetic studies on small numbers of anaplastic oligodendrogliomas and mixed gliomas have already described individual cases with structural alterations of 9p [46–47]. In the RFLP study of James et al. [80], 1 of 2 analyzed anaplastic oligodendrogliomas had lost alleles on 9p. Occasional cases of anaplastic oligodendrogliomas and mixed gliomas with deletions of chromosome 10 have been reported by several groups [39,51,81,82]. With regard to the genes involved in these progression-associated genetic alterations, recent studies suggest that homozygous loss of the *CDKN2* (*p16/MTS1*) gene on 9p21 appears to be the

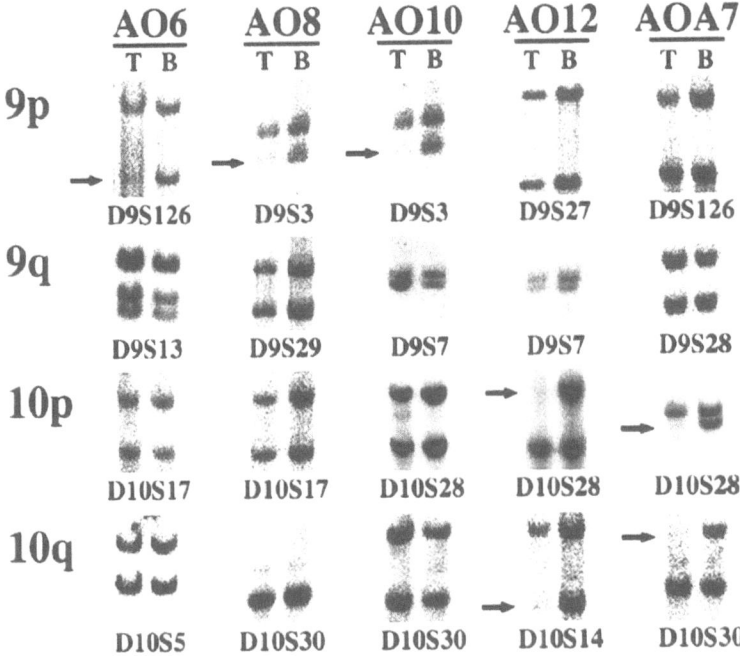

Fig. 2. Examples of LOH on 9p and 10 in anaplastic oligodendrogliomas and oligoastrocytomas. Case numbers appear at *top* of figure (*AO*, anaplastic oligodendroglioma; *AOA*, anaplastic oligoastrocytoma; *T*, tumor DNA; *B*, blood DNA; for details see Reifenberger et al. [43]). For each case and chromosome arm, the hybridization result obtained for one selected locus is shown. *Arrows* indicate constitutional alleles absent in corresponding tumor DNAs. Tumors AO6, AO8, and AO10 had LOH at loci on chromosome 9p while AO12 and AOA7 had lost alleles at all informative loci on chromosome 10

relevant event targeted for by allelic deletions on 9p in anaplastic astrocytomas and glioblastomas [35–38]. We assume that inactivation of this gene is also involved in the progression of oligodendroglial tumors; however, this hypothesis warrants experimental corroboration. Unfortunately, none of the suspected tumor suppressor genes on chromosome 10 associated with the progression of glial tumors has been identified so far.

In addition to specific chromosomal losses, anaplastic oligodendroglial tumors and mixed gliomas show an increased incidence of multiple allelic losses on several different chromosomes [43]. This apparent accumulation of genetic alterations associated with tumor progression has also been well documented for astroglial neoplasms [28]. Furthermore, anaplastic oligodendrogliomas and mixed gliomas may demonstrate amplification of certain cellular oncogenes [43]. In a series of 29 such tumors we found one anaplastic oligoastrocytoma with amplification of the *EGFR* gene, one anaplastic oligodendroglioma with a coamplification of *EGFR* and the renin gene, and one anaplastic oligodendroglioma with a coamplification of the *MYC* gene with *CDK4* and *SAS* (Fig. 3). Thus, the incidence of gene amplification in anaplastic oligodendroglial and mixed oligoastrocytomas of WHO grade III approximately equals the incidence of gene amplification reported for anaplastic astrocytomas of WHO grade III [28].

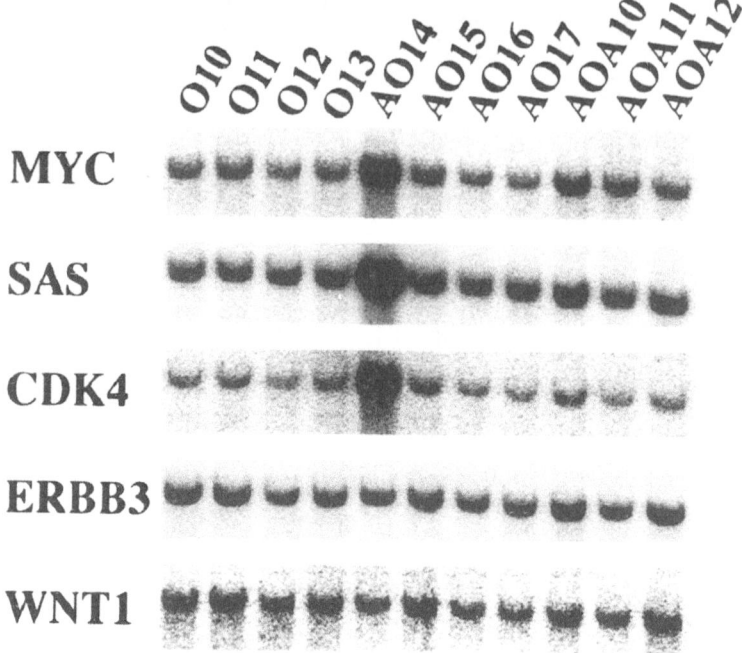

Fig. 3. Analysis of gene amplification in anaplastic oligodendrogliomas and oligoastrocytomas. These hybridization results were obtained on a Southern blot sequentially probed for the oncogenes *MYC*, *CDK4*, *SAS*, *WNT1*, and *ERBB3* in a series of oligodendroglial tumors and mixed gliomas. Case numbers appear at top of figure (only tumor DNA was loaded on this blot). Note gene amplification of *MYC*, *CDK4*, and *SAS* in tumor AO14. None of the tumors shows amplification of *WNT1* or *ERBB3*.

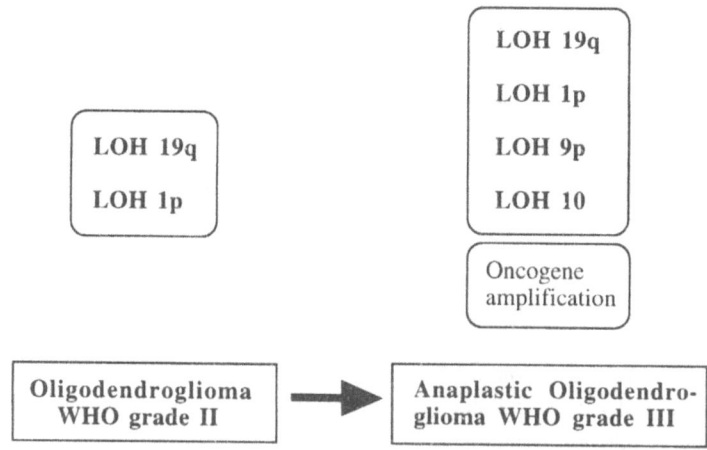

Fig. 4. Graphical summary of the molecular genetic alterations in oligodendroglial tumors. Oligodendrogliomas of WHO grade II typically show LOH on chromosome arms 19q and 1p. In anaplastic oligodendrogliomas of WHO grade III, additional allelic losses occur that most frequently affect the short arm of chromosome 9 and chromosome 10. Amplification of certain oncogenes such as *EGFR* or *CDK4/SAS* may occur in about 10% of anaplastic oligodendrogliomas

Conclusions

Recent studies have provided important new insights into the molecular genetic alterations associated with the development and progression of oligodendroglial tumors. As discussed in this review and summarized in Fig. 4, the present data suggest that the early events in the oncogenesis of oligodendroglial tumors are distinct from those associated with astroglial tumors and characteristically involve the loss of genetic information from 19q and 1p. The tumor suppressor genes targeted for by theses deletions remain to be identified. In contrast to astrocytic tumors, allelic loss on 17p and/or mutations of the *TP53* gene appear to be of minor significance in oligodendroglial neoplasms. However, similarities between molecular genetic alterations in astrocytic and oligodendroglial tumors are indicated by losses of alleles on 9p, 10, and amplification of the *EGFR* gene in the anaplastic tumors, suggesting the utilization of common pathways in the progression of glial tumors.

References

1. Robertson WF (1900) A microscopic demonstration of the normal and pathological histology of mesoglia cells. J Ment Sci 46:724
2. del Rio-Hortega P (1921) Estudios sobre la neuroglía. La glía de escasas radiaciones (oligodendroglía). Bol Soc Esp Hist Nat 21:63–92
3. Penfield W (1924) Oligodendroglia and its relation to classical neuroglia. Brain 47:430–452
4. Bailey P, Hiller G (1924) The interstitial tissues of the central nervous system: a review. J Nerv Ment Dis 59:337–361
5. Bailey P, Cushing H (1926) A classification of the tumors of the glioma group on a histogenetic basis with a correlated study of prognosis. Lippincott, Philadelphia
6. Bailey P, Bucy PC (1929) Oligodendrogliomas of the brain. J Pathol Bacteriol 32:735–751
7. Zülch KJ (1986) Brain tumors. Their biology and pathology, 3rd edn. Springer, Berlin Heidelberg New York Tokyo, pp 240–258
8. Russell D, Rubinstein LJ (1989) Pathology of tumors of the nervous system, 5th edn. Arnold, London, pp 172–187
9. Burger PC, Scheithauer BW (1994) Tumors of the central nervous system. Atlas of Tumor pathology, 3rd series, Fasc 10. Armed Forces Institute of Pathology, Washington, DC, pp 107–120
10. Kleihues P, Burger PC, Scheithauer B (1993) Histological typing of tumors of the central nervous system. Springer, Berlin Heidelberg New York Tokyo
11. Mørk SJ, Lindegaard KF, Halvorson TB, Lehmann EH, Solgaard T, Hatlevoll R, Harvei S, Ganz J (1985) Oligodendroglioma: incidence and biological behavior in a defined population. J Neurosurg 63:881–889
12. Chin HW, Hazel JJ, Kim TH, Webster JH (1980) A clinical study of cerebral oligodendrogliomas. Cancer 45:1458–1466
13. Ludwig CL, Smith MT, Godfrey AD, Armbrustmacher VW (1986) A clinicopathological study of 323 patients with oligodendrogliomas. Ann Neurol 19:15–21
14. Burger PC, Rawlings CE, Cox EB, McLendon RE, Schold SC, Bullard DE (1987) Clinicopathologic correlations in the oligodendroglioma. Cancer 59:1345–1352
15. Smith MT, Ludwig CL, Godfrey AD, Armbrustmacher VW (1983) Grading of oligodendrogliomas. Cancer 52:2107–2114
16. Mørk SJ, Halvorsen TB, Lindegaard KF, Eide GE (1986) Oligodendroglioma. Histologic evaluation and prognosis. J Neuropathol Exp Neurol 45:65–78
17. Motoi M, Yoshino T, Hayashi K, Nose S, Horie Y, Ogawa K (1985) Immunohistochemical

studies on human brain tumors using anti-Leu 7 monoclonal antibody in paraffin-embedded specimens. Acta Neuropathol 66:75–77

18. Nakagawa Y, Perentes E, Rubinstein LJ (1986) Immunohistochemical characterization of oligodendrogliomas: an analysis of multiple markers. Acta Neuropathol 72:15–22

19. Reifenberger G, Szymas J, Wechsler W (1987) Differential expression of glial- and neuronal-associated antigens in human tumors of the central nervous system. Acta Neuropathol 74:105–123

20. Reifenberger G (1991) Immunhistochemie der Tumoren des Zentralnervensystems. Springer, Berlin

21. Perentes E, Rubinstein LJ (1986) Immunohistochemical recognition of human neuroepithelial tumors by anti-Leu 7 (HNK-1) monoclonal antibody. Acta Neuropathol 69:227–233

22. Herpers MJHM, Budka H (1984) Glial fibrillary acidic protein (GFAP) in oligodendroglial tumors: gliofibrillary oligodendroglioma and transitional oligoastrocytoma as subtypes of oligodendroglioma. Acta Neuropathol 64:265–272

23. Nakagawa Y, Perentes E, Rubinstein LJ (1987) Non-specificity of anti-carbonic anhydrase C antibody as a marker in human neuro-oncology. J Neuropathol Exp Neurol 46:451–460

24. de la Monte SM (1989) Uniform lineage of oligodendrogliomas. Am J Pathol 135:529–540

25. Sun ZM, Genka S, Shitara N, Akanuma A, Takakura K (1988) Factors possibly influencing the prognosis of oligodendroglioma. Neurosurgery 22:886–891

26. Cairncross JG, Macdonald DR, Ramsay DA (1992) Aggressive oligodendroglioma: a chemosensitive tumor. Neurosurgery 31:78–82

27. Glass J, Hochberg FH, Gruber ML, Louis DN, Smith D, Rattner B (1992) The treatment of oligodendrogliomas and mixed oligodendroglioma-astrocytomas with PCV chemotherapie. J Neurosurg 76:741–745

28. Collins VP, James CD (1993) Gene and chromosomal alterations associated with the development of human gliomas. FASEB J 7:926–930

29. Wong AJ, Zoltick PW, Moscatello DK (1994) The molecular biology and molecular genetics of astrocytic neoplasms. Semin Onco 21:139–148

30. Batra SK, Rasheed BKA, Bigner SH, Bigner DD (1994) Oncogenes and anti-oncogenes in human central nervous system tumors. Lab Invest 71:621–637

31. Fults D, Brockmeyer D, Tullous MW, Pedone CA, Cawthon RM (1992) p53 mutation and loss of heterozygosity on chromosome 17 and 10 during human astrocytoma progression. Cancer Res 52:674–679

32. Frankel R, Bayonu W, Koslow M, Newcomb EW (1992) p53 mutations in human malignant gliomas: comparison of loss of heterozygosity with mutation frequency. Cancer Res 52:1427–1433

33. von Deimling A, Eibl RH, Ohagaki H, Louis DN, von Ammon K, Petersen I, Kleihues P, Chung RY, Wiestler OD, Seizinger BR (1992) p53 mutations are associated with 17p allelic loss in grade II and grade III astrocytoma. Cancer Res 52:2987–2990

34. Henson JW, Schnitker BL, Correa KM, von Deimling A, Fassbender F, Xu HJ, Benedict WF, Yandell DW, Louis DN (1994) The retinoblastoma gene is involved in malignant progression of astrocytomas. Ann Neurol 36:714–721

35. He J, Allen JR, Collins VP, Allalunis-Turner MJ, Godbout R, Day RS III, James CD (1994) CDK4 amplification is an alternative mechanism to p16 gene homozygous deletion in glioma cell lines. Cancer Res 54:5804–5807

36. Schmidt EE, Ichimura K, Reifenberger G, Collins VP (1994) CDKN2 (p16/MTS1) gene deletion or CDK4 amplification occurs in the majority of glioblastomas. Cancer Res 54:6321–6324

37. Jen J, Harper JW, Bigner SH, Bigner DD, Papadopoulos N, Markowitz S, Willson JKV, Kinzler KW, Vogelstein B (1994) Deletion of p16 and p15 genes in brain tumors. Cancer Res 54:6353–6358

38. Walker DG, Duan W, Popovic EA, Kaye AH, Tomlinson FH, Lavin M (1995) Homozygous deletions of the multiple tumor suppressor gene 1 in the progression of human astrocytomas. Cancer Res 55:20–23

39. Ransom DT, Ritland SR, Kimmel DW, Moertel CA, Dahl RJ, Scheitauer BW, Kelly

PJ, Jenkins RB (1992) Cytogenetic and loss of heterozygosity studies in ependymomas, pilocytic astrocytomas, and oligodendrogliomas. Genes Chromosomes & Cancer 5: 348–356

40. von Deimling A, Louis DN, von Ammon K, Petersen I, Wiestle OD, Seizinger BR (1992) Evidence for a tumor suppressor gene on chromosome 19q associated with human astrocytomas, oligodendrogliomas, and mixed gliomas. Cancer Res 52:4277–4279

41. von Deimling A, Nagel J, Bender B, Lenartz D, Schramm J, Louis DN, Wiestler OD (1994) Deletion mapping of a putative tumor suppressor gene on chromosome 19q associated with human gliomas. Int J Cancer 57:676–680

42. Bello MJ, Vaquero J, de Campos JM, Kusak ME, Sarasa JL, Saez-Castresana J, Pestana A, Rey JA (1994) Molecular analysis of chromosome 1 abnormalities in human gliomas reveals frequent loss of 1p in oligodendroglial tumors. Int J Cancer 57:172–175

43. Reifenberger J, Reifenberger G, Liu L, James CD, Wechsler W, Collins VP (1994) Molecular genetic analysis of oligodendroglial tumors shows preferential allelic deletions on 19q and 1p. Am J Pathol 145:1175–1190

44. Kraus JA, Koopmann J, Kaskel P, Maintz D, Brandner S, Schramm J, Louis DN, Wiestler OD, von Deimling A (1995) Shared allelic losses on chromosomes 1p and 19q suggest a common origin of oligodendroglioma and oligoastrocytoma. J Neuropathol Exp Neurol 54:91–95

45. Rubio M-P, Correa KM, Ueki K, Mohrenweiser HW, Gusella JF, von Deimling A, Louis DN (1994) The putative glioma suppressor gene on chromosome 19q maps between *APOC2* and *HRC*. Cancer Res 54:4760–4763

46. Bigner SH, Mark J, Burger PC, Mahaley MS, Bullard DE, Muhlbaier LH, Bigner DD (1988) Specific chromosomal abnormalities in malignant human gliomas. Cancer Res 88:405–411

47. Jenkins RB, Kimmel DW, Moertel CA, Schultz CG, Scheitauer BW, Kelly PJ, Dewald GW (1989) A cytogenetic study of 53 human gliomas. Cancer Genet Cytogenet 39:253–279

48. von Deimling A, Bender B, Jahnke R, Waha A, Kraus J, Albrecht S, Wellenreuther R, Fassbender F, Nagel J, Menon AG, Louis DN, Lenartz D, Schramm J, Wiestler OD (1994) Loci associated with malignant progression in astrocytomas: a candidate on chromosome 19q. Cancer Res 54:1397–1401

49. Ropers HH, Pericak-Vance MA, Siciliano MJ, Mohrenweiser HW (1992) Report of the second international workshop on human chromosome 19 mapping. Cytogenet Cell Genet 60:87–95

50. Ropers HH, Mohrenweiser H (1993) Report of the committee on the genetic constitution of chromosome 19. Genome Priority Rep 1:524–547

51. Venter DJ, Thomas DGT (1991) Multiple sequential molecular abnormalities in the evolution of human gliomas. Br J Cancer 63:753–757

52. Rey JA, Bello MJ, de Campos JE, Kusak ME, Moreno S (1987) Chromosomal composition of a series of 22 human low-grade gliomas. Cancer Genet Cytogenet 29:233–237

53. Griffin CA, Long PP, Carson BS, Brem H (1992) Chromosome abnormalities in low-grade central nervous system tumors. Cancer Genet Cytogenet 60:67–73

54. Brodeur GM, Fong CT (1989) Molecular biology and genetics of human neuroblastoma. Cancer Genet Cytogenet 41:153–174

55. Dracopoli NC, Harnett P, Bale SJ, Stanger BZ, Tucher MA, Housman DE, Kefford RF (1989) Loss of alleles from the distal short arm of chromosome 1 occurs late in melanoma progression. Proc Natl Acad Sci USA 86:4614–4618

56. Bigner SH, Mark J, Friedman HS, Biegel JA, Bigner DD (1988) Structural chromosomal abnormalities in human medulloblastoma. Cancer Genet Cytogenet 30:91–101

57. Mathew S, Murty VVVS, Bosl GJ, Chaganti RSK (1994) Loss of heterozygosity identifies multiple sites of allelic deletions on chromosome 1 in human male germ cell tumors. Cancer Res 54:6265–6269

58. Bello MJ, de Campos JM, Kusak ME, Vaquero J, Sarasa JL, Pestana A, Rey JA (1994) Allelic loss at 1p is associated with tumor progression of meningiomas. Genes Chromosomes Cancer 9:296–298

59. Lindblom A, Ruttledge M, Collins VP, Nordenskjold M, Dumanski JP (1994) Chromosomal deletions in anaplastic meningiomas suggest multiple regions outside chromosome 22 as important in tumor progression. Int J Cancer 56:354–357

60. Griffin CA, Hruban RH, Long PP, Miller N, Volz P, Carson B, Brem H (1994) Chromosome abnormalities in meningeal neoplasms: do they correlate with histology. Cancer Genet Cytogenet 78:46–52

61. Leister I, Weith A, Brüderlein S, Cziepluch C, Schlag P, Schwab M (1990) Human colorectal cancer: high frequency of deletions at chromosome 1p35. Cancer Res 50:7232–7238

62. Devilee P, van Vliet M, Bardoel A, Kievits T, Kuipers-Dijkshoorn N, Pearson PL, Cornelisse CJ (1991) Frequent somatic imbalance of marker alleles for chromosome 1 in human primary breast carcinoma. Cancer Res 51:1020–1025

63. Simon D, Knowles BB, Weith A (1991) Abnormalities of chromosome 1 and loss of heterozygosity on 1p in primary hepatomas. Oncogene 6:765–770

64. Bardi G, Pandis N, Fenger C, Kronborg O, Bomme L, Heim S (1993) Deletion of 1p36 as a primary chromosomal aberration in intestinal tumorigenesis. Cancer Res 53:1895–1898

65. Thiel G, Losanowa T, Kintzel D, Nisch G, Martin H, Vorpahl K, Witkowski R (1992) Karyotypes in 90 human gliomas. Cancer Genet Cytogenet 58:109–120

66. Ransom DT, Ritland SR, Moertel CA, Dahl RJ, O' Fallon JR, Scheitauer BW, Kimmel DW, Kelly PJ, Olopade OI, Diaz MO, Jenkins RB (1992) Correlation of cytogenetic analysis and loss of heterozygosity studies in human diffuse astrocytomas and mixed oligoastrocytomas. Genes Chromosomes & Cancer 5:357–374

67. Kim DH, Maeda T, Mohapatra G, Park S, Waldman FW, Graz JW, Feuerstein BG (1993) Molecular cytogenetics of malignant gliomas (abstract). J Neuro-Oncol 15:S13

68. James CD, Carlbom E, Dumanski JP, Hansen M, Nordenskjöld M, Collins VP, Cavenee WK (1988) Clonal genomic alterations in glioma malignancy stages. Cancer Res 48:5546–5551

69. Bièche I, Champème M-H, Matifas F, Cropp CS, Callahan R, Lidereau R (1993) Two distinct regions involved in 1p deletion in human primary breast cancer. Cancer Res 53:1990–1994

70. El-Azouzi M, Chung RY, Farmer GE, Martuza RL, Black RML, Rouleau GA, Hettlich C, Hedley-White ET, Zervas NT, Panagopoulos K, Nakamura Z, Gusella JF, Seizinger BR (1989) Loss of distinct regions on the short arm of chromosome 17 associated with tumorigenesis in human astrocytomas. Proc Natl Acad Sci USA 86:7186–7190

71. Fults D, Tippers RH, Thomas GA, Nakamura Z, White R (1989) Loss of heterozygosity for loci on chromosome 17p in human malignant astrocytoma. Cancer Res 49:6572–6577

72. James CD, Carlbom E, Nordenskjöld M, Collins VP (1989) Mitotic recombination of chromosome 17 in astrocytomas. Proc Natl Acad Sci USA 86:2858–2862

73. Ohgaki H, Eibl RH, Wiestler OD, Yasargil MG, Newcomb EW, Kleihues P (1991) p53 mutations in non-astrocytic human brain tumors. Cancer Res 51:6202–6205

74. Rasheed BKA, McLendon RE, Herndon JE, Friedman HS, Friedman AH, Bigner DD, Bigner SH (1994) Alterations of the TP53 gene in human gliomas. Cancer Res 54:1324–1330

75. Coles C, Thompson AM, Elder PA, Cohen BB, Mackenzie IM, Cranston G, Chettz U, Mackay J, MacDonald M, Nakamura Y, Hoyheim B, Steel CM (1990) Evidence implicating at least two genes on chromosome 17p in breast carcinogenesis. Lancet 336:761–763

76. Saylors RL III, Sidranski D, Friedman HS, Bigner SH, Bigner DD, Vogelstein B, Brodeur GM (1991) Infrequent p53 mutations in medulloblastomas. Cancer Res 51:4721–4723

77. Biegel JA, Burk CD, Barr FG, Emanuel BS (1992) Evidence for a 17p tumor related locus distinct from TP53 in pediatric primitive neuroectodermal tumors. Cancer Res 52:3391–3395

78. Saxena A, Clark WC, Robertson JT, Ikejiri B, Oldfield EH, Ali IU (1992) Evidence for the involvement of a potential second tumor suppressor gene on chromosome 17 distinct from p53 in malignant astrocytomas. Cancer Res 52:6716–6721

79. Chen P, Ellmore N, Weissman BE (1994) Functional evidence for a second tumor suppressor gene on chromosome 17. Mol Cell Biol 14:534–542

80. James CD, He J, Carlbom E, Nordenskjöld M, Cavenee WK, Collins VP (1991) Chromosome 9 deletion mapping reveals interferon α and interferon β-1 gene deletions in human glial tumors. Cancer Res 51:1684–1688

81. Wu JK, Folkerth RD, Ye Z, Darras BT (1993) Aggressive oligodendroglioma predicted by chromosome 10 restriction length polymorphism analysis. J Neuro-Oncol 15:29–35

82. Ye Z, Wu JK, Darras BT (1993) Loss of heterozygosity for alleles on chromosome 10 in human brain tumors. Neurol Res 15: 59–67

83. Fuller GN, Bigner SH (1992) Amplified cellular oncogenes in neoplasms of the human central nervous system. Mutat Res 276:299–306
84. Ekstrand AJ, James CD, Cavenne WK, Sekiger B, Pettersson RF, Collins VP (1991) Genes for epidermal growth factor receptor, transforming growth factor a, and epidermal growth factor and their expression in human gliomas in vivo. Cancer Res 51:2164–2172

Section 2. Expression of Oncogene and Growth Factor

The Correlation Between *flg* Gene Expression and the Progression of Glioma

Yoji Komatsu, Koji Tsuboi, Yoshihiko Yoshii, and Tadao Nose

Abstract. *flg* is a high-affinity receptor of basic fibroblast growth factor (bFGF) and a transmembrane protein that activates tyrosine kinase. The *flg* gene, as well as bFGF, expresses highly in astrocytic tumors. We investigated changes of bFGF and *flg* gene expression level in three cases of recurrent malignant astrocytic tumor by means of semiquantitative reverse transcriptase-polymerase chain reaction (RT-PCR). In all three cases, pathological examination showed malignant progression, especially in cellularity, cell pleomorphism, and mitosis. Both genes, bFGF and *flg*, had a higher level of expression in recurrent cases than in specimens of first-time occurrences. *flg* gene expression of recurrent specimens was 2.4- to 37.1 fold higher than in first-time specimens; bFGF expression changed only 1.0- to 3.3 fold. These results support our previous investigations in which we showed that the expression level of *flg* was significantly correlated to pathological grading in astrocytic tumors; however, bFGF is not statistically correlated. This suggests that *flg* plays a more important role in the progression of astrocytic tumors than bFGF does.

Key words. Basic FGF—*flg*—Astrocytic tumor—Tumor progression

Introduction

Basic fibroblast growth factor (bFGF) is a member of the FGF family and is a mitogen and differentiation factor for neuroectoderm-derived cells as well as a potent angiogenic factor [1–3]. Hyperexpression of the bFGF gene and its protein have been documented in human gliomas [4–8].

Biological responses to bFGF are mediated through specific transmembrane receptors; *flg* (bFGF receptor type I, FGFR-I) has the highest affinity. The hyperexpression of the *flg* gene has also been observed in human glioma cells [4–7]. Our prior investigations showed *flg* expression was more elevated than that of bFGF in malignant astrocytic tumors [6,7]. We consider that *flg* expression plays a more important role in progression of astrocytic tumors than does bFGF. To confirm this observation, we measured the expression of these genes and observed pathological changes in three recurrent glioma cases.

Department of Neurosurgery, University of Tsukuba, Tsukuba, Ibaraki 305, Japan

Methods

Samples were obtained from three patients who underwent therapeutic removal of malignant astrocytic tumors. In two cases, samples from the first surgery, and from the second surgery for recurrent tumors, were used. In another case, samples were obtained from the second and from the third surgery. Histopathological examination revealed that two patients had glioblastoma and the third had anaplastic astrocytoma. Normal brain tissue, which was obtained at a surgical procedure for intraventricle tumor, was also analyzed to provide a normal control.

Relative levels of gene expression of bFGF and flg were determined by reverse transcriptase-polymerase chain reaction (RT-PCR). Poly(A) mRNA was extracted using a Quick Prep Micro mRNA purification kit (Pharmacia P-L Biochemicals, Milwaukee, WI, USA). For analysis of human bFGF, we used nucleotide primers beginning with codon 20 at the 5' end of mRNA (5'-GCC-TTC-CCG-CCC-GGC-CAC-TTC-AAG-G-3') and complementary to codons 71–79 at the 3' end (5'-GCA-CAC-ACT-CCT-TTG-ATA-GAC-ACA-A-3') [9]. To analyze flg, we used nucleotide primers corresponding to nt 955–976 at the 5' end (5'-GAC-GCA-ACA-GAG-AAA-GAC-TTG-T-3') and complementary to nt 1594–1615 (5'-GCC-AGC-AGT-CCC-GCA-TCA-TCA-T-3') at the 3' end of mRNA [9]. We used β-actin as the inner control of RT-PCR, and primers (5'-TAC-ATG-GCT-GGG-GTG-TTG-AA-3') and (5'-AAG-AGA-GGC-ATC-CTC-ACC-CT-3') were synthesized. The amplification reaction mixtures (10 µl) consisted of 2.5 pmol each of upstream and downstream primers, 0.25 units of Taq DNA polymerase, and 0.20 mM deoxynucleoside triphosphate (dNTP).

Conditions for amplification were as follows: 94°C × 1 min (denaturation), 60°C × 1 min (primer annealing), and 72°C × 2 min plus 2 s in every cycle (primer extension). Sample of PCR products were taken from the reaction mixture every two cycles. The samples were visualized on 2.2% agarose gel developed in 1 × Tris acetate/borate buffer. The gel was stained with ethidium bromide and viewed on a UV light box. To measure the expression level of the genes, the cycles required for exponential phase and PCR efficiency were determined. Using normal human brain tissue as a control, gene expression was calculated as a value relative to normal brain tissue.

Pathological examinations were carried out using tissue specimens stained by hematoxylin-and-eosin and argyrophilic methods. Findings were classified in three degrees: class 1 indicates benign, and class 3 indicates malignant.

Tumor cells were observed using four points: cellularity, cell pleomorphism, mitosis, and necrosis. Classification criteria were as follows:

Cellularity: class 1, almost normal cellularity; class 2, more than 50% increase than normal brain tissue; class 3, more than 200% increase

Cell pleomorphism: class 1, mild; pleomorphism, class 2, moderate; class 3, remarkable pleomorphism

Mitosis: class 1, no mitosis was seen; class 2, one mitosis per a number of 100× fields; class 3, mitosis in every 100× field

Necrosis: class 1, no necrosis seen; class 3, necrosis was observed

Tumor vessels were classified using three points: vascularity, endothelial proliferation, and vascular pleomorphism.

Vascularity: class 1, fewer than 24 vessels in a 100× field; class 2, 25–49 vessels; class 3, more than 50 vessels

Endothelial proliferation: class 1, thickness of the endothelium was less than 24% of the outer diameter of the vessel; class 2, thickness 25%–49% of diameter; class 3, more than 50%

Vascular pleomorphism: class 1, mild; class 2, moderate; class 3, remarkable pleomorphism

Case Presentations

Case 1

A 26-year-old man was diagnosed as having anaplastic astrocytoma by a specimen of his second surgery in December 1990. Pathological classifications were as follows: cellularity, class 2; cell pleomorphism, class 2; mitosis, class 2; necrosis, class 1; vascularity, class 1; endotherial proliferation, class 1; and vascular pleomorphism, class 1. Chemotherapy and 50 Gy of proton radiation were administered after surgery. The tumor regrew and was surgically removed in August 1992. The tumor had progressed by the criteria of pathological cellularity, cell preomorphism, and vascularity (Fig. 1).

The bFGF gene had expressed 8 fold and the *flg* gene 50 fold higher than normal brain tissue at the second surgery. At the third surgery, bFGF was 8.2 fold and *flg* 120 fold higher than normal brain tissue (Fig. 2). (His first surgery was undergone in 1985; the pathological diagnosis was benign astrocytoma.)

Case 2

A 43-year-old man was diagnosed as having glioblastoma multiforme at the first surgery in July 1990. Pathological classification was categorized as follows: cellularity, class 2; cell pleomorphism, class 2; mitosis, class 2; necrosis, class 3; vascularity, class 3; endotherial proliferation, class 2; and vascular pleomorphism, class 2. Treatment was 67 Gy of irradiation and chemotherapy using (1,4-amino-2-methyl-5-pyrimidinyl)-methyl-3-(2-chloroethyl)-3-nitrosourea (ACNU). Recurrence was 2 years after the first surgery. In the pathological examination of a specimen of the second surgery, cellularity, cell pleomorphism, mitosis, and endotherial proliferation had progressed.

The bFGF gene was expressed 17 times and the *flg* gene 3.5 times as high as normal brain tissue at the first surgery. At the second surgery, bFGF was expressed 24 fold and *flg* 130 fold higher (Fig. 3).

Case 3

A 74-year-old woman was pathologically diagnosed as having glioblastoma multiforme by the specimen obtained in the first surgical procedure. Pathological classification was categorized as follows: cellularity, class 2; cell pleomorphism, class 3; mitosis, class 2; necrosis, class 3; vascularity, class 3; endothelial proliferation, class 3; and vascular pleomorphism, class 2. Radiation was tried until the total dose was 45 Gy; however, the tumor was progressive. At recurrence 2 months after the first surgery, tumor cellularity had progressed.

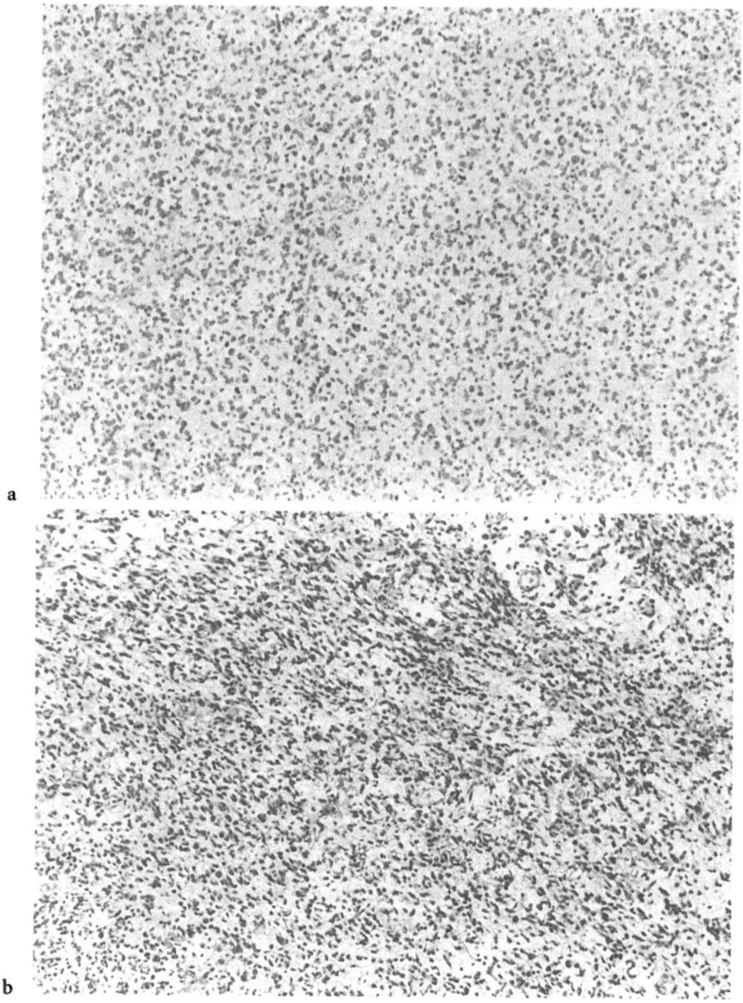

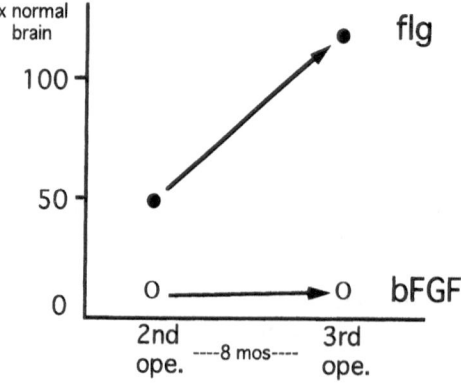

Fig. 1. Histopathological findings of specimen obtained by second surgery (**a**) and third surgery (**b**) of case 1. Hematoxylin and eosin stain, ×100

Gene expression level

Fig. 2. Basic fibroblast growth factor (bFGF) and *flg* gene expression levels in case 1

Fig. 3. bFGF and *flg* gene expression levels in case 2

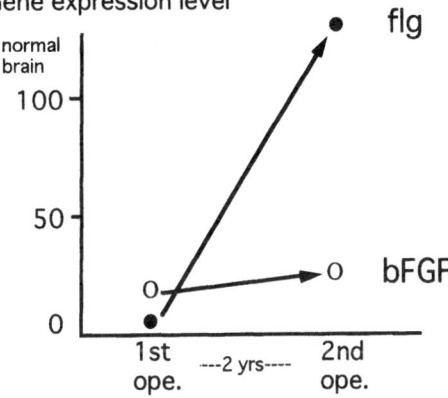

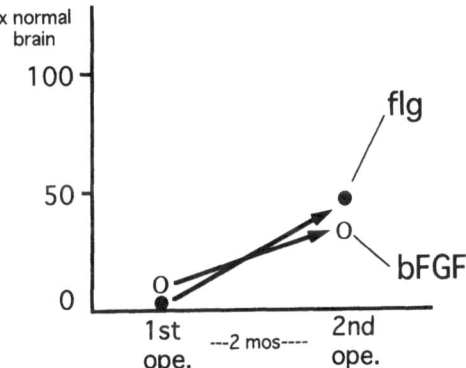

Fig. 4. bFGF and *flg* gene expression levels in case 3

bFGF was expressed 8.5 fold and *flg* 2.7 fold higher than normal brain tissue at the first surgery. These genes were expressed 28 fold and 42 fold, respectively, at the second surgery (Fig. 4).

Discussion

In all three cases, pathological classifications indicated deterioration in specimen at recurrence rather than in the initial tumors; notably, degenerative changes of tumor cell criteria were observed. Malignant progression as seen in our recurrent cases is frequently observed in astrocytic tumors. The expression level of both genes, bFGF and *flg*, was also elevated higher at the time of recurrence than in the initial specimens. bFGF gene expression level was elevated 1.0 to 3.3 fold higher at recurrence than at the first occurrence; *flg* gene expression level at recurrence was elevated 2.4 to 37.1 fold higher. The change of expression level between the first-time specimen and the recurrent one was remarkably significant in *flg* but not in bFGF.

We previously reported that the expression level of *flg* was significantly correlated with pathological grading in astrocytic tumors. However, the expression level of bFGF appeared in a wide range of grades and did not statistically correlate with pathological classification [6,7]. Although the bFGF gene was hyperexpressed frequently in astrocytic tumors, we consider that the *flg* gene, which encodes the high-affinity receptor of bFGF expression, was more strongly associated with malignant progression in astrocytic tumors. The gene expression level is numbered by cases; therefore, we measured the shift of the expression level between the initial occurrence and recurrence in three of the same patients. The results of these three cases suggest that *flg* plays a more important role in the progression of astrocytic tumors and support our conclusion.

bFGF and *flg* also have been implicated as regulators of the central nervous system (CNS) wounding response [2]. Surgical procedures and radiation therapy injure adjacent brain tissue, and it might be thought that these therapeutic injuries could cause increasing expression level. In vivo experiments by Logan et al. [10] have shown that a rapid, transient increase in bFGF mRNA and protein is readily detectable within 7 days of surgery, and increases in *flg* mRNA appear 7 days after injury and subside after 14 days in the injured brain. The interval between the first and second surgeries was 8 months in case 1, 2 years in case 2, and 2 months in case 3. In cases 1 and 2, the interval was so long that gene expression level was not affected by therapeutic injury; however, some effect may have occurred in case 3. The remarkable excess of *flg* expression level in cases 1 and 2 should be caused by tumor progression.

Ueba et al. [11] have examined the expression of *flg* in gliomas by means of immunohistochemistry. All glioma tissues were positively stained for *flg* protein, and gemistocytic tumor astrocytes showed relatively high immunoreactivity compared with fibrillary tumor astrocytes. This heterogeneity suggests the gene expression level of each tumor cell varied in a wide range, and therefore tumor cells that show a high expression of *flg* can grow more rapidly because of the effect of tumor-derived bFGF.

A splicing variant of FGF receptor type I (FGFR-1; flg) has been described [12]. The original form, named FGFR-1α, has three immunoglobulin-like disulfide loops in the extracellular domain; in contrast, FGFR-1β has only two loops; FGFR-1β exhibits a 10-fold greater affinity for bFGF than FGFR-1α. Malignant astrocytoma dominantly expresses FGFR-1β, whereas normal brain tissue expresses FGFR-1α [13]. Our PCR primers refer to the nucleotide between the third loop and transmembrane domain; therefore, we could not distinguish the two forms of *flg*. The receptor efficiency would dramatically increase under the condition of *flg* gene hyperexpression associated with the splicing pattern when it is shifted to FGFR-1β.

In summary, our data indicate that *flg* plays a more important role in the malignant progression of astrocytic tumor than does bFGF. This suggests that *flg* is an appropriate target of glioma therapy.

Acknowledgments. We are grateful to Miss Chizuko Nonaka for technical assistance. This work was supported by the Fund-in-Trust for Cancer Research from the Governor of Ibaraki Prefecture, Japan.

References

1. Folkman J, Klagsbrun M (1987) Angiogenic factors. Science 23:442–447
2. Gospodarowicz D (1990) Fibroblast growth factor. Chemical structure and biological func-

tion. Clin Orthop 257:231–248

3. Gross JL, Morrison RS, Eidsvoog K, et al (1990) Basic fibroblast growth factor: a potential autocrine regulator of human glioma cell growth. J Neurosci Res 27:689–696

4. Takahashi JA, Suzuki H, Yasuda Y, et al (1991) Gene expression of fibroblast growth factor receptors in the tissues of human gliomas and meningiomas. Proc Natl Acad Sci USA 177: 1–7

5. Takahashi JA, Fukumoto M, Igarashi K, et al. (1992) Correlation of basic fibroblast growth factor expression levels with the degree of malignancy and vascularity in human gliomas. J Neurosurg 76:792–798

6. Komatsu Y, Tsuboi K, Yoshii Y, Nose T (1993) Correlation of basic fibroblast growth factor expression level with the tumor vessels in astrocytic tumors. Neurol Med Chir (Tokyo) 33(Suppl):149 (in Japanese)

7. Komatsu Y, Tsuboi K, Yoshii Y, Nose T (1994) Correlation of basic fibroblast growth factor and its receptor (flg) gene expression level and pathological findings in astrocytic tumors. Brain Tumor Pathol 11(Suppl):75 (in Japanese)

8. Morrison RS, Yamaguchi F, Bruner JM, et al (1994) Fibroblast growth factor receptor gene expression and immunoreactivity are elevated in human glioblastoma multiforme. Cancer Res 54:2794–2799

9. Morrison RS (1991) Suppression of basic fibroblast growth factor expression by antisense oligodeoxynucleotides inhibits the growth of transformed human astrocytes. J Biol Chem 266:728–734

10. Logan A, Frautschy SA, Gonzalez AM, et al (1992) A time course for the focal elevation of synthesis of basic fibroblast growth factor and one of its high-affinity receptors (flg) following a localized cortical brain injury. J Neurosci 12:3828–3837

11. Ueba T, Takahashi JA, Fukumoto M, et al (1994) Expression of fibroblast growth factor receptor-1 in human glioma and meningioma tissues. Neurosurgery 34:221–226

12. Xu J, Nakahara M, Crabb JW, et al (1992) Expression and immunochemical analysis of rat and human fibroblast growth factor receptor (flg) isoforms. J Biol Chem 267:17792–17803

13. Yamaguchi F, Saya H, Bruner JM, Morrison RS (1994) Differential expression of two fibroblast growth factor-receptor genes is associated with malignant progression in human astrocytomas. Proc Natl Acad Sci USA 91:484–488

Expression of trk Proto-Oncogene Product in Medulloblastoma

Takashi Kokunai, Atsufumi Kawamura, Hideki Sawa, Ichirou Izawa, and Norihiko Tamaki

Abstract. The relationship between the expression of trk proto-oncogene product, which was examined using a monoclonal antibody (TGK1) specific for trk proto-oncogene product, and the survival period of 23 cases of medulloblastoma was analyzed. In the relationship between the tumor stage (by the Chang tumor staging system) and the expression of TGK1, cases of T_1 and T_2 stages showed high frequency of expression of TGK1. Good prognosis was obtained in TGK1-positive cases compared to the poor prognosis of TGK1-negative cases. The analysis of the expression of trk proto-oncogene was useful for prediction of the prognosis of medulloblastoma.

Key words. Medulloblastoma—trk Proto-oncogene—Nerve growth factor receptor—Nerve growth factor

Introduction

Meduloblastoma is the second most common neoplasm of the cerebellum, comprising about 20% of all brain tumors in children [1,2]. This tumor has carried a poor prognosis, and more recent studies reported 5-year survival rates of 40%–60% in spite of the development of radiation and chemotherapy [3,4]. Various factors have been evaluated for the prediction of prognosis of medulloblastoma, but these observations are still speculative and require further studies for acceptance [5].

Nerve growth factor (NGF), which has a major role in the development of the sympathetic nervous system [6,7], has both low-affinity (LNGFR) and high-affinity receptor [8], which is a product of the trk proto-oncogene [9]. It has been reported that the medulloblastoma cell line had LNGFR or trk proto-oncogene product and that the trk proto-oncogene product was a functional receptor for NGF in medulloblastoma cells [10,11]. In neuroblastoma, the abscence of proto-oncogene trk messenger RNA (mRNA) expression was associated with tumor progression, and mRNA expression of the trk proto-oncogene was found in patients with a favorable prognosis [12].

Department of Neurosurgery, Kobe University School of Medicine, Chuo-ku, Kobe 650, Japan

In this chapter, we report preparing the specific monoclonal antibody (mAb) against the product for trk proto-oncogene and analyzing the relationship between the prognosis of medulloblastoma and the expression of the trk proto-oncogene product.

Materials and Methods

Patients

We evaluated 23 cases of cerebellar medulloblastoma. Patient age ranged from 3 to 14 years (median age, 8 years), 15 cases were boys and 8 were girls. All patients were first treated, and were staged according to the Chang tumor staging system [13]. Tumor tissues were collected at the time of surgery in Kobe University Hospital. The tumors in 18 cases were located at the vermis, in 4 cases at the cerebellar hemisphere, and in 1 case at the fourth ventricle. Tumor tissues were subtotally or completely removed, and postoperative irradiation to the whole neuroaxial region were done in all cases. Pathological diagnosis of medulloblastoma was performed according to standard pathological criteria. Diagnosis was classical type in 18 cases and desmoplastic type in the other 5 cases. Survival curves of the two groups of patients, one bearing trk-positive and the other one trk-negative medulloblastomas, were constructed. Also, survival curves of patients were evaluated for the two groups of LNGFR-positive or LNGFR-negative medulloblastomas. The survival time from data of diagnosis to date of death was estimated by the Kaplan–Meier product limit method [14], and the outcomes were compared with the log rank statistic [15,16]. The follow-up period ranged from 8 to 157 months.

Preparation of Mouse Monoclonal Antibody (mAb)

BALB/c mice were immunized subcutaneously three times at 2-week intervals with 5×10^6 Mewo cells [17]. Four days after the final immunization, the spleen cells were fused with P3U1 mouse myeloma cells. The supernatant of each clone was screened for anti-trk proto-oncogene product by enzyme-linked immunosorbent assay (ELISA) using a synthetic oligopeptide with a C-terminal domain corresponding to residues of 776–790 (Ala, Leu, Ala, Asn, Ala, Pro, Pro, Val, Tyr, Leu, Asp, Val, Leu, Gly) as target. The clone detected in this assay was subcloned three times by limiting dilution. The immunoglobulin class of culture supernatants was determined with an Amersham immunoglobulin isotyping kit (Amersham, Buckinghamshire, England). The mAb was purified using MAPS-2 kit (Bio-Rad, Tokyo, Japan).

Immunoblotting

Mewo and PC-12 cells were solubilized with 500 μl of a cell lysis buffer containing 1% Triton X-100, 1% sodium deoxycholate, 0.01% sodium dodecylsulfate (SDS), 0.15 M NaCl, 50 mM Tris-HCl (pH 7.4), and 2 mM phenylmethyl sulfonyl fluoride. Lyophilized samples (1 mg/ml of protein concentration) were dissolved in a buffer containing 2.5% SDS, 5% 2-mercaptoethanol, and 0.01 M Tris-HCl (pH 8.0), and boiled for 5 min at 100°C. SDS-polyacrylamide gel electrophoresis essentially followed the method of Laemmli [18]. Electrophoresis was performed at room temperature for

4 h at 30 mA on a 0.4-mm-thick, 12% gel plate. Proteins were electrophoretically transferred onto nitrocellulose filters at a constant voltage of 10 V for 3 h as described by Towbin et al. [19]. The filters were blocked with 5% skim milk, then reacted with TGK1 antibody. Antibody binding to the filter was detected by the avidin—biotin—peroxidase system. Synthetic peptide of trk proto-oncogene was used for the absorption of TGK1 antibody for negative control.

Immunoperoxidase Staining

Paraffin-embedded sections (6 μm) were deparafinized with xylene and rehydrated with a graded ethanol and phosphate buffered saline (PBS) series (pH 7.4). Sections were preincubated with 0.03% H_2O_2 in methanol for 20 min and washed with PBS for 20 min. Sections were incubated with 5% goat normal serum in PBS for 30 min, then 10 μg/mL of monoclonal anti-NGFR antibody (low-affinity type) (clone ME20-4, IgG_1) (Amersham) or 1 μg/mL of TGK1 for 60 min at 37°C. After washing with PBS for 20 min, sections were incubated with biotinylated goat antimouse IgG for 30 min at 37°C. After PBS washing for 20 min, sections were incubated with avidin–biotin peroxidase complex for 30 min at 37°C. After PBS washing, the peroxidase reaction was initiated with 0.06% diaminobenzidine and 0.01% H_2O_2 in 50 mM Tris-HCl (pH 7.0) for 5 min. Nuclei were briefly counterstained with Meyer's hematoxylin. Negative control sections were incubated with nonimmunized mouse IgG instead of TGK1 or anti-NGFR antibodies.

Results

Summary of Cases

A total of 23 cases of medulloblastoma (Table 1) were evaluated, 13 male and 8 female patients. Age at diagnosis, sex, histological subgroup, location of tumor, gross total

Table 1. Summary of cases.

Patient information	trk (+)	trk (−)	LNGFR (+)	LNFGR (−)
Age at diagnosis (years) (mean ± SD)	7.4 ± 1.23	8.2 ± 2.31	7.6 ± 2.56	7.8 ± 1.48
Sex (M:F)	8:2	7:6	5:3	10:5
Histological subgroups				
Classical	8	10	6	12
Desmoplastic	2	3	2	3
Location				
Vermis	8	10	7	11
Hemisphere	2	2	1	3
Fourth ventricle	0	1	0	1
Gross total resection	52%	48%	49%	54%
Percent with chemotherapy	13%	12%	14%	8%
Radiation dose (cGy) (mean ± SD)				
Posterior fossa dose	5180 ± 384	5084 ± 282	4982 ± 183	5110 ± 294
Whole-brain dose	3050 ± 243	3180 ± 124	3240 ± 218	3042 ± 286
Spinal cord dose	1987 ± 228	2140 ± 184	2280 ± 224	2086 ± 142

trk (+), trk (−): trk positive or negative; LNGFR, low-affinity nerve growth factor receptor (positive or negative).

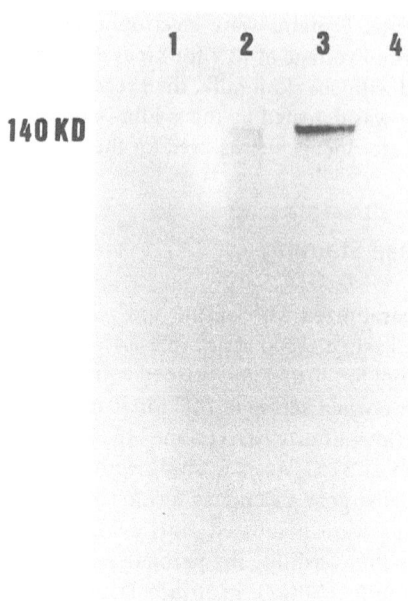

Fig. 1. Western blotting analysis of expression of trk proto-oncogene product by PC-12 (lane 2) and Mewo cells (lanes 1, 3, and 4). Lane 1, negative control using normal mouse IgG; lanes 2 and 3, reactivity by TGK1 monoclonal antibody (mAb); lane 4, absorption of TGK1 mAb by synthetic oligopeptide of trk proto-oncogene product

resection of tumor, percent with chemotherapy, and craniospinal radiation doses die not differ between trk-positive and trk-negative cases and between LNGFR-positive and LNGFR-negative cases.

Characterization of TGK1 mAb using Western Blotting

Figure 1 shows the result of Western blotting using the lysate of Mewo cells (lanes 1, 3, and 4) and PC-12 cells (lane 2). Lane 1 was incubated with nonimmunized mouse IgG instead of TGK1 mAb; lane 4 was incubated with TGK1 mAb absorbed with synthetic polypeptide specific for trk proto-oncogene product. TGK1 mAb detected the 140-kDa band (lane 2 and 3), and its reaction was absorbed with synthetic peptide of trk proto-oncogene product (lane 4), but did not absorb with that of LNGFR (data not shown).

Expression of TGK1 mAb in Tissues of Medulloblastoma

TGK1 mAb reacted the Purkinje cells in normal cerebellum of the adult human central nervous system (Fig. 2). TGK1 mAb reacted 10 of 23 cases (43.5%) of medulloblastoma, and 5 of the TGK1-positive cases also showed the expression of LNGFR, which was shown in 8 of 23 cases (34.8%) of medulloblastoma. The diffuse immunoreactivity of TGK1 mAb in medulloblastoma was shown (Fig. 3) compared to the localized reactivity of LNGFR in medulloblastoma (Fig. 4). The tissues treated with normal mouse IgG instead of TGK1 mAb (Fig. 5) showed only nuclear staining with hematoxylin.

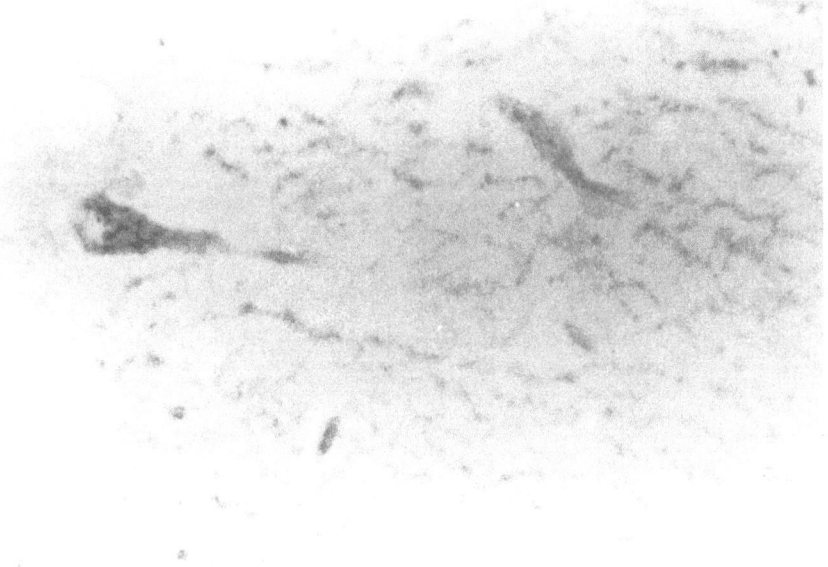

Fig. 2. Immunohistochemical analysis of the expression of trk proto-oncogene product in normal cerebellum. ×400

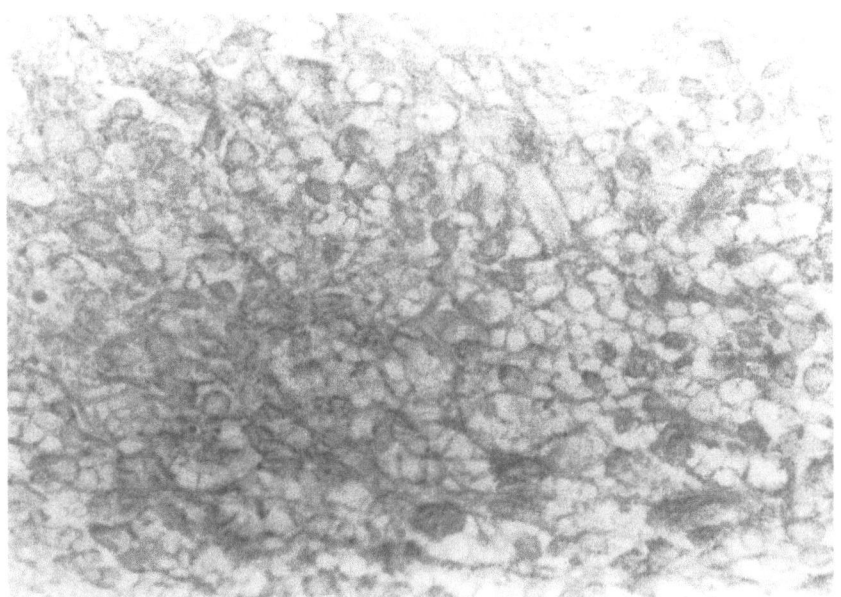

Fig. 3. Immunohistochemical analysis of the expression of trk proto-oncogene product in medulloblastoma. ×400

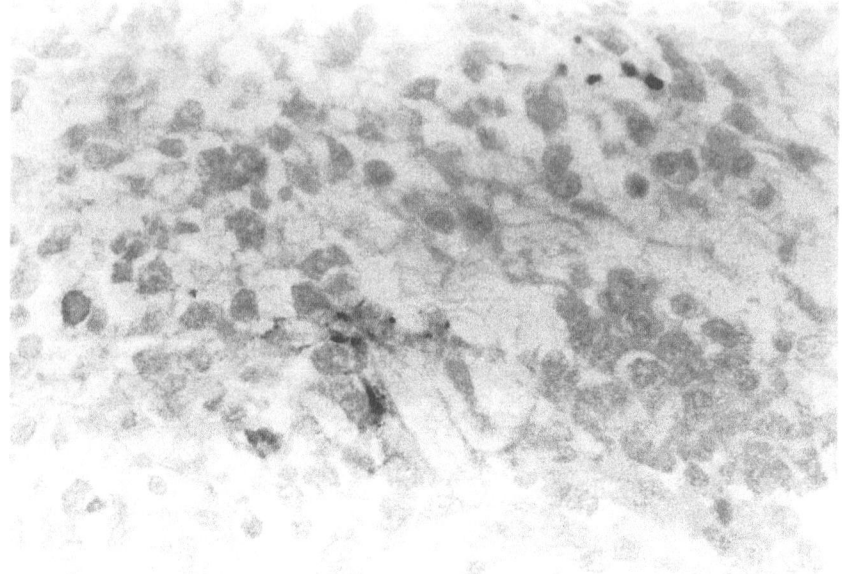

Fig. 4. Immunohistochemical analysis of the expression of low-affinity nerve growth factor receptor (LNGFR) in medulloblastoma. ×400

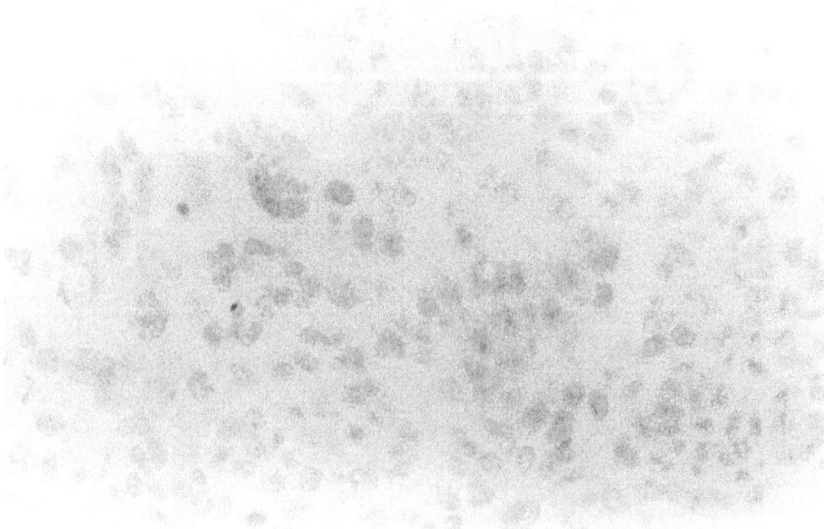

Fig. 5. Immunohistochemical analysis of medulloblastoma tissue (negative control). ×400

Expression of Product of trk Proto-Oncogene and LNGFR in Relationship to Clinical Stage

Figure 6 shows the relationship between the Chang tumor staging system and the expression of trk proto-oncogene product or LNGFR. The cases of T_1 and T_2 stages showed a high frequency of expression of TGK1 in contrast to the high frequency of TGK1-negative cases in the T_3 stage. There was no relationship between the tumor stage and the expression of LNGFR.

Expression of Product of trk Proto-Oncogene or LNGFR in Relationship to Prognosis of Medulloblastoma

Figure 7 shows the survival curves of trk-positive (10 cases) and trk-negative cases (13 cases) of medulloblastoma. The mean survival periods of trk-positive and trk-negative cases of medulloblastoma were 93.28 ± 28.30 and 33.54 ± 5.68 months, respectively. The survival curve of trk-positive cases was significantly different from trk-negative cases ($P < .05$). Figure 8 shows the survival curves of LNGFR-positive (8 cases) and LNGFR-negative cases (15 cases) of medulloblastoma. There were no differences between the survival periods of LNGFR-positive and LNGFR-negative cases.

Discussion

In this study, the relationship between the expression of trk proto-oncogene product, which was examined using the specific monolonal antibody (TGK1) for trk proto-oncogene product, and the survival time of 23 cases of medulloblastoma was analyzed. TGK1 mAb was specific for the product of trk proto-oncogene as analyzed

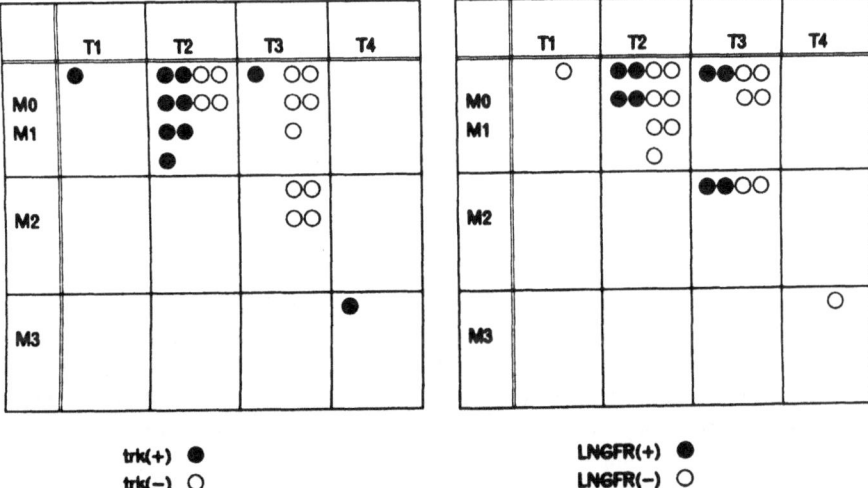

Fig. 6. Relationship between the Chang tumor staging system and the expression of trk proto-oncogene product or LNGFR

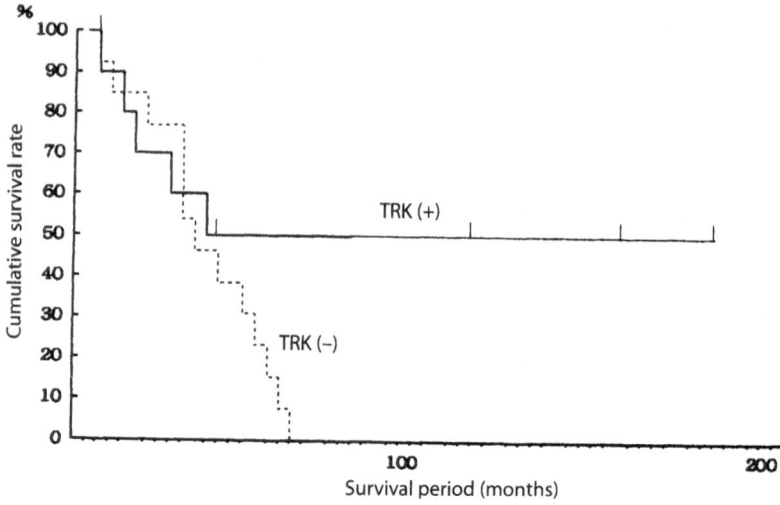

Fig. 7. Survival curves of trk-positive (10) and trk-negative (13) cases of medulloblastoma

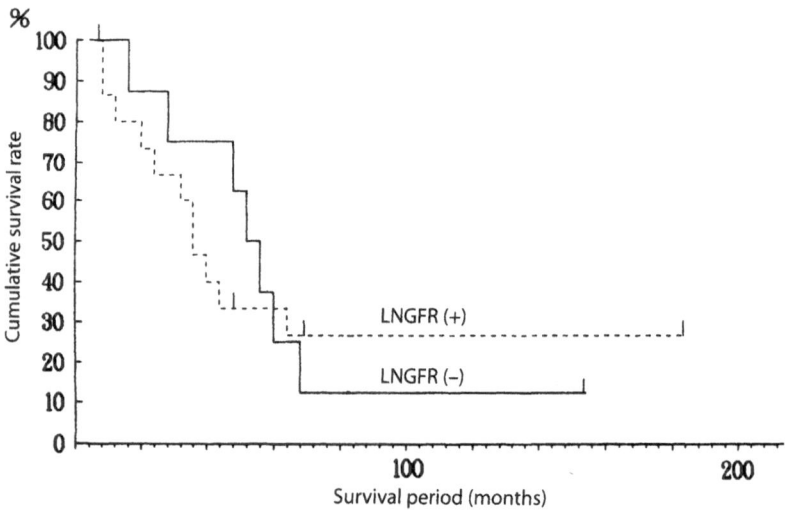

Fig. 8. Survival curves of LNGFR-positive (8) and LNGFR-negative (15) cases of medulloblastoma

by Western blotting, and reacted only the Purkinje cells in normal central nervous system tissues [20]. In medulloblastoma, 43.5% of the analyzed tumors expressed the product of trk proto-oncogene. In the relationship between the tumor stage by the Chang tumor staging system and the expression of TGK1, the cases of T_1 and T_2 stages showed high frequency of expression of TGK1. Good prognosis was obtained in TGK1-positive cases compared to the poor prognosis of TGK1-negative cases. There was no relationship between the tumor stage and the expression of LNGFR.

Various prognostic factors have been analyzed in medulloblastoma [5,21]. Patients with disseminated tumor have demonstrated a worse prognosis, and groups without metastasis (M_0), with smaller tumors (T_1 or T_2), and ages greater than 4 years have a favorable outcome [22]. Children with T_{3b} or T_4 tumors, or M1–M4 tumor spread, or more than 1.5 cm^3 of residual tumor on postoperative scan, are considered at high risk [23,24]. The analysis of DNA ploidy suggests that a worse prognosis is associated with diploid tumor [25]. But morphological, phenotypic, and genotypic parameters are not yet utilized to assign a standard or poor-risk classification. Also, the mechanisms responsible for the lack of expression of trk proto-oncogene product by medulloblastoma are unknown.

LNGFR is a transmembrane glycoprotein of approximately 75 000 daltons that binds NGF with kDa of 10^{-9} M [26,27]. However, high-affinity binding (kDa = 10^{-11} M) is necessary to mediate the biological action of NGF [8,9]. The proto-oncogene trk encodes a functional receptor for NGF, which is a 140 000-dalton protein belonging to the tyrosine kinase family of transmembrane receptors [9]. In neuroblastoma, trk expression is associated with an absence of N-*myc* amplification, lower disease stage, and favorable outcome, and the absence of trk mRNA expression is associated with tumor progression [12,28]. Furthermore, neuroblastoma cells with functional high-affinity NGF receptor show the extensive outgrowth of neurites and cessation of DNA synthesis after long-term treatment with NGF, suggesting terminal differentiation [29]. In normal central nervous system tissue, NGF mRNA is found in the cortex, hippocampus, pons, medulla, and spinal cord, of which astrocytes, neurons, and Schwann cells produce NGF [30,31]. It is speculated that medulloblastoma cells with the trk proto-oncogene product might be responsible for physiological NGF, and thus induce terminal differentiation with NGF.

References

1. Mori K, Kuriska M (1986) Brain tumors in childhood: statistical analysis of cases from the Brain Tumor Registry of Japan. Child's Nerv Syst 2:233–237
2. Matson DD (1969) Neurosurgery of infancy and childhood, edn 2. Thomas, Springfield, pp 448–456
3. Bellani FF, Gasparini M, Lombardi F, et al (1984) Medulloblastoma: results of a sequential combined treatment. Cancer 54:1956–1961
4. Bloom HJG, Wallace ENK, Henk JM (1969) The treatment and prognosis of medulloblastoma in children. A study of 82 certified cases. Am J Radiol 105:43–62
5. Caputy AJ, McCullough DC, Manz HJ, et al (1987) A review of the factors influencing the prognosis of medulloblastoma. The importance of cell differentiation. J Neurosurg 66:80–87
6. Levi-Montalcini R (1987) The nerve growth factor 35 years later. Science 237:1154–1162
7. Yanker B, Shooter EM (1982) The biology and mechanism of action of nerve growth factor. Annu Rev Biochem 51:845–868
8. Barbacid M (1993) Nerve growth factor. a tale of two receptors. Oncogene 8:2033–2042
9. Kaplan D, Hempstead B, Martin-Zanca D, et al (1991) The trk proto-oncogene product: a signal transducing receptor for nerve growth factor. Science 252:554–558
10. Kokunai T, Sawa H, Tatsumi S, et al (1994) Expression of nerve growth factor receptor by human primitive neuroectodermal tumors. Neurol Med Chir (Tokyo) 34:523–529
11. Kokunai T, Sawa H, Kawamura A, et al (1994) Analysis of NGF-receptor in medulloblastoma cell. Neuroimmunol Res 7:35–39
12. Suzuki T, Bogenmann E, Shimada H, et al (1993) Lack of high-affinity nerve growth factor receptors in aggressive neuroblastoma. J Natl Cancer Inst 85:377–384
13. Chang CH, Housepian EM, Herbert C Jr (1969) An operative staging system and a megavoltage radiotherapeutic technique for cerebellar medulloblastomas. Radiology 93:1351–1359

14. Kaplan EL, Meier P (1958) Non-parametric estimation from incomplete observations. J Am Stat Assoc 53:457–481
15. Cox DR (1972) Regression models and life tables. J R Stat Soc B 34:187–220
16. Peto R, Pike MC, Armitage P (1977) Design and analysis of randomized clinical trials requiring prolonged observation of each patient. II: Analysis and examples. Br J Cancer 35:1–39
17. Marchetti D, Menter D, Jin L, et al (1993) Nerve growth factor effects on human and mouse melanoma cell invasion and heparanase production. Int J Cancer 55:692–699
18. Laemmli UK (1970) Cleavage of structural proteins during the assembly of the head of bacteriophage T4. Nature 227:680–685
19. Towbin H, Staehelin T, Gordon J (1979) Electrophoretic transfer of proteins from polyacrylamide gels to nitrocellulose sheets; procedure and some applications. Proc Natl Acad Sci USA 76:4350–4354
20. Cohen-Cong S, Dreyfus CF, Black IB (1989) Expression of high- and low-affinity nerve growth factor receptors by purkinje cells in the developing rat cerebellum. Exp Neurol 105:104–109
21. Friedman HS, Oakes WJ, Bigner SH, et al (1991) Medulloblastoma: tumor biological and clinical perspectives. J Neurooncol 11:1–15
22. Evans AE, Jenkin RDT, Sposto R, et al (1990) The treatment of medulloblastoma. Results of a prospective randomized trial of radiation therapy with and wthout CCNU, vincristine, and prednisone. J Neurosurg 72:572–582
23. Berry MP, Jenkin RD, Keen CW, et al (1981) Radiation treatment for medulloblastoma. A 21-year review. J Neurosurg 55:43–51
24. Tait DM, Thornton-Jones H, Bloom HJG, et al (1990) Adjuvant chemotherapy for medulloblastoma: the first multicentre control trial of the International Society of Paediatric Oncology (SFOP). Eur J Cancer 26:464–469
25. Yasue M, Tomita T, Engelhard H, et al (1989) Prognostic importance of DNA ploidy in medulloblastoma of childhood. J Neurosurg 70:385–391
26. Johnson D, Lanahan A, Buck CR, et al (1986) Expression and structure of the human NGF receptor. Cell 47:545–554
27. Radeke MJ, Misko TP, Hsu C, et al (1987) Gene transfer and molecular cloning of the rat nerve growth factor receptor. Nature 325:593–597
28. Borrello MG, Bongarzone I, Pierotti MA, et al (1993) Trk and ret proto-oncogene expression in human neuroblastoma specimens: high frequency of trk expression in non-advanced stages. Int J Cancer 54:540–545
29. Matsushima H, Bogenmann E (1990) Nerve growth factor (NGF) induces neuronal differentiation in neuroblastoma cells transfected with the NGF receptor cDNA. Mol Cell Biol 10:5015–5020
30. Bandtlow CE, Heumann R, Schwab ME, et al (1987) Cellular localization of nerve growth factor synthesis by in situ hybridization. EMBO J 6:891–899
31. Spranger M, Lindholm D, Bandtlow C, et al (1990) Regulation of nerve growth factor (NGF) synthesis in the rat central nervous system: comparison between the effects of interleukin-1 and various growth factors in astrocyte cultures and in vivo. Eur J Neurosci 2:69–76

Differential Expression of FGF Receptor-1 and FGF Receptor-2 Is Associated with Malignant Progression of Gliomas

Fumio Yamaguchi[1,2], Richard S. Morrison[2], Hideyuki Saya[3], Janet M. Bruner[4], Hiroshi Takahashi[1], and Shozo Nakazawa[1]

Abstract. Human gliomas were examined for alternative splicing of extracellular domain of FGFR1 (fibroblast growth factor receptor-1). The expression of the 2 Ig domain form of FGFR1 (FGFR1-β) relative to the expression of the 3-Ig domain form of FGFR1 (FGFR1-α) was significantly elevated in glioblastoma multiforme (GBM). Although low-grade astrocytomas (LGAs) showed less FGFR1-β than GBMs but more than normal brains, anaplastic astrocytomas (AAs) had expression of FGFR1-β intermediate between GBMs and LGAs. The expression ratio of FGFR1-β and FGFR1-α had positive correlation with malignancy of gliomas. These results indicate that alternative RNA splicing of the FGFR1 may be associated with malignant progression of gliomas. We also analyzed the expression of FGFR2 transcript in normal brains and gliomas. GBMs showed no expression or a decreased level of FGFR2 transcript compared to adjacent normal brains. Because the FGFR2 gene localizes on chromosome 10q26, which is often lost in glioblastoma cells, and the tumor suppressor gene is inferred to exist in chromosome 10q24–q26, it is suggested that the putative tumor suppressor gene is correlated with the lack of FGFR2.

Key words. Brain tumor—Malignancy grading—Alternative splicing—Polymerase chain reaction—Astrocytoma

Introduction

Fibroblast growth factors (FGFs) are heparin-binding polypeptide mitogens that induce proliferation of a wide variety of cells and are known to participate in angiogenesis [1], differentiation [2–6], maintenance of survival of neurons [7], cell migration [1,8–10], and embryonal development [11–13]. The family of FGFs includes seven members that share a varying degree of homology at the protein level and most of which seem to have a very similar spectrum of action [14]. The receptors for them also constitute a gene family, which includes at least four members [15]. Variants of FGFR can be encoded by alternative RNA splicing of the same gene [16–19]. Alternative splicing of the second half of the third immunoglobulin (Ig-)like disulfide loop of

[1]Department of Neurosurgery, Nippon Medical School, Bunkyo-ku, Tokyo 113, Japan
Departments of [2]Neurosurgery, [3]Neuro-Oncology, and [4]Pathology, The University of Texas M.D. Anderson Cancer Center, Houston, TX 77030, USA

both FGFR1 and FGFR2 gives rise to two receptors that exhibit striking differences in their ligand-binding properties [20]. One of the other splicing variants exhibits differences in the external domains including the presence or absence of the first Ig-like loop and an acidic stretch of amino acids between the first and second Ig loop [21–23]. The expression of FGFRs is increased in many kinds of neoplasm. One of these is glioma [24–26], a brain tumor characterized by rapid tumor growth, extensive infiltration of tumor cells, and hypervascularity. In this study, we examined the differential expression of FGFR1 isoforms in clinical samples of glioma and established glioma cell lines by the reverse transcription-polymerase chain reaction (RT-PCR) Southern blot method. The more malignant gliomas appeared to express two Ig-like loop types of FGFR1 (FGFR1-β) predominantly. We describe here the characterization of alternative transcripts of FGFR1 in astrocytic tumors and the possibility that the ratio of FGFR1-β and FGFR1-α (β/α ratio of FGFR1) transcripts may be useful as a marker for assessing malignancy grade of glioma.

We also examined the expression of FGFR2 (BEK), one of the FGFR family members. FGFR2 has 72% homology with FGFR1 on the overall level of amino acids; however, it is a different human FGFR gene product from FGFR1. The FGFR2 gene is reported to overexpress in breast cancer as well as FGFR1 [27]. Its expression in glioma, however, has not yet been characterized to our knowledge. We observed no, or a barely detectable level of, FGFR2 transcripts in glioblastoma multiforme (GBM) samples from patients. FGFR2 expression is reported to correlate with glia; therefore, our result suggested that GBM may be modulated with its FGFR2 expression. We discuss here the transcriptional regulations of both FGFR1 and FGFR2 gene in gliomas.

Materials and Methods

Tissue Specimens

We studied 26 patients with gliomas who underwent therapeutic removal of the tumors: 15 glioblastoma multiformes (GBMs), 6 anaplastic astrocytomas (AAs), and 5 low-grade astrocytomas (LGAs). Brain adjacent to the tumor in 10 of 15 patients with GBM and 1 of 6 patients with AA was also examined and each case compared with the patient's tumor. Two samples of normal brain tissue obtained at surgical lobectomy for epilepsy management and one sample obtained at autopsy of a patient without brain disease were also analyzed.

Cell Lines

Three cell lines of human malignant gliomas, SNB-19, U373MG, and U251MG, were analyzed. Three × 10⁶ cells were harvested from subconfluent flasks and submitted to RT-PCR analysis.

Histology

The neuropathological classification of human glial tumors used in this study was based on the grading scheme of Burger et al. [28]. The population of tumor cells and normal cells in each area was assessed by microscopic examination of sequential sections stained with hematoxylin and eosin.

RT-PCR Analysis

The presence and relative expression levels of the α-form and β-form of FGFR1 transcripts in normal brain, tumor, brain adjacent to tumor, and established cell lines were determined by RT-PCR analysis. mRNA was extracted using the MicroFast Track kit (Invitrogen, San Diego, CA, USA). For tumor and adjacent brain, we extracted mRNA from 20 4-μm-thick frozen sections. First-strand cDNA was synthesized from mRNA with a cDNA cycle kit (Invitrogen). For analysis of human FGFR-1, nucleotide primers P1a (5′-CGAGCTCACTGTGGAGTATCCATG-3′), corresponding to nucleotides -67 to -44 at the 5′ end, and P1b (5′-GTTACCCGCCAAGCACGTATAC-3′), complementary to nucleotides 1014–1035 at the 3′ end of the mRNA for FGFR1 [29–31], were used. For analysis of human FGFR2, we used nucleotide primers P1a-R2 (5′-AAGTGTGCAGATGGGATTAACGTC-3′), corresponding to nucleotides 113–136 at the 5′ end, and P1b-R2 (5′-ATTACCCGCCAAGCACGTATAT-3′), complementary to 1196–1217 at the 3′ end of the mRNA for FGFR2 [32]. PCR was performed for 30 cycles at 96°C for 30 sec, 64°C for 15 sec, and 72°C for 60 sec with GeneAmp PCR system 9600 (Perkin Elmer Cetus, Norwalk, CT, USA). As a quantitative control, (glyceraldehyde-3-phosphate dehydrogenase) (GAPDH) was amplified using nucleotide primers corresponding to nucleotides 27–46 at the 5′ end (5′-ACGGATTTGGTCGTATTGGG-3′) and complementary to nucleotides 238–257 (5′-TGATTTTGGAGGGATCTCGC-3′) at the 3′ end of mRNA for GAPDH [33]. Conditions were the same as in the analysis for FGFR-1. The PCR product of GAPDH was labeled with [^{32}P]-dCTP (deoxy cytosine triphosphate) by two-cycle PCR, run on 6% acrylamide gel, and exposed to film. Reaction mixtures (25 μl) contained 10 mM Tris-HCl (pH 8.3), 1.5 mM MgCl$_2$, 50 mM KCl, 0.1 mg/ml gelatine, 0.8 units of Taq polymerase (Perkin-Elmer/Cetus), and 0.20 mM each of deoxyadenosine triphosphate (dATP), deoxycytosine triphosphate (dCTP), deoxythymidine triphosphate (dTTP), and 0.5 μM each of primers. To quantify the relative expression levels of α-form and β-form transcripts, PCR Southern blot analysis was performed by transferring PCR products separated on 1.5% agarose gels to nylon membrane filters (Hybond-N, Amersham, MA, USA), and then hybridizing to ^{32}P-labeled FGFR-1 oligonucleotide complementary to nucleotides 610–630 [30], which is from a sequence common to α, β, and γ isoformes (5′-ATAACGGACCTTGTAGCCTCC-3′). The intensity of each signal was measured directly from hybridized nylon membrane by PhosphorImager (Molecular Dynamics, Sunnyvale, CA, USA). For FGFR2, an oligonucleotide corresponding to nucleotides 192–212 (5′-GGTCGTTTCATCTGCCTGGTC-3′) [32], which does not have homology with FGFR1, was used as a probe for Southern blot.

Results

Distinct Alternative Splicing of FGFR1 in Gliomas of Various Grades of Malignancy

To determine which forms of extracellular domain of FGFR-1 transcript are expressed in brain tumors, PCR was carried out with a 5′ primer (P1a), which began 67 bp

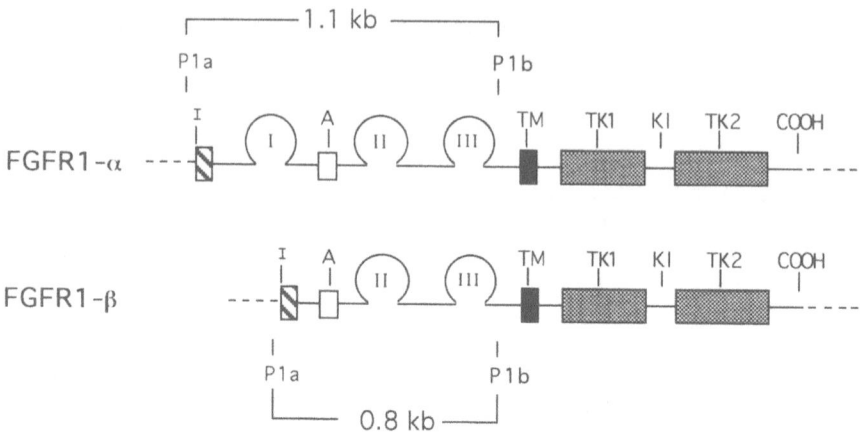

Fig. 1. Schematic of fibroblast growth factor receptor-1(FGFR1) mRNA and polymerase chain reaction (PCR) primer location. *I*, initiation start site; *I–III*, immunoglobulin-like disulfide loops; *A*, acidic box domain; *TM*, transmembrane domain; *TK1, TK2*, tyrosine kinase domain 1 and 2; *KI*, kinase insert region; *COOH*, carboxyl terminal; *Dotted lines*, nontranslated regions; *hatched box*, leader sequence. The PCR yielded 1.1-kb and 0.8-kb fragments encoding FGFR1-α and FGFR1-β, respectively. The 1.0-kb fragment for FGFR1-γ is also detected by this PCR (not shown in this schema)

upstream of the common translational initiation site in the α- and β-form cDNA, and a 3′ primer (P1b), which ended 111 bp downstream from the site having a single base pair T/C variant [19]. This PCR yielded 1.1-kb (1102-bp), 1.0-kb (979-bp), and 0.8-kb (835-bp) fragments encoding the α, γ, and β motifs, respectively, which were confirmed to be FGFR-1 (flg) cDNA by PCR Southern blot analysis (Fig. 1).

All GBMs expressed predominantly the β-form (Fig. 2A) while adjacent brain tissues showed low to nondetectable levels of FGFR1 expression. GAPDH signals showed that the amounts of mRNA from adjacent brains were as much as in the tumors themselves. LGAs expressed less β-form than GBMs, and AAs had intermediate expression of β-form (Fig. 3). Glioma cell lines showed predominantly the β-form, consistent with GBM specimens from the patients (Fig. 4). Figure 5 shows the relationship between the malignancy of gliomas and the expression ratio of β- and α-forms. The β/α ratio in GBMs varied from 1.52 to 4.95 [mean, 2.54 ± 0.32 (SEM); $n = 11$], while the ratio in LGAs appeared to range from 0.52 to 0.97 [mean, 0.72 ± 0.07, SEM; $n = 5$]. AAs displayed two receptor phenotypes, one similar to that of GBMs, the other similar to that of LGAs. Higher and lower subset of AAs showed the ratios of 1.70 ± 0.12 (SEM; $n = 3$) and 0.6 ± 0.12 (SEM; $n = 3$), respectively. The normal brain samples showed a low β/α ratio [mean, 0.53 ± 0.04 (SEM); n = 10].

FGFR2 Expression in Normal Brain and Gliomas

We analyzed FGFR2 expression in seven GBMs and their adjacent normal brains, four AAs, and three LGAs (see Figs. 2A, 7). PCR with P1a-R2 and P1b-R2 gave a 1.1-kb product of FGFR2-α (3 Ig form), a 0.9-kb product of FGFR2-β_1, and a 0.8-kb product of FGFR2-β_2 (2-Ig form lacking the acidic box). This FGFR2-β_2 is a novel form; the functional difference from FGFR2-β_1 is as yet unknown (Fig. 6). In GBMs, the expressions of FGFR2 were lost or much lower than that of their adjacent normal brains

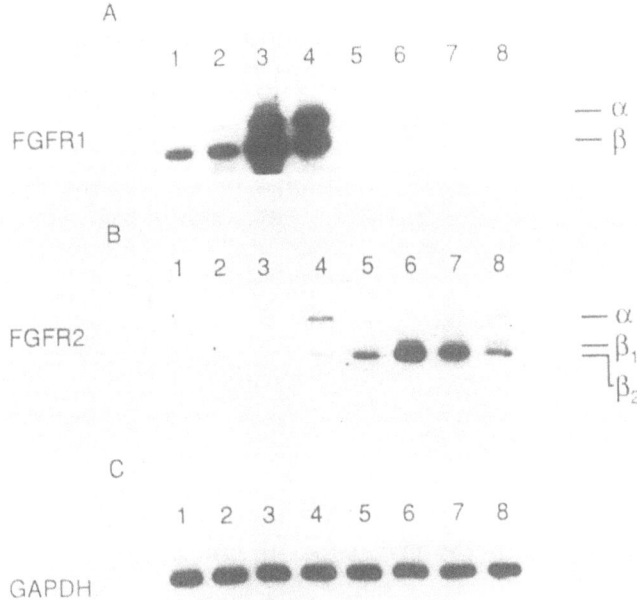

Fig. 2A–C. A Reverse transcription (RT-)PCR Southern blot analysis of FGFR1 expression in glioblastoma multiformes (1–4) and their adjacent normal brains (5–8). RT-PCR Southern blot analysis was performed as described in Materials and Methods. FGFR1 primers P1a and P1b gave FGFR1-α (1.1-kb), FGFR1-γ (1.0-kb), and FGFR1-β (0.8-kb) fragments. **B** Analysis of FGFR2 expression in glioblastoma multiforme (GBMs). FGFR2 primers P1a-R2 and P1b-R2 gave FGFR2-α (1.1-kb), FGFR2-β1 (0.9-kb), and FGFR2-β₂ (0.8-kb) fragments. **C** As a quantitative control, glyceraldehyde-3-phosphate dehydrogenase (GAPDH) was amplified for each specimen using the same amount of cDNA used in **A** and **B**. Amount of samples appeared to be at almost the same level as determined by GAPDH bands

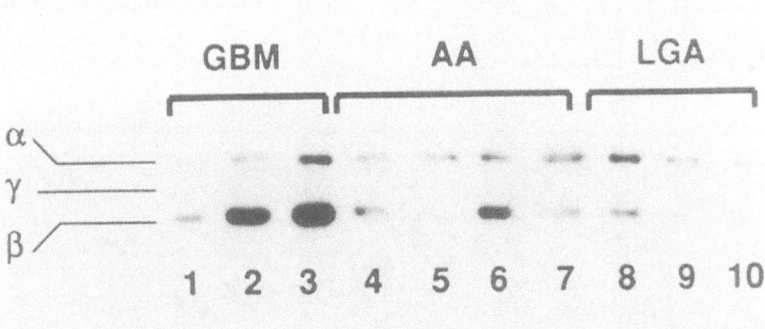

Fig. 3. FGFR1 expression in gliomas of various degrees of malignancy. Analysis was done as described. *Lanes 1–3*, GBM; *lanes 4–7*, anaplastic astrocytoma (AA); *lanes 8–10*, low-grade astrocytoma (LGA)

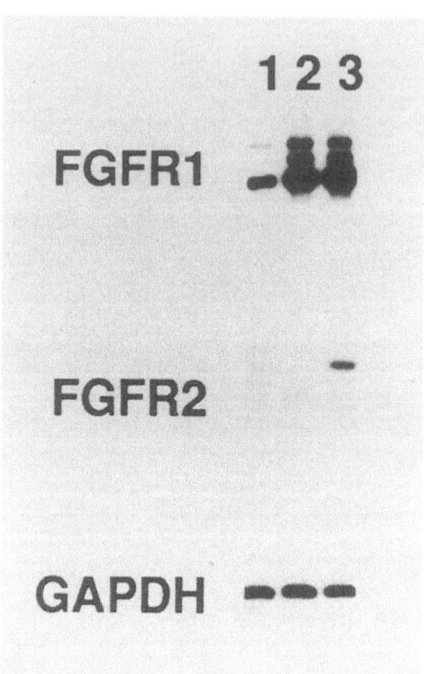

Fig. 4. Differential expression of FGFR1 variants in human glioma cell lines were examined by RT-PCR Southern blot. The same number of cells was used for analysis. *Lane 1*, SNB-19; *lane 2*, U373MG; *lane 3*, U251 MG

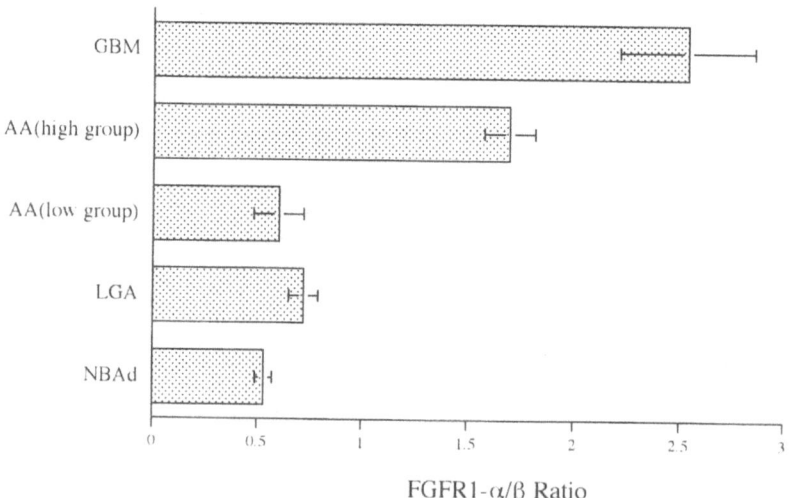

FGFR1-α/β Ratio

Fig. 5. FGFR1-β/FGFR1-α ratio in various tissues. Mean values ± SEM for FGFR1α/FGFR1β ratios were as follows: *GBM*, 2.54 ± 0.32 (*n* = 11); *AA*, 1.70 ± 0.12 (high group, *n* = 3) and 0.6 ± 0.12 (low group, *n* = 3); *LGA*, 0.72 ± 0.07 (*n* = 5); *normal adult brain (NBAd)*, 0.53 ± 0.04 (*n* = 10)

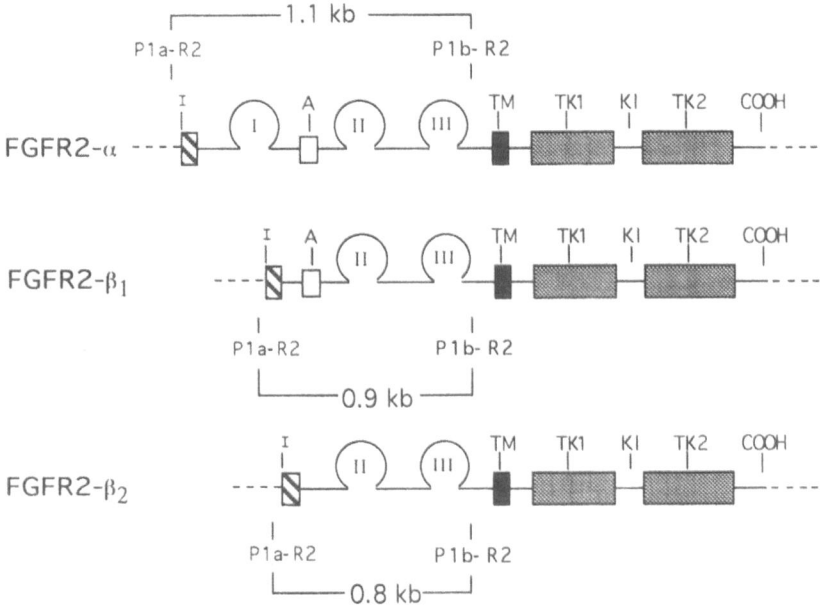

Fig. 6. Schematic of FGFR2 mRNA and PCR primer location. Symbols are as described in Fig. 1. The PCR yielded 1.1-kb, 0.9-kb, and 0.8-kb fragments encoding FGFR2-α, FGFR2-β$_1$ and FGFR2-β$_2$, respectively. FGFR2-β$_2$ is a novel 2-Ig form lacking an acidic box

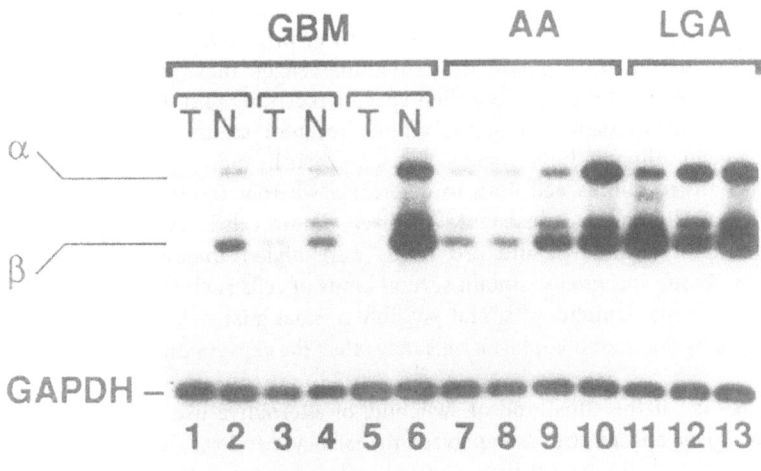

Fig. 7. FGFR2 expression in human gliomas different in their malignancy. FGFR2 cDNA was amplified as mentioned in Materials and Methods. *Lanes 1, 3, 5*, GBM; *lanes 2, 4, 6*, the adjacent brain of lanes 1, 3, 5; *lanes 7–10*, AA; *lanes 11–13*, LGA. GAPDH amplifications showed that the mRNA amounts in these samples are almost the same

whereas FGFR1 transcripts were overexpressed. On the other hand, AAs and LGAs showed strong amplificaions in all cases (Fig. 7).

Discussion

We have demonstrated here differential alternative splicing of FGFR1 in human gliomas. RT-PCR studies clearly showed predominant expression of FGFR1-β transcript in GBMs, the most malignant astrocytic brain tumors (see Fig. 2A). LGAs expressed predominantly FGFR1-α transcripts as well as normal adult cerebrums (see Fig. 3), while AAs, having malignancy intermediate between GBMs and LGAs, showed an intermediate expression pattern.

Several studies have indicated that alternative splicing of mRNA is responsible for generating the diverse receptor forms [22,35], and three amino-terminal domain motifs, two juxtamembrane motifs, and two intracellular carboxyl-terminal domain motifs combine to form a minimum of 6 and potentially 12 receptor forms [19]. A 144-bp substitution in place of the 267-bp sequence, which encoded the first Ig-like loop of FGFR1-α, gives rise to FGFR1-γ. This γ-form has two Ig-like domains but lacks a hydrophobic membrane translocation sequence (signal sequence); therefore, this is the putative intracellular receptor. It is reported that FGFR-γ transcript is increased in rat prostate tumors. Also, transfection of fibroblasts with an FGFR-γ expression vector exhibited an anchorage-independent transformed phenotype [36]. As to first-Ig domain the lack of 267-bp exon gives 2-Ig loop FGFR1, which was reported to have a tenfold higher affinity for its ligand than 3-Ig loop FGFR1 [37].

It is known that some transformed cells use alternative RNA splicing to modify growth factors (PDGF-A) [38], or adhesion molecules (CD44 [39,40]; Tenascin [41]; fibronectin [42]) or growth-regulatory genes (NF1 gene) [43,44] to obtain the malignant phenotype. Mitogenic signals provided by growth factors may be transmitted to the cell nucleus by the action of intracellular messengers that are activated through an interaction of growth factors and their specific receptors [45]. From this standpoint, the increased population of higher affinity receptor seems to give the cells great advantage in utilizing the mitogenic signal by their ligand.

We analyzed glioma cell lines to determine whether the trend found in clinical samples of glioma was consistent. All three glioma cell lines appeared to express predominantly FGFR1-β, and β/α ratios were higher than in tissue samples of gliomas. Tissue specimens contain several kinds of cells such as vascular endothelial cells, fibroblasts, lymphocytes, and possibly normal glial cells. Therefore the signal generated by these nonneoplastic cells may affect the expression pattern of neoplastic cells.

To assess whether this kind of switching of alternative use of exon is conserved within a given species, we also analyzed rat astrocyte and rat glioma cell lines. Interestingly, all rat glioma cell lines showed a β-dominant pattern similar to human glioma cell lines. Rat type-1 astrocytes expressed more FGFR1-α than FGFR1-β. Overall, the tendency for expression of FGFR1 of transformed cells to shift from α- to β-form is conserved between human and rat (unpublished data).

Developmentally, 3-Ig domain forms of FGFR1 are the predominant forms of receptor expressed during mouse embryogenesis [20,21]. Two-Ig domain forms were not detected by RNase protection analysis until after birth [46]. Following birth, 3-Ig and 2-Ig forms are simultaneously expressed at nearly levels in heart, lung, and muscle, but in brain, 3-Ig domain forms continue to be the predominant form [20].

Considering the report that FGFR1-β has higher affinity than FGFR1-α, more malignant cells may take a certain advantage by switching the expression of FGFR1 from 3-Ig form (FGFR1-α) to the 2-Ig form (FGFR1-β).

The relative increase in PCR amplification of FGFR1-β compared to that of FGFR1-α may provide a sensitive method for detecting malignant glial tumor cells in small biopsy specimens. Further studies, however, are required to assess whether the β/α ratio can be a useful marker for assessing malignancy grade of gliomas.

FGFR2 is a product of the human FGFR gene that differs from the FGFR1 gene [16]. FGFR1 and FGFR2 accept the common ligand members such as aFGF (FGF-1), bFGF (FGF-2), and K-FGF/HST (FGF-4); however, the functional difference between FGFR1 and FGFR2 is not clear. The two FGF receptors have distinct spatial expression in brain during development, and it is suggested that they may have a distinct role for the growth and differentiation of both neuron and glia. In the adult mouse central nervous system, FGFR1 is expressed preferentially in neuronal populations but FGFR2 localization is correlated with glia [34]. In our study, FGFR1 appeared to be expressed dominantly in cortex rather than white matter when obtained from adult humans; on the other hand, FGFR2 was expressed in both cortex and white matter. Considering that neurons exist preferentially in cortex and that glia exist in both cortex and white matter, our results were consistent with previous reports. Interestingly, GBMs showed no or very low expression of FGFR2, although they have been recognized to originate from glial cells. The gene of FGFR2 is reported to be localized on chromosome 10q26 [47]. It is known that chromosome 10 is frequently lost in tumor cells from GBMs and that the common region of deletion is in 10q24–q26 [48]. It is not clear whether decreased expression of FGFR2 is because there is a partial population of tumor cells with chromosome 10 deletion or because of suppressed transcription of FGFR2 gene. Supposing that chromosome 10 deletion took place, the putative tumor suppressor gene, which is inferred to localize in chromosome 10q24–q26, would lose its regulation with growth factor receptor expression. As the promoter sequence of FGFR1 is not homologous to that of the FGFR2 gene [49,50], these two genes may be controlled in different ways. In any case, overexpression of FGFR1-β and decrease of FGFR2 expression seem to be characteristic of GBMs. The functional roles of both receptors in glioma must be studied to assess the importance of FGFRs in tumor progression.

References

1. Folkman J, Klagsbrun M (1987) Angiogenic factors. Science 235:442–447
2. Serro G, Khoo JC (1982) An in vitro model to study adipose differentiation in serum-free medium. Anal Biochem 120:351–359
3. Broad TE, Ham RG (1983) Growth and adipose differentiation of sheep preadipocyte fibroblasts in serum-free medium. Eur J Biochem 135:33–39
4. Walcke P, Cowan WM, Ueno N, Baird A, Guillemin R (1986) Fibroblast growth factor promotes survival of dissociated hippocampal neurons and enhances neurite extension. Proc Natl Acad Sci USA 83:3012–3016
5. Togari A, Dickens G, Kuzuya H, Guroff G (1985) The effect of fibroblast growth factor on PC12 cells. J Neurosci 5:307–316
6. Wagner JA, D'Amore PA (1986) Neurite outgrowth induced by an endothelial cell mitogen isolated from retina. J Cell Biol 103:1363–1367
7. Morrison RS, Sharma A, De Vellis J, Bradshaw RA (1986) Basic fibroblast growth factor supports the survival of cerebral cortical neurons in primary culture. Proc Natl Acad Sci USA 83:7537–7541

8. Presta M, Moscatelli D, Joseph-Silverstein J, Rifkin DB (1986) Purification from a human hepatoma cell line of a basic fibroblast growth factor-like molecule that stimulates capillary endothelial cell plasminogen activator production, DNA synthesis, and migration. Mol Cell Biol 6:4060–4066

9. Armstrong RC, Harvath L, Dubois-Dalcq ME (1990) Type 1 astrocytes and oligodendrocyte-type 2 astrocyte gilal progenitors migrate toward distinct molecules. J Neurosci Res 27:400–407

10. Mignatti P, Morimoto T, Rifkin DB (1991) Basic fibroblast growth factor released by single, isolated cells stimulates their migration in an autocrine manner. Proc Natl Acad Sci USA 88:11007–11011

11. Kimelman D, Kirschner M (1987) Synergistic induction of mesoderm by FGF and TGF-β and the identification of an mRNA coding for FGF in the early Xenopus embryo. Cell 67:229–231

12. Slack JM, Darlington BG, Heath JK, Godsave SF (1987) Mesoderm induction in early Xenopus embryos by heparin-binding growth factors. Nature 326:197–200

13. Kimelman D, Abraham JA, Haaparanta T, Palisi TM, Kirschner MW (1988) The presence of fibroblast growth factor in frog egg: its role as a natural mesoderm inducer. Science 242:1053–1056

14. Burgess WH, Maciag T (1989) The heparin-binding (fibroblast) growth factor family of proteins. Annu Rev Biochem 58:575–606

15. Johnson DE, Williams LT (1993) Structural and functional diversity in FGF receptor multigene family. Advance Cancer Res 60:1–41

16. Dionne CA, Crumley G, Bellot F, Kaplow JM, Searfross G, Ruta M, Burgess WH, Jaye M, Schlessinger J (1990) Cloning and expression of two distinct high-affinity receptors cross-reacting with acidic and basic fibroblast growth factors. EMBO J 9:2685–2692

17. Keegan K, Johnson DE, Williams LT, Hayman MJ (1991) Isolation of additional member of the fibroblast growth factor receptor family, FGFR-3. Proc Natl Acad Sci USA 88:1095–1099

18. Partanen J, Makela TP, Erola E, Kohonen J, Hirvonen H, Claesson-Welsh L, Alitalo K (1991) FGFR-4, a novel acidic fibroblast growth factor receptor with a distinct expression pattern. EMBO J 10:1347–1354

19. Hou J, Kan M, McKeehan K, McBride G, Adams P, McKeehan WL (1991) Fibroblast growth factors from liver vary in three structural domains. Science 251:665–668

20. Werner S, Duan DSR, de Vries C, Peters KG, Johnson DE, Williams LT (1992) Differential splicing in the extracellular region of fibroblast growth factor receptor 1 generates receptor variants with different ligand-binding specificities. Mol Cell Biol 12:82–88

21. Reid HH, Wilks AF, Bernard O (1990) Two forms of basic fibroblast growth factor receptor-like mRNA are expressed in the developing mouse brain. Proc Natl Acad Sci USA 87:1596–1600

22. Johnson DE, Lu J, Chen H, Werner S, Williams LT (1991) The human Fibroblast growth factor receptor genes: a common structural arrangement underlies the mechanisms for generating receptor forms that differ in their third immunoglobulin domain. Mol Cell Biol 11:4627–4634

23. Eisemann A, Ahn JA, Graziani G, Tronick SR, Ron D (1991) Alternative splicing generates at least five different isoforms of the human basic FGF receptor. Oncogene 6:1195–1202

24. Takahashi JA, Suzui H, Yasuda Y, Ito N, Ohta M, Jaye M, Fukumoto M, Oda Y, Kikuchi H, Hatanaka M (1991) Gene expression of fibroblast growth factor receptors in the tissues of human gliomas and meningiomas. Biochem Biophys Res Commun 177:1–7

25. Morrison RS, Gross JL, Herblin WF, Reilly TM, La Sala PA, Alterman RL, Moskal JR, Kornblith PL, Deter DL (1990) Basic fibroblast growth factor-like activity and receptors expressed in a human glioma cell line. Cancer Res 50:2524–2529

26. Morrison RS, Yamaguchi F, Bruner JM, Tang M, McKeehan W, Berger MS (1994) Fibroblast growth factor receptor gene expression and immunoreactivity are elevated in human glioblastoma multiforme. Cancer Res 54:2794–2799

27. Adnane J, Gaudray P, Dionne CA, Crumley G, Jaye M, Schlessinger J, Jeanteur P, Birnbaum D, Theillet C (1991) BEK and FIG, two receptors to members of the FGF family, are amplified in subsets of human breast cancers. Oncogene 6:659–663

28. Burger PC, Scheithaner BW, Vogel FS (1991) Surgical pathology of the nervous system and its coverings, 3rd edn. Churchill Livingstone, New York, pp 193–437

29. Ruta M, Howk R, Ricca G, Drohan W, Zabelshansky M, Laureys G, Barton DE, Francke U, Schlessinger J, Givol D (1988) A novel protein tyrosine kinase gene whose expression is modulated during endothelial cell differentiation. Oncogene 3:9–15

30. Ruta M, Burgess W, Givol D, Epstein J, Neiger N, Kaplow J, Crumley G, Dionne C, Jaye M, Schlessinger J (1989) Receptor for acidic fibroblast growth factor is related to the tyrosine kinase encoded by the fms-like gene (FlG). Proc Natl Acad Sci USA 86:8722–8726

31. Issachi A, Bergonzoni L, Sarmientos P (1990) Complete sequence of a human receptor for acidic and basic fibroblast growth factors. Nucleic Acids Res 18:1906

32. Dionne CA (1990) Human bek mRNA for fibroblast growth factor receptor-BEK. GenBank, HUMFGFRBE, Accession: X52832

33. Ercolani L, Florence B, Denara M, Alexander M (1988) Isolation and complete sequence of a functional human glyceraldehyde-3-phosphate dehydrogenase gene. J Biol Chem 263:15335–15341

34. Peters KG, Werner S, Chen G, Williams LT (1992) Two FGF receptor genes are differentially expressed in epithelial and mesenchymal tissues during limb formation and organogenesis in the mouse. Development 114:233–243

35. Champion-Arnaud P, Ronsin C, Gilbert E, Gesnel MC, Houssaint E, Breathnach R (1991) Multiple mRNAs code for proteins related to the BEK fibroblast growth factor receptor. Oncogene 6:979–987

36. Yan G, Wang F, Fukabori Y, Sussman D, Hou J, McKeehan WL (1992) Expression and transforming activity of a variant of the heparin-binding fibroblast growth factor receptor (flg) gene resulting from splicing of the alpha exon at an alternate 3′-acceptor site. Biochem Biophys Res Commun 183:423–430

37. Shi E, Kan M, Xu J, Wang F, Hou J, McKeehan WL (1993) Control of fibroblast growth factor receptor kinase signal transduction by heterodimerization of combinatorial splice variants. Mol Cell Biol 13:3907–3918

38. Collins T, Bonthron DT, Orkin SH (1987) Alternative RNA splicing affects function of encoded platelet-derived growth factor A chain. Nature 328:621–624

39. Matsumura Y, Tarin D (1992) Significance of CD44 gene products for cancer diagnosis and disease evaluation. Lancet 340:1053–1058

40. Tanabe KK, Ellis LM, Saya H (1993) Expression of CD44R1 adhesion molecule is increased in human colon carcinomas and metastases. Lancet 341:725–726

41. Borsi L, Carnemolla B, Nicolo G, Spina B, Tanara G, Zardi L (1992) Expression of different tenascin isoforms in normal, hyperplastic and neoplastic human breast tissues. Int J Cancer 52:688–692

42. Oyama F, Hirohashi S, Shimosato Y, Titani K, Sekiguchi K (1990) Oncodevelopmental regulation of the alternative splicing of fibronectin pre-messenger RNA in human lung tissues. Cancer Res 50:1075–1078

43. Nishi T, Saya H (1991) Neurofibromatosis type-1 (NF1) gene: implication in neuroectodermal differentiation and genesis of brain tumors. Cancer Metastasis Rev 10:301–310

44. Mochizuki H, Nishi T, Bruner JM, Lee PSY, Levin VA, Saya H (1992) Alternative splicing of neurofibromatosis type 1 gene transcript in malignant brain tumors: PCR analysis of frozen-section mRNA. Mol Carcinog 6:83–87

45. Ullrich A, Schlessinger J (1990) Signal transduction by receptors with tyrosine kinase activity. Cell 61:203–212

46. Bernard O, Li M, Rei HH (1991) Expression of two different forms of fibroblast growth factor receptor 1 in different mouse tissues and cell lines. Proc Natl Acad Sci USA 88:7625–7629

47. Mattei M-G, Moreau A, Gesnel M-C, Houssaint E, Breathnach R (1991) Assignment by in situ hybridization of a fibroblast growth factor receptor gene to human chromosome band 10q26. Hum Genet 87:84–86

48. Rasheed BKA, Fuller GN, Friedman AH, Bigner DD, Bigner SH (1992) Loss of heterozygosity

for 10q loci in human gliomas. Genes Chromosomes & Cancer 5:75–82

49. Saito H, Kouhara H, Kasayama S, Kishimoto T, Sato B (1992) Characterization of the promoter region of the murine fibroblast growth factor receptor 1 gene. Biochem Biophys Res Commun 183:688–693

50. Avivi A, Skorecki K, Yayon A, Givol D (1992) Promoter region of the murine fibroblast growth factor receptor 2 (bek/KGFR) gene. Oncogene 7:1957–1962

Point Mutations of Epidermal Growth Factor Receptor Transcripts in Primary Human Malignant Gliomas

Noriaki Sugawa, Yoshio Nakagawa, and Satoshi Ueda

Abstract. Malignant gliomas, in particular glioblastomas, have various types of aberrant epidermal growth factor receptors (EGFR). The most common type of alteration of the EGFR in glioblastomas shows an aberrant mRNA lacking 801 bases that encode amino acids 30–297 of the extracellular domain of the receptor. Other types of aberrant EGFR lack amino acids 983–1067 and 983–1091 of the intracellular domain of the receptor. However, fewer than 40% of glioblastomas have these aberrant EGFRs. We estimated that malignant gliomas have other aberrant EGFRs that we could not detect using Northern blot analysis. Therefore, we examined the point mutation to find a new aberrant EGFR and were able to determine the point mutations of EGFR transcripts. One mutation, from Gly to Arg, occurred in codon 998; in the other mutation, cytocine was added at sense base 3366, the codons were changed from 1037 to 1054, and stop codon (TGA) appeared at 1055. These mutations were found among lack lesions of the intracellular domain of the aberrant EGFR that we previously reported in malignant gliomas.

Key words. Point mutation—Epidermal growth factor receptor (EGFR)—Malignant gliomas

Introduction

Aberrant epidermal growth factor receptors (EGFR) found in malignant gliomas have abnormalities in the extracellular and intracellular domains [1–3]. These abnormalities have been reported to be related to the malignancy of gliomas with tyrosine kinase activity. We previously analyzed 73 gliomas for expression and abnormalities of EGFR and found that aberrant transcripts were expressed in 35% of the glioblastomas, 17.6% of anaplastic gliomas, and 0% of low-grade gliomas. More than 50% of the malignant gliomas did not have these aberrant EGFRs, however, and therefore we examined new aberrant EGFR mRNA in human malignant gliomas without expression of these aberrant EGFRs.

Department of Neurosurgery, Kyoto Prefectural University of Medicine, Kyoto 602, Japan

Materials and Method

Tumor Materials

We used 13 primary glioblastomas, 3 anaplastic astrocytomas, and 3 medullo-blastomas. These samples did not have overexpression of normal EGFR, and the aberrant has been previously reported.

RNA Isolation

The tumor tissue was frozen for 1 week to 1 year at −80°C. A small fragment of each tumor piece studied was examined histopathologically. Total RNA was isolated from the frozen tumor tissue by homogenization in guanidinium isothiocyanate buffer followed by ultracentrifugation in a cesium chloride gradient.

Production of cDNA and Amplification by the Polymerase Chain Reaction

Single-stranded cDNA was produced using Moloney murine leukemia virus reverse transcriptase and random priming with hexanucleotides. The single-stranded cDNA was subjected to polymerase chain reaction (PCR) using appropriate primers (Fig.1). The PCR was standaridized to 30 cycles, each consisting of denaturation (94°C, 1 min), annealing (54°C, 1 min), and extension (72°C, 3 min).

Production of Single-Stranded DNA by PCR and Sequencing

Double-stranded cDNA was produced and amplified as described. The DNA was then electrophoresed and isolated from 1% agarose gel by freeze-thawing. cDNA was then used in an unbalanced PCR reaction (30 cycles as described previously) with primers PC135 (50 pM) and PC136 (1.5 pM) to produce a single-stranded sense cDNA template, which was isolated as described. Approximately 100 ng of this sense-stranded cDNA was then primed with PC145 (0.6 pM) and sequenced by the deoxy chain-termination method, according to the manufacturer's recommendations (Fig. 1).

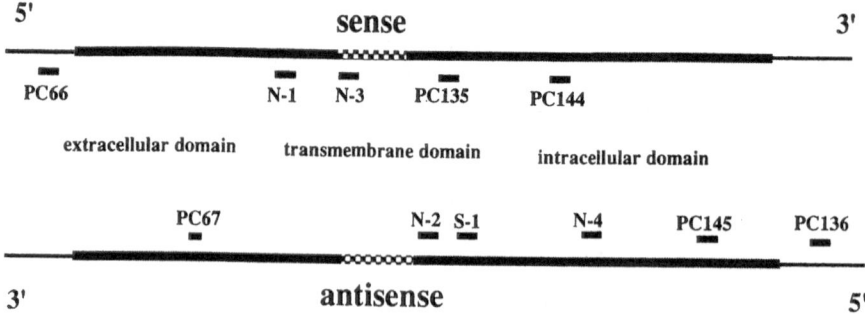

Fig. 1. Primers used for polymerase chain reaction of cDNA of epidermal growth factor receptor (EGFR)

Results

Case 1 (anaplastic astrocytoma) revealed a codon 998 mutation (Gly(CCG)-Arg(GCT)) in the intracellular domain of the EGFR mRNA. In the mutation of Case 2 (glioblastoma), cytocine was added at sense base 3366, the codons were changed from 1037 to 1054, and the stop codon (TGA) appeared at 1055 in the intracellular domain of the EGFR mRNA (Fig. 2).

Discussion

The most common type of alteration of the EGFR gene in human glioblastomas results in the synthesis of an aberrant mRNA lacking 801 bases that encode amino acids 6–273 of the receptor's extracellular domain [1,2,4]. This aberrant EGFR was reported to have tyrosine kinase activation without ligands [5,6]. For the intracellular domain, ligand-sensitized transformation has been conferred by constructs lacking sequences that encode a portion of the receptor important for receptor internalization and degradation (between residues 991 and 1022) and thus downregulation of the receptor [7,8]. These new mutations of EGFR mRNA in malignant gliomas occurred between the lost regions of the intracellular domain of the aberrant EGFR still reported in glioblastomas [3]. On the other hand, autophosphorylation is considered to be important in regulating the kinase activity for determining substrate specificity. The major autophosphorylation sites are located at Tyr-1068, -1148, and -1173, and the minor sites are located at Tyr-992 and -1086 in EGFR [9]. These new mutations were located

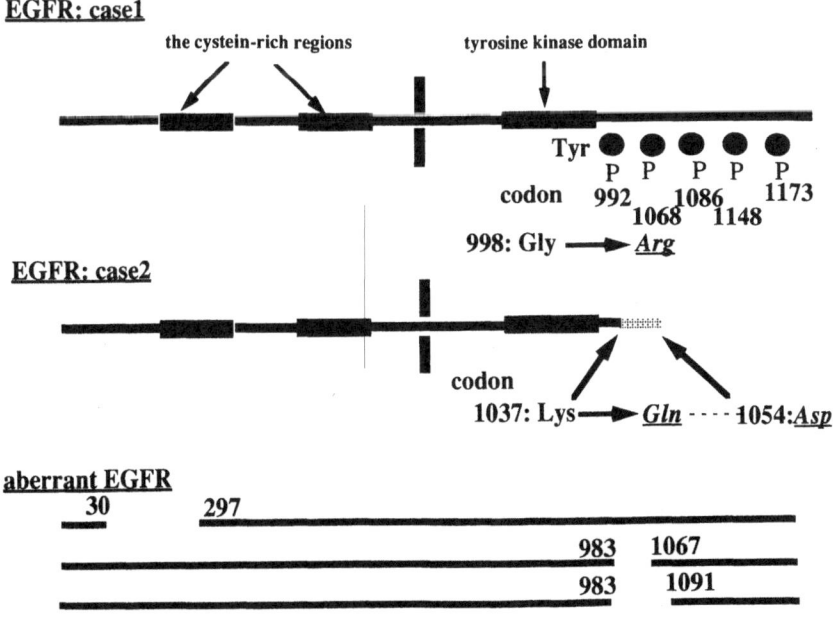

Fig. 2. Mutations of EGFR mRNA observed in cases 1 and 2

near these autophosphorylation sites. These findings suggest that these new mutations are important in the malignancy of gliomas.

References

1. Yamazaki H, Fukui Y, Ueyama Y, Tamaoki N, Kawamoto T, Taniguchi S, Shibuya M (1988) Amplification of the structurally and functionally altered epidermal growth factor receptor gene (c-erbB) in human brain tumors. Mol Cell Biol 8:1816–1820
2. Sugawa N, Ekstrand AJ, James CD, Collins VP (1990) Identical splicing of aberrant epidermal growth factor receptor transcript from amplified rearranged genes in human glioblastomas. Proc Natl Acad Sci USA 87:8602–8606
3. Ekstrand AJ, Sugawa N, James CD, Collins VP (1992) Amplified and rearranged epidermal growth factor receptor genes in human glioblastomas reveal deletions of sequences encoding portions of the N- and/or C-terminal tails. Proc Natl Acad Sci USA 89:4309–4313
4. Humphrey P, Wong AJ, Vogelstein B, Zalutsky MR, Fuller GN, Archer GE, Friedman HS, Kwatra MM, Bigner SH, Bigner DD (1990) Anti-synthetic peptide antibody reacting at the fusion junction of deletion-mutant epidermal growth factor receptors in human glioblastoma. Proc Natl Acad Sci USA 87(11):4207–4211
5. Yamazaki H, Ohba Y, Tamaoki N, Shibuya M (1990) A deletion mutation within the ligand binding domain is responsible for activation of epidermal growth factor receptor gene in human brain tumors. Jpn J Cancer Res 81:773–779
6. Ekstrand AJ, Longo N, Hamid ML, Olson JJ, Liu L, Collins VP, James CD (1994) Functional characterization of an EGF receptor with a truncated extracellular domain expressed in glioblastomas with EGFR gene amplification. Oncogene 1994(9):2313–2320
7. Chen WS, Lazar CS, Lund KA, Welsh JB, Chang CP, Walton GM, Der CJ, Wiley HS, Grill GN, Rosenfeld MG (1989) Functional independence of the epidermal growth factor receptor from a domain required for ligand induced internalization and calcium regulation. Cell 59:33–43
8. Wells A, Welsh JB, Lazar CS, Wiley HS, Gill GN, Rosenfeld MG (1990) Ligand-induced transformation by a noninternalizing epidermal growth factor receptor. Science 247:962–964
9. Schlessinger J, Ullrich A (1992) Growth factor signaling by receptor tyrosine kinases. Neuron 9:383–391

Expression of Vascular Endothelial Growth Factor in Human Brain Tumors In Vivo

Kiyonobu Ikezaki[1], Ken Samoto[1, 2], Takanori Inamura[1],
Tadahisa Shono[1, 2], Masashi Fukui[1], Mayumi Ono[2],
and Michihiko Kuwano[2]

Abstract. To examine the expression of vascular endothelial growth factor (VEGF), which may correlate with neovascularization in human brain tumors, the mRNA levels of the VEGF gene were determined by a Northern blot analysis in various human brain tumors, including gliomas, meningiomas, neurinomas, hemangioblastomas, hemangiopericytomas, and metastatic brain tumors. We obtained the VEGF mRNA expression index by dividing the VEGF mRNA levels by glyceraldehyde phosphate dehydrogenase (GAPDH) mRNA levels to compare the intensity of VEGF gene expression among tumors. In all brain tumors examined, the mRNA of VEGF was expressed at various levels. The mRNA levels of VEGF were significantly higher in gliomas and meningiomas. There was a significant difference between benign neuroepithelial tumors and malignant counterparts regarding the expression index of VEGF. However, the expression index showed similar values when anaplastic meningiomas were compared with meningotheliomatous meningiomas. The localization of VEGF protein was examined immunocytochemically. VEGF was specifically expressed on the endothelial cells in the tumor capillaries and also on the tumor cells surrounding them in various brain tumors. These findings suggest that VEGF is expressed in the wide range of brain tumors at various degrees and they may work on tumor angiogenesis in paracrine fashion to develop and maintain tumor vascularity. Furthermore, VEGF may work as an essential endothelial-specific mitogen in brain tumors.

Key words. Vascular endothelial growth factor—Angiogenesis—Brain neoplasm—Northern blot analysis—Endothelial cells

Introduction

Compared to the normal angiogenesis that has self-limiting and strict regulation, tumor angiogenesis appears to be deregulated and occurs to support tumor enlargement. Currently, various peptide growth factors have been identified in brain tumors and are considered to work in an autocrine fashion for tumor proliferation [1,2].

Departments of [1] Neurosurgery and [2] Biochemistry, Kyushu University Faculty of Medicine, Fukuoka 812-82, Japan

Some of these have also been known as angiogenic growth factors, which act on the endothelial cells with a paracrine mechanism and induce neovascularization in brain tumors (tumor angiogenesis) [3–5].

Basic fibroblast growth factor (bFGF), for example, shows a potent angiogenic activity [4,6,7], and a high level of bFGF production has been identified in human gliomas [8–11]. Epidermal growth factor (EGF) and its related family, transforming growth factor- (TGF-) α, also stimulate angiogenesis [12–14]. In contrast, the TGF-β family antagonizes the effects of bFGF [15–18]. TGF-α and -β are also produced at high levels in various tumor cells [2,19,20]. However, their roles as inducers of angiogenic growth may be limited to circumstances involving cell death and injury because they lack a signal peptide required for extracellular secretion in normal conditions [21]. It is also unclear whether any of these agents actually mediates angiogenesis in vivo.

On the contrary, vascular endothelial growth factor (VEGF), also known as vascular permeability factor, is an endothelial cell-specific mitogen. VEGF is a preferentially secreted 36- to 46-kDa dimeric heparin-binding glycoprotein and has been identified from the conditioned medium of several cell lines [22–24]. Molecular cloning of the complementary DNA (cDNA) has revealed four forms of VEGF in human cells to date. These forms, generated by alternative splicing of the VEGF gene [25,26], are designated $VEGF_{121}$, $VEGF_{165}$, $VEGF_{189}$, and $VEGF_{206}$. VEGF can induce neovascularization in vivo [27,28] and in in vitro angiogenesis models [29,30]. We investigated the in vivo expression of VEGF mRNA in various human brain tumors, and the responsibility of VEGF for tumor angiogenesis is discussed.

Materials and Methods

Samples

Surgically removed human specimens (Table 1), as prepared for histopathological diagnosis, Northern blot analysis, and immunocytochemical examination, formed the basis of this study. All surgical specimens were snap-frozen immediately after removal and stored at −80°C until processing. A human glioma cell line (IN301) was

Table 1. Vascular endothelial growth factor (VEGF) expression index.

Histology	Expression index
Astrocytoma grade II ($n = 5$)	0.197 ± 0.097
Oligodendroglioma ($n = 3$)	0.389 ± 0.185
Glioblastoma ($n = 5$)	0.555 ± 0.200*
Medulloblastoma + PNET ($n = 3$)	0.387 ± 0.049
Hemangioblastoma ($n = 4$)	0.328 ± 0.151
Hemangiopericytoma ($n = 3$)	0.170 ± 0.060
Anaplastic meningioma ($n = 4$)	0.406 ± 0.253
Meningotheliomatous meningioma ($n = 4$)	0.505 ± 0.158*
Metastasis ($n = 3$)	0.124 ± 0.069
Neurinoma ($n = 3$)	0.246 ± 0.171

Data are expressed as mean ± SD.
PNET, primitive neuroectodermal tumor.
*$P < .05$ when compared to other tumors.

utilized as a positive control, and a portion of normal brain, which was obtained at frontal lobectomy for astrocytoma and histologically confirmed tumor cell free, was the negative control.

Northern Blot Analysis

A human VEGF cDNA probe was kindly provided by Dr. H.A. Weich (Bio-technologische Forschung, Deptartment of Gene Expression, Braunschweig, Germany). Glyceraldehyde phosphate dehydrogenase (GAPDH) cDNA was donated from JCRB (Foundation for Promotion of Cancer Research, Tokyo, Japan). The Northern blot analysis was performed as described previously [31]. Briefly, the mRNA was purified by the acid guanidinium thiocyanate–phenol–chloroform method. The resulting RNA was fractionated through a 1% agarose gel containing $2.2\,M$ formaldehyde, transferred onto a nylon membrane (Hybond N+, Amersham, UK), and UV cross-linked using FLUO-LINK (Viler Lourmat, Marne-La-Vallee, France). The filter was hybridized to ^{32}P-labeled cDNA probes in Hybrisol (Oncor, Gaithersburg, MD, USA) for 24 hr at 40°C, and then washed first at room temperature in 2× standard saline-citrate (SSC) and 0.1% sodium dodecyl sulfate (SDS) and then in 0.2× SSC and 0.1% SDS. The mRNA levels were quantified by a densitometric analysis using a Fujix BAS 2000 bioimage analyzer (Fuji, Tokyo, Japan). The expression index of VEGF was presented when normalized by the GAPDH mRNA level in each sample.

Immunohistochemistry

For the immunocytochemical study, VEGF protein was stained as described previously [32]. The anti-VEGF antibody was purchased from Santa Cruz Biotechnology (Santa Cruz, CA, USA). After fixation with cooled acetone and the endogenous peroxidase block, the specimens were incubated with primary antibody at 4°C overnight. The streptavidin–biotin method was used with a Histofine SAB (R) kit (Nichirei, Tokyo, Japan). The sections were visualized by incubation with 300 µg/ml of diaminobenzidine tetrahydrochloride (Wako, Osaka, Japan) in $0.05\,M$ Tris buffer (pH 7.6) containing 0.003% hydrogen peroxide.

Statistics

The data were analyzed statistically by analysis of variance (ANOVA); the criterion for statistical significance was the 0.05 level.

Results

The Expression of VEGF mRNA in Various Brain Tumors

We carried out a Northern blot analysis to examine whether VEGF was expressed in brain tumors. An example of a Northern blot analysis of VEGF (3.9 kb) and GAPDH (internal control, 1.3 kb) mRNA in various tumor samples is presented in Fig. 1. Most tumor tissues expressed VEGF mRNAs at various degrees in addition to the histological diagnosis. As shown in Table 1, the mRNA levels of VEGF were then

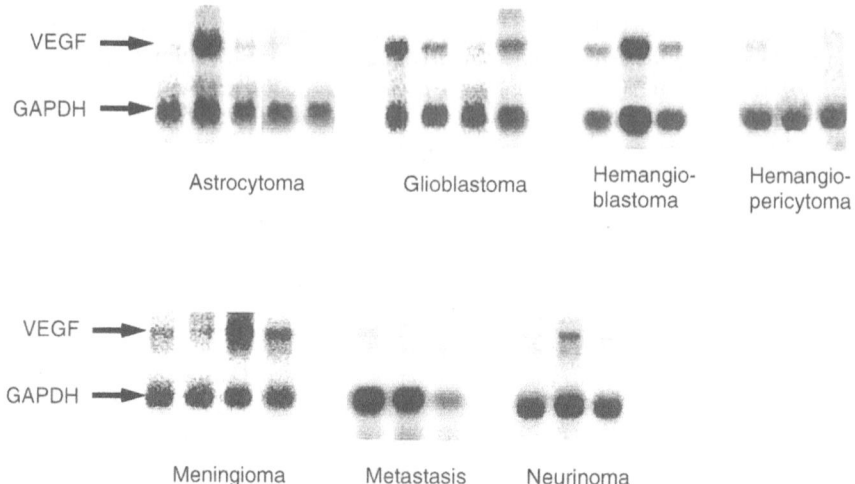

Fig. 1. Northern blot analysis of vascular endothelial growth factor (*VEGF*) in various brain tumors. Total RNA (15 μg) was electrophoresed on a 1% agarose-formaldehyde gel that was then transferred to a nylon membrane and hybridized with radio labeled VEGF cDNA probes. Control, glyceraldehyde phosphate dehydrogenase (*GAPDH*) cDNA probe (1.3 kb). Various mRNA levels of the VEGF gene were observed at 3.9 kb

determined when normalized by those of the GAPDH gene and shown as the expression indices.

Although the samples were limited in number, ANOVA revealed that the expression indices were significantly different ($P = .0017$) among histologically different tissues. There appeared to be some correlation between the histological tissue type and the level of VEGF mRNA expression. Glioblastomas and meningotheliomatous meningiomas expressed a significantly higher level of VEGF mRNA of 3.9 kb than that of others. Benign neuroepithelial tumors, including astrocytoma and oligodendroglioma, showed a significantly lower expression index (0.269 ± 0.158) when compared to that of malignant types, including glioblastomas and primary neuroectodermal tumors (0.492 ± 0.176). In the tumors arising from vascular components, hemangioblastomas showed a relatively higher index than hemangiopericytomas. However, there was no significant difference between these types. In astrocytoma, hemangiopericytoma, neurioma, and metastasis, VEGF mRNA was observed at a relatively lower level when compared to others. The human glioma cell line and the normal brain (positive and negative controls) showed a moderate (0.347) and minimum (0.072) level of VEGF expression index, respectively.

Immunohistochemical Detection of VEGF

To investigate whether VEGF protein is produced in certain cells or whether this protein is transported to its target cells, we incubated tissue sections with an antibody directed against human VEGF. In Fig. 2, showing a representative case of neurinoma, immunocytochemical staining for VEGF protein shows strong immunoreactivity in the vasculature. Tumor cells near the vasculature also showed strong immuno-

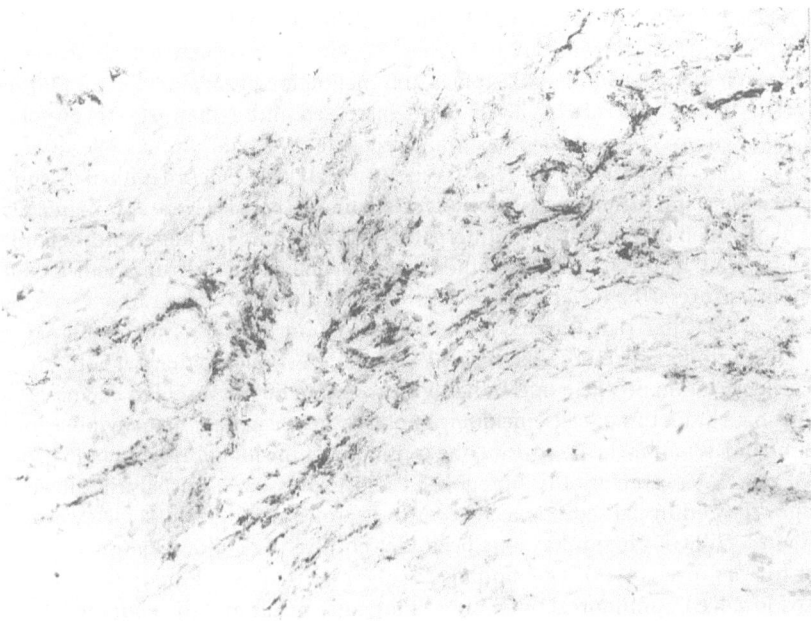

Fig. 2. Example of immunohistochemical staining of VEGF in a neurinoma using 6-μm frozen sections incubated with anti-VEGF antibody and detected with streptavidin–biotin. Localized expression of VEGF is noted on capillary endothelial cells in the tumor tissue and also on the tumor cells near the vasculature. ×180

reactivity. However, the tumor cells away from the vasculature showed only faint immunoreactivity indistinguishable from background levels. This immunostaining was totally inhibited by exclusion of the primary antibody.

Discussion

In some histologically distinct tissues and brain neoplasm, for example, in pituitary follicular cells [23,24,33], primary malignant gliomas [34–38], and human capillary hemangioblastomas [39], VEGF was found to be synthesized and secreted. We have shown direct and quantitative correlation between VEGF expression and neovascularization in vivo in human gliomas and meningiomas [31]. Among four angiogenic growth factors including VEGF, TGF-α and -β, and bFGF, only VEGF mRNA levels were statistically correlated with tumor vascularity in gliomas ($n = 17$; correlation coefficient $r = .499$; $P < .05$) and meningiomas ($n = 16$; $R = .779$; $P < .001$), although the mRNA of TGF-α, TGF-β, bFGF, and VEGF were expressed at various levels. VEGF was thus considered to be a strong candidate for a factor inducing angiogenesis in both human gliomas and meningiomas, while the other three growth factors were determined not likely to possess such an ability in vivo.

In this study, we determined that various brain tumors that have different histological features have the potential to release VEGF at various levels. Glioblastomas and meningiomas are known to be vascular-rich tumors; as we expected, they showed the highest VEGF expression index. Although hemangioblastomas and hemangi-pericytomas originate from vascular tissue, they showed a relatively lower expression index when compared to glioblastomas and meningiomas. Weindel et al. [36] have reported that VEGF mRNA levels were increased more than 20- to 50-fold in anaplastic gliomas or glioblastomas compared with low-grade gliomas. We also could observe that the VEGF mRNA levels in malignant neuroepithelial tumors [glioblastoma and primitive neuroectodermal tumors (PNET)] were approximately 2-fold higher than that in benign counterparts (astrocytomas and oligodendrogliomas). Weindel et al. also reported that other tumors, such as meningioma and medullo-blastoma, expressed a lower level of VEGF mRNA although these tumors have been known as vascular-rich tumors. In our examination, however, meningiomas and medulloblastomas also showed levels of VEGF mRNA similar to that of glioblastomas.

The localization of VEGF mRNA has been shown in highly vascular, edema-associated human brain tumor cells, including glioblastomas, capillary hemangioblastomas, meningiomas, and metastases using the technique of in situ hybridization [37,38,40]. VEGF mRNA is dramatically upregulated and expressed, especially in clusters of tumor cells and in palisade cells adjacent to necrotic areas [37,38,41]. However, the presence of VEGF protein has only been identified in the endothelial cells of malignant tumors in vivo [38]. Our findings, using a polyclonal antibody to VEGF, disclosed localized immunoreactivity in both the tumor cells and the endothelial cells.

Insufficient vascular supply and the resultant reduction in tissue oxygen tension often lead to neovascularization to satisfy the needs of the tissue. These in vivo findings were substantiated by in vitro experiments. VEGF is highly hypoxia inducible in glioma cells as compared with other angiogenic growth factors, and is considered to mediate hypoxia-initiated angiogenesis in brain tumors [37,38]. In a rat glioma model of tumor angiogenesis, the high-affinity tyrosine kinase receptor family for VEGF, *flt*-1 and *flk*-1, are specifically expressed in endothelial cells within the tumor and at the border between tumor and normal brain, while VEGF itself is expressed in the rat glioma cells [41]. Further, *flt* is not expressed in the normal brain endothelium but is upregulated in the endothelium of the human gliomas, which thus suggests a paracrine control by VEGF for angiogenesis in brain tumors [38].

These recent findings and our current data suggest that the VEGF/*flt* system may play an essential role in the angiogenesis of solid tumors, in particular brain tumors. Furthermore, modification of the VEGF/*flt* system might be implied for the treatment of brain tumors [42–44].

It remains to be established how various angiogenic growth factors work together [45] for tumor angiogenesis in vivo.

Acknowledgments. This work is supported in part by a grant from the Ministry of Education and the Ministry of Health and Welfare, Japan. We thank Dr. Etsuo Miyake (Miyake Neurosurgical Hospital) and Dr. Haruo Matsuno (Department of Neurosurgery, Iizuka Hospital) for providing some of the surgical specimens.

References

1. Todaro GJ, Fryling C, De LJ (1980) Transforming growth factors produced by certain human tumor cells: polypeptides that interact with epidermal growth factor receptors. Proc Natl Acad Sci USA 77:5258–5262
2. Roberts AB, Sporn MB (1985) Transforming growth factors. Cancer Surv 4:683–705

3. Klagsbrun M (1991) Angiogenic factors: regulators of blood supply-side biology. FGF, endothelial cell growth factors and angiogenesis: a keystone symposium, Keystone, CO, USA, April 1–7, 1991. New Biol 3:745–749

4. Rifkin DB, Moscatelli D (1989) Recent developments in the cell biology of basic fibroblast growth factor. J Cell Biol 109:1–6

5. Kuwano M, Ushiro S, Ryuto M, Samoto K, Izumi H, Ito K, Abe T, Nakamura T, Ono M, Kohno K (1994) Regulation of angiogenesis by growth factors. In: Kuwano M, Ushiro S, Ryuto M, Samoto K, Izumi H, Ito K, Abe T, Nakamura T, Ono M, Kohno K (eds) Gann monograph on cancer research in growth factors in cell growth, morphogenesis and transformation. Japan Scientific Societies Press (CRC Press, Boca Raton), pp 113–125

6. Lobb RR, Alderman EM, Fett JW (1985) Induction of angiogenesis by bovine brain derived class 1 heparin-binding growth factor. Biochemistry 24:4969–4973

7. Kandel J, Bossy WE, Radvanyi F, Klagsbrun M, Folkman J, Hanahan D (1991) Neovascularization is associated with a switch to the export of bFGF in the multistep development of fibrosarcoma. Cell 66:1095–1104

8. Abe T, Okamura K, Ono M, Kohno K, Mori T, Hori S, Kuwano M (1993) Induction of vascular endothelial tubular morphogenesis by human glioma cells. A model system for tumor angiogenesis. J Clin Invest 92:54–61

9. Zagzag D, Miller DC, Sato Y, Rifkin DB, Burstein DE (1990) Immunohistochemical localization of basic fibroblast growth factor in astrocytomas. Cancer Res 50:7393–7398

10. Takahashi JA, Mori H, Fukumoto M, Igarashi K, Jaye M, Oda Y, Kikuchi H, Hatanaka M (1990) Gene expression of fibroblast growth factors in human gliomas and meningiomas: demonstration of cellular source of basic fibroblast growth factor mRNA and peptide in tumor tissues. Proc Natl Acad Sci USA 87:5710–5714

11. Stefanik DF, Rizkalla LR, Soi A, Goldblatt SA, Rizkalla WM (1991) Acidic and basic fibroblast growth factors are present in glioblastoma multiforme. Cancer Res 51:5760–5765

12. Schreiber AB, Winkler ME, Derynck R (1986) Transforming growth factor-alpha: a more potent angiogenic mediator than epidermal growth factor. Science 232:1250–1253

13. Gospodarowicz D, Bialecki H, Thakral TK (1979) The angiogenic activity of the fibroblast and epidermal growth factor. Exp Eye Res 28:501–514

14. Ito K, Ryuto M, Ushiro S, Ono M, Sugenoya A, Kuraoka A, Shibata Y, Kuwano M (1995) Expression of tissue-type plasminogen activator and its inhibitor couples with development of capillary network by human microvascular endothelial cells on matrigel. J Cell Physiol 162:213–224

15. Sato Y, Rifkin DB (1989) Inhibition of endothelial cell movement by pericytes and smooth muscle cells: activation of a latent transforming growth factor-beta 1-like molecule by plasmin during co-culture. J Cell Biol 109:309–315

16. Pepper MS, Belin D, Montesano R, Orci L, Vassalli JD (1990) Transforming growth factor-beta 1 modulates basic fibroblast growth factor-induced proteolytic and angiogenic properties of endothelial cells in vitro. J Cell Biol 111:743–755

17. Okamura K, Morimoto A, Hamanaka R, Ono M, Kohno K, Uchida Y, Kuwano M (1992) A model system for tumor angiogenesis: involvement of transforming growth factor-alpha in tube formation of human microvascular endothelial cells induced by esophageal cancer cells. Biochem Biophys Res Commun 186:1471–1479

18. Tada K, Fukunaga T, Wakabayashi Y, Masumi S, Izumi H, Kohno K, Kuwano M (1994) Inhibition of tubular morphogenesis in human microvascular endothelial cells by co-culture with chondrocytes and involvement of transforming growth factor beta: a model for avascularity in human cartilage. Biochim Biophys Acta 1201:135–142

19. Massague J (1990) The transforming growth factor-beta family. Annu Rev Cell Biol 6:597–641

20. Moses HL, Yang EY, Pietenpol JA (1990) TGF-beta stimulation and inhibition of cell proliferation: new mechanistic insights. Cell 63:245–247

21. D'Amore PA (1990) Modes of FGF release in vivo and in vitro. Cancer Metastasis Rev 9:227–238

22. Favard C, Moukadiri H, Dorey C, Praloran V, Plouët J (1991) Purification and biological properties of vasculotropin, a new angiogenic cytokine. Biol Cell 73:1–6

23. Ferrara N, Henzel WJ (1989) Pituitary follicular cells secrete a novel heparin-binding growth factor specific for vascular endothelial cells. Biochem Biophys Res Commun 161:851–855

24. Gospodarowicz D, Abrahma J, Schilling J (1989) Isolation and characterization of a vascular endothelial cell mitogen produced by pituitary-derived folliculo stellate cells. Proc Natl Acad Sci USA 86:7311–7315

25. Houck KA, Ferrara N, Winer J, Cachianes G, Li B, Leung DW (1991) The vascular endothelial growth factor family: identification of a fourth molecular species and characterization of alternative splicing of RNA. Mol Endocrinol 5:1806–1814

26. Tischer E, Mitchell R, Hartman T, Silva M, Gospodarowicz D, Fiddes J, Abraham J (1991) The human gene for vascular endothelial growth factor. J Biol Chem 266:11947–11954

27. Wilting J, Christ B, Bokeloh M, Weich HA (1993) In vivo effects of vascular endothelial growth factor on the chicken chorioallantoic membrane. Cell Tissue Res 274:163–172

28. Connolly DT, Heuvelman DM, Nelson R, Olander JV, Eppley BL, Delfino JJ, Siegel NR, Leimgruber RM, Feder J (1989) Tumor vascular permeability factor stimulates endothelial cell growth and angiogenesis. J Clin Invest 84:1470–1478

29. Bikfalvi A, Sauzeau C, Moukadiri H, Maclouf J, Busso N, Bryckaert M, Plouet J, Tobelem G (1991) Interaction of vasculotropin/vascular endothelial cell growth factor with human umbilical vein endothelial cells: binding, internalization, degradation, and biological effects. J Cell Physiol 149:50–59

30. Pepper MS, Ferrara N, Orci L, Montesano R (1991) Vascular endothelial growth factor (VEGF) induces plasminogen activators and plasminogen activator inhibitor-1 in microvascular endothelial cells. Biochem Biophys Res Commun 181:902–906

31. Samoto K, Ikezaki K, Ono M, Shono T, Kohno K, Kuwano M, Fukui M (1995) Expression of vascular endothelial growth factor and its possible relation with neovascularization in human brain tumors. Cancer Res 55:1189–1193

32. Samoto K, Ikezaki K, Yokoyama N, Fukui M (1994) P-Glycoprotein expression in brain capillary endothelial cells after focal ischaemia in the rat. Neurol Res 16:217–223

33. Ferrara N, Leung DW, Cachianes G (1991) Purification and cloning of vascular endothelial growth factor secreted by pituitary folliculostellate cells. Methods Enzymol 198:391–405

34. Criscuolo G, Lelkes P, Rotrosen D, Oldfield E (1989) Cytosolic calcium changes in endothelial cells induced by a protein product of human gliomas containing vascular permeability factor activity. J Neurosurg 71:884–891

35. Bruce J, Criscuolo G, Merrill M, et al. (1987) Vascular permeability induced by protein product of malignant brain tumors: inhibition by dexamethasone. J Neurosurg 67:880–884

36. Weindel K, Moringlane JR, Marmé D, Weich HA (1994) Detection and quantification of vascular endothelial growth factor/vascular permeability factor in brain tumor tissue and cyst fluid: the key to angiogenesis? Neurosurgery 35:439–449

37. Shweiki D, Itin A, Soffer D, Keshet E (1992) Vascular endothelial growth factor induced by hypoxia may mediate hypoxia-initiated angiogenesis. Nature 359:843–845

38. Plate KH, Breier G, Weich HA, Risau W (1992) Vascular endothelial growth factor is a potential tumour angiogenesis factor in human gliomas in vivo. Nature 359:845–848

39. Morii K, Tanaka R, Washiyama K, Kumanishi T, Kuwano R (1993) Expression of vascular endothelial growth factor in capillary hemangioblastoma. Biochem Biophys Res Commun 194:749–755

40. Berkman RA, Merrill MJ, Reinhold WC, Monacci WT, Saxena A, Clark WC, Robertson JT, Ali IU, Oldfield EH (1993) Expression of the vascular permeability factor/vascular endothelial growth factor gene in central nervous system neoplasms. J Clin Invest 91:153–159

41. Plate KH, Breier G, Millauer B, Ullrich A, Risau W (1993) Up-regulation of vascular endothelial growth factor and its cognate receptors in a rat glioma model of tumor angiogenesis. Cancer Res 53:5822–5827

42. Van Meir E, Polverini P, Chazin V, Su Huang H-J, de Tribolet N, Cavenee W (1994) Release of an inhibitor of angiogenesis upon induction of wild type p53 expression in glioblastoma cell. Nat Genet 8:171–176

43. Kim EG, Kwon HM, Burrow CR, Ballermann BJ (1993) Expression of rat fibroblast growth factor receptor 1 as three splicing variants during kidney development. Am J Physiol 264:66–73

44. Millauer B, Shawver LK, Plate KH, Risau W, Ullrich A (1994) Glioblastoma growth inhibited in vivo by a dominant-negative FlK-1 mutant. Nature 367:576–579
45. Pepper MS, Ferrara N, Orci L, Montesano R (1992) Potent synergism between vascular endothelial growth factor and basic fibroblast growth factor in the induction of angiogenesis in vitro. Biochem Biophys Res Commun 189:824–831

Section 3. Tumor Suppressor Gene

Studies of Retinoblastoma and *p53* Gene Mutations in Human Astrocytomas

Toshihide Tsuzuki[1], Shigeru Tsunoda[2], Toshisuke Sakaki[1],
Noboru Konishi[3], Yoshio Hiasa[3], Hiroyuki Hashimoto[1],
Toru Yabuno[1], and Mitsutoshi Nakamura[1]

Abstract. Mutations in the retinoblastoma (*RB*) and *p53* genes of human gliomas were screened by single-strand conformation polymorphism (SSCP) analysis of polymerase chain reaction (PCR) products (PCR-SSCP analysis) and confirmed by dideoxy sequencing. Aberrations of the *RB* gene were found in 5 cases (21.7%) of 23 surgical specimens of human astrocytomas, including 3 of 6 (50%) grade 2 and 2 of 15 (13.3%) grade 4 astrocytomas. In 3 cases, mutation was found at either codon 754 in exon 22, codon 519 in exon 17, or codon 900 in exon 26. These mutational locations were all posterior portions associated with the functional domains of the *RB* gene. Aberrations of the *p53* gene were found in 4 cases (17.4%), including 1 of 6 (16.7%) grade 2 and 3 of 15 (20.0%) grade 4 astrocytomas. These mutations were found at codons 146 and 165 in exon 5, codon 73 in exon 4, and codon 313 in exon 9. *RB* and *p53* mutations in brain tumors occurred with a similar frequency, but in even lower grades of astrocytomas. No case with both *RB* and *p53* mutations was found in this study. These results lead us to suspect that mutations of the *RB* or *p53* genes may be necessary in the early stages of tumorigenesis but do not occur in combination. Some different genetic changes of the *RB* or *p53* gene may be involved in human astrocytomas.

Key words. RB gene—*p53* gene—Human astrocytomas—PCR-SSCP—Direct sequence analysis

Introduction

RB and *p53* genes are the most common tumor suppressor genes associated with the genesis of various human tumors [1,2]. The *p53* gene spans approximately 20 kb of DNA and consists of 11 exons including conserved domains in exons 5–8 (Fig. 1) [3,4]. Mutations are frequently found in exons 5 to 9. Restriction fragment length polymphysm (RFLP) analysis of gliomas has revealed a nonrandom loss of heterozygosity (LOH) for markers on chromosomes 9, 10, 13, and 17. Nigro et al. [5] indentified 4 of 5 gliomas that had lost one chromosome 17p allele. Fults et al. [6]

[1] Department of Neurosurgery, Nara Medical University, Kashihara, Nara 634, Japan
[2] Department of Health Science, College of Integrated Arts and Science, University of Osaka Prefecture, Osaka, Japan
[3] Second Department of Pathology, Nara Medical University, Kashihara, Nara 634, Japan

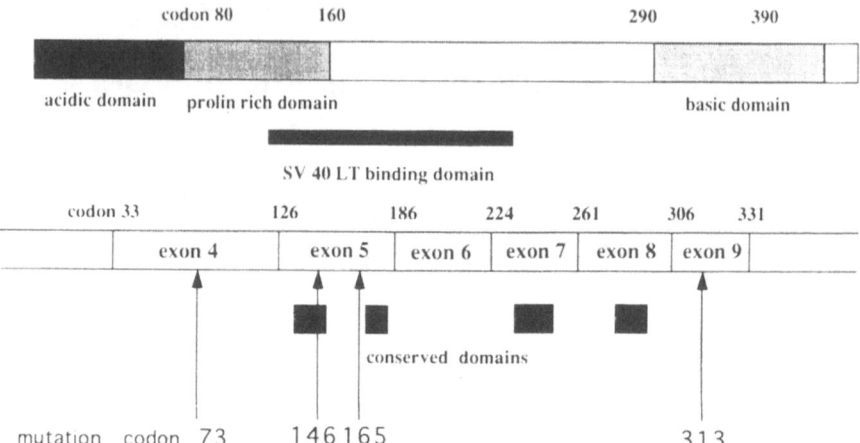

Fig. 1. Conserved regions of the *p53* gene and locations of mutations. Conserved regions of the *p53* gene are located in exons 5–9, and most mutations were found in these regions

reported that *p53* mutations were found in 8 of 13 malignant astrocytomas (62%) with LOH on chromosome 17p, 7 of 25 glioblastomas (28%), 5 of 14 anaplastic astrocytomas (36%), and in none of 6 low-grade astrocytomas examined in a series of 45 gliomas. von Deimling et al. [7] found *p53* mutations in 4 of 8 grade 2 astrocytomas (50%) and 7 of 14 grade 3 astrocytomas (50%), suggesting that *p53* mutations were not restricted to glioblastoma multiformes and might be important in the tumorigenesis of lower grade astrocytomas.

Another important tumor suppressor gene is the retinoblastoma (*RB*) gene, which was the first tumor suppressor gene identified in retinoblastomas [8]. The *RB* gene spans approximately 200 kb of DNA within human chromosome 13q14. The previously determind cDNA sequence comprises 27 exons [9]. Somatic mutations have been implicated in the formation of a variety of human cancers, especially retinoblastoma, osteosarcoma, small cell lung carcinoma, bladder cell carcinoma, and breast carcinoma [10–14]. However, little is known about *RB* gene mutations in human gliomas.

In this study, we examined 23 surgical specimens of human astrocytomas for mutations in the *RB* and *p53* genes by single-strand conformation polymorphism (SSCP) analysis and DNA sequencing. Exons 4 through 9, known mutational "hot spots," were examined in the *p53* gene. All the exons, 1 through 27, were examined in the *RB* gene because this gene has no known mutational hot spots [10–15].

Materials and Methods

Materials

Twenty-three brain tumor specimens were obtained during surgery at the Department of Neurosurgery, Nara Medical University. Six tumors were classified as grade 2, 2 tumors were grade 3, and 15 tumors were grade 4.

Polymerase Chain Reaction–
Single-Strand Conformational Polymorphism Analysis

Tumor tissues were digested with proteinase K, and high molecular weight genomic DNA was extracted using the phenol/chloroform method. Genomic DNA was subjected to polymerase chain reaction (PCR) using two synthetic oligonucleotide primers at each of the 27 exons of the *RB* gene as described by Hogg et al. [16] and at exons 4 through 9 of the *p53* gene [17]. Each 100 µl of the PCR mixture contained 1 µg of DNA template, 22.7 pmol of each primer pair, 1.5 mmol $MgCl_2$, 250 pmol/µl of each deoxyribonucleotide triphosphate, and 2.0 units of Taq polymerase. Thirty-five cycles of amplification were carried out using a thermal cycler (Perkin-Elmer Cetus, Norwalk, CT, USA) at 94°C for 30 s, 55°–62°C for 30 s, and 72°C for 1 min. These products were reamplified by PCR for SSCP using [γ-^{32}P]ATP-labeled primers. Although single base pair (bp) mutations can be detected by SSCP in PCR products up to 350 bp in size, the products generated in our reactions ranged from 212 to 625 bp, necessitating in some cases the use of appropriate restriction enzymes to generate shorter fragments suitable for SSCP analysis [16]. Samples were analyzed by electrophoresis in 5% polyacrylamide gel with 10% glycerol at 40 W, 25°C for 3–6 h.

Direct Sequence Analysis

The samples that showed abnormal mobility in the SSCP analysis were isolated and run on 2% agarose gels and purified using the Geneclean II kit (Bio 101, La Jolla, CA, USA) in preparation for sequencing. The sequencing reaction was performed by means of the dideoxy method [18] using the termination mixture supplied by the Circum Vent Thermal Cycle Sequencing Kit (New England Biolab, Beverly, MA, USA). Following the manufacturer's instrutions, 35 cycles of amplification were carrid out in a themal cycler with the addition of [γ-^{32}P]ATP to the samples. PCR products were electrophoresed on 8% polyacrylamide/7 *M* urea gels for 2–3 h at 1800 V. The gels were dried and exposed to Kodak X-ray film without intensifying screens at −70°C for 3–6 h.

Results

RB Gene Analysis

Aberrations of the *RB* gene, identified by both SSCP and sequence analysis, were found in 5 of 23 astrocytomas (21.7%), including 3 of 6 (50.0%) grade 2 and 2 of 15 (13.3%) grade 4 astrocytomas. All aberrations were point mutations. Case 3 of the grade 2 astrocytomas had a mutation at codon 900 in exon 26, where AAA (Lys) was changed to AGG (Arg). Case 4 of the grade 2 astrocytomas had a mutation at codon 519 in exon 17 (ACA→CCA transversion), resulting in a Thr to Pro substitution. Three cases, cases 6 (grade 2), 11 (grade 4), and 13 (grade 4), had a mutation at codon 754 in exon 22 (GTA→GGA transversion), resulting in a Val to Gly substitution (Table 1).

Table 1. Summary of results.

Case	Grade	RB gene				p53 gene			
		Exon	Codon	Mutation	Amino acid	Exon	Codon	Mutation	Amino acid
1	II								
2	II					5	146	TGG → GGG	Trp → Gly
3	II	26	900	AAA → AGG	Lys → Arg				
4	II	17	519	ACA → CCA	Thr → Pro				
5	II								
6	II	22	754	GTA → GGA	Val → Gly				
7	III								
8	III								
9	IV								
10	IV								
11	IV	22	754	GTA → GGA	Val → Gly				
12	IV								
13	IV	22	754	GTA → GGA	Val → Gly				
14	IV					4	73	GTG → GAG	Val → Glu
15	IV								
16	IV								
17	IV								
18	IV					5	165	CAG → CAT	Gln → His
19	IV								
20	IV					9	313	AGC → AAC	Ser → Asn
21	IV								
22	IV								
23	IV								

p53 Gene Analysis

Aberrations identified by both SSCP and sequence analysis were found in 4 of 23 astrocytomas (17.4%), which included 1 of 6 (16.7%) grade 2 and 3 of 15 (20.0%) grade 4 astrocytomas. All aberrations were point mutations. Case 14 of the grade 4 astrocytomas had a mutation at codon 73 in exon 4 (GTG→GAG transversion), resulting in a Val to Glu substitution. Case 20 of the grade 4 astrocytomas had a mutation at codon 313 in exon 9 (AGC→AAC transition), resulting in a Ser to Asn substitution. Cases 2 (grade 2) and 18 (grade 4) had a mutation at codons 146 and 165, respectively, in exon 5. Case 2 (TGG→GGG transversion) resulted in a Trp to Gly substitution, and case 18 (CAG→CAT transversion) resulted in a Gln to His substitution (see Table 1). Combined mutations of both RB and p53 genes were not detected in any of the cases.

Discussion

The p53 gene is the one of the best characterized genes in human gliomas. This gene is known to exhibit different mutational patterns from those typically found in other tumors such as coloretal carcinomas or small cell lung carcinomas. The frequency of p53 mutations increases with the loss of the 17p allele in colorectal carcinomas or small cell lung carcinomas [19], but no such correlation has been indentified in gliomas. It is suggested that p53 mutations occur before, or independent of, deletions in the 17p locus in a large proportion of gliomas [20]. In addition, a low frequency of loss of heterozygosity for chromosome 17p was observed, even in grade 4 astrocytomas. These findings also suggest that the progression of low-grade astrocytomas to high-grade gliomas occurs independently of 17p allele loss [7]. In our study, mutations of the *p53* gene were detected in 4 of 23 (17.4%) astrocytomas, 1 of 6 (16.7%) grade 2 astrocytomas, and 3 of 15 (20.0%) grade 4 astrocytomas. A lower frequency of mutations was found, even in the high-grade astrocytomas, than is found in colorectal carcinomas (70%–80%). This suggests that *p53* mutation is not the only specific fator closely linked to the malignant progression of human astrocytomas.

In this study, the *RB* gene was also examined in the same series of human astrocytomas, using PCR-SSCP analysis. Aberrations in the *RB* gene were identified by both SSCP and sequence analyses in 5 of 23 (21.7%) of the human astrocytomas. All aberrations were point mutations with changes in single amino acids that were located in the posterior parts of the *RB* gene (exons 17, 22, and 26). The DNA-binding region has been reported to span from codon 612 in exon 19 to codon 928 in exon 27 [15]. Mutations in these functional domains may have a profound effect on the *RB* gene (Fig. 2). Ishikawa et al. [21] suggested that the loss of *RB* gene function in bladder cancer most frequently involves mutations in both alleles with retention of heterozygosity at the *RB* gene locus rather than a mutation of one *RB* allele followed by LOH. This observation suggested that RFLP analysis for LOH on chromosome 13 is not sufficient to evaluate the *RB* gene function. Franckel et al. [20] examined the *RB* locus in 40 human gliomas using RFLP analysis and found no evidence of LOH at this locus. However, it is possible that mutations may occur within the *RB* gene that cause gene inactivation. The mutations detected in our study were located in the functional domains of the *RB* gene, suggesting a significant influence on gene function.

Two of the most common tumor suppressor genes, the *p53* and *RB* genes, were studied in the same series of tumors, but few cases were detected that had both *p53* and *RB* gene mutations in either bladder carcinomas or samll cell lung carcinomas

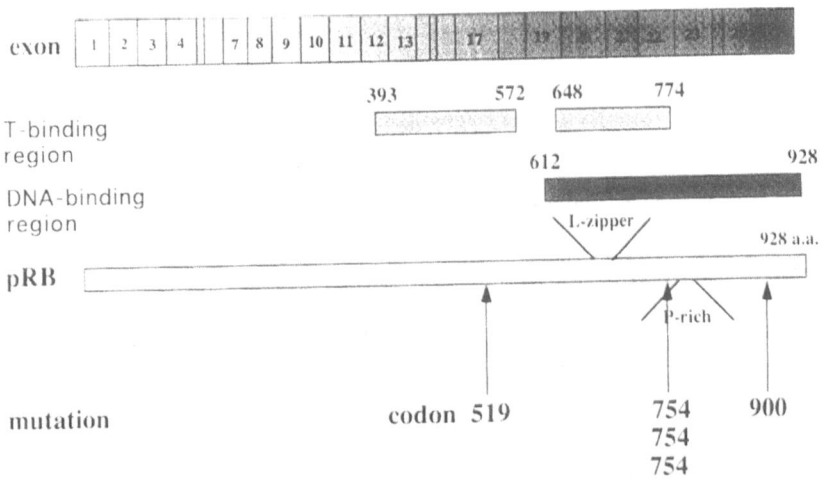

Fig. 2. Functional domains of the *RB* gene and locations of mutations. Lee [15] elucidated the functional domains of the *RB* gene and identified the DNA-binding site and the T-antigen-binding site. The DNA-binding site spans from codon 612 to codon 928 in exons 19–27

[22]. In our study, the frequency of *p53* mutations was almost the same as that of *RB* gene mutations, whereas no case of combined *p53* and *RB* mutations were found. These findings led us to speculate that genetic changes correlated with the genesis and progression of human gliomas may act through more than one pathway and that alternate routes should be considered in progression from low-grade astrocytomas to glioblastomas. Aberrations in the *p53* and *RB* genes may be included in these alternate pathways. The genesis and progression mechanisms in human gliomas will likely be resoved in future studies of genetic abnormalities in tumors. The *p53* and *RB* genes must be associated with other oncogenes or proto-oncogenes specific for gliomas.

References

1. Cavenee WK (1991) Recessive mutations in cancer predisposition and progression. In: Sudilovsky et al (eds) Boundaries between promotion and progression during Carcinogenesis. Plenum, New York, pp 171–181
2. Stanbridge EJ (1990) The evidence for human tumor suppressor genes. In: Knudson AG Jr, et al (eds) Genetic basis for carcinogenesis. Tayler and Francis, London, pp 3–13
3. Buchman VL, Chumakov PM, Ninkina NN, Samarina OP, Georgiev GP (1988) A variation in the structure of the protein-coding region of the human p53 gene. Gene 70:245–252
4. Chen PL, Chen Y, Bookstein R, Lee WH (1990) Genetic mechanism of tumor suppression by the human p53 gene. Science 250:1576–1580
5. Nigro JM, Baker SJ, Preisinger AC, Jessup JM, Hostetter R, Cleary K, Bigner SH, Davidson N, Baylin S, Devilee P, Glover T, Collins FS, Weston A, Modali R, Harris CC, Bogelstein B (1989) Mutations in the p53 gene occur in diverse human tumor types. Nature 342:705–708
6. Fults D, Brockmeyer D, Tullous MW, Pedone CA, Cawthon RM (1992) p53 mutation and loss of heterozygosity on chromosomes 17 and 10 during human astrocytoma progression. Cancer Res 52:674–679
7. von Deimling A, Eibl RH, Ohgaki H, Louis DN, von Ammon K, Petersen I, Kleihues P, Chung RY, Wiestler OD, Seizinger BR (1992) p53 mutations are associeted with 17p allelic loss in grade II and grade III astrocytoma. Cancer Res 52:2987–2990
8. Lee WH, Bookstein R, Hong F, Young LJ, Shew JY, Lee EY-HP (1987) Human retinoblastoma susceptibility gene: cloning, identification and sequence. Science 235:1349–1399
9. McGee TL, Yandell DW, Dryja TP (1989) Structure and partial genomic sequence of the human retinoblastoma susceptibility gene. Gene 80:119–128
10. Harbour JW, Lai S-L, Whang-Peng J, Gazdar AF, Minna JD, Kaye FJ (1988) Abnormalities in structure and expression of the human retinoblastoma gene in SCLC. Science 241:353–357
11. Friend SH, Horowitz JM, Gerber MR, Wang XF, Bogenmann E, Frederick PL, Weinberg RA (1987) Deletions of a DNA sequence in retinoblastomas and mesenchymal tumors: organization of the sequence and its encoded protein. Proc Natl Acad Sci USA 84:9059–9063
12. Horowitz JM, Yandell DW, Park SH, Whyte SCP, Harlow E, Weinberg RA, Dryja TP (1989) Point mutational inactivation of the retinoblastoma anti-oncogene. Science 243:937–940
13. Murakami Y, Hayashi K, Hirohashi S, Sekiya T (1991) Aberrations of the tumor suppressor p53 and RB genes in human hepatocellular carcinomas. Cancer Res 51:5520–5525
14. Lee EY-HP, To H, Shew J-Y, Bookstein R, Scully P, Lee W-H (1988) Inactivation of the retinoblastoma susceptibility gene in human breast cancers. Science 241:218–221
15. Lee WH (1990) The molecular basis of cancer suppression by the retinoblastoma gene. In: Knudson AG Jr, et al (eds) Genetic basis for carcinogenesis. Taylor and Francis, London, pp 159–170
16. Hogg A, Onadim Z, Baird PN, Cowell JK (1992) Detection of heterozygous mutations in the RB1 gene in retinoblastoma patients using single-strand conformation polymorphism analysis and polymerase chain reaction sequencing. Oncogene 7:1445–1451
17. Lehman TA, Bennett WP, Metcalf RA, Welsh JA, Ecker J, Modali RV, Ullrich S, Romano JW, Appella E, Testa JR, Gerwin BI, Harris CC (1991) p53 mutations, *ras* mutations, and p53-

heat shock 70 protein complex in human lung carcinoma cell lines. Cancer Res 51:4090–4096

18. Sanger F, Nicklen S, Coulson AR (1977) DNA sequencing with chain terminating inhibitor. Proc Natl Acad Sci USA 74:5463–5467
19. Baker SJ, Fearon ER, Nigro JM, Hamilton SR, Preisinger AC, Jessup JM, van Tuinen P, Ledbetter DH, Barker LD, Nakamura Y, White R, Vogelstein B (1990) p53 gene mutations occur in combination with 17p allelic deletions as late events in colorectal tumorigenesis. Cancer Res 50:7717–7722
20. Frankel R, Bayona W, Koslow M, Newcomb EW (1992) p53 mutations are in human malignant gliomas: comparison of loss of heterozygosity with mutation frequency. Cancer Res 52:1427–1433
21. Ishikawa J, Xu H-J, Hu S-X, Yandell DW, Maeda S, Kamidono S, Benedict WF, Takahashi R (1991) Inactivation of the retinoblastoma gene in human bladder and renal cell carcinomas. Cancer Res 51:5736–5743
22. Presti JC, Reuter VE, Galan T, Fair WR, Cordon-Cardo C (1991) Molecular genetic alterations in superficial and locally advanced human bladder cancer. Cancer Res 51:5405–5409

Immunohistochemical Assessments of P53 Protein Accumulation and Tumor Growth Fraction During the Progression of Astrocytomas

Kunihiko Watanabe[1,3,4], Nobuyoshi Ogata[2], Klaus von Ammon[2], Yasuhiro Yonekawa[2], Masakatsu Nagai[3], Hiroko Ohgaki[4], and Paul Kleihues[1,4]

Abstract. P53 protein accumulation and growth fraction were assessed immunohistochemically in primary and recurrent astrocytoma with malignant progression. The tumors analyzed were diffusely infiltrating astrocytomas of the cerebral hemispheres and they were graded according to the World Health Organization (WHO) criteria into low grade astrocytoma (grade II), anaplastic astrocytoma (grade III), and glioblastoma (grade IV). The fraction of P53-positive cases, i.e., biopsies containing P53 immunoreactive cells, significantly increased during progression, in group II→III from 65% to 90%, in group II→IV from 68% to 95%, and in group III→IV from 69% to 100%. None of the initially P53-positive cases became P53 negative after progression. During progression, the P53 labeling index (LI)increased significantly in groups II→III (3.5%→9.8%) and II→ IV (3.3%→13%), suggesting that P53 immunoreactive glioma cells may have a growth advantage. The mean proliferating cell index (PI), analyzed by monoclonal antibody MIB-1, increased significantly in groups II→III (2.5%→11%), II→IV (2.9%→19%), and III→IV (8.7%→16%). Gemistocytes showed a significantly lower PI than the average of all tumor cells.

Key words. P53 protein—MIB-1—Immunohistochemistry—Astrocytoma—Tumor progression

Introduction

Astrocytomas are the most common of primary brain tumors, accounting for more than 50% of all central nervous system (CNS) neoplasms. According to the histopathologic classification of the World Health Organization (WHO), diffusely infiltrating cerebral astrocytomas comprise a spectrum of increasing anaplasia from low-grade (usually fibrillary or gemistocytic) astrocytoma (grade II), anaplastic astrocytoma (grade III), to glioblastoma (grade IV) [1,2]. Thus, glioblastomas frequently develop from lower-grade astrocytomas (secondary glioblastomas), but may also arise de novo after a short clinical history without evidence of a less malignant precursor lesion (primary glioblastoma) [3].

Institute of Neuropathology, [1] Department of Pathology and [2] Department of Neurosurgery, University Hospital, 8091, Zürich, Switzerland
[3] Department of Neurosurgery, Dokkyo University School of Medicine, Mibu, Tochigi 321-02, Japan
[4] International Agency for Research on Cancer, 69372 Lyon Cedex 08, France

Molecular genetic analyses have shown that inactivation of the *p53* tumor suppressor gene may play an important role in the evolution of human gliomas. Gene mutations have been identified at an overall incidence of 25%–40% in low-grade astrocytoma, anaplastic astrocytoma, and glioblastoma [4–10], indicating that astrocytic tumors of different grades of malignancy do not differ significantly with respect to the frequency of *p53* mutations. This observation does not exclude the possibility that these mutations play a role in the progression of gliomas. One study suggests that glial cells with *p53* mutations outgrow non-mutated neoplastic astrocytes and that this parallels the emergence of an increasingly malignant pheno-type [11]. To date, the number of cases is rather limited in which the frequency of *p53* gene alterations and/or P53 protein accumulation has been studied in the same pa-tients, i.e., at initial operation and in recurrences with histopathological evidence of progression [5,6,11,12].

Cell kinetic analyses with Ki-67 and/or MIB-I antibodies have shown that higher grade astrocytomas tend to show a higher proliferation index (PI) [13–15]. However, little is known about the PI in individual cellular components of astrocytoma. In this study, we assessed the P53 protein accumulation and the proliferating activity of individual cellular components of astrocytoma in a large cohort of 52 patients with recurrent astrocytoma with histological evidence of progression.

Materials and Methods

Tumor Samples

Surgical specimens were obtained from patients treated in the Department of Neuro-surgery, University Hospital, Zürich, Switzerland between 1974 and June 1994. A total of 52 patients with astrocytomas were found to have experienced at least one recur-rence with histologically verified progression.

Definition of Tumor Groups

The astrocytomas were graded according to WHO criteria into low grade (usually fibrillary or gemistocytic) astrocytoma (grade II), anaplastic astrocytoma (grade III), and glioblastoma (grade IV) [1,2]. The patients were classified into three groups: progression from low-grade astrocytoma to anaplastic astrocytoma (II→III; 20 pa-tients), from low-grade astrocytoma to glioblastoma (II→IV; 19 patients), and from anaplastic astrocytoma to glioblastoma (III→IV; 13 patients). In patients with recur-rences showing the same grade as the previous biopsy, the primary tumor (first surgical intervention) and the tumor that showed progression for the first time were analyzed and compared.

P53 Immunohistochemistry

A mouse anti-human P53 protein monoclonal antibody (PAb 1801) [16] was diluted 1:300 in phosphate-buffered saline (PBS) and applied to representative formalin-fixed paraffin-embedded sections. Tissue sections were deparaffinized and dehy-drated through xylene and graded alcohol. Normal rabbit serum (X902 [Dako,

Glostrup, Denmark] diluted 1:10 in PBS) was applied to each tissue section for 15 min to block non-specific binding. Sections were incubated with the primary antibody for 1h and then the reaction was visualized using biotinylated rabbit anti-mouse immunoglobulins (Dako) and avidin and biotinylated horseradish peroxidase (Dako), followed by diaminobenzidine solution. Sections were counterstained with Harris' hematoxylin. Formalin-fixed, paraffin-embedded sections of glioblastoma, which had previously been found to contain *p53* point mutations by sequence analysis, were used as positive controls.

MIB-I Immunohistochemistry

A mouse mAb MIB-I [17,18] against recombinant parts of the Ki-67 antigen was purchased from Dianova Hamburg (Raboisen 5, D-2000 Hamburg 1, Germany). Pretreatment of cleaned microscopic glass slides was carried out with 3-aminopropyltriethoxysilane. After deparaffinization, the slides were incubated in 10mM citrate buffer three times, for 5min each time, in a 750W microwave oven. After cooling, the sections were reacted for 1h with mAb MIB-1 diluted 1:50 in PBS countering 1% normal rabbit serum (Dako).

P53 Labeling Index and MIB-1 Proliferating Cell Index

The fractions of PAb 1801 and MIB-1 immunoreactive tumor cells were quantified at high-power magnification (×400) on five to ten visual fields, using an ocular with a square graticule. The data from different tumor areas were pooled, with at least 1000 counted cells in each specimen. The percentage of PAb 1801-positive tumor nuclei was recorded as the P53-labeling index (LI) and that of MIB-1 reactive tumor nuclei was recorded as the proliferating cell index (PI).

Cell Component Analyses

Immunoreactivity with PAb 1801 and MIB-1 was analyzed separately in the various cellular components of astrocytoma, including gemistocytes, multinuclear giant cells (MNGC), mitotic cells, and endothelial cells in normal tumor vessels and those in proliferated tumor vessels. These cellular components were selected from more than 100 visual fields with high-power magnification. For each cell type, the percentage of P53-positive cells was again defined as P53-LI and that of MIB-1 positive cells as PI.

Results

P53 Immunohistochemistry

Twenty-six of 39 tumors (67%) progressing from low-grade astrocytoma (II→III and II→IV) and 9 of 13 (69%) anaplastic astrocytomas (III→IV) were P53-positive at the initial operation. Fourteen of 17 cases of low-grade or anaplastic astrocytomas which were initially P53-negative became P53-positive after progression. The fraction of P53-positive cases significantly increased during progression, in group II→III from 65% to 90%, in group II→IV from 68% to 95%, and in group III→IV from 69% to

100%. The Wilcoxon signed rank test showed a value of $P < 0.05$ for each group. None of the initially P53-positive cases became negative after recurrence.

P53 Labeling Index

The mean P53-LI was 3.2% in low-grade astrocytomas, 8.2% in anaplastic astrocytomas, and 12.2% in glioblastomas. In the P53-positive cases, the P53-LI increased significantly during progression from low-grade astrocytomas: in group II→III (Fig. 1a,b) from 3.5% to 9.8% ($P < 0.05$) and in group II→IV from 3.3% to

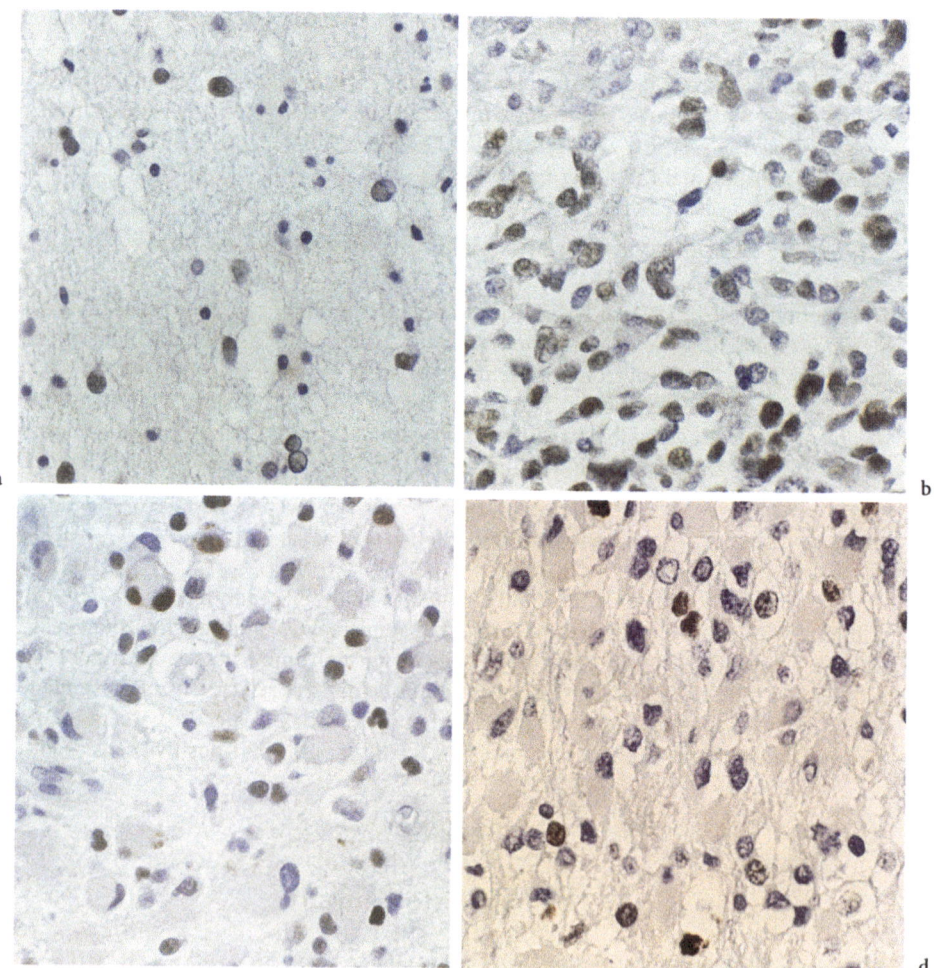

Fig. 1a–d. Photomicrographs of P53 with **a–c** PAb 1801 and **d** MIB-I immunostaining (×410). Low grade astrocytoma, **a** before progression (mean P53 labeling index; *LI*, 4%) and **b** after progression (mean P53 LI, 27%) to anaplastic astrocytoma. **c** Low-grade gemistocytic astrocytoma. Note the high P53 LI of gemistocytes. **d** Gemistocytic component of an anaplastic astrocytoma. Note the absence of MIB-1 immunoreactivity in gemistocytes

Table 1. Growth fraction (MIB-1) and p53 labeling index of cellular components of astrocytoma.

Cell type	Grade II		Grade III		Grade IV	
	MIB-1 (%)	P53 (%)	MIB-1 (%)	P53 (%)	MIB-1 (%)	P53 (%)
All tumor cells	2.7	3.2	9.5	8.2	17.5	12.2
Gemistocytes	0.6*	7.0*	1.6*	6.6	2.1*	8.8
Multinuclear giant cells	ND	ND	9.7	29.0*	14.6	31.4*
Mitotic cells	99.4*	0.4	96.4*	2.5	96.3*	3.4*
Normal endothelial cells	1.0	0.3*	1.7*	0.2*	2.5*	0.2*
Prolif. endothelial cells	ND	ND	8.8	2.4	12.2	0.7*

*Significantly different from the mean of all tumor cells of the same grade ($P < .05$).
ND, not detected.

12.9% ($P < 0.01$, Student's paired t-test). No significant increase was observed in tumors progressing from anaplastic astrocytoma to glioblastoma (6.6% vs 8.5%).

Proliferating Cell Index (PI)

The average PI was 2.7% (range, 1.2–4.7) in low-grade astrocytomas, 9.5% (range, 1.0–30.3) in anaplastic astrocytomas, and 17.5% (range, 5.9–43.0) in glioblastomas, and the difference was significant in each grade ($P < 0.001$, Scheffe's test). The PI increased significantly during progression in group II→III, from 2.5% to 11.1%, in group II→IV, from 2.9% to 18.7% ($P < 0.01$), and in group III→IV, from 8.7% to 16.0% ($P = 0.01$, Student's paired t-test).

Cell Component Analysis

The P53 labeling index (LI) and the growth fraction, as determined by immunoreactivity to MIB-1, was determined for the various cellular components (Table 1).

Discussion

Inactivation of the normal *p53* function is a common event in the development of a wide variety of human neoplasms. In astrocytic human brain tumors, the overall incidences of *p53* mutations and P53 accumulation have been reported to be 25%–40% [4–10] and 25%–50% [4–6,8,10,12,19–24], respectively. There was no evidence of a significant difference in the incidence of *p53* abnormalities among different grades of astrocytomas. However, these data represent mean values for different groups of patients, and more direct evidence of the role of *p53* in glioma progression requires the analysis of *p53* abnormalities in neoplasms of the same patient at different stages of the disease. The results in this study showed a high incidence of P53-positivity in both initially low-grade astrocytomas (67%) and initially anaplastic astrocytomas (69%). This high incidence of *p53* abnormalities prior to progression suggests that *p53* abnormalities may contribute to the histological progression of astrocytomas.

The mechanism of progression of astrocytic gliomas has been explained by several hypotheses. Cells that undergo a genetic change may acquire a selective growth advantage [25], resulting in the clonal expansion of *p53* mutant cells, which are considered more likely to acquire additional genetic alterations [11]. A two-step model for inactivation of the *p53* gene in astrocytoma was proposed by del Arco et al. [26]. According to this proposal, a *p53* mutation occurs in the initial stage of astrocytoma tumorigenesis and subsequent loss of the remaining wild-type allele appears to be associated with progression towards a more malignant phenotype. Lack of *p53*-associated G_1 arrest and the inability to induce DNA repair can lead to the replication of damaged DNA and to genomic instability. This facilitates further genetic alterations, including loss of tumor suppressor function or oncogene amplification. Furthermore, inability to induce differentiation or apoptotic pathways serves to bypass essential cellular checkpoints against neoplastic transformation [27,28].

In this and previous reports involving astrocytoma recurrence, no initial P53-positive case became P53-negative after progression, Moreover, in five cases reported by Iuzzolino et al. [12], as well as in 39 of our cases which progressed from low-grade astrocytoma (II→III and II→IV), P53-LIs increased significantly during progression. This suggests that P53-positive glioma cells may have a growth advantage. A clonal expansion of neoplastic astrocytes with *p53* mutations during tumor progression has previously been reported [11].

Since the presence of gemistocytes in glial tumors is considered a sign of poor prognosis [29,30] and up to 80% of gemistocytic astrocytomas have been reported to convert to glioblastomas [31], it has been suggested that gemistocytic astrocytomas may be biologically equivalent to anaplastic astrocytomas [29]. However, previous cell kinetic studies with small numbers of samples, using tritiated thymidine (^{3}H-T) ($n = 7$) [32] and bromodeoxyuridine (BrdU) ($n = 8$) [29,33], have shown that gemistocytes have a low proliferating activity. Since the mAb MIB-I recognizes the nuclei of cells in all phases of the cell cycle (G_1, S, G_2, and M-phase), cells with negative immunostaining with mAb MIB-I are considered as those that remain in G_0-phase. In 109 cases, we clearly showed that the MIB-1 PI of gemistocytes was significantly lower than the PI of each tumor. Despite the finding that the PI increased significantly during histological progression, no significant change was observed in the LI of gemistocytes. Furthermore, in tumor areas with a high PI, and which contained gemistocytes, most MIB-1 reacted cells were anaplastic astrocytes or mitotic cells; the gemistocytes did not react with MIB-1. There is a hypothesis that fibrillary or protoplasmic astrocytes convert to gemistocytes when they leave the mitotic cycle and convert again to highly anaplastic small cells when they move into the cell cycle [32,34]. Our results show that gemistocytic cells have a lower than average proliferative activity, while P53 immunoreactivity is higher or similar to that of other tumor cells. Thus, P53 immunoreactivity may not necessarily indicate loss of growth control.

Acknowledgments. The authors are grateful to Beatrice Pfister, Ursula Recher, Marianne König, and Angelica Ruf for their excellent technical assistance.

References

1. Kleihues P, Burger PC, Scheithauer BW (1993) The new WHO classification of brain tumours, Brain Pathol 3:255–268
2. Kleihues P, Burger PC, Scheithauer BW (1993) Histological typing of tumours of the central nervous system. World Health Organization International Histological Classification of Tumours, 2nd edn. Springer, Berlin Heidelberg New York Tokyo
3. Scherer H (1940) Cerebral astrocytomas and their derivatives. Am J Cancer 40:159–198

4. Aka K, Bruner JM, Bondy ML, Ligon K, Nishi T, del Giglio A, Moser RP, Levin VA, Saya H (1993) Detection of *p53* alterations in human astrocytomas using frozen tissue sections for the polymerase chain reaction. J Neurooncol 16:125–133

5. Chozick BS, Weicker ME, Pezzullo JC, Jackson CL, Finkelstein SD, Ambler MW, Epstein MH, Finch PW (1994) Pattern of mutant *p53* expression in human astrocytomas suggests the existence of alternate pathways of tumorigenesis. Cancer 73:406–415

6. Kraus JA, Bolln C, Wolf HK, Neumann J, Kindermann D, Fimmers R, Forster F, Baumann A, Schlegel U (1994) TP53 alterations and clinical outcome in low grade astrocytomas. Genes Chromosom Cancer 10:143–149

7. Lang FF, Miller DC, Pisharody S, Koslow M, Newcomb EW (1994) High frequency of p53 protein accumulation without *p53* gene mutation in human juvenile pilocytic, low grade and anaplastic astrocytomas. Oncogene 9:949–954

8. Louis DN, von Deimling A, Chung RY, Rubio MP, Whaley JM, Eibl RH, Ohgaki H, Wiestler OD, Thor AD, Seizinger BR (1993) Comparative study of *p53* gene and protein alterations in human astrocytic tumors. J Neuropathol Exp Neurol 52:31–38

9. Ohgaki H, Eibl RH, Schwab M, Reichel MB, Mariani L, Gehring M, Petersen I, Holl T, Wiestler OD, Kleihues P (1993) Mutations of the *p53* tumor suppressor gene in neoplasms of the human nervous system. Mol Carcinog 8:74–80

10. Rasheed BK, McLendon RE, Herndon JE, Friedman HS, Friedman AH, Bigner DD, Bigner SH (1994) Alterations of the TP53 gene in human gliomas. Cancer Res 54:1324–1330

11. Sidransky D, Mikkelsen T, Schwechheimer K, Rosenblum ML, Cavanee W, Vogelstein B (1992) Clonal expansion of *p53* mutant cells is associated with brain tumor progression. Nature 355:846–847

12. Iuzzolino P, Ghimenton C, Nicolato A, Giorgiutti F, Fina P, Doglioni C, Barbareschi M (1994) p53 protein in low-grade astrocytomas : A study with long-term follow up. Br J Cancer 69:586–591

13. Karamitopoulou E, Perentes E, Diamantis I, Maraziotis T (1994) *Ki-67* immunoreactivity in human central nervous system tumors: A study with MIB 1 monoclonal antibody on archival material. Acta Neuropathol (Berl) 87:47–54

14. Montine TJ, Vandersteenhoven JJ, Aguzzi A, Boyko OB, Dodge RK, Kerns BJ, Burger PC (1994) Prognostic significance of Ki-67 proliferation index in supratentorial fibrillary astrocytic neoplasms. Neurosurgery 34:674–679

15. Shibuya M, Ito S, Miwa T, Davis RL, Wilson CB, Hoshino T (1993) Proliferative potential of brain tumors. Analyses with Ki-67 and anti-DNA polymerase alpha monoclonal antibodies, bromodeoxyuridine labeling, and nuclear organizer region counts. Cancer 71:199–206

16. Banks L, Matlashewski G, Crawford L (1986) Isolation of human p53-specific monoclonal antibodies and their use in the studies of human p53 expression. Eur J Biochem 159:529–534

17. Gerdes J, Becker MH, Key G, Cattoretti G (1992) Immunohistological detection of tumor growth fraction (Ki-67 antigen) in formalin-fixed and routinely processed tissues, J Pathol 168:85–86

18. Key G, Becker MH, Baron B, Duchrow M, Schluter C, Flad HD, Gerdes J (1993) New Ki-67-equivalent murine monoclonal antibodies (MIB 1-3) generated against bacterially expressed parts of the Ki-67 cDNA containing three 62 base pair repetitive elements encoding for the Ki-67 epitope. Lab Invest 68:629–636

19. Barbareschi M, Iuzzolino P, Pennella A, Allegranza A, Arrigoni G, Dalla-Palma P, Doglioni C (1992) p53 protein expression in central nervous system neoplasms. J Clin Pathol 45:583–586

20. Bruner JM, Saya H, Moser RP (1991) Immunocytochemical detection of p53 in human gliomas. Mod Pathol 4:671–674

21. Ellison DW, Gatter KC, Steart PV, Lane DP, Weller RO (1992) Expression of the p53 protein in a spectrum of astrocytic tumors. J Pathol 168:383–386

22. Haapasalo H, Isola J, Sallinen P, Kalimo H, Helin H, Rantala I (1993) Aberrant p53 expression in astrocytic neoplasms of the brain: Association with proliferation. Am J Pathol 142:1347–1351

23. Jaros E, Perry RH, Adam L, Kelly PJ, Crawford PJ, Kalbag RM, Mendelow AD, Sengupta RP, Pearson AD (1992) Prognostic implications of p53 protein, epidermal growth factor receptor, and Ki-67 labelling in brain tumours. Br J Cancer 66:373–385

24. Karamitopoulou E, Perentes E, Diamantis I (1993) p53 protein expression in central nervous system tumors: An immunohistochemical study with CM1 polyvalent and DO-7 monoclonal antibodies. Acta Neuropathol (Berl) 85:611–616

25. Nowell PC (1976) The clonal evolution of tumor cell populations. Science 194:23–28

26. del Arco A, Garcia J, Arribas C, Barrio R, Blazquez MG, lzquierdo JM, lzquierdo M (1993) Timing of p53 mutations during astrocytoma tumorigenesis. Hum Mol Genet 2:1687–1690

27. Kuerbitz SJ, Plunkett BS, Walsh WV, Kasten MB (1992) Wild-type p53 is a cell cycle checkpoint determinant following irradiation. Proc Natl Acad Sci USA 89:7491–7495

28. Lane DP (1992) *p53*, guardian of the genome. Nature 358:15–16

29. Krouwer HG, Davis RL, Silver P, Prados M (1991) Gemistocytic astrocytomas: A reappraisal.J Neurosurg 74:399–406

30. Schiffer D, Chio A, Giordana MT, Leone M, Soffietti R (1988) Prognostic value of histologic factors in adult cerebral astrocytoma. Cancer 61:1386–1393

31. Russell DS, Rubinstein LJ (1989) Pathology of tumors of the nervous system. 5th edn. Edward Arnold, London, pp.95–161

32. Hoshino T, Wilson BC, Ellis WG, (1975) Gemistocytic astrocytes in gliomas. An autoradiographic study. J Neuropathol Exp Neurol 34:263–281

33. Onda K, Davis RL, Wilson CB, Hoshino T (1994) Regional differences in bromodeoxyuridine uptake, expression Ki-67 protein, and nucleolar organizer region counts in glioblastoma multiforme. Acta Neuropathol (Berl) 87:586–593

34. Bruner JM (1994) Neuropathology of malignant gliomas. Semin Oncol 21:126–138

Homozygous Deletion of the p16 Gene in Malignant Glioma

Shuichi Izumoto, Norio Arita, Takanori Ohnishi, Shoju Hiraga, Takuyu Taki, and Toru Hayakawa

Abstract. The short arm of chromosome 9 is frequently rearranged or deleted in melanoma, lung cancer, glioma, and a variety of human tumors, strongly suggesting that this subchromosomal region includes a tumor suppressor gene. Because the gene for p16 (also known as CDK4I or MTS1) lies on chromosome 9p21 and loss of its function may activate the G_1 cyclin function, the p16 gene is a strong candidate for a novel tumor suppressor gene. To investigate the frequency of homozygous deletions of the p16 gene in human glioma tissues and cultured cell lines, DNA samples were amplified by the polymerase chain reaction (PCR), and homozygous deletions of the p16 gene were determined by the absence of PCR products of the p16 gene. As a result, the p16 gene PCR products were absent in 6 of 6 human glioma cell lines and 4 of 12 glioblastoma tissues. Homozygous deletion of the p16 gene was not detected, however, in any of 6 anaplastic astrocytoma tissues or 5 astrocytoma tissues. Deletions of the p16 gene were more common in cultured glioma cell lines than in glioma tissues. These results indicate that p16 gene deletions may provide an additional growth advantage to some glioblastomas.

Key words. p16 gene—CDK4I—Glioma—Tumor suppressor gene

Introduction

Many tumor suppressor genes have been identified, for example, p53, retinoblastoma (RB), WT1, and NF1, and alterations such as mutations or deletions of these genes in a wide variety of human cancers have been reported. Previous molecular studies identified a distinct region on the short arm of chromosome 9 as the likely location of a tumor suppressor gene, because a portion of 9p21-22 around the INFA cluster is often homozygously deleted in human cancers [1-5]. Nobori et al. [6] and Kamb et al. [7] have recently reported that the p16 gene, which lies on chromosome 9p21, is a novel candidate tumor suppressor gene. The p16 gene, also called CDK4I or MTS1, negatively regulates the cell cycle through specific inhibition of cyclin-dependent kinase4 (CDK4) [8] and is frequently deleted in cultured cell lines of melanoma, glioma, lung cancer, and leukemia [6,7].

Because the proteins of the CDK family promote normal cell-cycle passage and regulate cell proliferation, p16, which inhibits these process, is a plausible tumor

Department of Neurosurgery, Osaka University Medical School, Osaka, 565 Japan

263

suppressor gene candidate. Loss of the p16 function might therefore push cells into uncontrolled division. Frequent losses of heterozygosity on 9p have been known to occur in malignant gliomas, and homozygous deletions of the p16 gene in glioma cell lines have been reported [9,10]. Although p16 deletions are indeed frequent in tumor cell lines, they were recently reported to be much less common in tumor tissues of many types [11]. Thus, we have examined the frequency of homozygous deletions of the p16 gene in a series of cultured glioma cell lines and surgical specimens of gliomas to elucidate whether this gene is a tumor suppressor gene for gliomas.

Materials and Methods

Cell Lines, Tumor Samples, and DNA Isolation

Six human glioma cell lines (T98G, U373MG, U251MG, U87MG, A172, and KNS-3) were cultured in Dulbecco's modified Eagle's medium with 10% fetal bovine serum or in Eagle's minimal essential medium (MEM) with nonessential amino acids, sodium pyruvate, and 10% fetal bovine serum. All the cells were scraped, collected in sample tubes, and stored at −80°C until use. Twelve glioblastomas, 6 anaplastic astrocytomas, and 5 astrocytomas were used for analysis; all specimens were frozen in liquid nitrogen immediately after resection and stored at −80°C until use. DNA was extracted from cultured cells or frozen tissues with proteinase K and phenol/chloroform as described previously [12] and diluted in 1 × TE. DNA from healthy human lymphocyte was used as normal control.

DNA Amplification and Deletion Analysis

The p16 gene was amplified by the polymerase chain reaction (PCR) method. The G3PDH gene was coamplified as a internal control for amplification. The primers of both genes are as follows: p16 forward primer, 5′-GAGAGGCTCTGAGAAACCTC -3′; p16 reverse primer, 5′-CCTGAGCTTCCCTAGTTCAC-3′; G3PDH forward primer, 5′-TGGTATCGTGGAAGGACTCATGAC-3′; G3PDH reverse primer, 5′-ATGCCAGTGAGCTTCCCGTTCAGC-3′. The PCR reaction was performed with 1 × PCR buffer (10 mM Tris-HCl, 50 mM KCl, 1.5 mM MgCl$_2$), 250 nM of each forward and reverse primer of both genes, 200 μM of each deoxynucleotide triphosphate, 2.5 units of Taq DNA polymerase (Takara Shuzo, Kyoto, Japan), and 200 ng of template DNA. Amplification was carried out in a Perkin-Elmer (Norwalk, CT, USA) Cetus thermocycler for 25 cycles at 94°C for 1 min, 60°C for 1 min, and 72°C for 2 min. The PCR products were separated by electrophoresis on 1.5% agarose gel containing 0.5 μg/ml ethidium bromide.

Results

In the control, a band of approximately 380 bp, which is the p16 PCR product, was detected as well as a band of 190 bp, which is the G3PDH PCR product. No other bands were detected with this PCR condition. No p16 PCR product was detected in any of the six glioma cell lines, but a single band of 190 bp, the G3PDH-PCR product, was detected. All six glioma cell lines were judged to have homozygous deletions in the p16 gene (Fig. 1). No p16 PCR product was detected in 4 of 12 glioblastoma tissues, indicating that 33.3% of the glioblastoma tissues in our study have homozygous deletions in the p16 gene (Fig. 2). In all 6 anaplastic astrocytoma tissues, a band of the p16 PCR product was detected, demonstrating that none of anaplastic astrocytoma tissues tested had a homozygous deletion in the p16 gene (Fig. 3A). In all 5 astrocytoma tissues, a band of the p16 PCR product was detected as well (Fig. 3B). A 190-bp band of the G3PDH PCR product, used as an internal control, was detected in

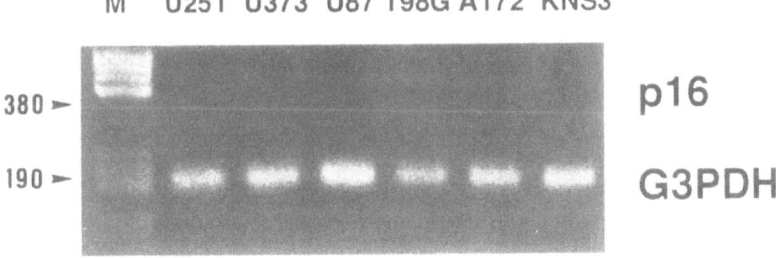

Fig. 1. Polymerase chain reaction (PCR) analysis of six glioma cell lines with a set of primers of the p16 gene and a set of primers of the G3PDH gene. Note that no band of p16 PCR product was detected; however, a 190-bp band of G3PDH PCR product was detected in all samples. M, DNA marker

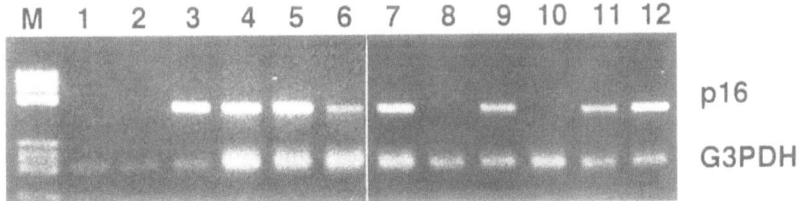

Fig. 2. PCR analysis of 12 glioblastoma tissues with a set of primers of the p16 gene and a set of primers of the G3PDH gene. Note no band of p16 PCR product was detected in lanes 1,2,8, and 10, indicating homozygous deletion of the p16 gene. In lanes 3,4,5,6,7,9,11, and 12, however, a 380-bp p16 PCR product was detected

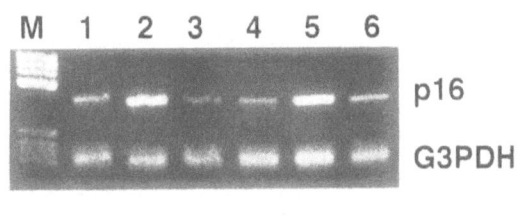

Fig. 3. PCR analysis of six anaplastic astrocytoma tissues (**A**) and five astrocytoma tissues (**B**) with a set of the p16 gene primers and a set of the G3PDH gene primers. Note a 380-bp p16 PCR product was detected in all lanes (**A** and **B**)

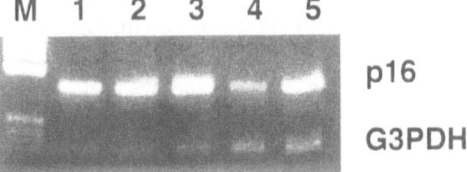

all the glioma tissues. All the p16 PCR products detected in various grade of gliomas were the same size as the normal control.

Discussion

The cell division cycle is regulated in the G_1 phase by G_1 cyclin such as cyclin C, D, and E, which are regulated by a number of kinases known as cyclin-dependent kinases (CDKs). The complex formed by CDK4 and cyclin D have been strongly implicated in controlling cell proliferation during the G_1 phase. Serrano et al. [8] reported the p16 protein, which binds to CDK4 and inhibits the catalytic activity of the CDK4/cyclin D enzymes. On the other hand, two groups have independently identified a new candidate for a tumor suppressor gene that is located between the INFA gene cluster and MTAP on 9p21. Sequence analysis demonstrated that this gene is identical to the p16 gene [6,7]. The reports that the p16 gene is homozygously deleted in a wide variety of human tumor cell lines seem to strongly support the idea that it is a novel tumor suppressor gene [6,7]. To confirm that, we analyzed the frequency of homozygous deletions of the p16 gene in glioma cell lines and in glioma tissues by the PCR method.

In our study, one-third of the glioblastoma tissues had the p16 gene deletions, while no deletion was detected in anaplastic astrocytoma and astrocytoma tissues. Overall, 17.4% of the glioma had the p16 gene deletions. In contrast, it seems remarkable that all six cultured cell lines had homozygous deletions of the p16 gene. Our study on cultured cells supported the idea that the p16 was a tumor suppressor in glioma cell lines as well as in a wide variety of other tumor cells. All samples in which the p16 PCR product was absent were amplified with different experimental conditions, changing the cycling time to 35 or changing the annealing temperature to 55°C. As a result, no p16 PCR product was detected by other methods, confirming that homozygous deletion of the p16 gene occurs in these samples.

In our study, homozygous deletions of the p16 gene are less frequent in glioma tissues than in the glioma cell lines. Cairns et al. [11] suggested that the gene alterations of p16 may give a selective growth advantage to cultured cells because they did not find homozygous deletion in 75 surgical tumor specimens. We did however detect homozygous deletions of the p16 gene in glioblastoma tissues although the frequency is lower than in cultured cell lines. The p16 gene deletion may activate the G_1 cyclin function and therefore provide an additional growth advantage to some of the glioma tissues as well as cultured cells. In tissue samples, homozygous deletions of the p16 gene were detected in about one-third of glioblastomas but not in lower grade gliomas, suggesting that loss of the p16 function may contribute to the development of de novo glioblastomas.

The frequency of p16 gene alterations varies with the type of tumor. Homozygous deletions of the p16 gene were reported in 6 of 31 bladder cancers [13] and in 4 of 72 leukemia patients [14]; mutations or deletions of the p16 gene were found in about 75% of human pancreatic cancers [15]. Mutations of the p16 gene were reported in 14 of 27 esophageal squamous cell carcinomas [16], in 11 of 68 head and neck squamous cell carcinomas [17] and in 19 of 64 non-small-cell lung carcinomas [18], but no mutation was detected in melanomas [19] and breast carcinomas [20]. In our study of gliomas, the frequency of p16 gene alterations was relatively higher than in other tumors.

In this study, we did not examine whether point mutations of the p16 gene were present in glioma cells or in tissues in which no homozygous deletion of the p16 gene was found. There is also a possibility that other mechanisms which inactivate the p16 function might occur in glioma tissues. Amplification of the CDK4 gene has been reported in glioma [21]. Therefore, the balance of protein functions between CDK4, CDK4I, and CDK4-activating kinase [22] might be important for G_1 cyclin, in other words, for tumor growth in malignant gliomas.

Conclusion

Frequency of homozygous deletions of the p16 gene, which is believed to be a tumor suppressor gene, was analyzed in glioma cell lines and tissues by PCR. Homozygous deletions of the p16 gene were detected in all the glioma cell lines and one-third of glioblastoma tissues but not in anaplastic astrocytoma and astrocytoma tissues. These results suggest that loss of the p16 function may activate the G_1 cyclin function and provide an additional growth advantage to some of the gliomas.

References

1. Fountain JW, Karayiorgou M, Ernstoff MS, Kirkwood JM, Vlock DR, Titus-Ernstoff L, Bouchard B, Vijayasaradhi S, Houghton AN, Lahti J, Kidd VJ, Housman DE, Dracopoli NC (1992) Homozygous deletions within human chromosome band 9p21 in melanoma. Proc Natl Acad Sci USA 89:10557–10561
2. Olopade OI, Buchhagen DL, Malik K, Sherman J, Nobori T, Bader S, Nau MM, Gazda AF, Minna JD, Diaz MO (1993) Homozygous deletion of the interferon genes defines the critical region on 9p that is deleted in lung cancers. Cancer Res 53:4761–4763
3. Olopade OI, Jenkins RB, Ransom DT, Malik K, Pomykala H, Nobori T, Cowan JM, Rowley JD, Diaz MO (1992) Molecular analysis of deletions of the short arm of chromosome 9 in human gliomas. Cancer Res 52:2523–2529
4. Diaz MO, Rubin CM, Harden A, Ziemin S, Larson RA, Le-Beau MM, Rowley JD (1990) Deletions of interferon genes in acute lymphoblastic leukemia. N Engl J Med 322:77–82
5. Cheng JQ, Jhanwar SC, Lu YY, Testa JR (1993) Homozygous deletions within 9p21-p22 identify a small critical region of chromosomal loss in human malignant mesotheliomas. Cancer Res 53:4761–4763
6. Kamb A, Gruis NA, Weaver-Feldhaus J, Liu Q, Harshman K, Tavtigian SV, Stockert E, Day RS III, Johnson BE, Skolnick MH (1994) A cell cycle regulator potentially involved in genesis of many tumor types. Science 264:436–440
7. Nobori T, Miura K, Wu DJ, Lois A, Takabayashi K, Carson DA (1994) Deletions of the cyclin-dependent kinase-4 inhibitor gene in multiple human cancers. Nature 368:753–756
8. Serrano M, Hannon GJ, Beach D (1993) A new regulatory motif in cell-cycle control causing specific inhibition of cyclin D/CDK4. Nature 366:704–707
9. James CD, He J, Collins VP, Allalunis-Turner MJ, Day RS III (1993) Localization of chromosome 9p homozygous deletions in glioma cell lines with markers constituting a continuous linkage group. Cancer Res 53:3674–3676
10. Ichimura K, Schmidt EE, Yamaguchi N, James CD, Collins VP (1994) A common region of homozygous deletion in malignant human gliomas lies between the IFNa/w gene cluster and the D9S171 locus. Cancer Res 54:3127–3130
11. Cairns P, Mao L, Merlo A, Lee DJ, Schwab D, Eby Y, Tokino K, van der Riet P, Blaugrund JE, Sidransky D (1994) Rates of p16 (MTS1) mutations in primary tumors with 9p loss. Science 265:415–416
12. Madisen L, Holar DI, Holroyd CD, Crisp M, Hodes ME (1987) DNA banking: the effects of storage of blood and isolated DNA on the integrity of DNA. Am J Med Genet 27:379–390

13. Spruck CH III, Gonzalez-Zulueta M, Shibata A, Simoneau AR, Lin MF, Gonzales F, Tsai YC, Jones PA (1994) p16 gene in uncultured tumors. Nature 370:183–185
14. Ogawa S, Hirano N, Sato N, Takahashi T, Hangaishi A, Tanaka K, Kurokawa M, Tanaka T, Mitani K, Yazaki Y, Hirai H (1994) Homozygous loss of the cyclin-dependent kinase 4-inhibitor (p16) gene in human leukemias. Blood 84:2431–2435
15. Caldas C, Hahn SA, daCosta LT, Redston MS, Schutte M, Seymour AB, Weinstein CL, Hruban RH, Yeo CJ, Kern SE (1994) Frequent somatic mutations and homozygous deletions of the p16 (MTS1) gene in pancreatic adenocarcinoma. Nature Genet 8:27–32
16. Igaki H, Sasaki H, Kishi T, Sakamoto H, Tachimori Y, Kato H, Watanabe H, Sugimura T, Terada M (1994) Highly frequent homozygous deletion of the p16 gene in esophageal cancer cell lines. Biochem Biophys Res Commun 203:1090–1095
17. Zhang SY, Klein-Szanto AJP, Sauter ER, Shafarenko M, Mitsunaga S, Nobori T, Carson DA, Ridge JA, Goodrow TL (1994) Higher frequency of alterations in the p16/CDKN4 gene in squamous cell carcinoma cell lines than in primary tumors of the head and neck. Cancer Res 54:5050–5053
18. Hayashi N, Sugimoto Y, Tsuchiya E, Ogawa M, Nakamura Y (1994) Somatic mutations of the MTS (multiple tumor suppressor) 1/CDK4I (cyclin-dependent kinase-4 inhibitor) gene in human primary non-small cell lung carcinomas. Biochem Biophys Res Commun 202:1426–1430
19. Ohta M, Nagai H, Shimizu M, Rasio D, Berd D, Mastrangelo M, Singh AD, Shields JA, Shiels CL, Croce CM, Huebner K (1994) Rarity of somatic and germline mutations of the cyclindependent kinase 4 inhibitor gene, CDK4I, in melanoma. Cancer Res 54:5269–5272
20. Xu L, Sgroi D, Sterner CJ, Beauchamp RL, Pinney DM, Keel S, Ueki K, Rutter JL, Buckler AJ, Louis DN, Gusella JF, Ramesh V (1994) Mutational analysis of CDKN2 (MTS1/p16[ink4]) in human breast carcinomas. Cancer Res 54:5262–5264
21. Reifenberger G, Reifenberger J, Ichimura K, Meltzer PS, Collins VP (1994) Amplification of multiple genes from chromosomal region 12q13–14 in human malignant gliomas: preliminary mapping of the amplicons shows preferential involvement of CDK4, SAS, and MDM2. Cancer Res 54:4299–4303
22. Kato J, Matsumoto M, Strom D, Sherr CJ (1994) Regulation of cyclin D-dependent kinase 4 (cdk4) by cdk4-activating kinase. Mol Cell Biol 14:2713–2721

Detection of Binding Proteins of Merlin, the NF2 Tumor Suppressor Gene Product

Hideo Takeshima[1] and Hideyuki Saya[2]

Abstract. The neurofibromatosis type 2 (*NF2*) gene was recently identified, and the protein it encodes, designated merlin, is similar in sequence to members of the band 4.1 superfamily that link cytoskeletal components with proteins in the cell membrane. To elucidate the function of merlin as a tumor suppressor gene, we tried to identify the merlin-binding proteins that might form a protein complex and transmit the cell contact signaling. For this aim, we created a bacterially expressed fusion protein consisting of glutathione S-transferase and merlin. The protein-binding assay detected five merlin-binding cellular proteins, designated p165, p145, p125, p85, and p70. Immunoprecipitation showed that only p85 constitutively bound the native form of merlin. Although the entire merlin-ezrin-radixin-moesin (MERM) homology domain of merlin was found to be essential for binding to all five proteins, the MERM homology domains of ezrin and moesin did not bind to any of the five proteins. Because most NF2 mutations that have been reported are in the region we determined was necessary for binding, the mutations probably impair binding. Therefore, the formation of the protein complex is probably one of the crucial steps for tumor suppression.

Key words. NF2—Binding protein—Tumor suppressor—Merlin

Introduction

Neurofibromatosis type 2 (NF2) is an autosomal, dominantly inherited disorder with an incidence of about 1 in 37 000 individuals [1]. NF2 is strongly associated with the development of benign intracranial tumors including bilateral vestibular schwannomas and meningiomas [2]. The *NF2* gene was isolated recently using positional cloning methods [3,4] and shown to have mutations both in the germline DNA of NF2 patients and in sporadically occurring meningiomas and schwannomas [4].

The *NF2* gene has been reported to have 16 exons and is expected to encode a protein composed of 595 amino acids that has been called merlin [3] (and, alternatively, schwannomin [4]). Merlin was found to be strikingly similar to the moesin-

[1] Department of Neuro-Oncology, University of Texas M.D. Anderson Cancer Center, Houston, TX 77 030, USA
[2] Department of Oncology, Kumamoto University Medical School, Kumamoto 860, Japan

ezrin-radixin (MER) family of cytoskeleton-associated proteins. The MER family proteins are known to belong to the band 4.1 superfamily, which includes erythrocyte protein 4.1, talin, and the protein tyrosine phosphatases. Each of these members contains a homologous domain of about 200–300 amino acids near the N-terminus, followed by a segment that is predicted to be a long α-helix and a highly charged C-terminal domain. Some of the members of the band 4.1 superfamily have been studied extensively and are believed to act as links between cell membrane proteins and cytoskeletal proteins. For example, protein 4.1 binds to the transmembrane glycophorin at the homologous N-terminal domain [5] and to the spectrin–actin complex of the cytoskeleton at the long α-helix [6]. Talin binds integrins [7] as well as with vinculin [8].

MER family proteins have been reported to work as molecular linkers between CD44 and actin-based cytoskeleton [9]. These proteins have been postulated to act as mediators between plasma membrane proteins and cytoskeletal proteins, regulating cell-surface structure and dynamics as well as cytoplasmic responses to growth factors and other external stimuli. Accordingly, it is reasonable to speculate that merlin also forms a complex with cell membrane protein and cytoskeletal protein and is involved in cell–cell and cell–matrix contact signaling. Alterations in or absence of merlin may affect the contact growth-inhibition signal and so result in continuous growth of cells and development of benign tumors in NF2 patients. Therefore, identifying the molecules that interact and form protein complexes with merlin may clarify the biological function of merlin itself and give a clue for elucidating the mechanism of tumorigenesis in NF2 patients.

Detection of Cellular Proteins That Interact with GST-Merlin Fusion Protein

To investigate the interaction of merlin with cellular proteins, a fusion protein that contains glutathione S-transferase (GST) and nearly the entire merlin was expressed in bacteria using the pGEX-2TH expression vector system [10,11]. The cDNA encoding the human merlin was isolated, using the reverse transcription-polymerase chain reaction (PCR) method, from human neuroblastoma SH-SY5Y cells. Whole-cell lysates of SH-SY5Y cells metabolically labeled with [^{35}S] methionine were incubated with either GST or the GST–merlin fusion protein immobilized on reduced glutathione (GSH) beads. Sodium dodecyl sulfate (SDS) polyacrylamide gel electrophoresis (PAGE) analysis of the binding complex revealed that five prominent bands with relative molecular masses of 165, 145, 125, 85, and 70 kDa appeared to bind only to the GST–merlin fusion protein [12] (Fig. 1). There bands were designated p165, p145, p125, p85, and p70, respectively.

To delineate the regions required for the interaction of merlin with these five binding proteins, we made a series of merlin deletion mutants (Fig. 2). The protein-binding assay with various deletion mutants of merlin in addition to the expression pattern of various cell lines showed that these five binding proteins can be grossly categorized into three groups, as follows.

The first group of the proteins consists of p165 and p125, which were expressed ubiquitously and abundantly in all the cell lines examined [12]. The deletion study revealed that the large region spanning N-terminal residues 20 to 339, which includes

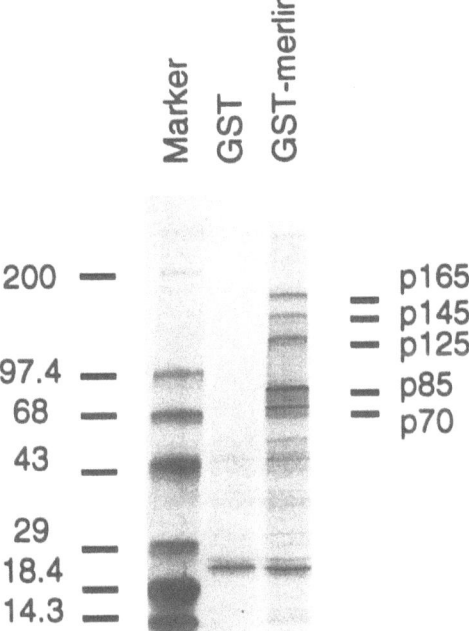

Fig. 1. Detection of merlin-binding proteins. Lysates of [35S] methionine-labeled SH-SY5Y cells were incubated with either glutathione S-transferase (GST) or the GST–merlin fusion protein immobilized on reduced glutathione (GSH) beads. The bound proteins were washed, subjected to 8–16% sodium dodecyl sulfate-polyacrylamide gel electrophoresis (SDS-PAGE) and visualized by fluorography. The positions of p165, p145, p125, p85, and p70 are indicated on the *right*. The positions of the 14C-labeled protein standards and their sizes (in kilodaltons, kDa) are shown on the *left*. (From [12], with permission)

most of the merlin-ezrin-radixin-moesin (MERM) homology domain, was necessary for p165 and p125 binding.

The second kind of merlin-binding protein is p145, which was detected only in the neuroblastoma cell line SH-SY5Y [12]. p145 could only bind the deletion mutants that bound to p165 and p125. This suggests that p145 forms a complex with p165 or p125 (or both) in certain types of cells and may be involved in tissue-specific signaling.

The third group of merlin-binding proteins includes p85 and p70, which were widely expressed in the various human cell lines [12]. The deletion study showed that not only the long α-helical domain but also most of the MERM homology domain was essential for the binding of p85 and p70.

Specific Binding of p165, p145, and p125 with Merlin But Not with Ezrin and Moesin

The MERM homology domain of merlin is as much as 63% identical to the other MERM family members at the amino acid level [3,4]. Although no conserved structural motifs important for the protein–protein interaction have been found in the

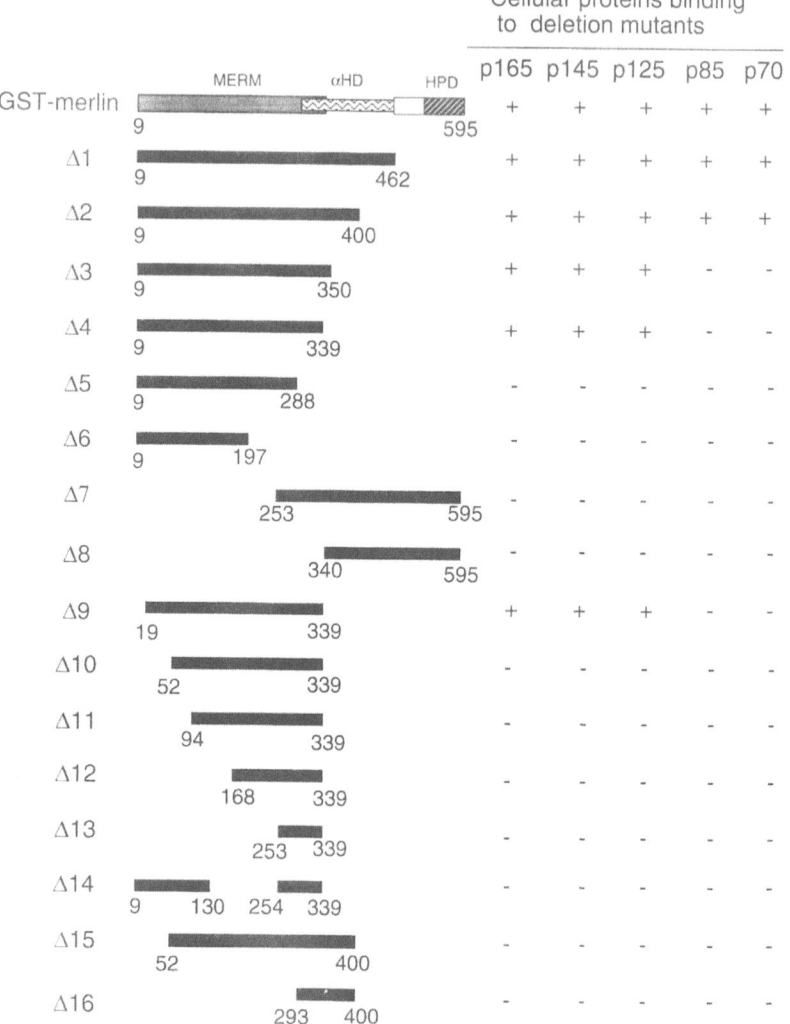

Fig. 2. Schematic presentation of association of cellular proteins with GST-merlin deletion mutants. The structure of human merlin, with the N-terminus at the left, is shown on the *top*. The merlin-ezrin-radixin-moesin (MERM) family homology domain (*MERM*), the long α-helical domain (*αHD*) and the hydrophilic domain (*HPD*) are indicated. The blocks below the model merlin structure represent the portions of human merlin retained in the deletion mutants; the deleted portion of each mutant is shown as a gap. The numbers under the blocks indicate the actual residues retained. The GST region of the fusion proteins is not shown. The columns on the *right* summarize binding activity to each cellular protein. (From [12], with permission)

MERM homology domain, the striking similarity throughout this domain implies that this region is functionally important, especially for protein binding. Therefore, we have to consider the possibility that p165, p145, and p125 do not bind specifically with merlin but also bind other MERM family members. To test this, we created GST-ezrin and GST-moesin fusion proteins that had the same deletion as merlin deletion mutant

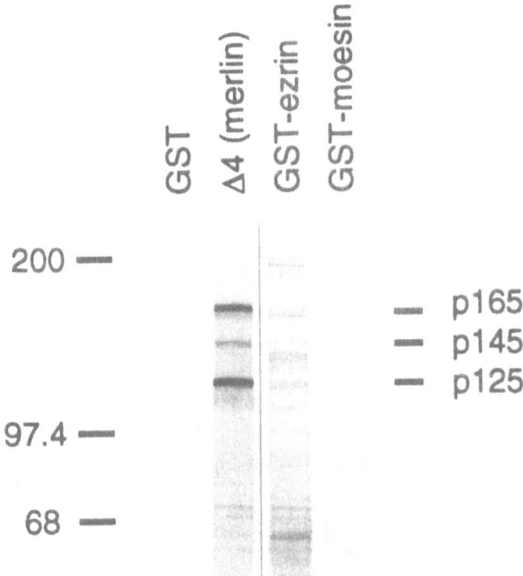

Fig. 3. Association of p165, p145, and p125 with MERM family proteins. Lysates were prepared from [³⁵S] methionine-labeled SH-SY5Y cells, and a protein-binding assay was performed. The GST-ezrin and GST-moesin fusion proteins used had the same deletion as merlin mutant Δ4. The positions and molecular sizes (in kilodaltons) of the ¹⁴C-labeled protein standards are shown to the *left* of the gel and the positions of p165, p145, and p125 are on the *right*. (From [12], with permission)

Δ4. The nucleotide sequence of human radixin has not been reported to date. Although merlin mutant Δ4 bound p165, p145, and p125, the GST-ezrin and GST-moesin proteins did not (Fig. 3) [12]. This result suggests that p165, p145, and p125 specifically bind to merlin.

The overall tertiary structure of the MERM homology domain is probably essential for the protein–protein interaction, and the seemingly small amino acid variation within the MERM homology domain of merlin provides the basis for the specific binding, which may be associated with merlin-specific cellular signaling.

Ezrin was found to be a substrate in vivo for both epidermal growth factor (EGF) receptor and platelet-derived growth factor (PDGF) receptor, and was rapidly phosphorylated on tyrosine in response to treatment with both growth factors. Radixin was phosphorylated only by the PDGF receptor, and moesin by neither receptor. We found that merlin and p165 were constitutively phosphorylated on serine or threonine residues [12]. To determine whether merlin was also regulated by growth factors, we stimulated U-251 MG cells with both EGF and PDGF. However, neither the level of phosphorylation of merlin nor that of p165 changed significantly (unpublished data). The two major tyrosine phosphorylation sites in ezrin were recently identified [13]. One of the sites, Tyr-145, lies in the MERM homology domain and is conserved throughout the band 4.1 superfamily members with the exception of talin. The other site, Tyr-353, is localized within a long α-helix domain and is unique to ezrin. Neither of these tyrosine residues is conserved in merlin. These data suggest that merlin participates in a different signal transduction pathway from ezrin.

Detection of Merlin and Merlin-Binding Proteins with Anti-Merlin Antibody

To determine whether the five proteins that bound bacterially expressed merlin also interacted with endogenous merlin, rat antiserum was raised against the GST-merlin fusion protein. Western blot analysis of various cell lines with the antiserum showed a specific protein of 72kDa [12].

The antiserum was then immunoprecipitated with [35S] methionine-labeled U-251 MG cell lysates to detect the binding proteins, and a 72-kDa band corresponding to merlin was revealed. It is interesting that p165 and p125 were not coprecipitated with endogenous merlin (Fig. 4). Instead, we found a prominent band of 85kDa that was not detected by Western blotting. To determine if this 85-kDa protein was identical to the p85 detected in the protein-binding assay, both bands were excise from the gels and subjected to V8 proteolytic peptide mapping. The two bands had very similar proteolytic patterns [12], suggesting that endogenous merlin as well as recombinant merlin interacted with p85.

The reason the native form of merlin interacted with p85 but not with the other four proteins that could associate with bacterially expressed merlin is still unclear. One possibility is that posttranslational modification of merlin, such as phosphorylation and glycosylation, negatively regulates its interaction with p165, p145, p125, and p70. For instance, the binding of band 4.1 protein with glycophorin is known to be regulated by the phosphorylation of the band 4.1 protein [14].

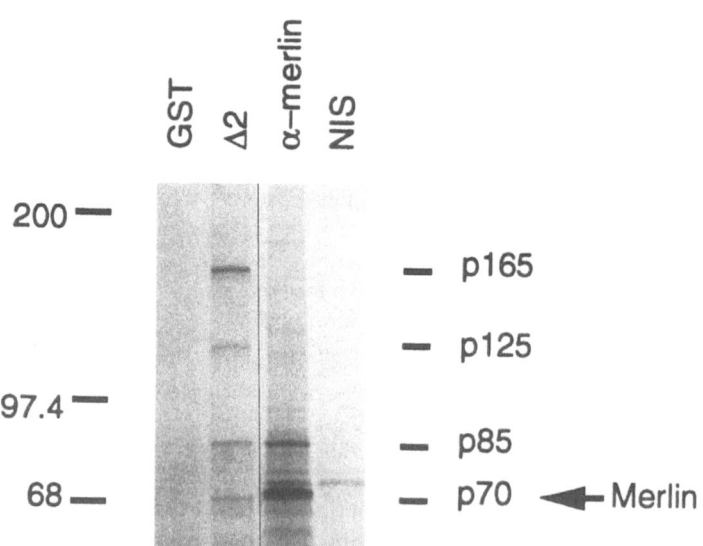

Fig. 4. Coprecipitation of p85 with endogenous merlin by anti-merlin antibody. U-251 MG cells were [35S] methionine labeled, and the cellular protein constitutively associated with merlin was coimmunoprecipitated with endogenous merlin by anti-merlin antibody (α-merlin). Rat nonimmune serum served as a background control (*NIS*). The protein complexes generated from the protein-binding assay of the same cell lysates with GST and deletion mutant Δ2 were included for comparison. (From [12], with permission)

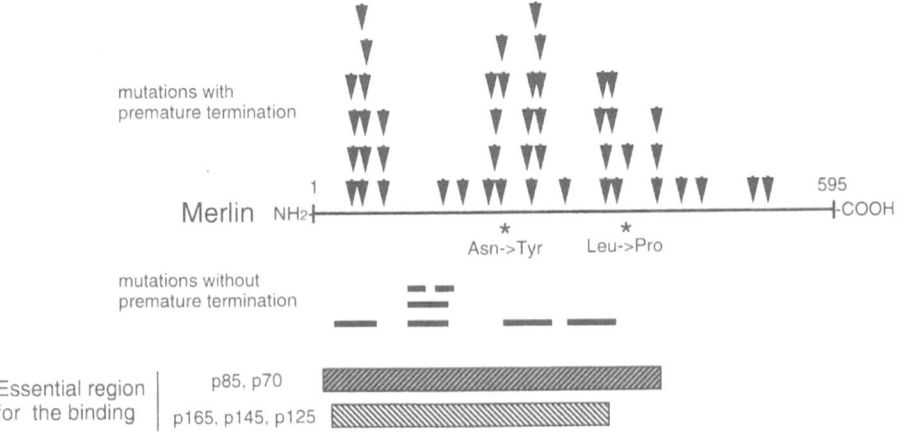

Fig. 5. Correlation between merlin mutations and the regions essential for protein binding. The positions of the *NF2* mutations in NF2 patients and NF2-related tumors reported to date [3,4,15,16, 17] are shown. The termination points caused by the generation of stop codons and the positions of frameshift mutations are indicated by *arrowheads*. The amino acid substitutions caused by two point mutations, which do not produce a truncated form of merlin, are indicated by *asterisks*. *Solid lines* represent in-frame deletions. The regions essential for the binding to p165, p145, and p125, and to p85 and p70, are indicated by *hatched boxes*. (From [12], with permission)

Correlation Between Merlin Mutation and the Regions Essential for Protein Binding

NF2 gene mutations recently have been reported in NF2 patients and NF2-related sporadic tumors such as acoustic schwannomas and meningiomas [3,4,15–17]. The majority of mutations were nonsense mutations or frameshifts that resulted in premature termination of merlin. The results of our deletion study indicate that more than 90% of the merlin mutations reported to truncate the protein will disrupt binding with p85 (Fig. 5), which was shown to make a protein complex with native form of merlin. Moreover, all nine in-frame mutations that do not result in premature termination of merlin were found in the region essential for binding to p85. Therefore, impaired binding of proteins with merlin may disrupt cell membrane–cytoskeleton signaling and so cause tumorigenesis in NF2 patients and NF2-related tumors. If the formation of the complex is crucial for tumor suppression, alterations in the merlin-binding proteins as well as in merlin itself may cause tumorigenesis. Identifying and characterizing these binding proteins therefore should provide insight into the normal cellular signaling related to cell–cell contact growth inhibition and into aberrant pathways that lead to benign tumors in nervous tissues.

References

1. Tos M, Thomsen J (1984) Epidemiology of acoustic neuromas. J Laryngol Otol 98:685–692
2. Martuza RL, Eldridge R (1988) Neurofibromatosis 2 (bilateral acoustic neurofibromatosis). N Engl J Med 318:684–688

3. Trofatter JA, MacCollin MM, Rutter JL, Murrell JR, Duyao MP, Parry DM, Eldridge R, Kley N, Menon AG, Pulaski K, Haase VH, Ambrose CM, Munroe D, Bove C, Haines JL, Martuza RL, MacDonald ME, Seizinger BR, Short MP, Buckler AJ, Gusella JF (1993) A novel moesin-, ezrin-, radixin-like gene is a candidate for the neurofibromatosis 2 tumor suppressor. Cell 72:791–800

4. Rouleau GA, Morel P, Lutchman M, Sanson M, Zucman J, Marineau C, Hoang-Xuan K, Demczuk S, Desmaze C, Plougastel B, Pulst SM, Lenoir G, Bijlsma E, Fashold R, Dumanski J, de Jong P, Parry D, Eldridge R, Aurias A, Delattre O, Thomas G (1993) Alteration in a new gene encoding a putative membrane-organizing protein causes neurofibromatosis type 2. Nature 363:515–521

5. Anderson RA, Marchesi VT (1985) Regulation of the association of membrane skeletal protein 4.1 with glycophorin by polyphosphoinositide. Nature 318:295–298

6. Correas I, Leto TL, Speicher DW, Marchesi VT (1986) Identification of the functional site of erythrocyte protein 4.1 involved in spectrin-actin associations. J Biol Chem 261:3310–3315

7. Horwitz A, Duggan K, Buck C, Beckerle MC, Burridge K (1986) Interaction of plasma membrane fibronectin receptor with talin—a transmembrane linkage. Nature 320:531–533

8. Burridge K, Mangeat P (1984) An interaction between vinculin and talin. Nature 308:744–746

9. Tsukita S, Oishi K, Sato N, Sagara J, Kawai A, Tsukita S (1994) ERM family members as molecular linkers between the cell surface glycoprotein CD44 and actin-based cytoskeletons. J Cell Biol 126:391–401

10. Maruta H, Holden J, Sizeland A, D'Abaco G (1991) The residues of Ras and Rap proteins that determine their GAP specificities. J Biol Chem 266:11 661–11 668

11. Smith DB, Johnson KS (1988) Single-step purification of polypeptides expressed in Escherichia coli as functions with glutathione S-transferase. Gene 67:31–40

12. Takeshima H, Izawa I, Lee PSY, Safdar N, Levin VA, Saya H (1994) Detection of cellular proteins that interact with the NF2 tumor suppressor gene product. Oncogene 9:2135–2144

13. Krieg J, Hunter T (1992) Identification of the two major epidermal growth factor-induced tyrosine phosphorylation sites in the microvillar core protein ezrin. J Biol Chem 267:19258–19265

14. Danilov YN, Fennell R, Ling E, Cohen CM (1990) Selective modulation of Band 4.1 binding to erythrocyte membranes by protein kinase C. J Biol Chem 265:2556–2562

15. MacCollin M, Mohney T, Trofatter J, Wertelecki W, Ramesh V, Gusella J (1993) DNA diagnosis of neurofibromatosis 2. Altered coding sequence of the merlin tumor suppressor in an extended pedigree. JAMA 270:2316–2320

16. Ruttledge MH, Sarrazin J, Rangaratnam S, Phelan CM, Twist E, Merel P, Delattre O, Thomas G, Nordenskjöld M, Collins VP, Dumanski JP, Rouleau GA (1994) Evidence for the complete inactivation of the NF2 gene in the majority of sporadic meningiomas. Nature Genet 6:180–184

17. Bianchi AB, Hara T, Ramesh V, Gao J, Klein-Szanto AJP, Morin F, Menon AG, Trofatter JA, Gusella JF, Seizinger BR, Kley N (1994) Mutation in transcript isoforms of the neurofibromatosis 2 gene in multiple human tumor types. Nature Genet 6:185–192

Mutations and Loss of Heterozygosity of the von Hippel-Lindau Tumor Suppressor Gene in Sporadic Central Nervous System Hemangioblastomas

Susumu Ito[1], Hiroshi Kanno[1], Keiich Kondo[2], Taro Shuin[2], Masahiro Yao[2], Masahiko Hosaka[2], Satoshi Fujii[1], and Isao Yamamoto[1]

Abstract. Hemangioblastomas are tumors of the central nervous system (CNS), predominantly located in the cerebellum. In some cases, the tumor manifests as von Hippel-Lindau (VHL) disease. The VHL gene was recently isolated and identified as the VHL tumor suppressor gene. However, somatic mutations and allelic loss of the VHL gene have not been detected in sporadic CNS hemangioblastomas. We investigated 16 sporadic CNS hemangioblastomas to detect mutations of the VHL tumor suppressor gene with single-strand conformation polymorphism (SSCP) analysis and loss of heterozygosity (LOH) with microsatellite probes located close to the VHL gene. Abnormal SSCP patterns were detected in 8 of 16 hemangioblastomas (50%), and LOH in 4 of 6 informative cases (67%). We identified mutations in 3 tumors by direct sequencing; 2 were missense mutations and 1 was a microdeletion. However, we were unable to sequence 6 paraffin-embedded tumor samples, and only 7 frozen samples could be analyzed for LOH, probably because the DNA was of poor quality and because contamination by undetected substances inhibited polymerase chain reaction (PCR) amplification. These data suggest that inactivation of the VHL tumor suppressor gene is one of the major molecular mechanisms in the development of sporadic CNS hemangioblastomas.

Key words. von Hippel-Lindau Disease gene—Tumor suppressor gene—Loss of heterozygosity—Sporadic hemangioblastoma

Introduction

Hemangioblastomas are tumors that originate in the central nervous system (CNS) and are predominantly located in the cerebellum, with a reported incidence of 1.1%–2.4% of all intracranial tumors [1]. In about 20% of cases, this tumor occurs as a manifestation of von Hippel-Lindau (VHL) disease, an autosomally dominant inherited tumor syndrome [1,2]. The VHL gene region was recently isolated at human chromosome 3p 25–26 and identified as the VHL tumor suppressor gene [3,4]. Mutations of the VHL gene were frequently detected both in familial and sporadic renal cell

Departments of [1] Neurosurgery and [2] Urology, Yokohama City University School of Medicine, Yokohama, 232 Japan

carcinomas [5,6]. However, mutations and loss of heterozygosity (LOH) of the VHL gene have rarely been reported in sporadic CNS hemangioblastomas [7]. We have analyzed mutations of the VHL tumor suppressor gene and allelic loss of chromosome 3p to investigate the tumorigenetic mechanisms of sporadic hemangioblastomas.

Materials and Methods

Materials

Sixteen sporadic CNS hemangioblastomas and 15 matched peripheral blood samples were obtained from patients operated on at Yokohama City University and its affiliated hospitals. Seven tumor specimens were frozen and the remaining 9 tissues were paraffin embedded. None of the patients had a family history or clinical manifestations of VHL disease, as was evaluated from physical and opthalmological examination and from abdominal ultrasound and radiological imaging.

DNA Extraction

DNA was extracted from 7 frozen tumors and 15 peripheral blood samples by standard procedures. DNA of 9 tumors was extracted from paraffin-embedded sections by the following method. Paraffin-embedded tissues were cut into 5 μm sections and the paraffin removed with xylene. The tissues were then washed with ethanol. Eight hundred microliters of TE buffer (10 mM. Tris, 1 mM. EDTA, pH 8.3) and 0.8 mg of proteinase K were added to the tissues, which were digested at 50°C for 48 h. DNA was then extracted with 500 μl of phenol, followed by chloroform/isoamylalcohol. After the administration of 0.1 vol of $3 M$ ammonium acetate, DNA was precipitated by adding absolute ethanol at −20°C for 24 h. After centrifugation at 15 000 rpm, the supernatant was removed and the DNA was washed with 70% ethanol. DNA was rehydrated in distilled water, and concentrations were determined using a UV microspectrophotometer.

Single-Strand Conformation Polymorphism Analysis and DNA Sequencing

Polymerase chain reactions (PCR) with the six sets of primers and Single-Strand conformational polymorphism (SSCP) analysis were performed as described previously [6]. When abnormal SSCP patterns were detected, the PCR products were directly sequenced according to the manufacturer's protocol (United States Biochemical, Cleveland, OH, USA) using Dynabeads (Dynai, Oslo, Norway).

Loss of Heterozygosity Analysis

We analyzed the allelic loss of heterozygosity (LOH) of chromosome 3p with microsatellite probes located close to the VHL gene. PCR amplification of two types of microsatellite probes (D3S1317 [8]; D3S1038 [9]) was performed using 100 ng genomic DNA, 10 × Taq buffer (Takara Shuzo, Kyoto, Japan), 12.5 pM of each primer,

500 μM concentrations each of dGTP, dATP, dTTP, dCTP with 0.04 μl [³²P]dATP of 10 mCi/ml (Amersham, Buckinghamshire, UK), and 0.5 units of Taq polymerase (Takara Shuzo, Kyoto, Japan) for a total volume of 10 μl. The PCRs were performed on a DNA thermal cycler (Perkin-Elmer Cetus, Norwalk, CT) with an initial denaturing step of 5 min at 94°C, 4 cycles of 10 s at 94°C, 10 s at 60°C, and 20 s at 72°C, followed by 16 cycles of 10 s at 94°C, 10 s at 56°C, and 20 s at 72°C. PCR products were run on a 6% polyacrylamide sequencing gel, followed by autoradiography. For informative cases, LOH was scored if the radiographic signal of one allele was at least 50% decreased in the tumor DNA as compared with the corresponding normal allele in the blood sample.

Results

The SSCP analysis showed abnormal electrophoresis patterns in 8 of 16 hemangioblastomas (50%); 3 were detected in exon 1, 3 in exon 2, and 2 in exon 3, respectively (Fig. 1). However, all 15 cases of the DNA extracted from peripheral blood showed normal SSCP patterns. In addition, we identified the presence of mutations in 3 of 8 tumors by direct sequencing: 2 were missense mutations and 1 was a microdeletion. We were unable however to sequence the other 5 tumor DNAs extracted from paraffin blocks. Furthermore, 4 of 6 informative cases (67%) obtained from frozen tumor samples showed LOH (Fig. 2).

From the clinical data (Table 1), in 4 of 16 patients the tumor recurred after 8–20 years following the first operation. Abnormal SSCP patterns were detected in 3 of these 4 recurrent cases.

Discussion

In this study, we found abnormal SSCP patterns of the VHL tumor suppressor gene in 8 of 16 cases (50%), and mutations were identified in 3 of these 8 tumors by direct sequencing. However, all peripheral blood samples showed normal SSCP patterns. These data suggest that mutations of the tumors are somatic. We identified LOH in 4 of 6 cases (67%).

We were unable to sequence five paraffin-embedded tumor samples, and only seven frozen tumors could be analyzed for LOH. We speculate this is probably because the DNA was of poor quality and because contamination by undetected substances inhibited PCR amplification in the paraffin-embedded samples.

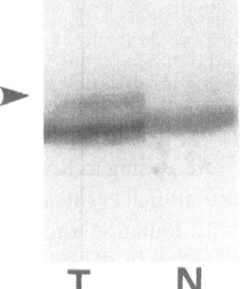

Fig. 1. Single-strand conformational polymorphism (SSCP) analysis of DNAs from tumor (*T*) and peripheral blood (*N*) in case 4 using primer set for exon 2. An abnormal band was detected only in the polymerase chain reaction (PCR) products from tumor tissue (*arrowhead*)

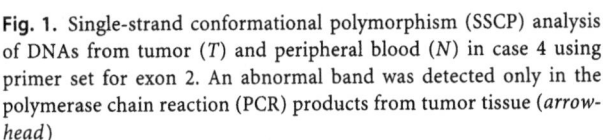

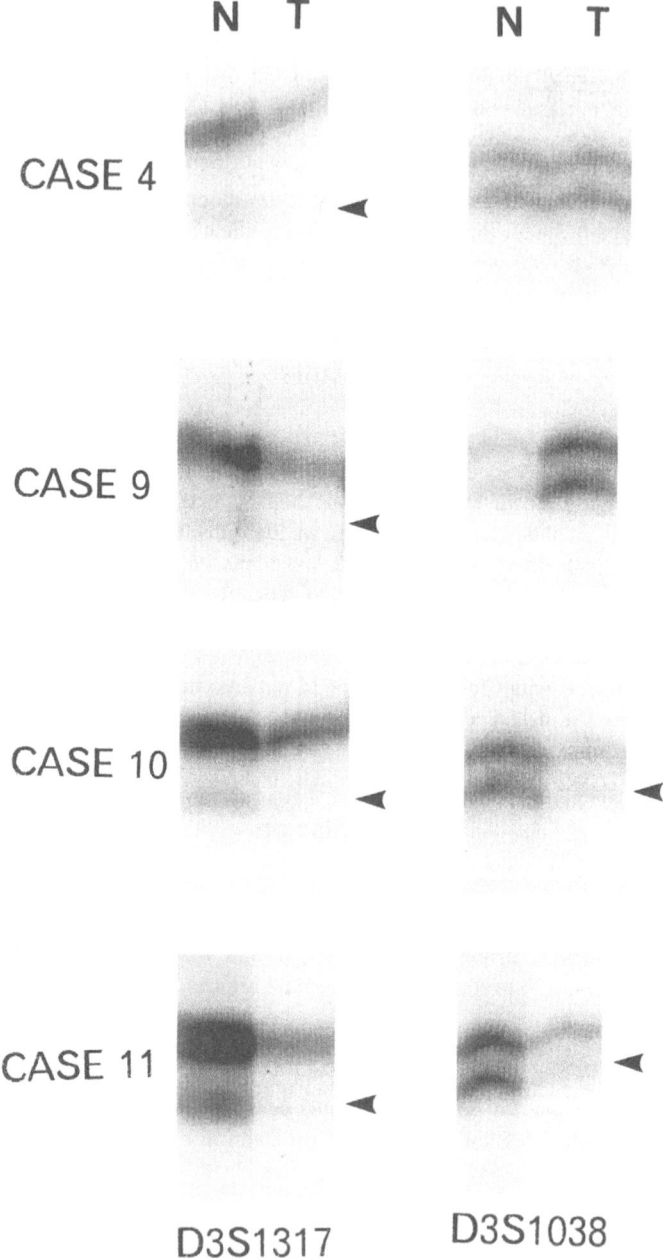

Fig. 2. Analysis of loss of heterozygosity (LOH) in paired peripheral blood (*N*) and tumor (*T*) DNAs with primer sets for D3S1317 and D3S1038. *Arrowheads* indicate alleles exhibiting LOH

According to Knudson's theory, in the nonhereditary form of retinoblastomas two mutational events occur in somatic cells [10]. In this study, one case (case 4) showed both mutation and LOH in the VHL gene. However, only SSCP abnormalities were detected in the other seven cases, and three of four informative cases showed only LOH without SSCP changes. Although these differences cannot be fully explained,

Table 1. Summary of the cases.

Case no.	Age	Location	Tumor sample	Site of SSCP change	VHL gene mutation	LOH D3S1317	LOH D3S1038	Recurrence (years from first surgery)
1	40	Cerebellum	P	Exon 1	476: G → C[a]			
2	58	Cerebellum	F	Exon 1	ND	ND	ND	
3	66	Cerebellum	P	Exon 1	ND			
4	68	Cerebellum	F	Exon 2	663: T del.	+	ND	+(20)
5	51	Cerebellum	P	Exon 2	618: A → C[b]			+(8)
6	50	Brainstem	F	Exon 2	ND	ND	NI	
7	65	Cerebellum	P	Exon 3	ND			
8	38	Cerebellum	P	Exon 3	ND			+(8)
9	26	Cerebellum	F	ND		+	ND	
10	71	Cerebellum	F	ND		+	+	
11	26	Cerebellum	F	ND		+	+	
12	72	Cerebellum	F	ND		NI	NI	
13	53	Cerebellum	P	ND				
14	28	Cerebellum	P	ND				
15	55	Cerebellum	P	ND				
16	42	Spinal	P	ND				+(11)

SSCP, single-strand conformational polymorphism; VHL, von Hippel-Lindau; LOH, loss of heterozygosity; P, paraffin-embedded; F, frozen; ND, not detected; NI, not informative; del, deletion.
[a] Point mutation resulted in amino acid change, tryptophan to serine.
[b] Point mutation resulted in amino acid change, leucine to phenylalanine.

SSCP analysis possibly does not elucidate mutations of the VHL gene in cases with only LOH. Other strategies may be needed to identify the VHL gene abnormalities in those cases.

Hemangioblastoma in the CNS is usually a benign tumor [1], and cure of the disease can be expected by total resection. However, tumor recurrences have been reported, and the mean rate was 16% in reviewed cases [11]. Four of 16 patients had recurrences in our series (25%), and 3 of 4 recurrent cases showed abnormal SSCP patterns. One of these cases had multicentric tumors, and mutations of the VHL gene may be one of the risk factors for tumor recurrence.

These data suggest that inactivation of the VHL tumor suppressor gene is one of the major molecular mechanisms in the development of sporadic CNS hemangioblastomas. Further study is necessary to elucidate the tumorigenesis of hemangioblastomas.

Acknowledgments. The authors gratefully acknowledge Yoshinobu Inada, M.D., Yasuhiro Tiba, M.D., Kazuhiko Fujitsu, M.D., and Yuusuke Ishiwata, M.D., who provided tumor and blood samples, and thank Dr. Berton Zbar for technical support.

References

1. Russel DS, Rubinstein LJ (1989) Pathology of tumors of the nervous system. Arnold, London, pp 639–657
2. Neumann HPH, Eggert HR, Weigel K, Friedburg H, Wiestler OD, Schollmeyer P (1989) Hemangioblastomas of the central nervous system. J Neurosurg 70:24–30

3. Latif F, Tory K, Gnarra J, Yao M, Duh FM, Orcutt ML, Stackhouse T, Kuzmin I, Modi W, Geil L, Schmidt L, Zhou F, Li H, Wei MH, Chen F, Glenn G, Choyke P, Walther MM, Weng Y, Duan DSR, Dean M, Galavac D, Richards FM, Crossey PA, Ferguson-Smith MA, Paslier DL, Chumakov I, Cohen D, Chinault AC, Maher ER, Linehan WM, Zbar B, Lerman MI (1993) Identification of the von Hippel-Lindau disease tumor suppressor gene. Science 260:1317–1320

4. Seizinger BR, Smith DI, Filling-Katz MR, Neumann H, Green JS, Choyke PL, Anderson KM, Freiman RN, Klauck SM, Whaley J, Decker HJH, Hsia YE, Collins D, Halperin J, Lamiell JM, Oostra B, Waziri MH, Gorin MB, Scherer G, Drabkin HA, Aronin N, Schinzel A, Martuza RL, Gusella JF, Haines JL (1991) Genetic flanking markers refine diagnostic criteria and provide insights into the genetics of Von Hippel-Lindau disease. Proc Natl Acad Sci USA 88:2864–2868

5. Gnarra JR, Tory K, Weng Y, Schmidt L, Wei MH, Li H, Latif F, Liu S, Chen F, Duh FM, Lubensky I, Duan DR, Florence C, Pozzatti R, Walther MM, Bander NH, Grossman HB, Brauch H, Pomer S, Brooks JD, Issacs WB, Lerman MI, Zbar B, Linehan WM (1994) Mutations of the VHL tumour suppressor gene in renal carcinoma. Nature Genet 7:85–90

6. Shuin T, Kondo K, Torigoe S, Kishida T, Kubota Y, Hosaka M, Nagashima Y, Kitamura H, Latif F, Zbar B, Lerman MI, Yao M (1994) Frequent somatic mutations and loss of heterozygosity of the von Hippel-Lindau tumor suppressor gene in primary human renal cell carcinomas. Cancer Res 54:2852–2855

7. Kanno H, Kondo K, Ito S, Yamamoto I, Fujii S, Torigoe S, Sakai N, Hosaka M, Shuin T, Yao M (1994) Somatic mutations of the von Hippel-Lindau tumor suppressor gene in sporadic central nervous system hemangioblastomas. Cancer Res 54:4845–4847

8. Li H, Schmidt L, Duh FMC, Wei MH, Latif F, Stackhouse T, Lerman MI, Zbar B, Tory K (1993) Three polymorphic dinucleotide repeats near the von Hippel-Lindau (VHL) disease gene on human chromosome 3:D3S587; D3S1317; D3S1435. Hum Mol Genet 2:1326

9. Jones MH, Yamakawa K, Nakamura Y (1992) Isolation and characterization of 19 dinucleotide repeat polymorphisms on chromosome 3p. Hum Mol Genet 1:131–133

10. Knudson AG (1971) Mutation and cancer: Statistical study of retinoblastoma. Proc Natl Acad Sci USA 68:820–823

11. Constans JP, Meder F, Maiuri F, Donzelli R, Spaziante R, de Divitiis E (1986) Posterior fossa hemangioblastomas. Surg Neurol 25:269–275

Section 4. Apoptosis

Anti-Fas Antibody Induces Apoptosis in Cultured Glioma Cells by Activation of the Sphingomyelin Pathway

Tetsuya Shiraishi, Setsuko Nakagawa, Keisuke Toda, Shun-ichi Kihara, Yan Ju, and Kazuo Tabuchi

Abstract. We have previously demonstrated that apoptosis occurs spontaneously in brain tumors. The Fas antigen is a cell-surface protein that can trigger apoptosis in a variety of cell types on the binding of anti-Fas monoclonal antibody (Fas mAb). In this study, we investigated the role of the Fas antigen–Fas ligand system in human glioblastoma cell lines (T98G, U251, and A172) and the potential involvement of a sphingomyelin signaling process in the induction of apoptosis by Fas mAb. Immunohistochemical and flow cytometrical analyses revealed that all three cell lines expressed Fas antigen highly; however, apoptotic changes such as nuclear fragmentation, the DNA ladder pattern on gel electrophoresis, and reduction of viable cells were observed only in T98G cells by treatment of Fas mAb (50 ng/ml). The fraction of sphingomyelin of T98G was markedly decreased 15 min after the treatment with Fas mAb, indicating hydrolysis of sphingomyelin to ceramide. Exposure to exogenous C2 ceramide, which is a cell-permeable synthetic ceramide, induced apoptotic cell death in T98G. These results demonstrate that a sphingomyelin signaling system might be involved in Fas mAb-induced apoptosis in T98G.

Key words. Apoptosis—Fas antigen—anti-Fas monoclonal antibody—Sphingomyelin—Glioma

Introduction

Apoptosis plays an essential role in the physiological processes of cell death occurring in embryogenesis, tissue atrophy, and immune regulation [1]. It was first described as a morphological pattern of cell death, characterized by cell shrinkage, membrane blebbing, chromatin condensation, and presence of apoptotic bodies. The nuclear changes secondary to apoptosis are associated with the activation of a specific endogenous endonuclease that breaks the double-stranded DNA of the chromatin at the internucleosomal linker DNA [2]. On gel electrophoresis, these DNA cleavage products display a ladder pattern of multiples of 180–200 base pairs (bp), which is considered to represent a useful biochemical indicator of apoptosis [3].

Department of Neurosurgery, Saga Medical School, Saga, 849 Japan

Apoptosis has recently become the focus of interest in oncology [4]. A variety of stimuli are known to induce apoptosis in many kinds of tumor [5,6], but little is known about apoptosis on brain tumors. The Fas antigen is a novel cell-surface receptor that mediates apoptosis when ligated with the Fas monoclonal antibody (Fas mAb) [7]. The aims of this study were to examine expression of the Fas antigen and to determine the effect of Fas mAb on cultured glioma cells. A recent study revealed that the sphingomyelin pathway mediated tumor necrosis factor- (TNF-) α-induced apoptosis in hematopoietic cells [8]; therefore, we also investigated the potential involvement of a sphingomyelin signaling process in Fas mAb-induced apoptosis.

Materials and Methods

Cell Culture

Human glioma cell lines (T98G, U251, and A172), obtained from the Japanese Cancer Research Resources Bank (Tokyo, Japan), were maintained in minimum essential medium (MEM) supplemented with 7.5% gentamycin (Schering-Plough, Osaka, Japan), and 10% (vol/vol) heat-inactivated fetal bovine serum (Nalgene, Victoria, Australia) in a water-saturated 5% CO_2 atmosphere at 37°C. Exponentially growing cells were studied.

Immunohistochemistry

Cells cultured on the chamber slides (Nunc, Naperville, IL, USA) were fixed in 3.5% paraformaldehyde. The slides were incubated with 10% rabbit serum for 15 min to block nonspecific binding. The slides were then covered with mouse anti-Fas monoclonal antibody (Fas mAb) (IgG class; MBL, Nagoya, Japan) at a concentration of 20 μg/ml. Immunohistochemical staining was performed using a labeled streptavidin–biotin method as previously described [9].

Flow Cytometric Analysis

Cells suspended with 0.1% EDTA in phosphate buffered saline (PBS) were reacted with 0.1 ml of PBS containing 50 ng/ml of Fas mAb (IgG class) at 4°C for 60 min. Non-specific mouse IgG (Dako, Kyoto, Japan) was used as a negative control. The cells were then washed twice and incubated with fluorescein isothiocyanate- (FITC-) conjugated goat anti-mouse IgG antibody (Vector, Burlingame, CA, USA) at room temperature for 30 min. Finally, cells were washed twice and analyzed using a FACScan (Becton-Dickinson, Mountain View, CA, USA).

Cell Treatment and Cytocidal Activity

Fas mAb (IgM class; MBL) or C2-ceramide (Matreya, Pleasant Gap, PA, USA) at various concentrations was added to the medium and incubated for as long as 60 h. C2-ceramide was dissolved in ethanol and diluted to final concentrations in serum-free medium at 37°C. At the time indicated the cells were suspended with 0.05% trypsin and 0.1% EDTA in PBS. Viable cells were determined by trypan blue exclusion.

Morphological Study

Cells were collected and fixed in 2% cacodylate buffered glutaraldehyde (pH 7.2) for 60 min, washed with 0.01 M cacodylate buffer, and postfixed in 1% osmium tetroxide for 60 min. After dehydration in a graded series of ethanol and embedment in epon medium, thin sections were prepared. The sections were examined under a light microscope after staining with toluidine blue.

In Situ DNA Double-Strand Break Staining

To detect DNA double-strand breaks of glioma cells in situ, we applied the in situ nick end-labeling method established by Gavrieli et al. [10] with a slight modification as described previously [11].

DNA Fragmentation

Genomic DNA was extracted by a salting-out procedure [12] using a DNA extraction kit (Toyobo, Osaka, Japan) and analyzed by 2% agarose gel electrophoresis, stained with ethidium bromide, and photographed under ultraviolet light. As a positive control of DNA fragmentation, we used genomic DNA digested with 1 unit of micrococcal endonuclease (Sigma, St. Louis, MO, USA) for 30 min.

Sphingomyelin Hydrolysis

The lipid substrates were purified from treated cells with chloroform/methanol (2:1 vol/vol), vortexed, and spun at 3000 rpm for 10 min to pellet insoluble material. Fractions of sphingomyelin, phosphatidyl choline, and phosphatidyl ethanolamine were measured by the method of Kano et al. [13].

Results

Expression of Fas Antigen

Almost all T98G cells were positively stained immunocytochemically with Fas mAb (IgG), mainly at the cytoplasm (Fig. 1A). Fas antigen was highly expressed on T98G by flow cytometry (Fig. 1B). U251 and A172 showed a similar staining pattern and expression of Fas antigen (Fig. 1C,D).

Cytocidal Effect of Fas mAb

To determine the optimum concentration of the Fas mAb (IgM) for cytocidal activity, Fas mAb of various concentrations was added to the cells and incubated for either 48 or 60 h. The number of viable cells were significantly decreased in a dose- and time-dependent manner (Fig. 2A). From these data, we chose a concentration of 50 ng/ml for the assay of cytocidal activity. In T98G, Fas mAb-induced cell death became apparent after 24 h of culture and all cells eventually died after 60 h

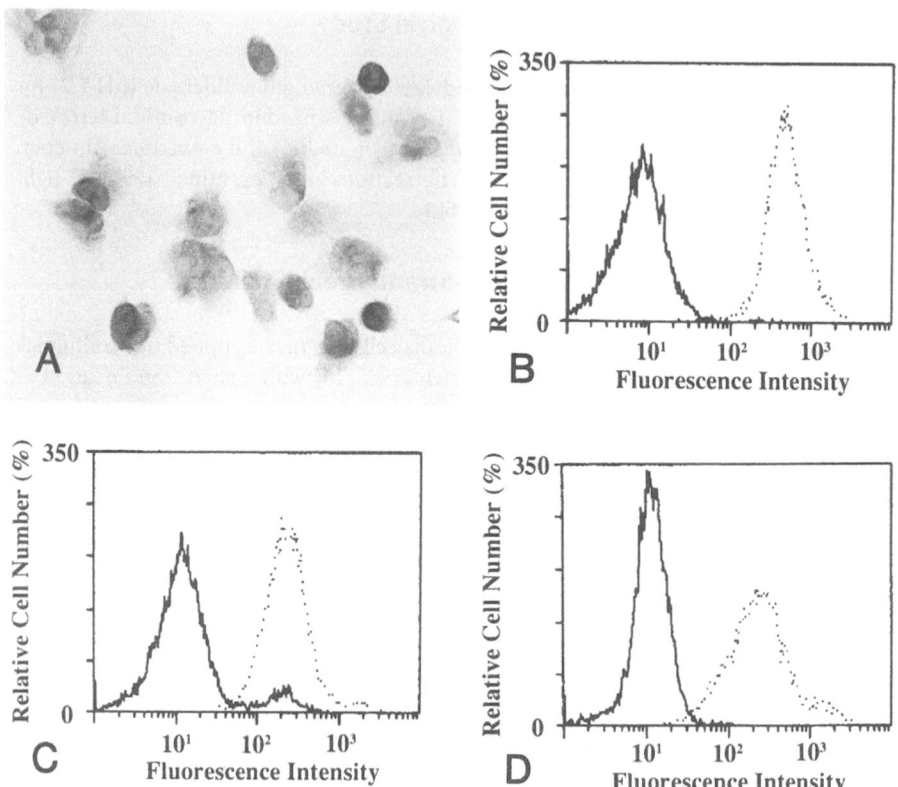

Fig. 1A–D. Expression of Fas antigen. Immunoperoxidase staining of T98G (A); almost all cells are positively stained, mainly at the cytoplasm (×400). Flow cytometric analysis of T98G (B), U251 (C), and A172 (D). *Dashed lines*, Fas antigen-positive cells; *thick lines*, control using nonspecific mouse IgG

(Fig. 2B). U251 cells were partially affected by anti-Fas mAb (Fig. 2C), whereas A172 cells were resistant to the anti-Fas mAb treatment (Fig. 2D). Normal mouse IgM, used as an isotype control, showed no effect on the growth of these three cell lines.

Morphological Changes and DNA Fragmentation

Nontreated T98G cells had a large nucleoplasm with prominent nucleoli (Fig. 3A). T98G cells treated with the anti-Fas mAb (IgM) for 36h displayed condensation of chromatin, fragmentation of the nucleus, and formation of apoptotic bodies under a light microscope (Fig. 3B). At 12h of incubation with Fas mAb, approximately 4% of nuclei were stained clearly by in situ DNA strand break staining (Fig. 3C). At 48h of incubation, more than 50% of cells displayed condensation of chromatin, shrinkage, and fragmentation of nuclei that were stained by in situ DNA strand break staining (Fig. 3D). Gel electrophoresis of the DNA extracted from T98G cells treated with anti-Fas mAb (IgM) for 36–48h showed characteristic DNA fragmentation with a ladder pattern similar to the positive control. This ladder of DNA fragments was not observed until 36h of incubation. Most of the genomic DNA extracted from the cells treated with nonspecific IgM remained at high molecular weight (Fig. 4).

Ceramide-Induced Apoptosis and Sphingomyelin Hydrolysis

Exogenous membrane-permeable N-acyl-sphingosine (C2-ceramide [14]) induced a dose- and time-dependent decrease in viable cells (Fig. 5A) and the DNA ladder characteristic of apoptosis (data not shown). The fraction of sphingomyelin of T98G was markedly decreased 15 min after treatment with Fas mAb, indicating hydrolysis of sphingomyelin to ceramide (Fig. 5B).

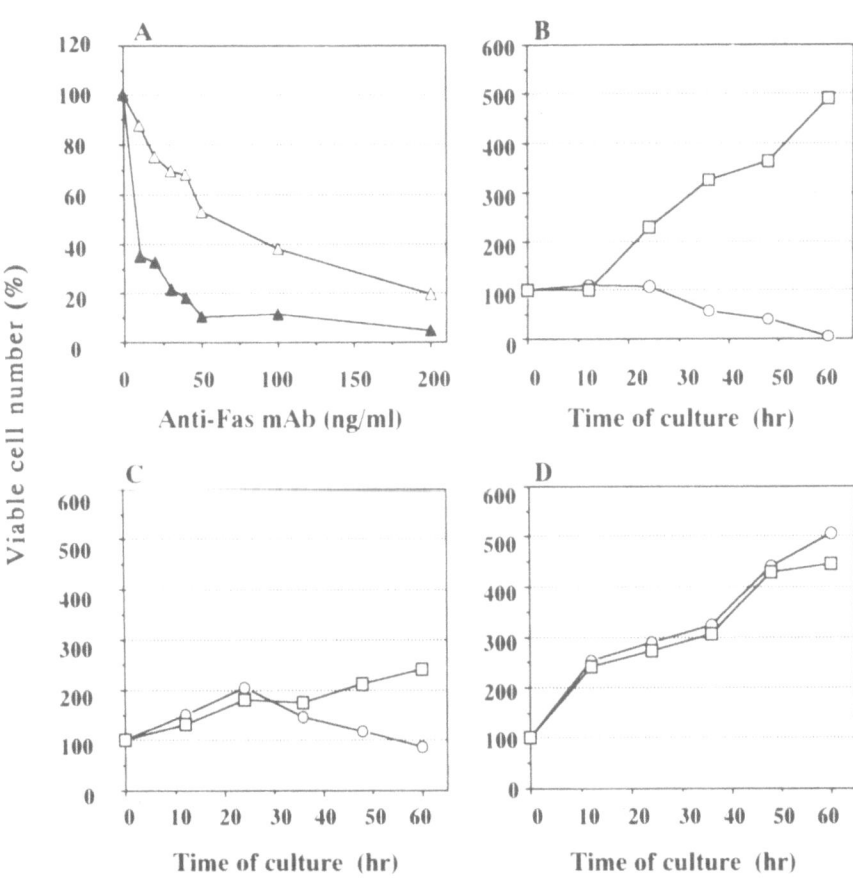

Fig. 2A–D. Cytocidal effect of anti-Fas mAb (IgM) on glioma cells. A Cells are cultured with various concentrations of anti-Fas IgM for 48h (*open triangle*) or 60h (*solid triangle*). Number of viable cells are considerably decreased in dose- and time-dependent manner. T98G (**B**), U251 (**C**), or A172 (**D**) cells are cultured in the presence of either 50ng/ml anti-Fas IgM (*circles*) or control IgM (*squares*). Each point is the average of triplicate determinations. Y axis, percentage of viable cell number compared to 0h

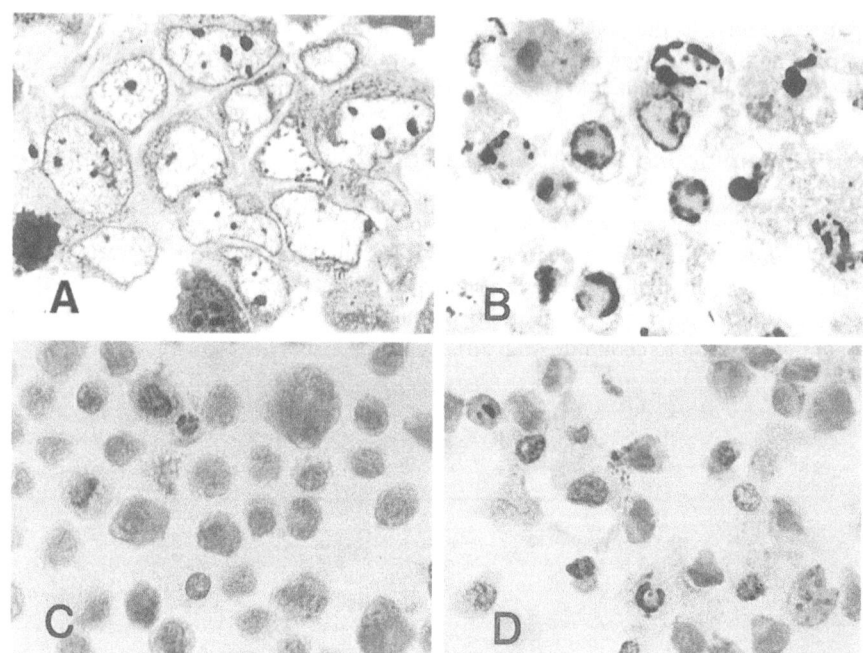

Fig. 3A–D. Morphological changes and DNA strand breaks. T98G cells without treatment show large nucleoplasm and prominent nucleoli (**A**). T98G cells treated with anti-Fas IgM for 48 h reveal marginal condensation and fragmentation of chromatin; apoptotic bodies are also seen (**B**) (×1000). In situ DNA strand break staining of T98G treated with Fas mAb for 12 h (**C**) or 48 h (**D**) (×400)

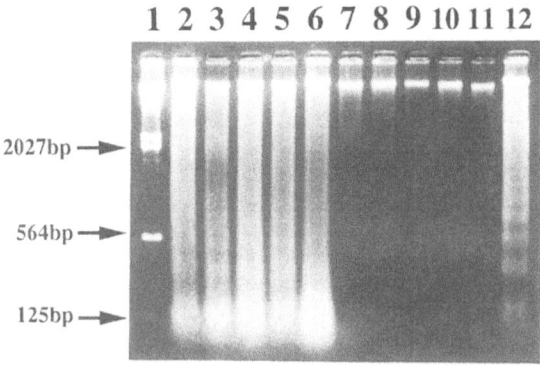

Fig. 4. DNA fragmentation induced by anti-Fas IgM in T98G glioma cells. T98G cells were incubated with either anti-Fas IgM (lanes 2–6) or control IgM (lanes 7–11). After incubation for 32 h (lanes 2 and 7), 36 h (lanes 3 and 8), 40 h (lanes 4 and 9), 44 h (lanes 5 and 10), or 48 h (lanes 6 and 11), total DNA was prepared from cells and electrophoresed on 2% agarose gel in the presence of 0.5 mg/ml ethidium bromide. Genomic DNA digested with micrococcal endonuclease (lane 12) as positive control and molecular weight markers (lane 1) are also given

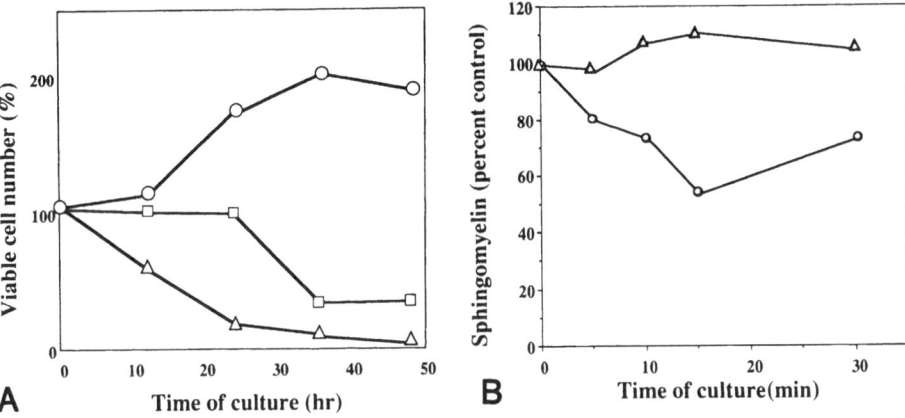

Fig. 5A. Cytocidal effect on T98G of 50 μM C2-ceramide (*circle*) or 100 μM C2-ceramide (*triangle*); *square* is control. Induction of sphingomyelin hydrolysis by anti-Fas monoclonal antibody in T98G (**B**). Each point is the mean of duplicate determinations of results of three independent experiments

Discussion

The Fas monoclonal antibody (Fas mAb) produced by Yonehara et al. [7] is reported to kill Fas antigen-expressing human cells by a process known as apoptosis. The Fas antigen gene encodes a 48-kDa glycoprotein containing a single transmembrane domain [15]. The extracellular domain is rich in cysteine residue, similar to that of the nerve growth factor (NGF)/tumor necrosis factor (TNF) receptor superfamily [15]. The cytoplasmic region contains a cell-killing domain that may play a major role in the induction of apoptosis [16].

Recent investigations have clarified the physiological function of Fas antigen in the regulation of immune processes. Fas antigen has been proposed to play important roles in negative selection of autoreactive T cells in the thymus [17] and autoimmune diseases [18]. The natural ligand of Fas antigen has been recently identified in rats [19] and humans [20]. Human Fas ligand cDNA, which is approximately 1.9 kb and encodes 281 amino acids, is a type II integral membrane protein homologous to TNF [20]. Fas ligand expressed on the surface of T cells is reported to bind to Fas antigen in target cells and to cause apoptotic cell death [21,22]. It is supposed that this Fas antigen–Fas ligand lytic system plays an important part in T-cell-mediated cytotoxicity [22]. In this study, we demonstrated that Fas mAb can kill Fas antigen-expressing T98G cells by the apoptotic pathway through the activation of the sphingomyelin signaling system. We have also reported that Fas antigen is expressed highly in biopsied glioblastoma and is well correlated with the incidence of apoptosis [23,24]. These results lead us to speculate that the Fas ligand could be one of the treatment modalities for gliomas.

However, there are two major problems to be solved before clinical use. First, because Fas expression has been demonstrated in various normal tissues [25], intravenous administration will cause severe damage to normal organs. In fact, the intraperitoneal administration of Fas mAb into mice rapidly caused fulminant hepatitis by inducing apoptosis in hepatocytes [26]. Although the expression of Fas antigen in brain is thought to be low [27], the safety of local administration of Fas ligand into brain should be thoroughly investigated.

Second, the difference in susceptibility to the Fas mAb is not fully understood. From our data and recent reports, the difference may be well explained from four independent points of view: (1) synthesis of a protective protein against apoptosis, such as Bcl-2 [9,28] and Bcl-2-related proteins (Bax [29], Bcl-x [30,31]); (2) different expression of functional Fas antigen on the cell surface [32]; (3) blocking the interaction of Fas antibody with Fas antigen by soluble form of Fas antigen, which lacks a transmembrane domain [33]; and (4) alterations in Fas intracellular signaling pathways including the sphingomyelin pathway.

The future elucidation of detailed mechanisms of anti-Fas-induced apoptosis in glioma cells may contribute to establishing a new treatment modality for brain tumors.

Acknowledgments. We thank Mrs. Yumiko Oh-ishi for her assistance in this research. This study was supported by a Grant-in-Aid for Scientific Research from the Ministry of Education, Science and Culture, Japan.

References

1. Wyllie AH, Kerr JFR, Currie AR (1980) Cell death: the significance of apoptosis. Int Rev Cytol 68:251–306
2. Duke RC, Chervenak R, Cohen JJ (1983) Endogenous endonuclease induced DNA fragmentation: an early event in cell mediated cytolysis. Proc Natl Acad Sci USA 80:6361–6365
3. Wyllie AH (1980) Glucocorticoid-induced thymocyte apoptosis is associated with endogenous endonuclease activation. Nature 284:555–556
4. Williams GT (1991) Programmed cell death: apoptosis and oncogenesis. Cell 65:1097–1098
5. Forster TH, Allan DJ, Gobe GC, Harmon BV, Walsh TP, Kerr JF (1992) Beta-radiation from tracer doses of ^{32}P induces massive apoptosis in a Burkitt's lymphoma cell line. Int J Radiat Biol 61:365–367
6. Bertrand R, Kerrigan D, Sarang M, Pommier Y (1991) Cell death induced by topoisomerase inhibitors: role of calcium in mammalian cells. Biochem Pharmacol 42:77–85
7. Yonehara S, Ishii A, Yonehara M (1989) A cell-killing monoclonal antibody (anti-Fas) to a cell surface antigen co-downregulated with the receptor of tumor necrosis factor. J Exp Med 169:1747–1756
8. Jarvis WD, Kolesnick RN, Fornari FA, Traylor RS, Gewirtz DA, Grant S (1994) Induction of apoptotic DNA damage and cell death by activation of the sphingomyelin pathway. Proc Natl Acad Sci USA 91:73–77
9. Kihara S, Shiraishi T, Nakagawa S, Tabuchi K (1994) Induced expression and subcellular localization of the Bcl-2 protein in cultured glioma cells. Brain Tumor Pathol 11:161–167
10. Gavrieli Y, Sherman Y, Ben SS (1992) Identification of programmed cell death in situ via specific labeling of nuclear DNA fragmentation. J Cell Biol 119:493–501
11. Nakagawa S, Shiraishi T, Kihara S, Tabuchi K (in press) Detection of DNA strand breaks associated with apoptosis in human brain tumors. Virchows Arch
12. Miller SA (1988) A simple procedure for extracting DNA from human nucleated cells. Nucleic Acids Res 16:1215
13. Kano M, Teshima T, Tanaka M, Sugizaki M, Narukawa M, Itoh K, Ueda H, Okada J, Mizuguchi K, Tadano J (1976) The use of Thinchrograph for the determination of serum phospholipids fractions in hyperlipidemic patients. Mod Med 31:2002–2009
14. Okazaki TO, Bielawska A, Bell RM, Hannun YA (1990) Role of ceramide as a lipid mediator of 1α-2,5-dihydroxyvitamin D_3-induced HL-60 cell differentiation. J Biol Chem 265:15813–15823

15. Itoh N, Yonehara S, Ishii A, Yonehara M, Mizushima S, Sameshima M, Hase A, Seto Y, Nagata S (1991) The polypeptide encoded by the cDNA for human cell surface antigen Fas can mediate apoptosis. Cell 66:233–243

16. Itoh N, Nagata S (1993) A novel protein domain required for apoptosis. Mutational analysis of human Fas antigen. J Biol Chem 268:10932–10937

17. Andjelic S, Drappa J, Lacy E, Elkon KB, Nikolic-Zugic J (1994) The onset of Fas expression parallels the acquisition of CD8 and CD4 in fetal and adult alpha beta thymocytes. Int Immunol 6:73–79

18. Watanabe-Fukunaga R, Brannan CI, Copeland NG, Jenkins NA, Nagata S (1992) Lymphoproliferation disorder in mice explained by defects in Fas antigen that mediates apoptosis. Nature 356:314–317

19. Suda T, Takahashi T, Golstein P, Nagata S (1993) Molecular cloning and expression of the Fas ligand, a novel member of the tumor necrosis factor family. Cell 75:1169–1178

20. Mita E, Hayashi N, Iio S, Takehara T, Hijioka T, Kasahara A, Fusamoto H, Kamada T (1994) Role of Fas ligand in apoptosis induced by hepatitis C virus infection. Biochem Biophys Res Commun 204:468–474

21. Kagi D, Vignaux F, Ledermann B, Burki K, Depraetere V, Nagata S, Hengartner H, Golstein P (1994) Fas and perforin pathways as major mechanisms of T cell-mediated cytotoxicity. Science 265:528–530

22. Hanabuchi S, Koyanagi M, Kawasaki A, Shinohara N, Matsuzawa A, Nishimura Y, Kobayashi Y, Yonehara S, Yagita H, Okumura K (1994) Fas and its ligand in a general mechanism of T-cell-mediated cytotoxicity. Proc Natl Acad Sci USA 91:4930–4934

23. Shiraishi T, Nakagawa S, Kihara S, Toda K, Tabuchi K (1994) Detection of DNA strand breaks associated with apoptosis in human brain tumors (in Japanese). Igaku No Ayumi (Journal of Clinical and Experimental Medicine) 170:775–776

24. Toda K, Shiraishi T, Nakagawa S, Kihara S, Ju Y, Tabuchi K (1995) Relationship between Fas antigen expression and apoptosis in glial tumors. Neuroimmunology 7:125–128

25. Watanabe-Fukunaga R, Brannan CI, Itoh N, Yonehara S, Copeland NG, Jenkins NA, Nagata S (1992) The cDNA structure, expression, and chromosomal assignment of the mouse Fas antigen. J Immunol 148:1274–1279

26. Ogasawara J, Watanabe-Fukunaga R, Adachi M, Matsuzawa A, Kasugai T, Kitamura Y, Itoh N, Suda T, Nagata S (1993) Lethal effect of the anti-Fas antibody in mice. Nature 364:806–809

27. Leithäuser F, Dhein J, Mechtersheimer G, Koretz K, Brüderlein S, Henne C, Schmidt A, Debatin K-M, Krammer PH, Möller P (1993) Constitutive and induced expression of APO-1, a new member of the nerve growth factor/tumor necrosis factor receptor superfamily, in normal and neoplastic cells. Lab Invest 69:415–429

28. Hockenbery D, Nunez G, Milliman C, Schreiber RD, Korsmeyer SJ (1990) Bcl-2 is an inner mitochondrial membrane protein that blocks programmed cell death. Nature 348:334–336

29. Oltvai ZN, Milliman CL, Korsmeyer SJ (1993) Bcl-2 heterodimerizes in vivo with a conserved homolog, Bax, that accelerates programmed cell death. Cell 74:609–619

30. Boise LH, Gonzalez-Garcia M, Postema CE, Ding L, Lindsten T, Turka LA, Mao X, Nunez G, Thompson CB (1993) bcl-x, a bcl-2-related gene that functions as a dominant regulator of apoptotic cell death. Cell 74:597–608

31. Shiraishi T, Nakagawa S, Toda K, Tabuchi K (1994) Immunohistochemical expression of Bcl-2 and Bcl-x in various brain tumors (in Japanese). Bull Jpn Neurochem Soc 33:646–647

32. Owen-Schaub LB, Radinsky R, Kruzel E, Berry K, Yonehara S (1994) Anti-Fas on nonhematopoietic tumors: levels of Fas/APO-1 and bcl-2 are not predictive of biological responsiveness. Cancer Res 54:1580–1586

33. Cheng J, Zhou T, Liu C, Shapiro JP, Brauer MJ, Kiefer MC, Barr PJ, Mountz JD (1994) Protection from Fas-mediated apoptosis by a soluble form of the Fas molecule. Science 263:1759–1762

Induction of Apoptosis in Malignant Glioma Cells by Anti-Fas Antibody

Cheho Park, Osamu Tachibana, Yoshikazu Okamoto, Yutaka Hayashi, Tetsumori Yamashima, and Junkoh Yamashita

Abstract. The Fas antigen belongs to the TNF (tumor necrosis factor)/NGF (nerve growth factor) receptor family and can mediate apoptosis. Also, the anti-Fas antibody induces apoptosis in cells expressing the Fas antigen. It has been reported that the apoptotic signal can be inhibited by Bcl-2. This study revealed that rat C6 glioma cells expressed the Fas antigen and that anti-Fas antibody induced apoptosis in C6 cells both in vivo and in vitro. Anti-Fas antibody caused no direct cytotoxic damage to neurons expressing Bcl-2. We concluded that anti-Fas antibody could safely be administered directly into the brain for therapeutic purposes.

Key words. Apoptosis—Anti-Fas antibody—C6 glioma cell—Local injection—Bcl-2

Introduction

Apoptosis plays an important role in regulating the cell number in a wide variety of tissues during development [1]. The Fas antigen (APO-1) is a 45-kDa protein belonging to the TNF (tumor necrosis factor)/NGF (nerve growth factor) receptor family and can mediate apoptosis [2,3]. Fas antigen is expressed in the thymus, liver, heart, lung, and ovary in mice [4]. Anti-Fas antibody induces apoptosis in cells expressing the Fas antigen [5,6].

On the other hand, it is also well known that the proto-oncogene *bcl-2* inhibits apoptotic and necrotic neural cell death and that Bcl-2 expression can prevent apoptosis in certain hematopoietic cells [7]. In this study, we investigated whether apoptosis is inducible in rat C6 glioma cells, in which the Fas antigen is expressed, by anti-Fas antibody in vitro and in vivo.

We also performed a histological examination of the direct effects of intracerebral anti-Fas antibody injection on normal rat brain tissue, taking into consideration the expression of Bcl-2 protein that blocks apoptosis.

Department of Neurosurgery, Kanazawa University School of Medicine, 13-1, Takaramachi, Kanazawa 920, Japan

Materials and Methods

Cell Culture Study

C6 rat glioma cells obtained from a human tumor cell bank were cultured in chamber slides and fixed in 70% ethanol. They were subjected to immunohistochemical staining using anti-human Fas antibodies (MBL, Nagoya, Japan; clone UB2, diluted 1:100) and anti Bcl-2 antibodies (DAKO, Kyoto, Japan; diluted 1:40).

C6 glioma cells, 4×10^5, were grown in F-10 medium (Gibco, Grand Island, NY, USA) supplemented with 15% horse serum (Gibco) and 2.5% fetal bovine serum (Gibco) in 4 ml of culture medium on 60-mm-diameter dishes. The cells were grown in a humid atomosphere of 95% air/5% CO_2 at 37°C for 96 h. After 24, 48, 72, and 96 h of incubation with anti-Fas antibody (100 ng/ml) (clone CH-11; MBL), cell viability was assessed by trypan blue dye exclusion, and cytocentrifuge preparations were made for morphological analysis of apoptotic cells. Cells were centrifuged at 2000 × g for 5 min, and fixed in 4% paraformaldehyde in phosphate buffered saline (PBS, pH 7.4) for 4 h and embedded in octocompound. Frozen sections (4 μm thick) were cut with a microtome. The sections were stained with hematoxylin and eosin (H&E) for light microscopy. An in situ nick end labeling method was also used for investigation of DNA by light microscopy [8].

For ultrastructural analysis, centrifuged and pelleted (as just described) C6 cells were fixed with 2.5% glutaraldehyde in cacodylate buffer for 24 h and postfixed with 2% osmium tetroxide for 2 h. The fixed specimens were then dehydrated through a graded series of ethanol, dried, and embedded in Epon 812 and Araldite mixture. Ultrathin sections were made on an ultratome NOVA (LKB, Bromma, Sweden) and stained with uranyl acetate and lead citrate. An electron microscope (H-600, Hitachi, Tokyo, Japan) was used.

For DNA extraction from tumor cells, the cells were lysed overnight at 50°C in 400 μl of a solution containing 0.15 M NaCl, 0.1 M EDTA (pH 8), 0.015 M sodium acetate, 1% (wt/vol) sodium dodecyl sulfate, and 100 μg/ml proteinase K (Nippon Gene, Tokyo, Japan). The cell lysate was extracted in phenol-chloroform-isoamyl alcohol (25:24:1, vol/vol) followed by chloroform. DNA was precipitated with 10 M ammonium acetate and ethanol, resuspended in 100 μl of TE buffer (1 mM EDTA, 10 mM Tris, pH 7.8), and treated with ribonuclease at 37°C for 3 h. The DNA (10 μg) was then electrophoresed for approximately 2 h at 70 V in 1.5% agarose gels (Nippon Gene). Marker 4 (Takara, Osaka, Japan) was used as a marker for DNA fragment sizes. The gels were stained with ethidium bromide (Nippon Gene) and were photographed under ultraviolet light.

Induction of Apoptosis in C6 Glioma Cell-Implanted Rat Brains

Wistar rats, 6–8 weeks old, were anesthetized with 5% chloral hydrate (0.01 ml/kg) and placed in a stereotaxic frame. A burrhole was drilled in the skull 4 mm lateral to the bregma with a 1.5-mm burr to expose the dura. Using a microliter syringe (Hamilton, NV, USA) fitted with a 26-gauge needle and connected to the manipulating arm of the stereotaxic frame, 1×10^6 C6 glioma cells in 3 ml of F-10 medium were injected during 5 min into the caudate nucleus at a depth of 5 mm from the dura. The needle was left in place for 10 min and then withdrawn over 3 min. Fourteen days after tumor injection, the same coordinates were used for injection of 1000 ng anti-Fas antibody (clone CH 11, IgM) diluted with 3 ml F-10 medium. The animals were killed 17 or 21 days after tumor injection and fixed by intracardial perfusion of 4% paraformaldehyde in PBS. The brains were removed and incubated for 24 h in 4% paraformaldehyde. The brains were then embedded in paraffin, and 4-mm sections were cut with a microtome. The sections were stained with hematoxylin and eosin (H&E) and examined by light microscopy.

Histopathological Study of Rat Brain After Intracerebral Anti-Fas Antibody Injection

To evaluate the direct effects of intracerebral anti-Fas antibody (clone CH 11), 1000 ng of anti-Fas antibody diluted with 3 ml F-10 medium was injected into the brain of normal rats using the same stereotactic coordinates as already indicated. Mouse IgM (1000 ng; ZYMED, San Francisco, CA, USA) diluted with 3 ml F-10 medium was used for intracerebral injection in a sham-treated control group.

The animals were killed 3 or 7 days after the antibody injection and fixed by intracardial perfusion of 4% paraformaldehyde in PBS. Each brain was submitted for histological processing. Samples of 4-μm-thick sections paraffin-embedded tissue were stained with standard H&E.

Immunohistochemistry for light microscopy was performed by the streptoavidin-biotin–peroxidase complex technique, using mouse anti-human glial fibrally acidic protein (GFAP), monoclonal antibody (MAb), and mouse anti-human neurofilament (NF) MAb.

Results

Mortality, Morphological Changes, and DNA Changes of C6 Glioma Cells Treated with Anti-Fas Antibodies

Immunohistochemical studies using anti-human Fas antibodies (clone UB2, diluted 1:100) and anti-Bcl-2 antibodies (1:40) demonstrated that C6 glioma cells were positive for anti-human Fas antibodies and negative for anti-Bcl-2 antibodies (Fig. 1).

Loss of cell viability was observed after as few as 48 h of treatment with anti-Fas antibodies, and further incubation resulted in about 90% cell death in 72 h (Fig. 2a,b). In contrast, more than 95% of C6 cells without anti-Fas antibodies remained viable in the same culture conditions during the observation period of 72 h. DNA strand breaks were assessed by an in situ nick end labeling method. In situ labeling of fragmented nuclear DNA showed stained cells after 72 h of incubation (Fig. 2d). Ultrastructural analysis revealed morphological alterations consistent with various stages of apoptotic cell death (Fig. 3). Agarose gel electrophoresis of extracted DNA from C6 cells showed a ladder-type pattern that is characteristic of apoptosis (Fig. 4).

Induction of Apoptosis in Implanted C6 Cells

The brains ($n = 10$) were examined microscopically, and local administration of anti-Fas antibody was found to induce apoptosis in implanted C6 cells (Fig. 5).

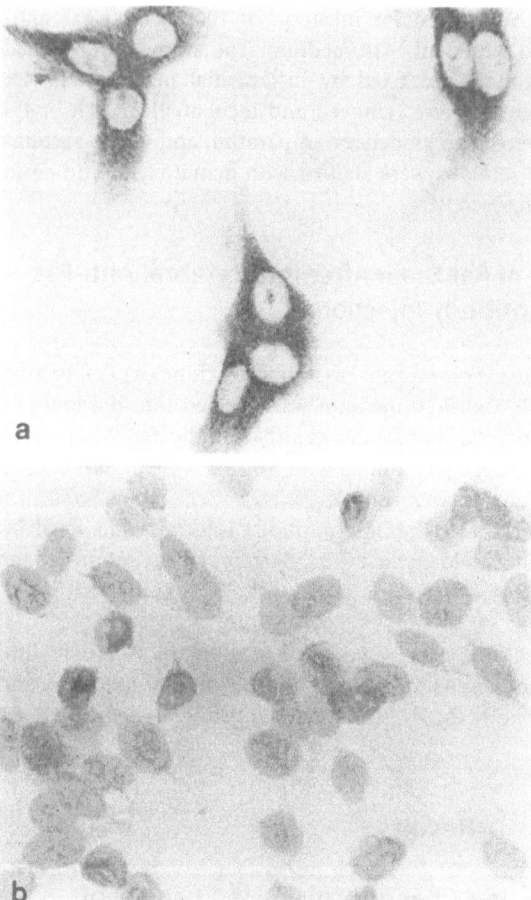

Fig. 1a,b. Immunostaining of cultured C6 cells (**a**) with anti-Fas antibodies (×400) and (**b**) with anti Bcl-2 antibodies (×400). C6 cells were positive for anti-Fas antibodies and negative for anti Bcl-2 antibodies

Histopathological Findings in Rat Brain After Anti-Fas Antibody Injection

Following the intracerebral injections, no significant difference in the incidence of motor weakness or absence of weight gain was observed between the anti-Fas antibody-treated ($n = 27$) and the sham-treated control groups ($n = 6$). Standard histological examination with H&E staining showed reactive gliosis, a small hemorrhage from the direct injection, and a small amount of lymphoid cell infiltration along the needle track (Fig. 6a).

Immunohistochemical investigation was pursued on specimens that showed histological evidence of a reactive gliosis (data not shown) or tissue destruction with intracerebral hemorrhage caused by direct injection. Most gliotic reactions stained positively with anti-GFAP antibodies. In addition, immunohistochemical study with anti-NF protein antibodies revealed little difference before or after intracerebral injections of anti-Fas antibodies in the basal ganglia (Fig. 6b). This suggested that anti-Fas antibody caused little direct cytotoxic damage to the central nervous system.

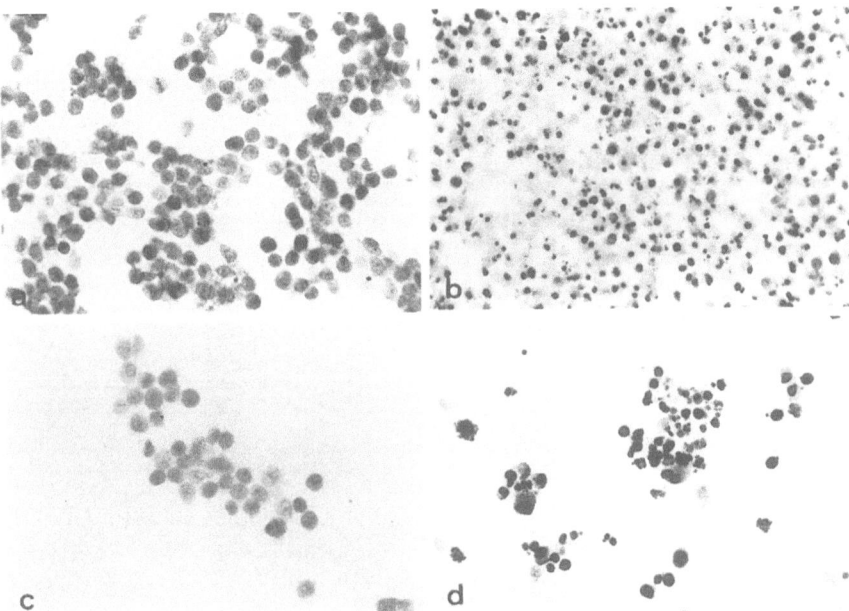

Fig. 2a–d. Appearance of C6 cells incubated with anti-Fas antibodies at 100 ng/ml. **a** At 24 h after incubation, none of the cells are in apoptosis. Hematoxylin and eosin (H&E), ×400. **b** At 72 h after incubation, most of the cells are in early stages of apoptosis. H&E, ×400. **c** At 24 h after incubation, no apoptotic nuclei were detected. In situ nick end labeling method, ×400. **d** At 72 h after incubation, apoptotic nuclei were detected, in almost all cells. In situ nick end labeling method, ×400

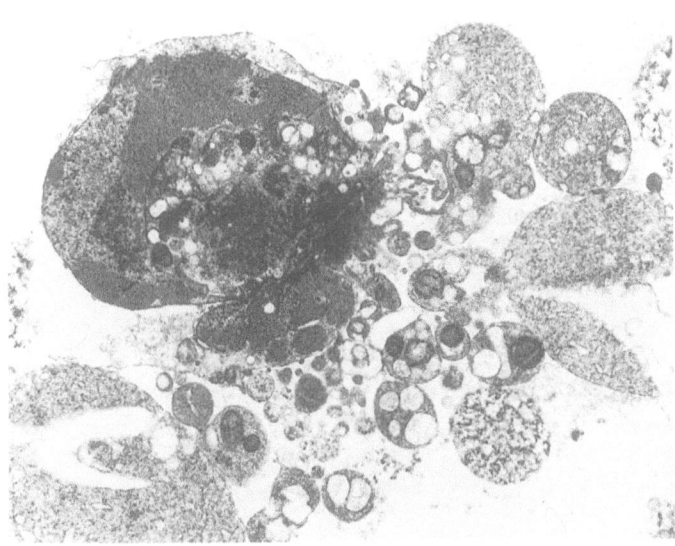

Fig. 3. Electron microscopic appearance of apoptotic changes in C6 cells. Note the discrete nuclear fragments with characteristic segregation of compacted chromatin, the crowding organelles, and the marked convolutions of the cellular surface. ×4500

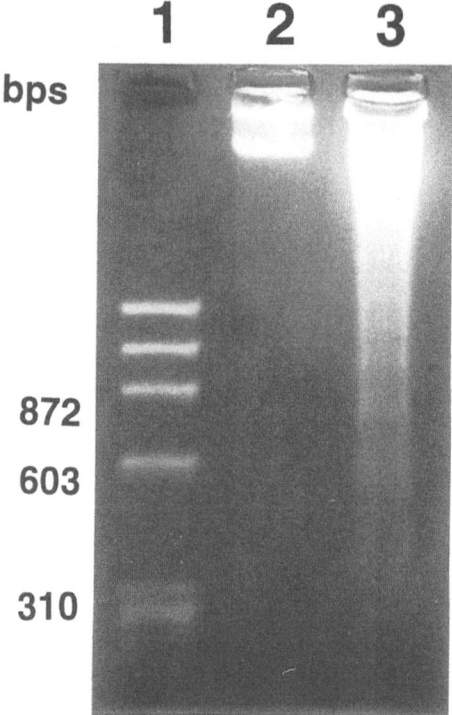

Fig. 4. Agarose gel electrophoresis of DNA extracted from cultured C6 cells. Lane 1, DNA fragment size marked, marker 4. Lane 2, DNA extracted from control cells at 72 h after start of incubation with anti-Fas antibody. Lane 3, DNA extracted from cells at 72 h after incubation with anti-Fas antibody. DNA fragmentation in C6 cells is indicated

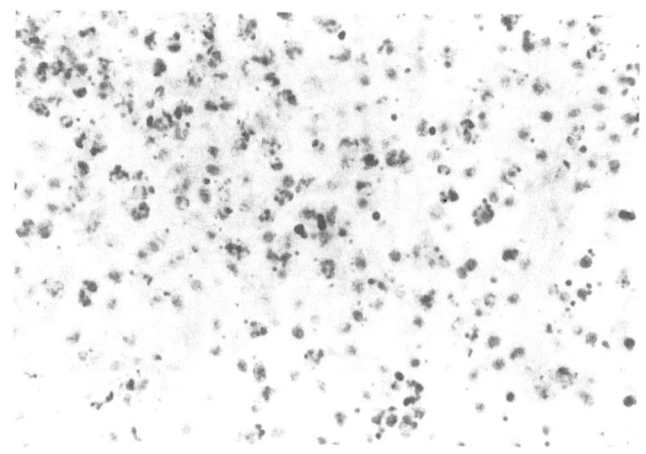

Fig. 5. Photomicrograph of apoptotic cells in the implanted tumor 3 days after injection of anti-Fas antibodies into the rat brain. H&E, ×400

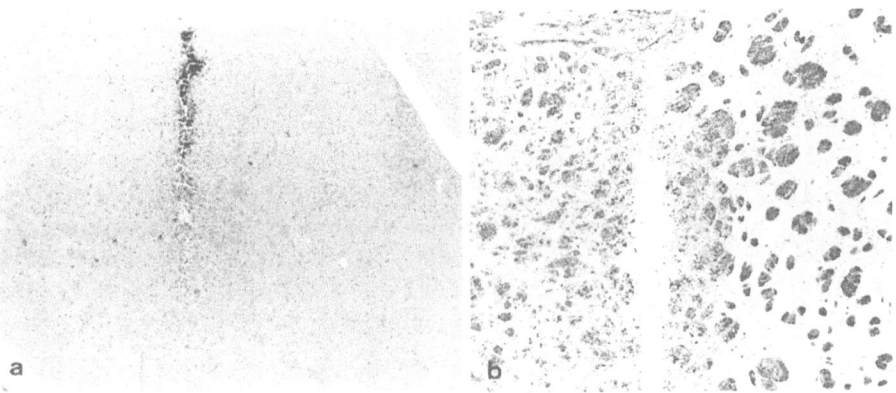

Fig. 6a,b. Photomicrographs of rat brain tissue obtained 1 week after intracerebral infusion of anti-Fas antibodies show (**a**) hemosiderin deposits along the injection pathway (H&E, ×100) and (**b**) immunostaining with antineurofilament antibodies (H&E, ×400)

Discussion

Human malignant gliomas are among the most malignant tumors and are resistant to all available therapies. Despite tremendous efforts by neurosurgeons and oncologists, the prognosis for malignant gliomas has changed very little during the past two decades [9].

Cell death can occur via either of two morphologically distinct models: necrosis or apoptosis [10]. Apoptosis is a more physiological cell death associated with no inflammatory reaction, so it is important to investigate the possibility of its usefulness for the treatment of gliomas.

Yonehara et al. [5], as well as Krammer and his colleagues [6], isolated mouse-derived, anti-human MAb that elicted apoptosis in various human cell lines; the cell-surface antigen against which it was directed was designated Fas or APO-1. In further investigations, Nagata and Yonehara concluded that Fas transmits the apoptotic signal into cells, and that the anti-Fas antibody acts as an agonist. The apoptotic signal is induced by binding of anti-Fas antibody to Fas, indicating that anti-Fas antibody is a death factor and Fas its recepter. Fas does not carry an enzymic domain such as kinase in the cytoplasmic region. A domain of about 80 amino acids homologus to the TNF type I receptor in the cytoplasmic region of Fas is responsible for the apoptotic signal transduction [9], and this signal can be partially inhibited by *bcl-2* [2].

To assess the potential usefulness of anti-Fas antibody for glioma therapy, we tested human and rat glioma cell lines for expression of the Fas antigen and susceptibility to anti-Fas antibody-induced apoptosis. The aim of this study was to investigate the induction of apoptosis in glioma cells. The results clearly showed that rat C6 glioma cells express Fas antigen.

In vitro induction of apoptosis was observed in cells treated with anti-Fas antibody after a 72-h incubation. In our study histological, in situ nick end labeling, electron microscopic analyses, and agarose gel electrophoresis revealed apoptosis and DNA fragmentation. In vivo induction of apoptosis was also observed in implanted C6 cells in the brain.

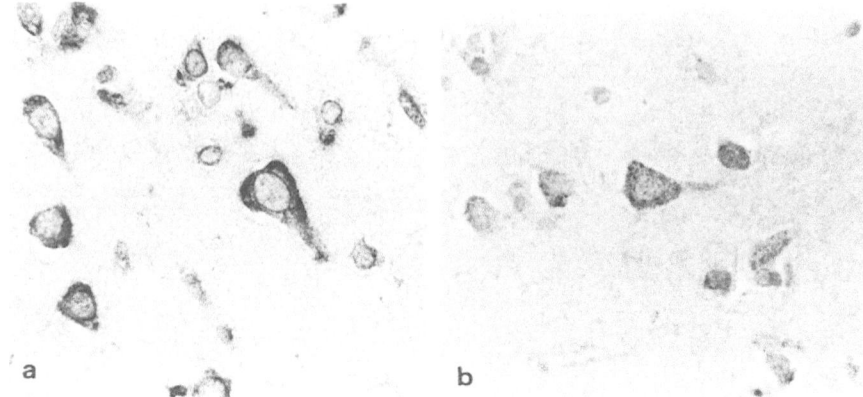

Fig.7. Immunostaining of an autopsied human brain that has been irradiated. Neurons are positively stained with (**a**) anti-Fas antibodies (×400) and (**b**) anti Bcl-2 antibodies (×400)

Intracerebral injection of anti-Fas antibody was undertaken to ascertain whether pathological changes or toxic reactions were induced by anti-Fas antibody when injected into normal brain tissue. The results of histological and immunohistochemical examinations revealed that the antibody produces no particular toxicity in normal rat brain tissues. Although local mononuclear and neutrophilic cell infiltration was seen, and some hemorrhage caused by the direct injection occurred along the needle pathway, there were no other pathological effects of anti-Fas antibody on glial and neuronal cells.

On the basis of our results, we concluded that anti-Fas antibody may safely be administered directly into the brain. Furthermore, it should be stressed that direct intratumoral injection might be more efficacious and more readily tolerated than a systemic infusion.

It has been reported that the apoptotic signal can be inhibited by *bcl-2* [7]. Our present study showed that most irradiated neurons in the human and rat central nervous system were immunostained not only with anti-Fas antibody but also with anti-*bcl-2* antibody (Fig. 7). We speculate that *bcl-2* may also block apoptosis induced by anti-Fas antibody in neurons.

We are investigating whether local anti-Fas antibody therapy might be useful for malignant tumors including gliomas, where survival after relapse is short and no other therapeutic possibilities are available. In summary, our data suggest that anti-Fas antibody might be useful for local therapy for malignant gliomas.

Conclusions

1. Anti-Fas antibody induces apoptosis in C6 cells in vitro as well as in vivo without causing any direct cytotoxic damage to neurons expressing Bcl-2.
2. Accordingly, anti-Fas antibody may safely be administered directly into the brain.
3. Further investigations will be necessary to evaluate the in vivo antitumor efficacy of local injection therapy of anti-Fas antibody for malignant gliomas.

References

1. Raff MC (1992) Social controls on cell survival and cell death. Nature 356:397–400
2. Itoh N, Yonehara S, Ishii A, Yonehara M, Mizushima S-I, Sameshima M, Hase A, Seto Y, Nagata S (1991) The polypeptide encoded by the cDNA for human cell surface antigen Fas can mediate apoptosis. Cell 66:233–243
3. Oehm A, Behrmann I, Falk W, Pawlita M, Maier G, Klas C, Li-Weber M, Richards S, Dhein J, Trauth BC, Ponstingl H, Krammer PH (1992) Purification and molecular cloning of the APO-1 cell surface antigen, a member of the tumor necrosis factor/nerve growth facter recepter superfamily: sequence identity with the Fas antigen. J Biol Chem 267:10709–10715
4. Watanabe-Fukunaga R, Brannan C, Itoh N, Yonehara S, Copeland NG, Jenkins NA, Nagata S (1992) The cDNA structure, expression, and chromosomal assignment of the mouse Fas antigen. J Immunol 148:1274–1279
5. Yonehara S, Ishii A, Yonehara M (1989) A cell-killing monoclonal antibody (anti-Fas) to a cell surface antigen co-downregulated with the recepter of tumor necrosis factor. J Exp Med 169:1747–1756
6. Trauth BC, Klas C , Peters AM, Matzku S, Moller P, Falk W, Debatin KM, Krammer PH (1989) Monoclonal antibody mediated tumor regression by induction of apoptosis. Science 245:301–305
7. Itoh N, Tsujimoto Y, Nagata S (1993) Effect of bcl-2 on Fas antigen-mediated cell death. J Immunol 151:621–627
8. Gavrieli Y, Sherman Y, Ben-Sasson SA (1992) Identification of programmed cell death in situ via specific labeling of nuclear DNA fragmentation. J Cell Biol 119:493–501
9. Peterson DL, Sheridan PJ, Brown WE (1994) Animal models for brain tumors: historical perspectives and future directions. J Neurosurg 80:865–876
10. Wyllie AH, Kerr JFR, Currie AR (1980) Cell death: the significance of apoptosis. Int Rev Cytol 68:251–306
11. Itoh N, Nagata S (1993) A novel protein domain required for apoptosis. Mutational analysis of human Fas antigen. J Biol Chem 268:10932–10937

References

Part IV
Advances of Novel Therapeutic Approaches
—BRM Therapy and
Gene Therapy on Malignant Brain Tumors

Section 1. BRM Therapy
(Basic and Clinical Studies)

Monocyte Chemoattractant Protein-1 (MCP-1) Derived from Brain Tumors: Its Significance and Clinical Application

Jun-ichi Kuratsu[1], Hideo Takeshima[1], Toru Nishi[1], Kyoichi Sato[1], Kimio Yoshizato[1], Shigeo Yamashiro[1], Yukitaka Ushio[1], and Teizo Yoshimura[2]

Abstract. The presence of macrophages within tumor tissue is one of the histological characteristics of malignant gliomas. Although the infiltration of macrophages suggests a possible immunological reaction by the host, the mechanisms and biological meaning of macrophage infiltration in malignant gliomas remain to be defined. A human monocyte chemoattractant protein-1 (MCP-1) was purified from the culture fluid of human glioma cell lines. MCP-1 is a 76-amino acid protein. MCP-1 is chemotactic for monocytes, but not for macrophages with an immunophenotype of the tissue-fixed, resident type. Expression and production of MCP-1 in glioma tissues and meningioma tissues were found, and there was a positive correlation between the degree of macrophage infiltration and the level of MCP-1 expression by tumor cells. Transplantation of tumor cells transfected by MCP-1 cDNA exhibited a lower growth rate than parental cells. Therefore, we speculate that tumor-associated macrophages have a suppressive effect on the growth of tumors. For clinical application of MCP-1, we measured MCP-1 concentration in cerebrospinal fluid (CSF) by enzyme-linked immunosorbent assay (ELISA). High concentration of MCP-1 was found in the CSF from malignant glioma patients with subarachnoid dissemination. Thus, measuring MCP-1 concentration in CSF may lead us to more accurate diagnosis of malignant glioma and detection of subarachnoid dissemination of the tumor cells. Further study on MCP-1 is warranted for its possible clinical applications.

Key words. Brain tumor—Macrophage—Chemotaxis

Introduction

The presence of macrophages within malignant tumors has been well established [1,2]. To account for macrophage infiltration, it has been postulated that a chemotactic factor is produced, either by T lymphoctes as part of the host immune response against tumors or by tumor cells themselves [3–8]. Bottazzi et al. [8] found monocyte chemotactic activity (MCA) in the culture supernatants of murine and

[1] Department of Neurosurgery, Kumamoto University Medical School, Kumamoto 860, Japan
[2] Immunopathology Section, Laboratory of Immunobiology, National Cancer Institute, Frederick, MD, USA

human tumor cells. There was a correlation between the amount of MCA in culture supernatants and the number of tumor-associated macrophages found when the cultured mouse tumor cells were transplanted into mice. Malignant glioma is one of the brain tumors in which macrophage infiltration is frequently observed [9–11]. In the current study, we investigated the mechanism and significance of macrophage infiltration into brain tumors.

Identification and Purification of MCP-1

We found that a human malignant glioma cell line, U-105 MG, produced large amounts of MCA [12,13]. Therefore, we initiated purification of MCA from large volumes of U-105 MG cell culture fluid. The human monocyte chemoattractant protein-1 (MCP-1) was purified from serum-free U-105 MG culture fluid in three steps: dye–ligand chromatography on orange-A agarose, carboxymethyl (CM) high pressure liquid chromatography (HPLC), and reversed phase (RP) HPLC [14]. The cation-exchange column separated MCP-1 into two well-defined peaks. On sodium dodecyl sulfate-polyacrylamide gel electrophoresis (SDS-PAGE), they migrated as 15- and 12-kDa proteins (MCP-1α and -β). The two MCP-1s represent a single gene product, and the difference resulted from O-linked glycosylation. Both forms of MCP-1 were precipitated by a rabbit antibody induced by pure MCP-1β or anti-MCP-1 mouse monoclonal antibodies induced by a mixture of MCP-1α and MCP-1β. MCP-1α and -β have also been isolated from the culture fluid of phytohemagglutinin- (PHA-) stimulated human blood mononuclear cells [15].

Amino Acid Sequence and Primary Structure of MCP-1

MCP-1β is composed of a single 76-residue protein chain. The amino acid sequence of MCP-1β has been completely analyzed [16]. There are four half-cystines in MCP-1, at positions 11, 12, 36, and 52. The four half-cystines are the basis for assigning MCP-1 to a family of proteins that are now called "chemokines," with amino acid sequence similarity and half-cystines in identical locations. It is likely that paired disulfide loops are required for biological activity. As noted, MCP-1α is glycosylated. However, glycosylation is not required for chemotactic activity because recombinant MCP-1, which is expressed in bacteria and is not glycosylated, showed equivalent activity to natural MCP-1 in multi-well chemotaxis chambers.

MCP-1 Gene

The amino acid sequence was confirmed by full-length cDNA cloning of MCP-1 from a glioma cell line library [15]. The cDNA open-reading frame codes for a 99-residue protein. The last 76 residues correspond to MCP-1. Hydrophobicity of the first 23 residues is typical of a signal peptide, which is consistent with the fact that MCP-1 is a secreted protein. Homologs of human MCP-1 have been purified or cloned from baboon [17], bovine [18], guinea pig [19], mouse [20,21], rat [22,23], and rabbit [24].

Human genomic MCP-1 DNA has also been cloned [25]. The gene is constituted of three exons of 45, 118, and 478bp in length and two introns of 800 and 385bp in length. The MCP-1 gene has been mapped on the human chromosome 17 [26].

Biological Activity of MCP-1

MCP-1 is a chemoattractant for human monocytes. Approximately 30% of input monocytes respond at the optimal agonist concentration of $10^{-9} M$ [15]. The migratory response to MCP-1 is primarily chemotactic rather than chemokinetic. Human neutrophils do not migrate to MCP-1 concentrations as high as $3 \times 10^{-8} M$ [15]. Basophils respond to MCP-1; the optimal concentration is about $10^{-9} M$ [15]. There is no detectable activity for eosinophils. Chemotactic activity for T lymphocytes was recently reported [27]. In vivo, intradermal injection of MCP-1 causes monocyte infiltration into the injected site [19].

The Role of MCP-1 in the Recruitment of Tumor-Associated Macrophages

Macrophages found in human or animal tumors [28] are called tumor-associated macrophages (TAM). TAMs secrete various mediators involved in tumor growth and regulation (progression and regression), angiogenesis, fibrin deposition, invasion and metastasis, and local or systemic immunosuppression. They consist of heterogeneous subpopulations differing in location, morphology, phenotype, and function [29]. The recent application of macrophage-specific monoclonal antibodies has made it possible to study the distribution, location, number, and phenotype of macrophage subpopulations not only in normal tissues [30] but also in various pathological conditions [31–33]. Various monoclonal antibodies against rat macrophages such as RM-1, ED-1, ED2, ED3, TRPM-3, and Ki-M2R have been used as markers for discriminating macrophage subpopulations. TRPM-3 recognizes monocyte-derived exudate macrophages and their activated form [34,35].

Yamashiro et al. [36] examined the distribution pattern of macrophages within and around tumors using various anti-rat macrophage monoclonal antibodies noted previously and found that TRPM-3-positive macrophages infiltrated into 9L-transplanted tumors, which produced a large amount of MCP-1. Furthermore, in transplanted tumors of four MT-P/MCP-1 cell lines established by transfecting MT-P parent cells by rat MCP-1 cDNA, the levels of MCP-1 production correlated well with the numbers of intratumorally infiltrated TRPM-3-positive macrophages. Takeshima et al. [37] recently reported that the majority of macrophages in the glioma tissue are monocyte derived rather than relatively proliferated microglias originally contained in brain tissue. The results described here and by others [38,39] strongly suggest that MCP-1 produced by tumor cells induces intratumoral infiltration of monocyte-derived macrophages but not macrophages with the immunophenotype of tissue-fixed, resident type.

Expression of MCP-1 in Malignant Gliomas

We examined the in vivo expression and localization of MCP-1 in glioma tissues using Northern blot analysis and immunohistochemistry. The samples tested consisted of 11 glioma cell lines and eight specimens of human malignant glioma. MCP-1 mRNA was detected by Northern blot analysis in 6 (55%) of the glioma cell lines and in all tumor specimens examined (Figs. 1 and 2). In vivo expression of MCP-1 mRNA and

MCP-1

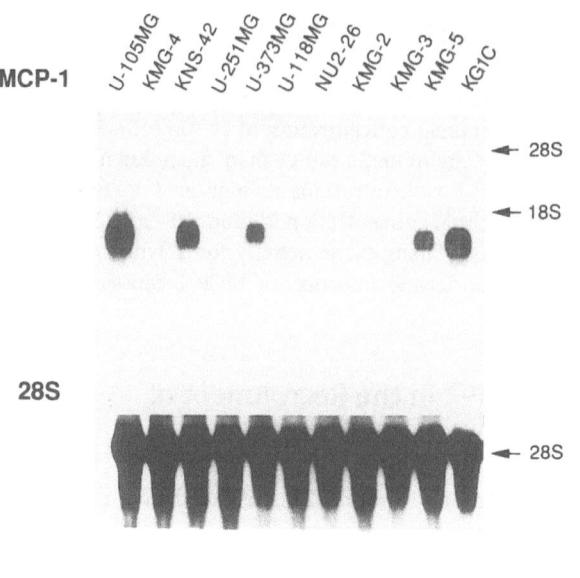

Fig. 1. Northern blot analysis of monocyte chemoattract protein-1 (MCP-1) mRNA in various human glioma cell lines. MCP-1 mRNA was detected in 6 (55%) of the 11 cell lines examined. *Arrows* show the position rRNA in 28S and 18S

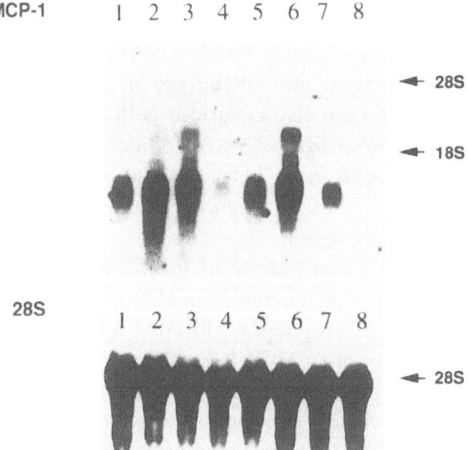

Fig. 2. Northern blot analysis of MCP-1 mRNA isolated from the eight surgical malignant glioma specimens. Expression of MCP-1 mRNA was detected in all tumor specimens; the intensity of the signal determined by densitometry differed among specimens by a factor of 10. *Arrows* show the position of rRNA in 28S and 18S

protein was found predominantly in glioma cells with large and pleomorphic nuclei rather than in areas of small nucleated glioma cells. Adjacent brain tissue did not produce a significant level of MCP-1 mRNA or protein. Macrophages were found among the glioma cells, and the degree of macrophage infiltration was grossly correlated with the level of MCP-1 expression. This study suggested that MCP-1 produced by the glioma cells may mediate macrophage infiltration into the glioma tissue [37].

Expression of MCP-1 in Meningiomas

Meningiomas, like malignant gliomas, contain a high number of infiltrating macrophages [9,40]. Wood and Morantz [11] reported that meningiomas had a mean macrophage content of 42% (range, 50%–80%) and glioblastomas had 41% (range,

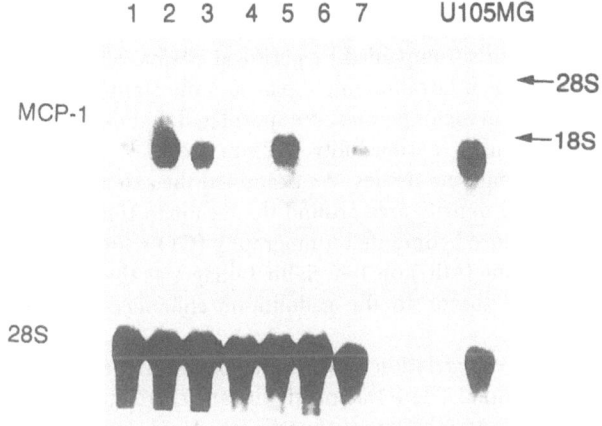

Fig. 3. Northern blot analysis of MCP-1 mRNA in meningiomas. Seven cases with positive expression of MCP-1 are shown. U-105 MG was used as a positive control. *Arrows* show the position of rRNA in 28S and 18S

5%–78%). To investigate the mechanism of macrophage infiltration in meningiomas, we examined, using Northern blot analysis and immunohistochemistry, the expression and localization of MCP-1 in 16 meningioma specimens obtained by surgery. MCP-1 mRNA was detected in 7 of 16 meningiomas (Fig. 3). Differences occurred in the mRNA expression levels for MCP-1 among the tumor specimens. The intensity of the signal determined by densitometry differed among specimens by a factor of 10. The MCP-1 protein was immunohistochemically detected in the same 7 cases that were positive by Northern blot analysis and was expressed diffusely in the cytoplasm of meningioma cells. The degree of macrophage infiltration was also grossly correlated with the level of MCP-1 expression. This study suggested that MCP-1 produced by the meningioma cells may mediate macrophage infiltration into the meningioma tissues [41].

Platelet-derived growth factor (PDGF) has been shown to stimulate MCP-1 expression in fibroblasts [42]. Because meningioma cells secrete PDGF-like molecules that stimulate their own growth in an autocrine manner [43], MCP-1 expression may be regulated by PDGF-like molecules produced by the meningioma. It will be interesting to study if PDGF stimulates meningioma cells to express MCP-1 and if there is a correlation between MCP-1 expression and PDGF expression in meningiomas.

Biological Significance of MCP-1 in Brain Tumors

It has been reported that when human tumor cells were added to monolayers of human monocytes, thymidine incorporation after 68h in culture was inhibited if MCP-1 was added at the beginning of the culture period [44]. This report suggests that MCP-1 not only attracts monocytes to the site of its release but also causes cellular activation for specific functions related to host defense. Thus, macrophages recruited by MCP-1 may play other roles in brain tumors.

Cerebral edema results from the disruption of the blood–brain barrier with increased vascular permeability and excessive interstitial fluid accumulation. Bruce et al. [45] reported that brain tumors produced and released a specific substance that evoked cerebral edema by increasing vascular permeability. It has been known that some meningiomas are accompanied by perifocal edema. Shinonaga et al. [46] suggested that macrophage infiltration might play an important role in the pathogenesis of peritumoral edema in meningiomas. We speculated that the perifocal edema might be caused by vascular permeability factors released by MCP-1-stimulated macrophages in meningioma tissues. We examined the extent of peritumoral edema as the ratio of the low-density area around the tumor to the enhanced high-density area by contrast-enhanced computed tomography (CT) scans [47] and also by magnetic resonance imaging (MRI) on T_2-weighted images as the ratio of the high-intensity area around the tumor to the gadolinium-enhanced high-intensity area in T_1-weighted images.

We then studied the correlation between the extent of edema and MCP-1 expression level in meningioma. There was no significant correlation between the MCP-1 mRNA expression level and the extent of perifocal edema. Therefore, MCP-1 does not appear to be directly involved in perifocal edema formation in meningioma. Other factors including tumor size, tumor location, and the extent of vascularity must be examined to understand the pathogenesis of perifocal edema in brain tumors.

Application of MCP-1 to the Diagnosis of Brain Tumors

We studied whether an MCP-1 enzyme-linked immunosorbent assay (ELISA) could be used in a clinical setting (1) to differentiate malignant gliomas from benign gliomas or nontumor disorders of the central nervous system or (2) to detect subarachnoid

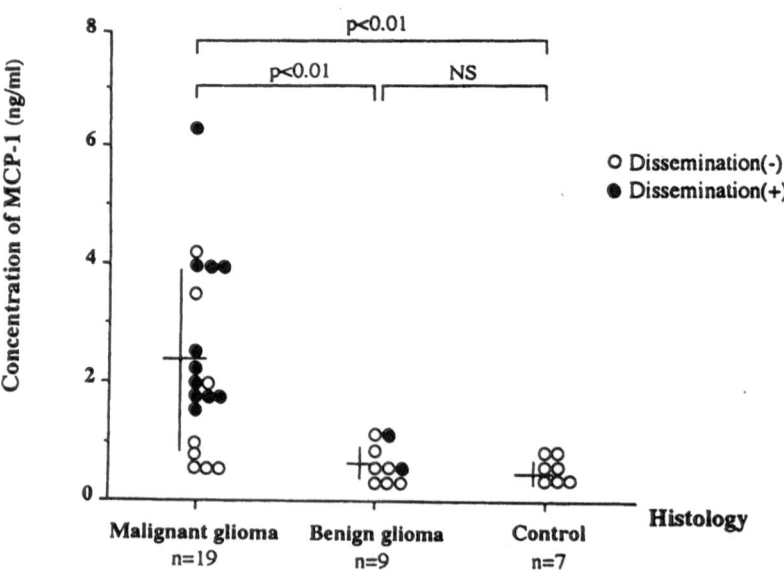

Fig. 4. MCP-1 concentrations in cerebrospinal fluid (CSF) samples obtained from 19 patients with malignant glioma and 9 patients with benign glioma. CSF samples from 7 patients with nontumor disorders of the central nervous system were used as controls

dissemination of glioma cells. Cerebrospinal fluid (CSF) was obtained from 19 patients with malignant gliomas, 9 patients with benign glioma, and 7 patients with nontumor disorders of the central nervous system (CNS). Cyst fluids from malignant glioma patients were also tested. As shown in Fig. 4, the MCP-1 concentration in CSF from patients with malignant glioma was significantly higher than that from patients with benign glioma or from patients with no tumor. Furthermore, CSF from patients with subarachnoid disemination of malignant glioma contained significantly higher amounts of MCP-1 than that from patients without dissemination. All cyst fluids contained high concentrations of MCP-1. These results suggest that measuring MCP-1 concentration in the CSF may lead to more accurate diagnosis of malignant glioma and detection of subarachnoid dissemination of the tumor cells so as to provide patients with appropriate therapies [48].

Conclusions

Since 1989 when MCP-1 was first purified and cloned, knowledge about MCP-1 has accumulated. As we have discussed in this chapter, it is clear that MCP-1 is expressed and produced in tumors including brain tumors and plays a role in recruiting blood monocytes into tumors. Clinically we found high concentration of MCP-1 in CSF from malignant glioma patients and suggested a possible use of MCP-1 ELISA in clinical diagnosis. Our goal is to further study the roles of MCP-1 in vivo and to develop clinical applications of MCP-1 to provide better treatments for patients who suffer from brain tumors.

References

1. Evans R (1972) Macrophages in syngeneic tumors. Transplantation 14:468–473
2. Evans R, Haskill S (1983) Activities of macrophages within and peripheral to the tumor mass. In: The reticuloendothelial system. Plenum, New York, p 155
3. Meltzer M, Stevenson MM, Leonard EJ (1977) Characterization of macrophage chemotaxins in tumor cell cultures and comparison with lymphocyte-derived chemotactic factors. Cancer Res 37:721–725
4. Hifumi M, Hayashi H (1983) Immunological function of adhesive protein from rat ascites hepatoma cells: production of macrophage chemotactic lymphokine. Immunology 49:245–253
5. Wang JM, Cianciolo GJ, Snyderman R, Mantovani A (1986) Coexistence chemotactic factor and a retroviral P15E-related chemotaxis inhibitor in human tumor cell culture supernatants. J Immunnol 137:2726–2732
6. Bottazzi B, Polentarutti N, Balsari A, Boraschi D, Ghezzi P, Salmona M, Mantovani A (1983) Chemotactic activity for mononuclear phagocytes of culture supernatants from murine and human tumor cells: evidence for a role in the regulation of the macrophage content of neoplastic tissues. Int J Cancer 31:55–63
7. Bottazzi B, Ghezzi P, Taraboletti G, Salmona M, Colombo N, Bonazzi C, Mantovani A (1985) Tumor-derived chemotactic factor(s) from human ovarian carcinoma: evidence for the regulation of macrophage content of neoplastic tissues. Int J Cancer 36:167–173
8. Bottazzi B, Polentarutti N, Acero R, Balsari A, Boraschi D, Ghezzi P, Salmona M, Mantovani A (1983) Regulation of the macrophage content of neoplasms by chemoattractant. Science 220:210–212
9. Phillips JP, Eremin O, Anderson JR (1982) Lymphoreticular cells in human brain tumours and in normal brain. Br J Cancer 45:61–69

10. von Hanwehr RI, Hofman F, Tayler C, Apuzzo MLJ (1984) Mononuclear lymphoid populations infiltrating the microenvironment of primary CNS tumors. Characterization of cell subsets with monoclonal antibodies. J Neurosurg 60:1138–1147

11. Wood GW, Morantz RA (1979) Immunological evaluation of the lymphoreticular infiltrate of human central nervous system tumors. J Natl Cancer Inst 62:485–491

12. Kuratsu J, Leonard EJ, Yoshimura T (1989) Production and characterization of human glioma cell-derived monocyte chemotactic factor. J Natl Cancer Inst 81:347–351

13. Yoshimura T, Leonard EJ (1992) Interleukin 8 (NAP-1) and related chemotactic cytokines. In: Baggiolini M, Song C (eds) Cytokines, Vol 4. Karger, Basel, pp 131–152

14. Yoshimura T, Robinson E, Tanaka S, Appella E, Kuratsu J, Leonard E (1989) Purification and amino acid analysis of two human glioma-derived monocyte chemoattractants. J Exp Med 169:1449–1459

15. Yoshimura T, Robinson E, Tanaka S, Appella E, Leonard EJ (1989) Purification and amino acid analysis of two human moncyte chemoattractants produced by phytohemagglutinin-stimulated human blood mononuclear leukocytes. J Immunol 142:1956–1962

16. Robinson EA, Yoshimura T, Leonard EJ, Tanaka S, Griffin PR, Shabanowitz J, Hunt DF, Appella E (1989) Complete amino acid sequence of a human monocyte chemoattractant, a putative mediator of cellular immune reactions. Proc Natl Acad Sci USA 86:1850–1854

17. Valente AJ, Graves DT, Vialle-Valentin CE, Delgado R, Schwartz CJ (1988) Purification of a monocyte chemotactic factor secreted by nonhuman primate vascular cells in culture. Biochemistry 27:4162–4168

18. Wempe F, Henschen A, Scheit KH (1991) Gene expression and cDNA cloning identified a major basic protein constituent of bovine seminal plasma as bovine monocyte chemoattractant protein-1 (MCP-1). DNA Cell Biol 10:671–679

19. Yoshimura T (1993) cDNA cloning guinea pig monocyte chemoattractant protein-1 and expression of the recombinant protein. J Immunol 150:5025–5032

20. Rollins BJ, Morrison ED, Stiles CD (1988) Cloning and expression of JE, a gene inducible by a platelet-derived growth factor and whose product has cytokine properties. Proc Natl Acad Sci USA 85:3738–3742

21. Kawahara RS, Deuel TF (1989) Platelet-derived growth factor-inducible gene JE is a member of a family of small inducible gene related to platelet factor 4. J Biol Chem 264:679–682

22. Timmers HTM, Pronk GJ, Bos J, van der Eb AJ (1990) Analysis of the rat JE gene promotor identifies an AP-1 binding site essential for basal expression but not for TPA induction. Nucleic Acid Res 18:23–34

23. Yoshimura T, Takeya M, Takahashi K (1991) Molecular cloning of rat chemoattractant protein-1 (MCP-1) and its expression in rat spleen cells and tumor cell lines. Biochem Biophys Res Commun 174:504–509

24. Yoshimura T, Takeya M, Takahashi K, Kuratsu J, Leonard EJ (1991) Production and characterization of mouse monoclonal antibodies against human monocyte chemoattractant protein-1. J Immunol 147:2229–2233

25. Shyy Y-J, Li Y-S, Kolattukudy PE (1990) Structure of human monocyte chemotactic protein gene and its regulation by TPA. Biochem Biophys Res Commun 169:346–351

26. Mehrabian M, Sparkes RS, Mohandas T, Fogelman AM, Lusis AJ (1991) Localization of monocyte chemotactic protein-1 gene (SCYA2) to human chromosome 17q11.2-q21.1. Genomics 9:200–203

27. Carr MW, Roth SJ, Luther E, Rose SS, Springer TA (1994) Monocyte chemoattractant protein 1 acts as a T-lymphocyte chemoattractant. Proc Natl Acad Sci USA 91:3652–3656

28. Fulton AM (1988) Tumor-associated macrophages. In: Hepper G, Fulton A (eds) Macrophages and cancer. CRC Press, Boca Raton, pp 98–111

29. Morahan P, Volkman A, Melnicoff M, Dempsey W (1988) Macrophage heterogeneity. In: Hepper G, Fulton A (eds) Macrophages and cancer. CRC Press, Boca Raton, pp 2–25

30. Dijkstra C, Döpp E, Joling P, Kraal G (1985) The heterogeneity of mononuclear phagocytes in lymphoid organs. Distinct macrophage subpopulations in the rat recognized by monoclonal antibodies ED1, ED2, and ED3. Immunology 54:580–598

31. Polman CH, Dijkstra CD, Sminia T, Koetsier JC (1986) Immunohistological analysis of macrophages in the central nervous system of Lewis rats with acute experimental allergic encephalomyelitis. J Neuroimmunol 11:215–222

32. Verschure PJ, van Noorden JF, Dijkstra CD (1989) Macrophages and dendritic cells during the early stages of antigen-induced arthritis in rats. Immunohistochemical analysis of cryostat sections of the whole knee joint. Scand J Immunol 29:371–381

33. Dijkstra CD, Döpp EA, Vogels IMC, van Noorden CJF (1987) Macrophages and dendritic cells in antigen-induced arthritis. An immunohistochemical study using cryostat sections of the whole knee joint of rat. Scand J Immunol 26:513–523

34. Miyamura S, Naito M, Takeya M, Okumura H, Takahashi K (1988) Analysis of rat peritoneal macrophages with combined ultrastructural peroxidase cytochemistry and immunoelectron microscopy using anti-rat macrophage monoclonal antibodies. J Clin Electron Microsc 21:545–546

35. Takeya M, Hsiao L, Takahashi K (1987) A new monoclonal antibody, TRPM-3, binds specifically to certain rat macrophage populations. Immunohistochemical and immunoelectron macroscopic analysis. J Leukocyte Biol 41:187–195

36. Yamashiro S, Takeya M, Nishi T, Kuratsu J, Yoshimura T, Takahashi K (1994) Tumor-derived monocyte chemoattractant protein-1 induces intratumoral infiltration of monocyte-derived macrophage subpopulation in transplanted rat tumors. Am J Pathol 145:856–867

37. Takeshima H, Kuratsu J, Takeya M, Yoshimura T, Ushio Y (1994) Expression and localization of messenger RNA and protein for monocyte chemoattractant protein-1 in human malignant glioma. J Neurosurg 80:1056–1062

38. Rollins BJ, Sunday M (1991) Suppression of tumor formation in vivo by expression of the JE gene in malignant cells. Mol Cell Biol 11:3125–3131

39. Walter S, Bottazzi B, Govoni D, Colotta F, Mantovani A (1991) Macrophage infiltration and growth of sarcoma clones expressing different amounts of monocyte chemotactic protein/JE. Int J Cancer 49:431–435

40. Morantz RA, Wood GW, Foster M, Clark M, Gollahon K (1979) Macrophages in experimental and human brain tumors. J Neurosurg 50:305–311

41. Sato K, Kuratsu J, Takeshima H, Yoshimura T, Ushio Y (1995) Expression of monocyte chemoattractant protein-1 (MCP-1) in meningioma. J Neurosurg 82:874–878

42. Cochran BH, Reffel AC, Stiles CD (1983) Molecular cloning of gene sequences regulated by platelet-derived growth factor. Cell 33:939–947

43. Todo T, Adams E, Fahlbusch R (1993) Inhibitory effect of trapidil on human meningioma cell population via interruption of autocrine growth stimulation. J Neurosurg 78:463–469

44. Matsushima K, Larsen CG, DuBois GC, Oppenheim JJ (1989) Purification and characterization of a novel monocyte chemotactic and activating factor produced by a human myelomonocytic cell line. J Exp Med 169:1485–1490

45. Bruce JN, Criscuolo GR, Merrill MJ, Moquin RR, Blacklock JB, Oldfield EH (1987) Vascular permeability induced by protein product of malignant brain tumors: inhibition by dexamethasone. J Neurosurg 67:880–884

46. Shinonaga M, Chang CC, Suzuki N, Sato M, Kawabara T (1988) Immunohistological evaluation of macrophage infiltrates in brain tumors. J Neurosurg 68:259–265

47. Kunishio K, Maeshiro T, Matsushima T, Mishima M, Tsuno K, Shigematsu H, Matsumoto K, Furuta T, Nishimoto A (1992) Study on the extent of peritumoral edema in glioma: its correlation with the proliferative potential and tumor-infiltrating mononuclear cells. Neurol Surg 20:39–44 (in Japanese)

48. Kuratsu J, Yoshizato K, Yoshimura T, Leonard EJ, Takeshima H, Ushio Y (1994) Quantitative study of monocyte chemoattractant protein-1 (MCP-1) in cerebrospinal fluid and cyst fluid from patients with malignant glioma. J Natl Cancer Inst 85:1836–1839

Experimental Analysis of Proto-Oncogene and Histocompatibility Antigen Gene Expression During Brain Tumor Progression

Toshiki Yamasaki, Kouzo Moritake, Yasuhiko Akiyama,
Masako Fukuda, and Seiichi Nagao

Abstract. The relationship between expression of proto-oncogenes (N-*myc* and c-*src*) and the major histocompatibility complex (MHC, H-2 in mice) antigen gene was investigated at the molecular level in two mouse neuroblastoma cell lines (NB-1, H-2 class I-positive; NB-V, H-2 class I-negative) derived from the spontaneously occurring C-1300 neuroblastoma cell line. In addition, the role of interactions between these genes in brain tumor progression was examined by an in vivo tumorigenicity assay. Molecular analysis showed that H-2 class I antigen expression on NB-1 cells was modulated by transcriptional regulation of the H-2 gene. In contrast, the lack of H-2 expression on NB-V cells was caused by a block in intracytoplasmic glycosylation of the H-2 heavy chain. Neither amplification nor rearrangement of the N-*myc* and c-*src* genes was identified in either cell line. Dimethyl sulfoxide (DMSO) treatment (1.5% vol) induced the neuronal differentiation of both lines. A nuclear run-on transcription assay revealed that the N-*myc* gene underwent posttranscriptional downregulation after DMSO-induced differentiation, while the c-*src* gene showed transcriptional upregulation. An in vitro cytotoxicity assay showed that H-2-positive NB-1 cells were susceptible to cytotoxic T-lymphocyte- (CTL-) mediated lysis and resistant to natural killer cell- (NK-) mediated lysis, while NB-V cells were refractory to both CTL- and NK-mediated lysis. An in vivo rapid elimination assay indicated that NK-mediated natural resistance was absent in the brain. An in vivo brain tumorigenicity assay showed that NB-1 was less tumorigenic than NB-V. These findings suggested that the N-*myc* and c-*src* genes might be linked to the proliferation and differentiation of neuronal tumors and that H-2 class I antigen expression may directly influence antitumor immunosurveillance in the brain.

Key words. Brain tumor—Major histocompatibility antigen gene—Defense immunosurveillance—Proto-oncogene—Tumor progression

Introduction

The development of malignant tumors may represent the failure of host defenses not only to eliminate aberrant cells but also to prevent neoplastic transformation [1,2].

Department of Neurosurgery, Shimane Medical University, Izumo 693, Japan

Effective immunosurveillance requires not only an immunocompetent host but also the appropriate expression of major histocompatibility complex (MHC; H-2 in the mouse) antigens along with tumor neoantigens. It has been demonstrated in several experimental models that tumor immunogenicity depends on the state of MHC class I antigen expression [3,4]. Oncogene activation in tumors has been documented along with neoplastic transformation, and there is ample evidence that malignant transformation can lead to aberrant MHC antigen expression by tumor cells [5]. To our knowledge, however, there has been no study asssessing reciprocal control between proto-oncogenes and MHC antigen genes during brain tumor progression.

In the present study, we examined the regulation of two proto-oncogenes (N-*myc* and c-*src*) and MHC class I antigen gene expression during the process of brain tumor differentiation and progression, using mouse H-2 class I-positive and -negative neuroblastoma cell lines.

Materials and Methods

Mice

A.BY(H-2^{b}K^{b}D^b) and A/Sn(H-2^{a}K^{k}D^d) inbred mice aged 4–8 weeks were used. The A.BY strain is congenic with the A strain, differing only at the segment of chromosome 17 containing H-2, but otherwise sharing the same genetic background. In the in vivo brain tumorigenicity assay, natural killer cell- (NK-) depleted and T-cell-depleted mice were used, as described elsewhere [6].

Tumor Cell Lines

Two sublines (NB-1 and NB-V) of a spontaneously occurring neuroblastoma derived from the A/J Ax (H-2^{a}K^{k}D^d) mouse (C-1300) were used. It was confirmed that there was no difference of in vitro growth between them. The in vitro cytotoxicity assay employed a Moloney-leukemia virus-induced T-cell lymphoma line (YAC-1) of A/Sn mouse origin, which is NK sensitive. All the cell lines used in this study were checked to exclude *Mycoplasma* contamination.

Molecular Analysis

Immunoprecipitation, sodium dodecyl sulfate-polyacrylamide gel electrophoresis (SDS-PAGE), Northern blotting, and Southern blotting were performed. For analysis of the H-2 gene, an *Eco*RI-*Kpn*I fragment of the complementary deoxyribonucleic acid (cDNA) corresponding to the first two exons and part of the third exon of the K gene (clone ph-2-33) was used as a class I heavy chain probe. Two *Pst*I-*Pst*I fragments (0.3 kilobase pairs, kbp, each) of the pAG69 cDNA clone, corresponding to the entire β2-microglobulin messenger ribonucleic acid (mRNA), were used as a β2-microglobulin probe. For oncogene analysis, the following cloned DNA fragments were used as hybridization probes: N-myc (mouse) (pNbl); c-myc (mouse) (pMC-54); v-src (mouse) (Pvull E); actin (mouse) (pAm91); and histone (mouse) (pCH3-3E). All probes were used as unexcised inserts into pBR 322 plasmids. The state of intracytoplasmic glycosylation of the H-2 class I heavy chain was assessed using endo-beta-N-acetyl-glycoseamidase H (Endo H), an enzyme that removes asparagine-linked core sugar moieties provided that final trimming and terminal glycosylation in the Golgi complex have not occurred.

Fluorescence-Activated Cell Sorter (FACS) Analysis

The appropriate monoclonal antibodies for H-2 class I antigens (hybridoma supernatants, H-2 K^k from 11-4.1 and H-2 D^d from 34-1-2S) and rabbit antiserum against mouse β 2-microglobulin were used.

In Vitro Cytotoxicity Assay

Specific anti H-2^a and H-2^b (as a control) cytotoxic T-lymphocyte (CTL) effectors were generated in one-way mixed lymphocyte culture using A.BY anti-A/Sn and A/Sn anti-A.BY spleen cells, respectively. The radioactivity released from ^{51}Cr-labeled target cells into the culture supernatant was measured, and calculation was according to the following formula: % specific ^{51}Cr release = (test cpm—spontaneous cpm/total cpm—spontaneous cpm) × 100. Spontaneous release was determined by the addition of only culture medium to the target cells, and total (maximum) release was determined by placing target cells into distilled water.

In Vivo Rapid Elimination Assay

Tumor cells were labeled with [^{125}I]-5-iodo-2′-deoxyuridine ([^{125}I]IUdR) for 12–24 h, extensively washed at least four times in phosphate buffered saline (PBS), and then injected intravenously or intracerebrally into mice at various different doses. The radioactivity in various organs, such as lung and brain, was measured after 24 h using an LKB gamma counter, and the percent radioactivity of the amount injected was calculated for each organ.

In Vivo Brain Tumorigenicity Assay

A tumor cell suspension was prepared by digesting monolayer cultures with trypsin. The cells were washed, adjusted to the specified concentrations, and then injected into the right cerebral hemispheres of H-2-compatible mice. The cumulative tumor take was recorded as the tumor-bearing rate (TBR, %), and the median survival time was also calculated (MST, days).

Induction of Neuritogenesis by Dimethyl Sulfoxide

It is known that the parental C-1300 cells differentiate into neuronal cells after treatment with dimethyl sulfoxide (DMSO) [7], and it was confirmed that neuronal differentiation of NB-1 and NB-V cells could also be induced by DMSO treatment. The normally round cells extended neurite processes after DMSO treatment (Fig. 1), and immunohistochemical examination revealed that both the cytoplasm and processes were stained by antineurofilament antibodies. Medium containing 6% DMSO (100 ml) was prepared weekly, and lower concentrations of DMSO were obtained by dilution of

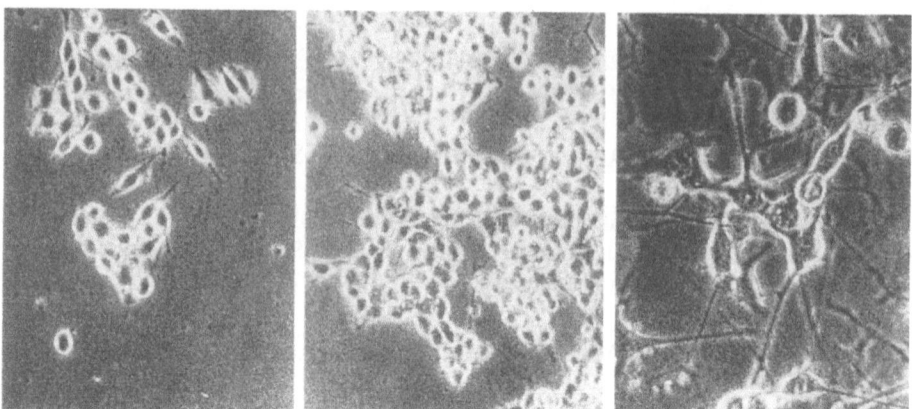

a,b

c

Fig. 1a–c. Photomicrographs show NB-1 cells after 2 days (**a**) and 5 days (**b**) of subculture with complete medium, and after of 1.5% dimethyl sulfoxide treatment (7 days) has induced neuronal differentiation (**c**)

this stock. Cells were propagated in medium containing 1.5% DMSO for 1–2 weeks, because this concentration was optimal for inducing differentiation without influencing the growth rate [7].

Results

Comparison of Proto-Oncogene Expression Between NB-1 and NB-V Cells

It was confirmed by Southern blot analysis that both NB-1 and NB-V cells contained a single copy of N-*myc* DNA (Fig. 2). Neither amplification nor rearrangement of the N-*myc* gene was identified in either cell line. Northern blot analysis of both cell lines indicated that the number of transcripts of the N-*myc* gene decreased after DMSO-induced neuronal differentiation. In contrast, the c-*src* gene showed an increase of transcripts of more than fourfold in each cell line after DMSO treatment. To examine N-myc and c-src mRNA synthesis, a nuclear run-on transcription assay was performed. It was found that the transcription rate of the N-*myc* gene remained unchanged, whereas there was rapid accumulation of c-*src* gene transcripts after the start of DMSO treatment (Fig. 3). These results suggested that N-*myc* may be down-regulated at the posttranscriptional level by DMSO-induced cellular differentiation, while primary up-regulation of the c-*src* gene occurred at the transcriptional level.

MHC Class I Antigen Gene Expression by NB-1 and NB-V Cells

The amount of H-2 DNA in both NB-1 and NB-V cells was found to be a single copy by Southern blot analysis, and there was no amplification, deletion, or rearrangement of the H-2 class I gene in either cell line. After DMSO-induced neuronal differentiation, an increase of H-2 and β 2-microglobulin gene transcripts was identified in both cell lines by Northern blot analysis (Fig. 4a). On the other hand, immunoprecipitation

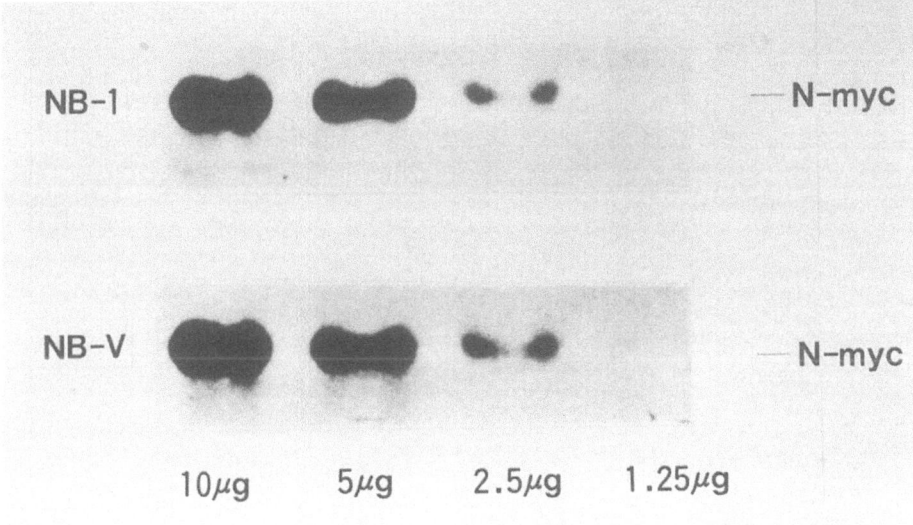

Fig. 2. Southern blot analysis of N-*myc* in genomic DNA shows a single copy of the N-*myc* gene in both NB-1 and NB-V cells. In lanes 1, 2, 3, and 4, the DNA corresponds to 10, 5, 2.5, and 1.25 µg, respectively

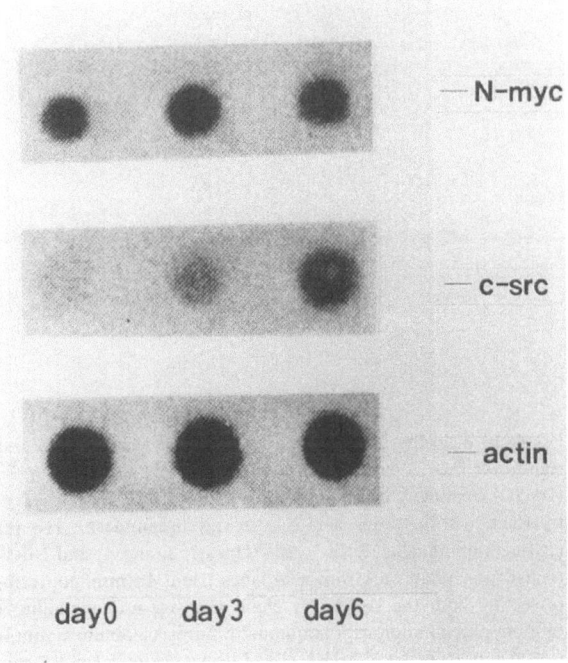

Fig. 3. Nuclear run-on transcription assay of cells undergoing dimethyl sulfoxide treatment shows an increase of c-*src* transcripts on days 3 and 6 in lanes 2 and 3, respectively, when compared to untreated cells (lane 1). No significant alterations are seen in the N-*myc* and actin probes

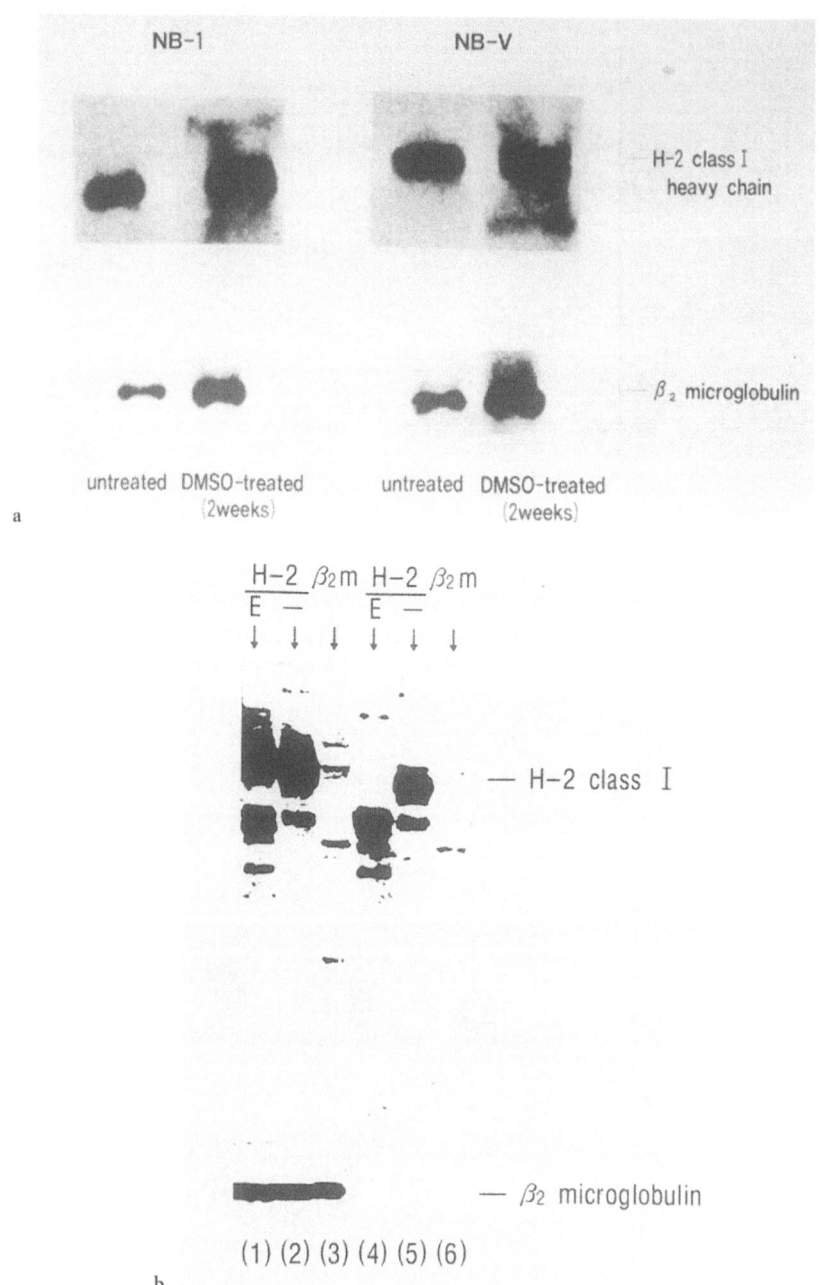

Fig. 4a,b. **a** Northern blot analysis of H-2 heavy chain mRNA and β 2-microglobulin mRNA shows a significant increase of transcripts in both NB-1 and NB-V cells on day 14 of dimethyl sulfoxide (DMSO) treatment. **b** Immunoprecipitation of H-2 class I heavy chain and β 2-microglobulin after treatment with endo-beta-*N*-acetyl-glycoseamidase H (Endo-H). Detergent lysates of [³⁵S]methionine-labeled NB-1 cells (lanes 1, 2, and 3) and NB-V cells (lanes 4, 5, and 6). Endo H-treated precipitates are shown in lanes 1 and 4. Immunoprecipitation with antimouse H-2 serum (detecting both the H-2 heavy chain and β 2-microglobulin) is shown in lanes 1, 2, 4, and 5. Immunoprecipitation with antimouse β 2-microglobulin serum (detecting β 2-microglobulin alone) is shown in lanes 3 and 6. H-2, class I heavy chain; β 2 m, β 2-microglobulin; E, endo-beta-*N*-acetyl-glycoseamidase H; (−), no treatment

revealed that the H-2 heavy chain and β 2-microglobulin bands remained unchanged in NB-1 cells after Endo H treatment, while NB-V cells showed alteration of the H-2 heavy chain band and deficiency of β 2-microglobulin band (Fig. 4b). This indicated that terminal glycosylation normally occurred in the Golgi apparatus of NB-1 cells, which demonstrated cell-surface expression of H-2 (Fig. 5), while NB-V cells were not only susceptible to enzyme Endo H treatment but were also impaired in the process of β 2-microglobulin synthesis and thus exhibited no surface H-2 expression (Fig. 5).

Relationship of MHC Class I Antigen Expression by NB-1 and NB-V Cells to CTL- and NK-Mediated Lysis

FACS analysis demonstrated that NB-1 cells exhibited both H-2 class I antigen and β 2-microglobulin expressions, while NB-V cells expressed neither of these cell surface antigens (see Fig. 5). Anti-H-2a CTL showed a great killing activity against NB-1 cells than NB-V cells (Table 1). Anti-H-2b CTL (as a control) had no cytotoxicity for either tumor cells. A correlation was found between H-2 class I expression and susceptibility to CTL-mediated lysis in H-2-positive NB-1 cells, while CTL showed no cytotoxicity against H-2-negative NB-V cells. On the other hand, both NB-1 and NB-V cells were quite resistant to NK-mediated lysis (Table 1), indicating that H-2 expression was not related to this type of cell lysis. As reported previously [8], there was an inverse correlation between H-2 class I expression and NK sensitivity in the case of NK-sensitive, H-2-positive YAC-1 cells.

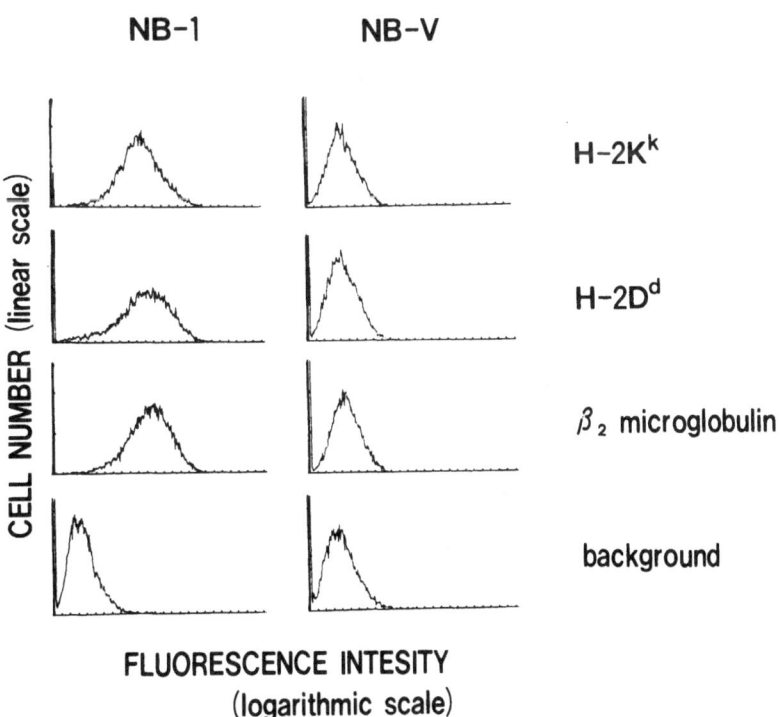

Fig. 5. Fluorescence-activated cell sorter (FACS) analysis of H-2 class I antigen expression by NB-1 and NB-V cells

Possible Absence of NK-Mediated Antitumor Immunosurveillance in the Brain

The in vivo survival and distribution of NB-1 and NB-V cells were studied by monitoring the residual radioactivity in various organs over 24h after the intravenous or intracerebral injection of [^{125}I]IUdR-labeled tumor cells. [^{125}I]IUdR is rapidly released from dead cells, so the amount of radioactivity remaining in each organ indicated the distribution of surviving cells. It has already been demonstrated that the lung is the optimal organ for this assay 4–24h after the intravenous injection of labeled tumor cells [9]. The assay using NK-sensitive YAC-1 cells revealed that the residual radioactivity in lung was higher in NK-depleted mice than in sham-operated controls (Table 2). This suggests that NK-sensitive YAC-1 cells were cleared from the lungs where NK-mediated immunosurveillance exists. On the other hand, there was no significant elimination of either NB-1 or NB-V cells from the lungs (Table 2). The reason why both neuroblastoma cell lines persisted in lung tissue remains unclear, but it may be partly because they are highly NK-resistant. Furthermore, it was noted that NB-1, NB-V, and YAC-1 cells were not cleared from the brain after intracerebral injection (Table 2). Thus, it seems possible that NK-mediated antitumor immunosurveillance may be absent in the brain.

Table 1. Differences in sensitivity of NB-1 and NB-B cells to cytotoxic T-lymphocyte- (CTL-) and natural killer cell- (NK-) mediated lysis.

Target	E/T ratio	^{51}Cr Release assay (% lysis)	
		H-2^a CTL-mediated lysis	NK-mediated lysis
NB-1	40:1	38.9 ± 4.6*	6.6 ± 1.8**
	20:1	20.1 ± 2.9*	4.0 ± 1.0**
NB-V	40:1	2.8 ± 1.0*	**8.2 ± 1.4
	20:1	1.9 ± 0.8*	**4.6 ± 1.2
YAC-1^a	40:1	43.6 ± 6.2	36.8 ± 4.2
	20:1	26.8 ± 3.9	21.6 ± 3.0

E/Tratio, effector to tumor cell ratio.
*, $P < .01$; **, $P < .05$.
^{a} YAC-1 cells were used as a control because they are reported to be NK-sensitive and to exhibit H-2 class I-positive expressions [8]. P values are significant statistically.

Table 2. In vivo rapid elimination assay with [^{125}I-] iododeoxyuridine-labeled tumor cells in natural killer cell-depleted mice and sham-operated control.

Injection route	Organ	Remaining radioactivity (%)^a					
		Natural killer cell-depleted mice			Sham control		
		YAC-1	NB-1	NB-V	YAC-1	NB-1	NB-V
Intravenous	Lung	1.95 ± 0.46	13.1 ± 4.2	14.8 ± 3.9	0.48 ± 0.09*	12.5 ± 3.6	14.1 ± 4.2
Intracerebral	Brain	20.32 ± 4.6	21.6 ± 3.9	20.6 ± 4.3	18.6 ± 2.9	20.8 ± 4.2	21.4 ± 4.2

*, $P < .01$.
^{a} Remaining radioactivities of lung and brain were measured 24 h after intravenous or intracerebral injection of the labeled cells, respectively. P value is significant statistically.

Table 3. Difference in intracerebral tumorigenicity between NB-1 and NB-V cells after intracerebral inoculation of various numbers of cells.

Tumor	Cell Dose	Intracerebral inoculation	
		TBR (%)	MST (days)
NB-1	10^4 cells	17/23 (73.9%)	18.3 ± 2.4
	10^3 cells	13/28 (46.4%)* ⎤	24.6 ± 4.3
NB-V	10^4 cells	19/20 (95.0%) ⎥	16.4 ± 3.2
	10^3 cells	13/18 (72.2%) ⎦	26.2 ± 4.8

TBR, tumor-bearing rate; MST, mean survival time. *P* value is significant statistically.
*, $P < .05$.

Table 4. Effects of T-cell and natural killer cell depletion on intracerebral tumorigenicity after intracerebral inoculation of 10^3 tumor cells.

Tumor	Intracerebral inoculation of 10^3 cells					
	T-Cell depletion		Natural killer cell depletion		Sham control	
	TBR (%)	MST (days)	TBR (%)	MST (days)	TBR (%)	MST (days)
NB-1	13/16* (81.3%)	16.9 ± 3.2	6/14 (42.9%)	23.9 ± 4.4	11/24 (45.8%)	22.8 ± 3.8
NB-V	11/13 (84.6%)	15.8 ± 2.9	10/12 (83.3%)	25.0 ± 4.0	11/14 (78.6%)	24.6 ± 4.1

TBR, tumor-bearing rate; MST, mean survival time. *P* value is significant statistically.
*, $P < .05$.

Comparison of Intracerebral Tumor Progression Between NB-1 and NB-V Cells

The in vitro proliferation rate did not differ between NB-1 and NB-V cells (data not shown). An in vivo brain tumorigenicity assay was therefore performed to determine whether H-2 class I expression is linked to tumor formation. It was found that NB-V was more tumorigenic than NB-1 in untreated mice (Table 3). In T-cell-depleted mice, however, there was no difference of tumor progression between the two cell lines, while NK-depleted mice showed results similar to those of untreated mice (Table 4). Because both NB-1 and NB-V cells were highly NK-resistant and because NK-mediated antitumor immunosurveillance is apparently absent in the brain, it was suggested that in vivo clearance of NB-1 from brain tissue may be closely associated with an H-2 class I-restricted, CTL-mediated natural resistance mechanism.

Discussion

Factors Influencing the Malignancy of Brain Tumors

Most normal brain cells show a very low level of MHC expression, and this might have favored the evolution of a specific barrier against the entry of immunocompetent cells into the brain [10,11]. Our experimental results suggest that NK-mediated natural antitumor immunosurveillance may be absent in the brain. This is consistent with other reports that NK cells are usually absent or are found only in small numbers in some brain tumors [12–14]. On the other hand, T-cell-mediated immune reactions occur in the brain, although the entry or function of the effector cells shows some limitations [13,15–17]. Thus, the lack of MHC molecules may facilitate the proliferation of tumor cells in the brain because of escape from a T-cell-mediated resistance mechanism. Accordingly, intracerebral MHC-deficient tumor cells may be sheltered from both host T-cell- and NK-mediated rejection systems.

Our study revealed the existence of immunosurveillance against H-2 class I-positive NB-1 cells in the brain, while H-2-negative NB-V cells escaped and developed tumors after intracerebral inoculation. Natural resistance against highly H-2 class I-positive cells was thus found to be thymus-dependent, making it likely that cell-surface MHC class I expression significantly affects the immunogenicity or tumorigenicity of neoplastic cells in hosts bearing brain tumors.

It should be stressed that in the immunologically privileged brain the level of MHC class I antigen expression by tumor cells may contribute mainly to in vivo tumorigenicity, irrespective of whether a high level of expression or amplification of tumor-related oncogenes is closely linked to in vitro tumor cell proliferation and differentiation.

Proto-Oncogene and MHC Class I Gene Interactions in Brain Tumor Growth

Our molecular analysis suggested that up-regulation of MHC class I antigen gene expression may be a consequence of deregulated N-*myc* gene expression after DMSO-induced cellular differentiation, contrasting with up-regulation of the c-*src* gene. It could be suggested that the combined products of these two proto-oncogenes (N-*myc* and c-*src*) contribute to the malignant phenotype of neuroblastoma cells, but the relationship between them remains unclarified. Furthermore, it seems that neuroblastoma cells may show down-regulation of N-*myc* mRNA and up-regulation of c-*src* mRNA in the process of neuronal differentiation. It is unclear, however, whether the changes of both genes are a trigger or a consequence of neuronal differentiation, and thus further investigation is warranted.

Acknowledgments. We thank Prof. George Klein, Prof. Klas Karre, and Dr. Hans-Gustaf Ljunggren of the Karolinska Institute (Sweden) for helpful advice.

References

1. Barbacid M (1986) Human oncogenes. In: Important advances in oncology. Lippincott, Philadelphia, pp 3–22
2. Ramsay GM, Moscovici G, Moscovici C (1990) Neoplastic transformation and tumorigenicity by the human proto-oncogene MYC. Proc Natl Acad Sci USA 87:2102–2106
3. Bernards R (1987) Suppression of MHC gene expression in cancer cells. Trends Genet 3:298–301
4. Goodenow RS, Vogel JM, Linsk RL (1985) Histocompatibility antigens on murine tumors. Science 230:777–783

5. Tanaka K, Isselbacher KJ, Khoury G (1985) Reversal of oncogenesis by the expression of a major histocompatibility complex class I gene. Science 228:26–30

6. Yamasaki T, Ljunggren HG, Ohlen C (1989) Enhanced H-2 expression and T-cell-dependent rejection after intracerebral transplantation of the murine lymphoma YAC-1. Cell Immunol 120:387–395

7. Kimhi Y, Palfrey C, Spector I (1976) Maturation of neuroblastoma cells in the presence of demethylsulfoxide. Proc Natl Acad Sci USA 73:462–466

8. Piontek GE, Taniguchi K, Ljunggren HG (1985) YAC-1 MHC class I variants reveal an association between decreased NK sensitivity and increased H-2 expression after interferon treatment of in vivo passage. J Immunol 135:4281–4288

9. Gorelik E, Herberman RB (1981) Radioisotope assay for evaluation of in vivo natural killer cell-mediated resistance of mice to local transplantation of tumor cells. Int J Cancer 27:709–720

10. Rossi ML, Hughes JT, Esiri MM (1987) Immunohistological study of mononuclear cell infiltrate in malignant gliomas. Acta Neuropathol 74:269–277

11. Stevens A, Kloter I, Roggendorf W (1988) Inflammatory infiltrates and natural killer cell presence in human brain tumors. Cancer 61:738–743

12. Circolo A, Bianchi R, Nardelli B (1982) Mouse brain: an immunologically privileged site for natural resistance against lymphoma cells. J Immunol 128:556–562

13. Ljunggren HG, Yamasaki T, Collins P (1988) Selective acceptance of MHC class I-deficient tumor grafts in the brain. J Exp Med 167:730–735

14. Satoh J, Kim SU, Kastrukoff LF (1990) Absence of natural killer (NK) cell activity against oligodendrocytes in multiple sclerosis. J Neuroimmunol 26:75–80

15. Aarli JA (1983) The immune system and the nervous system. J Neurol 229:137–154

16. Wekerle H, Linington C, Lassmann H (1988) Cellular immune reactivity within the CNS. Trends Neurosci 9:271–277

17. Yamasaki T, Handa H, Yamashita J (1983) Charactristic immunological responses to an experimental mouse brain tumor. Cancer Res 43:4610–4617

Suppressed Expression of T-Cell Costimulatory Molecules B7 and B70 in Human Glioblastomas In Vivo

Mitsuhiro Tada, Annie-Claire Diserens, Marie-France Hamou, Rehana Jaufeerally, Erwin G. van Meir, and Nicolas de Tribolet

Abstract. The question of whether tumor cells can be recognized by the host immune system in an antigen-specific manner that is also major histocompatibility complex-(MHC-) restricted is a major issue in immunotherapy of glioblastomas. It was recently found that interaction of B7/B70 costimulatory molecules with their T-cell counterstructures CD28/CTLA-4 is essential for T-cell activation of both recognition phase and effector phase. To know whether proper T-cell activation can take place in glioblastomas in situ, we studied the expression of B7 (B7–1) and B70 (B7–2) molecules in vitro and in vivo. In vitro Northern blot analysis showed that five glioblastoma cell lines and six primary cultures did not express mRNA for B7 or B70 molecules. Cultured human fetal astrocytes either with or without interferon-γ did not express the mRNA. Immunocytochemistry demonstrated that fetal astrocytes and glioblastoma cell lines are negative for B7 and B70 immunoreactive proteins. Interferon-γ increased HLA-DR (MHC class II) expression but did not induce B7/B70 molecules. In vivo, 21 glioblastoma tissues were studied with immunohistochemistry. Glioblastoma cells were found to be completely negative for both B7 and B70. At the tumor boundary or necrotic area, numerous macrophages (CD68+) were found positive for B7/B70. However, macrophages deep inside tumors almost invariably lacked B7/B70 expression. Northern blot analysis showed that 10 glioblastoma tissues did not express mRNA for B7/B70. The suppression of B7/B70 expression in both tumor cells and tumor-associated macrophages seems to be one mechanism of tumor evasion of host immune surveillance.

Key words. Glioblastoma multiforme—T-cell costimulatory molecules—B7 and B70 molecules—Tumor-associated macrophages—Biological response modification

Introduction

The activation of T cells in response to interactions between T-cell receptors (TCR) and antigens presented on major histocompatibility complex (MHC) molecules requires second or costimulatory signals because of interactions between receptors and ligands on the T cells and antigen-presenting cells (APC) [1,2]. Ligand–receptor pairs

Department of Neurosurgery, University Hospital, Lausanne, CH-1011, Switzerland mediating costimulatory signals include ICAM-1/LFA-1, VCAM-1/VLA-4, LFA-3/CD2, and B7 (B7-1)/CD28 and CTLA4 [3,4]. Although most of these molecules are more important for cell-to-cell adhesion than they are for signaling to T cells, signaling through B7 and CD28/CTLA4 interactions is essential for T-cell activation. In the absence of this costimulation, the MHC class II-restricted activation of both naive CD4+ Th cells and the antigen-specific Th1 clone does not take place, and the T cells go into an inactivated status called "anergy" or clonal deletion. It has been shown that B7 costimulation can also function at the effector phase mediated by MHC class I-restricted CD8+ cytotoxic T lymphocytes (CTL) [5], MHC class II-restricted CD4+ CTL [6], and MHC-unrestricted natural killer cells [7]. B70 (B7-2), a second costimulatory ligand for CTLA4, was recently described demonstrating the potential complexity of costimulatory interactions [4,8,9].

Several studies have suggested that B7-mediated costimulation plays an important role in tumor immunity. Murine melanoma cells transfected with the B7 gene were able to induce CD8+ T-cell-mediated rejection of wild-type cells in vivo [5,10,11]. It was also shown that expression of the B7 gene in murine sarcoma and melanoma cells can cause CD4+ T-cell-dependent tumor rejection [12,13]. Negative expression of B7 molecules on tumor cells together with decreased expression of class I and enhanced expression of class II MHC molecules may be a cause of tumor evasion of host immune surveillance [14]. Our study examines whether B7 and B70 molecules are expressed on glioblastoma cells and tumor-associated immune cells.

Materials and Methods

Cells and Culture

Six established glioblastoma cell lines (LN18, LN229, LN382, LN428, LN443, and LN827) were cultured and maintained in Dulbecco's modified minimal essential medium supplemented with 1 mM sodium pyruvate, 0.1 mM L-glutamine, 100 U/ml penicillin, and 5% heat-inactivated fetal calf serum (FCS) (DMEM-5) [15]. Five primary cultures of glioblastoma cells (LN835, LN963, LN966, LN971, and LN975) were also cultured in the same DMEM-5. All the glioblastoma cell lines and primary cultures were positive for glial fibrillary acidic protein (GFAP) (monoclonal antibody from Dako, Glostrup, Denmark). Two B-cell lymphoma cell line (Daudi and Raji) were maintained in RPMI-1640 media plus 10% FCS, 4 mM L-glutamine, and 100 U/ml penicillin (RPMI-10). Mononuclear cells were isolated from human peripheral blood obtained from the University Hospital Blood Center (Lausanne, Switzerland) by Ficoll/Hypaque gradient centrifugation. Monocytes were enriched by adherence to plastic culture flasks for 2 h at 37°C, 5% CO_2 in RPMI-10 media.

Tumor Tissue

Twenty-one glioblastoma tissue specimens were obtained from patients during standard surgical procedures, snap-frozen in liquid nitrogen, and stored at −80°C until use.

Monoclonal Antibodies and Cytokines

Anti-CD68 monoclonal antibody (MAb) M814 and anti-HLA-DR MAb M746 were purchased from Dako. Anti-B7 (B7–1) MAb L310 and anti-B70 (B7–2) MAb IT-2 were gifts of Dr. L.L. Lanier (DNAX Research, San Francisco, CA, USA) and Dr. M. Azuma (Department of Immunology, Juntendo University, Tokyo, Japan). Recombinant human interferon-γ (IFN-γ) was a gift of Biogen (Geneva, Switzerland).

Immunocytochemical Stainings

Immunostains on cover slip specimens of cell lines and frozen sections of tumor tissues were performed by an avidin–biotin staining kit (Vector, Burlinghame, CA, USA). Cells were grown to subconfluent state on cover slips placed in plastic petri dishes. Frozen specimens of human glioblastoma tissues were cut in 8-μm-thick sections. The cover slips and frozen sections were fixed in methanol and stained with M814, M746, L310, or IT-2 as the primary antibody (45 min) and biotinylated anti-mouse IgG rabbit antibody (Vector) as the secondary antibody (20 min), followed by a 20-min incubation with peroxidase-labeled streptavidin. The chromogen used was 3-amino-9-ethylcarbazole (5 min; Sigma, St. Louis, MO, USA). Nuclear counterstain was obtained with hematoxylin.

RNA Isolation

RNA isolation was performed according to the method previously described [16]. Cells were grown in culture flasks and washed twice with phosphate buffer. Glioblastoma tissues and cultured cells were lysed in GITC-containing lysis buffer (4 M guanidine isothiocyanate, 0.5% N lauroyl sarcosyl, 25 mM sodium citrate, 0.1 M O-mercaptoethanol) and homogenized with a Bounce homogenizer. Lysate was added with 1:10 volume of 2 M sodium acetate (pH 4.0), transferred to a polypropylene tube, and extracted with phenol/chloroform/isoamyl alcohol; RNA was precipitated in 60% ethanol with 1:20 volume of 7.5 M ammonium acetate. After a second precipitation with ethanol, the RNA pellet was washed with 70% ethanol twice and resuspended in diethylpyrocarbonate-treated water, analyzed by agarose gel electrophoresis, and quantified spectrophotometrically (OD_{260}/OD_{280}).

Northern Blot Analysis

Each 10 μg of RNA was electrophoresed on a 1% agarose formaldehyde gel and blotted onto a nitrocellulose membrane (Hibond N, Amersham, Arlington Heights, IL, USA). The blots were hybridized with the 1.5-kbp EcoRI fragment of the pBJ (B7) cDNA [17] or 1.5-kbp XhoI–NotI fragment of pJFE14 (B70) cDNA [8], and labeled by random primed DNA labeling (Boelinger, Mannheim, Germany). The hybridization buffer contained 4 × SSC (150 mM NaCl, 15 mM sodium citrate), 1.5 × Denhardt's solution, 0.5% sodium dodecyl sulphate, single-stranded salmon sperm DNA (0.2 mg/ml), and 20 mM sodium phosphate, pH 7.0. The blots were then washed in serial dilutions of SSC. Exposure to x-ray films was performed at −70°C with an intensifying screen for 1–8 days.

Results

In Vitro Northern Blot Analysis

To determine whether cultured normal fetal astrocytes and cultured glioblastoma cells express mRNA for B7 or B70 molecules, a Northern blot analysis was performed with B7 and B70 cDNA probes. The fetal astrocytes, either with or without stimulation with interferon-γ (1000 IU/ml, 48 h), did not express mRNA for B7 or B70 molecules, but Raji and Daudi B-cell lymphoma cell lines expressed four alternative splice forms (10, 4.2, 2.9, and 1.7 kb) of B7 mRNA and two forms (2.9 and 1.7 kb) of B70 mRNA (Fig. 1). None of the permanent culture glioblastoma cell lines (LN18, LN229, LN382, LN428, LN443, LN827) or the primary cultures (LN835, LN963, LN966, LN971, LN975) expressed mRNA for B7 or B70 molecules (data not shown).

In Vitro Immunocytochemistry

Both Raji and Daudi cells expressed B7 and B70 immunoreactive proteins. The fetal astrocytes and the permanent culture glioblastoma cell lines were negative for B7 and B70. The majority of the cells in the primary glioblastoma cultures (LN835, LN963,

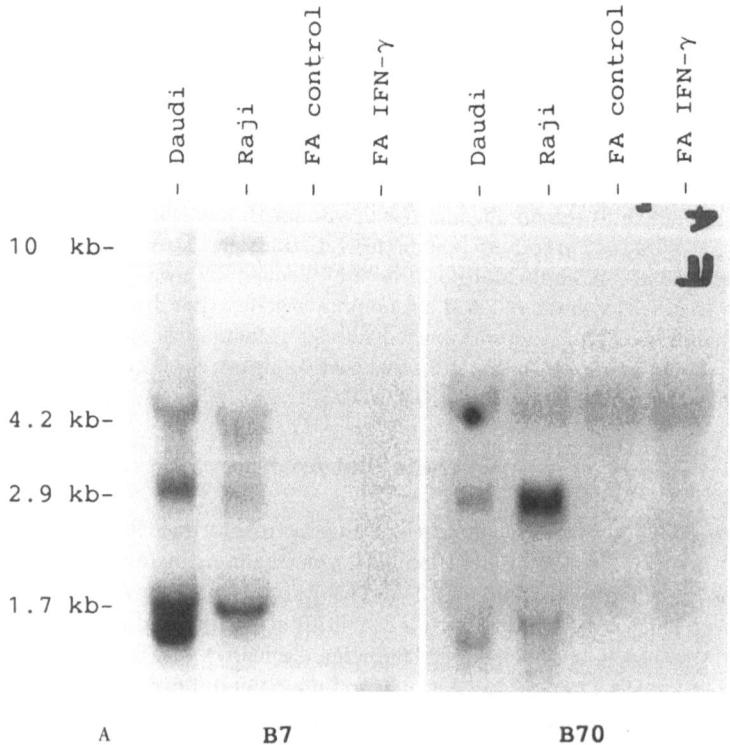

Fig. 1A,B. Northern blot analysis for mRNA expression of (A) B7 and (B) B70 molecules in Daudi and Raji B-cell lymphoma cells, unstimulated fetal astrocytes, and stimulated fetal astrocytes with 1000 IU/ml interferon-γ (IFN-γ)

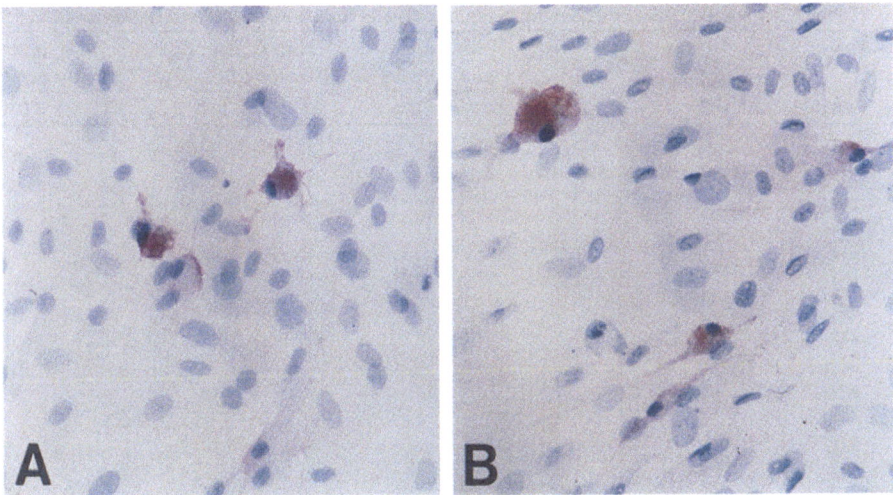

Fig. 2A,B. Immunocytochemistry with (**A**) anti-B7 monoclonal antibody (MAb) and (**B**) anti-B70 MAb in a primary culture of a glioblastoma (LN-966). Note that positive cells have round eccentric nuclei and plump cytoplasm, which are characteristic of central nervous system macrophages

LN966, LN971, LN975) did not express B7 and B70 proteins, but all contained a small number of positive cells that were positive for both B7 and B70 immunoreactive proteins (Fig. 2A,B). The positive cells had a plump cytoplasm and a round nucleus that were distinct from those of the tumor cells. They were also positive for CD68, indicating that they were macrophage-lineage cells. CD68 was negative in the permanent culture glioblastoma cell lines and the fetal astrocytes. With stimulation by IFN-γ (1000 IU/ml, 48h), neither the fetal astrocytes nor the glioblastoma cell lines changed in immunoreactivity to anti-B7 or -B70 antibodies, although HLA-DR expression was markedly enhanced.

In Vivo Immunohistochemistry

Twenty-two glioblastoma tissues were stained with anti-B7 MAb L310 and 19 glioblastoma tissues with anti-B70 MAb IT-2 (Table 1). None of the glioblastoma tissues contained tumor cells positive for B7 or B70 immunoreactivity. At the tumor boundary, which was present occasionally, numerous cells were found positive for B7 (2 of 6 cases) or B70 (5 of 6 cases) (Fig. 3A,B). The cells were considered to be macrophages but not normal astrocytes or glioblastoma cells, because they were positive for CD68 an negative for GFAP (Fig. 3C,D). Although the proliferating tumor center also contained CD68-positive macrophages except in a few cases, the tumor cells were completely negative for B7 an B70 molecules (Fig. 4A–C). However, in the necrotic areas, the macrophages occasionally stained positive for B7 or B70.

In Vivo Northern Blot Analysis

Total RNA from ten glioblastoma tissues was tested in a Northern blot analysis. None of the glioblastomas expressed mRNA for B7 or B70 molecules (data not shown).

Table 1. B7 and B70 immunoreactivity in tumor cells and tumor-associated macrophages (CD68+).

Case number	Tumor B7	Cells B70	MAb at tumor border[a] B7	B70	MAb among tumor cells[b] B7	B70	MAb in necrotic area[a] B7	B70
724	−	−			−	−	−	+
735	−	−			−	−		
769	−	−			−	−	−	−
817	−	−			−	−	−	−
827	−	−	+	+	−	−		
829	−	−			−	−		
832	−	−			−	−	−	+
835	−	−					+	+
849	−	−					−	−
859	−	−			−	−	+	+
887	NT[c]	−	NT	+	NT	−	NT	
894	−	−			−	−		
902	−	−			−	−	−	−
906	−	−	−	+	−	−		
912	−	−	−	+	−	−	−	−
913	−	−	−	−	−	−		
929	−	−			−	−	−	+
943	−	−			−	−		
946	−	−	+	+	−	−	−	−
963	−	NT		NT	−	NT	−	NT
966	−	NT	−	NT	+	NT	+	NT
971	−	NT		NT			−	NT
975	−	NT		NT	−	NT	−	NT
Total[c]	0/22	0/19	2/6	5/6	1/22	0/19	3/15	5/11

MAb, monoclonal antibody; NT, not tested.

[a] Blank indicates that there was no evaluable tumor border or necrotic area in the tissue specimen tested.

[b] Blank indicates that no CD68+ macrophages were observed.

[c] Total of positive cases/evaluated cases.

Discussion

The T-cell costimulatory molecules B7 and B70 have been demonstrated to play quite important roles in both recognition and effector phases of immunological response [4]. However, expression of these molecules in the central nervous system (CNS) has not been studied to date.

It was previously considered that astrocytes were capable of presenting antigen and stimulating helper T cells [18]. Astrocytes have a phagocytotic activity and express MHC class II molecules, at least in vitro. However, there has been no direct evidence that astrocytes can present antigen to T cells in a class II MHC-restricted manner, and thus this idea has recently been questioned [19]. The inability of astrocytes to express the B7/B70 costimulatory molecules, as was shown by the current results, further indicates that astrocytes do not function as professional antigen-presenting cells (APC). It appears that macrophages and microglial cells, instead of astrocytes, can present antigens to helper T cells in the CNS. In addition to the ability to present an antigen on MHC class II molecules [20], our results demonstrate that macrophages/

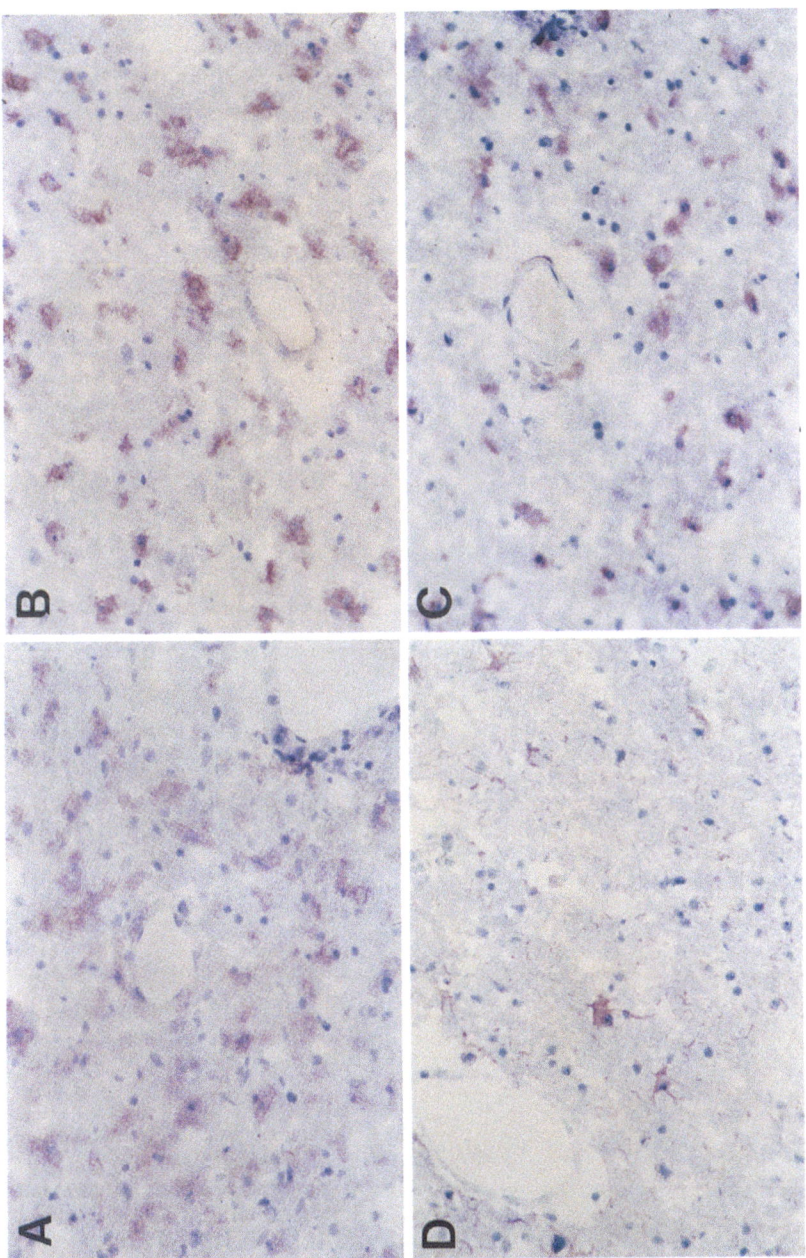

Fig. 3A–D. Immunohistochemistry at the border zone of a glioblastoma with (A) anti-B7 MAb, (B) anti-B70 MAb, (C) anti-CD68 MAb, and (D) anti-GFAP (glial fibrally active protein) MAb. Note that the staining pattern of B7 and B70 molecules is the same as that of C68, but different from that of GFAP, indicating that positive cells are macrophages

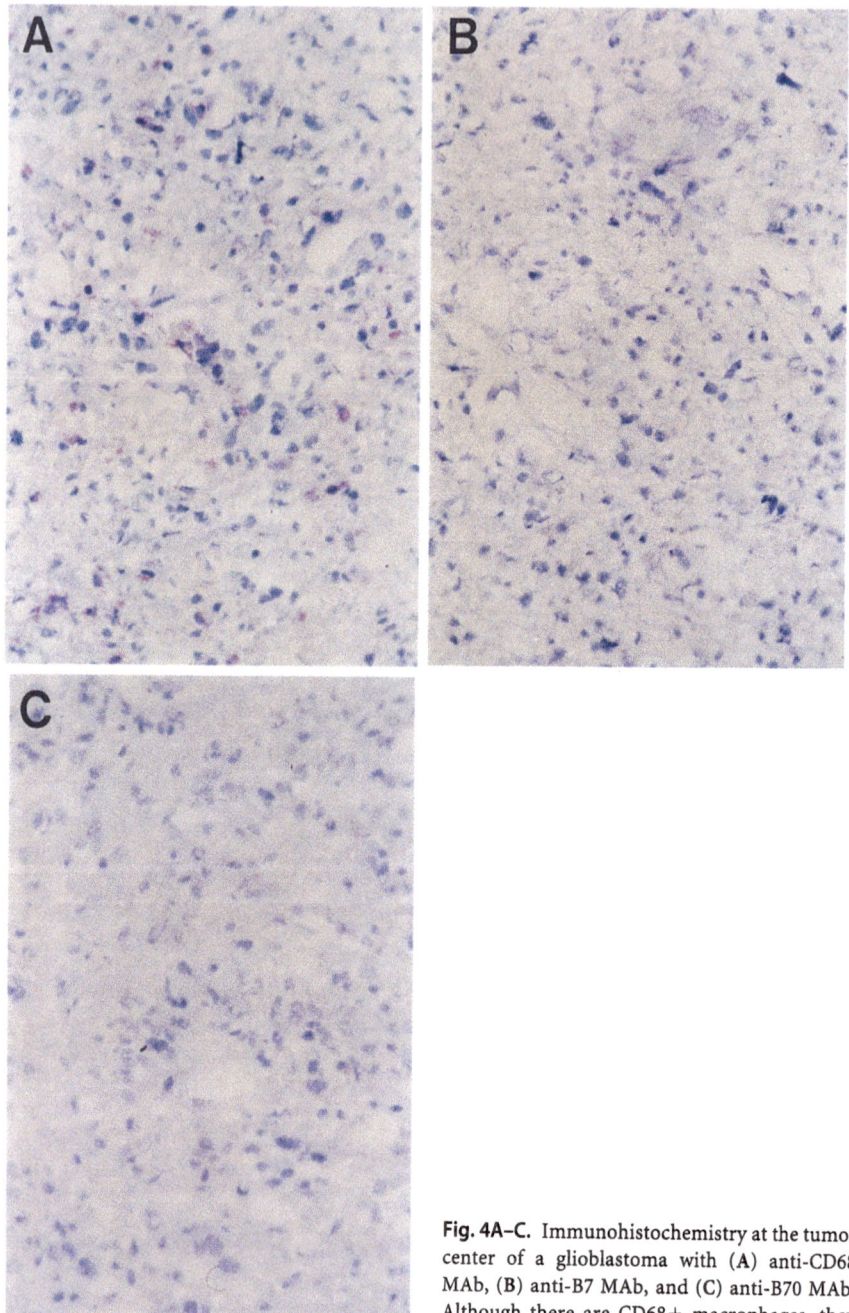

Fig. 4A–C. Immunohistochemistry at the tumor center of a glioblastoma with (A) anti-CD68 MAb, (B) anti-B7 MAb, and (C) anti-B70 MAb. Although there are CD68+ macrophages, they are negative for B7 and B70 molecules

microglial cells can express B7/B70 costimulatory molecules at least in the tumor border or necrotic area of glioblastomas.

It was found, however, that the CD68+ macrophages associated with the proliferating glioblastoma cells did not express either B7 or B70 molecules, suggesting a profound suppression of the expression. Although regulation of B7/B70 expression is not yet well known, it has been reported that interleukin 10 (IL-10) strongly suppresses the expression of B7 molecule in monocytes and macrophages [21]. It is known that glioblastoma cells express IL-10 mRNA in vitro and in vivo [22,23]. Thus, it is possible that certain glioblastoma-derived cytokines including IL-10 cause the suppression of B7/B70 expression in macrophages at the proliferating center of glioblastomas.

A variety of mechanisms by which glioblastomas evade host immune surveillance are known [24], and production of transforming growth factor-β_2 (TGE-β_2) is the most significant of these. TGF-β profoundly suppresses the systemic immunity of glioblastoma patients. It is known that there is a selective depletion of T lymphocytes, especially CD4+/CD45RA+ naive helper T cells, in the peripheral blood of the patients [25], as well as in the population of tumor-infiltrating T lymphocytes. Antigen presentation by APC to helper T cells in glioblastomas is thus compromised from both the APC side (suppressed B7/B70) and the T-cell side.

Glioblastoma cells express MHC class II molecules (HLA-DR) in vitro and in vivo (about 40%) [26,27]. Glioblastoma cells are at least partially capable of presenting antigen in an MHC class II-dependent manner [28]. However, it is unlikely that glioblastoma cells, which lack B7/B70 expression, present self-antigens effectively to helper T cells. Contrarily, it might induce an anergic state of T cells [29]. The expression of MHC class II molecules in glioblastoma cells seems to be a negative prognostic factor [30]. On the other hand, CD8+ cytotoxic T lymphocytes (CTL) need an antigen presented on MHC class I and engagement of CTLA4 or CD28 by B7/B70 molecules to recognize and kill target cells [5]. CTL cannot kill the tumor cells that do not express the MHC class I molecule [31]. In gliomas, in vivo expression of MHC class I molecules (heavy chains HLA-A, -B, -C) is very low [26,32]. Thus, this effector phase also does not seem to work effectively in glioblastomas. It is concluded that the future direction of immunotherapy of glioblastomas should include a modification of these defects in host immunity by means of biological response modifiers or gene therapy.

References

1. Schwartz RH (1990) A cell culture model for T lymphocyte clonal anergy. Science 248:1349–1356
2. Mueller DL, Jenkins MK, Schwartz RH (1989) Clonal expansion versus functional clonal inactivation: a costimulatory signaling pathway determines the outcome of T cell antigen receptor occupancy. Annu Rev Immunol 7:445–480
3. van Seventer GA, Shimizu Y, Shaw S (1991) Roles of multiple accessory molecules in T-cell activation: bilateral interplay of adhesion and costimulation. Curr Opin Immunol 3:294–303
4. June CH, Bluestone JA, Nadler LM, Thompson CB (1994) The B7 and CD28 receptor families. Immunol Today 15:321–331
5. Ramarathinam L, Castle M, Wu Y, Liu Y (1994) T cell costimulation by B7/BB1 induces CD8 T cell-dependent tumor rejection: an important role of B7/BB1 in the induction, recruitment, and effector function of antitumor T cells. J Exp Med 179:1205–1214
6. Azuma M, Cayabyab M, Phillips JH, Lanier LL (1993) Requirements for CD28-dependent T cell-mediated cytotoxicity. J Immunol 150:2091–2101

7. Azuma M, Cayabyab M, Buck D, Phillips JH, Lanier LL (1992) Involvement of CD28 in MHC-unrestricted cytotoxicity mediated by a human natural killer leukemia cell line. J Immunol 149:1115–1123

8. Azuma M, Ito D, Yagita H, Okumura K, Phillips JH, Lanier LL, Somoza C (1993) B70 antigen is a second ligand for CTLA-4 and CD28. Nature 366:76–79

9. Freeman GJ, Gribben JG, Boussiotis VA, Ng JW, Restivo VA Jr, Lombard LA, Gray GS, Nadler LM (1993) Cloning of B7-2: a CTLA-4 counterreceptor that costimulates human T cell proliferation. Science 262:909–911

10. Chen L, Asha S, Brady WA, Hellstroem I, Ledbetter JA, McGowan P, Linsley PS (1992) Co-stimulation of anti-tumor immunity by the B7 counter-receptor for the lymphocyte molecules CD28 and CTLA-4. Cell 71:1093–1102

11. Townsend SE, Allison JP (1993) Tumor rejection after direct co-stimulation of CD8+ T cells by B7-transfected melanoma cells. Science 259:368–370

12. Baskar S, Ostrand-Rosenberg S, Nabavi N, Nadler LM, Freeman GJ, Glimcher LH (1993) Constitutive expression of B7 restores immunogenicity of tumor cells expressing truncated major-histocompatibility-complex-class-II molecules. Proc Natl Acad Sci USA 90:5687–5690

13. Li Y, McGowan P, Hellstroem I, Hellstroem KE, Chen L (1994) Costimulation of tumor-reactive CD4+ and CD8+ T lymphocytes by B7, a natural ligand for CD28, can be used to treat established mouse melanoma. J Immunol 153:421–428

14. Garrido F, Cabrera T, Concha A, Glew S, Ruiz-Cabello F, Stern PL (1993) Natural history of HLA expression during tumour development. Immunol Today 14:491–499

15. Zuber P, Accolla RS, Carrel S, Diserens AC, de Tribolet N (1988) Effects of recombinant human tumor necrosis factor-α on the surface phenotype and the growth of human malignant glioma cell lines. Int J Cancer 42:780–786

16. Chomczynski P, Sacchi N (1987) Single-step method of RNA isolation by acid guanidinium thiocyanate-phenol-chloroform extraction. Anal Biochem 162:156–159

17. Azuma M, Cayabyab M, Buck D, Phillips JH, Lanier LL (1992) CD28 interaction with B7 co-stimulates primary allogeneic proliferative responses and cytotoxicity mediated by small, resting T lymphocytes. J Exp Med 175:353–360

18. Sun D, Wekerle H (1986) Ia-restricted encephalitogenic T lymphocytes mediating EAE lyse autoantigen-presenting astrocytes. Nature 320:70–72

19. Mucke L, Eddleston M (1993) Astrocytes in infectious and immune-mediated diseases of the central nervous system. FASEB J 7:1226–1232

20. Frei K, Lins H, Schwerdel C, Fontana A (1994) Antigen presentation in the central nervous system. The inhibitory effect of IL-10 on MHC class II expression and production of cytokines depends on the inducing signals and the type of cell analyzed. J Immunol 152:2720–2728

21. Willems F, Marchant A, Delville JP, Gerard C, Delvaux A, Velu T, de Boer M, Goldman M (1994) Interleukin-10 inhibits B7 and intercellular adhesion molecule-1 expression on human monocytes. Eur J Immunol 24:1007–1009

22. Merlo A, Juretic A, Zuber M, Filgueira L, Luscher U, Caetano V, Ulrich J, Gratzl O, Heberer M, Spagnoli GC (1993) Cytokine gene expression in primary brain tumours, metastases and meningiomas suggests specific transcription patterns. Eur J Cancer 29A:2118–2125

23. Nitta T, Hishii M, Sato K, Okumura K (1994) Selective expression of interleukin 10 gene within glioblastoma multiforme. Brain Res 649:122–128

24. Tada M, de Tribolet N (1993) Recent advances in immunobiology of brain tumors. J Neuro-oncol 17:261–271

25. Bhondeley MK, Mehra RD, Mehra NK, Mohapatra AK, Tandon PN, Roy S, Bijlani V (1988) Imbalances in T cell subpopulations in human gliomas. J Neurosurg 68:589–593

26. Lampson LA, Hickey WF (1986) Monoclonal antibody analysis of MHC expression in human brain biopsies: tissue ranging from "histologically normal" to that showing different levels of glial tumor involvement. J Immunol 136:4054–4062

27. Couldwell WT, de Tribolet N, Antel JP, Gauthier T, Kuppner MC (1992) Adhesion molecules and malignant gliomas: implications for tumorigenesis. J Neurosurg 76:782–791

28. Daeubener W, Zennati SS, Wernet P, Bilzer T, Fischer HG, Hadding U (1992) Human glioblastoma cell line 86HG39 activates T cells in an antigen-specific major histocompatibility complex class II-dependent manner. J Neuroimmunol 41:21–28
29. Lanzavecchia A (1993) Identifying strategies for immune intervention. Science 260:937–944
30. Jennings MT, Ebrahim SAD, Thaler HT, Jennings VDL, Asadourian LLH, Shapiro J (1989) Immunophenotypic differences between normal glia, astrocytomas and malignant gliomas: correlation with karyotype, natural history and survival. J Neuroimmunol 25:7–28
31. Main EK, Monos DS, Lampson LA (1988) IFN-treated neuroblastoma cell lines remain resistant to T cell mediated allo-killing and susceptible to non-MHC restricted cytotoxicity. J Immunol 141:2943–2950
32. Morioka T, Baba T, Black KL, Streit WJ (1992) Immunophenotypic analysis of infiltrating leukocytes and microglia in an experimental rat glioma. Acta Neuropathol 83:590–597

Clinical Trials with Interferon-Alpha as a Chemosensitizer in Gliomas

Jan C. Buckner

Abstract. To assess the efficacy of recombinant interferon-alpha (IFN-rα) combined with carmustine (BCNU) and other agents, we performed four prospective clinical trials. Of 35 patients with recurrent glioma who were given BCNU and IFN-rα, 29% experienced regression with a median duration of 10.1 months; 37% of nonresponders remained stable for more than 6 months. By contrast, the combination of IFN-rα and alpha-dimethylornithine (DFMO) produced no responses in 29 patients with recurrent glioma. We then completed a phase I study of 15 patients with newly diagnosed grade 3 or 4 glioma [World Health Organization (WHO) classification] treated with radiation, BCNU, and IFN-rα. In that study, IFN-rα 12×10^6 units/m^2 s.c. on days 1–3 of each week produced excessive fatigue, weight loss, and confusion, but patients could tolerate IFN-rα at 12×10^6 units/m^2 given on days 1–3 of weeks 1, 3, and 5 of each 7-week cycle with BCNU given at $150\,mg/m^2$ on day 3 every 7 weeks. Eight patients had grade 4 gliomas and 7 had grade 3 gliomas. For the 4 evaluable grade 4 patients, the mean survival time was 24.6 months (range, 12.6–44.7 months); 3 of the 7 grade 3 patients remained alive for 50.2+ to 55.5+ months without tumor recurrence. We are conducting a prospective phase III trial in which all patients first receive radiation plus BCNU then are randomized to BCNU alone or BCNU plus IFN-rα. To date, 383 patients have been registered on the study and 274 have been randomized. Toxicity with the IFN-rα regimen has been pronounced, consisting of flu-like symptoms, confusion, and somnolence. Survival data are not yet sufficiently established to be reported.

Key words. Brain neoplasm—Interferon—BCNU—Difluoromethylornithine—Radiotherapy

Introduction

The interferons are a diverse group of glycoproteins with antiviral, antiproliferative, immunomodulatory, and cytotoxic properties [1]. Clinical trials with interferon-alpha as a single agent have suggested some activity in glioma patients. Nakagawa et al. [2] reported responses in two of eight patients with recurrent glioblastoma given intratumoral interferon-alpha via an Ommaya reservoir. Subsequently, Nagai and

Department of Oncology, Division of Medical Oncology, Mayo Clinic and Foundation, Mayo Medical School, Rochester, MN 55905, USA

Arai [3] reported responses in 8 of 20 patients with residual or recurrent high-grade glioma who were given intratumoral or systemic beta interferon, 1 of 3 patients given intramuscular lymphoblastoid interferon (which is composed predominantly of interferon-alpha), and 2 of 9 patients given intramuscular recombinant human alpha interferon (IFN-rα). Then, Mahaley et al. [4] performed a phase II study in patients with recurrent gliomas in which lymphoblastoid interferon was administered either intravenously or intramuscularly in escalating doses daily for 3 consecutive days each week, then for 5 consecutive days each week. With this schedule, the authors reported objective responses in 7 of 17 evaluable patients. These studies suggested at least modest antitumor activity of interferon-alpha in recurrent glioma.

Preclinical investigations identified therapeutic synergism of interferons when combined with carnustine (BCNU) in murine leukemia [5] as well as in melanoma and renal carcinoma cell lines [6]. In a phase I trial, Creagan et al. [6] demonstrated that near-maximal doses of BCNU and IFN-rα could be safely administered to patients with various malignancies, even in the face of prior chemotherapy and radiation. In that study, patients received IFN-rα at 12×10^6 units/m^2 intramuscularly three times a week with BCNU doses up to $150\,mg/m^2$ every 4 weeks. Dose-limiting toxicities were fatigue, related to interferon, and myelosuppression, related predominantly to BCNU.

Combinations of IFN-rα with other agents have also demonstrated additive or synergistic antiproliferative effects. In particular, preclinical studies using cell culture techniques as well as studies of tumor xenografts in nude mice have suggested synergy of IFN-rα and alpha-difluoromethylornithine (DFMO), a reversible inhibitor of ornithine decarboxylase [7–10]. Subsequently, two phase I studies identified clinically tolerable treatment regimens [11,12].

On the basis of the preclinical data and phase I studies just mentioned, we performed two phase II clinical trials in patients with recurrent glioma, using first IFN-rα plus BCNU, then IFN-rα plus DFMO. Subsequently, we conducted a phase I trial in patients with newly diagnosed high-grade gliomas to determine the tolerability, safety, and utility of IFN-rα with BCNU and radiation therapy. Based upon these results, we recently completed a phase III trial comparing radiation and BCNU with radiation, BCNU, and IFN-rα in patients with high-grade glioma. We review the results of each of these trials separately.

Phase II Evaluation of Recombinant Interferon-Alpha and BCNU in Recurrent Glioma

Because BCNU is one of the most active single agents available for the treatment of patients with gliomas, we attempted to improve its efficacy by adding IFN-rα as a chemosensitizer. Using the phase I results of Creagan et al. [6], we initiated a clinical trial for patients with recurrent glioma [13]. To be eligible for this trial, patients must be 18 years of age or older, with histological confirmation of astrocytoma, oligodendroglioma, or oligoastrocytoma of any grade with computed tomography (CT) or magnetic resonance imaging (MRI) scan evidence of tumor progression following radiation therapy, but no prior chemotherapy. Measurable or evaluable tumor on CT or MRI scan was required. If patients required corticosteroids, the dose must have been stable for at least 1 week before entry into the study. Patients also must have had adequate bone marrow, hepatic, and renal function.

Our hypothesis, at the time the study began, was that IFN- rα was acting primarily as a chemosensitizer of BCNU. Therefore, treatment consisted of IFN-rα at 12×10^6 units/m² intramuscularly days on 1–3; this was followed by BCNU, 150 mg/m² intravenously, on day 3. Cycles were repeated every 6 weeks for 1 year, then every 10 weeks for a second year. Treatment was discontinued at the time tumor progression or if excessive toxicity occurred or after 2 years if there was no evidence of tumor progression.

Assessment of response was based upon CT or MRI scans, which were obtained before every second treatment, and by neurological examination. Complete regression was defined as disappearance of all visible tumor. Partial regression was defined as greater than 50% reduction in the product of perpendicular diameters of the clearly demarcated contrast-enhancing mass. Patients with tumors that were not bidimensionally measurable, but which were clearly evaluable for response to therapy, were considered to have a regression if there was unequivocal reduction in the size of contrast enhancement or decrease in mass effect. Patients must have remained on a stable or decreased dose of corticosteroids and must have remained neurologically stable or improved to qualify for regression. Progression indicated an increase of more than 25% in the product of perpendicular diameters of the mass, unequivocal increase in the size of the contrast-enhancing lesion, or increase in the mass effect. Neurological worsening despite two sequential stable CT or MRI scans also constituted progression.

Between October 1986 and August 1988, 35 patients from ten institutions were entered into this study. Patient characteristics are given in Table 1. Of note, most of the patients entered into this trial had low-grade or anaplastic astrocytoma. Slightly fewer than one-fourth of patients had either oligodendroglioma or oligoastrocytoma. Two of the 10 patients with well-circumscribed measurable lesions and 8 of the

Table 1. Characteristics of patients in recurrent glioma study.

Characteristic	n (%)
Gender	
Male	24 (69)
Female	11 (31)
ECOG performance score	
0–1	26 (74)
2–3	9 (26)
Age (years)	
<40	13 (37)
40–60	18 (51)
>60	4 (12)
Tumor grade at diagnosis	
1–2	20 (57)
3	9 (26)
4	5 (14)
Biopsy at recurrence only	1 (3)
Tumor histology	
Astrocytoma	27 (77)
Oligodendroglioma	1 (3)
Mixed astrocytoma/oligodendroglioma	7 (20)

ECOG, Eastern Cooperative Oncology Group.

remaining 25 patients with evaluable lesions experienced tumor regression for an overall response rate of 29% (10/35) and a 95% confidence interval estimate of 4%–40%. Thirteen additional patients (37%) remained stable for more than 6 months following study entry. Only 2 patients (6%) evidenced tumor progression at the time of the first evaluation at 6 weeks. Progressive disease was diagnosed for the remaining 10 patients at intervals ranging from 11 weeks to 5.8 months after study entry. In the 10 responders, the time from study entry to tumor progression ranged from 5.3 months to more than 5.6 years, with a median of 10.1 months. For the 10 responders, the minimum survival was 6.5 months; half (5 patients) lived less than 1.4 years while the other half lived more than 2.7 years.

Toxicity was quite acceptable, consisting primarily of moderate myelosuppression, vomiting, and venous irritation from BCNU and the expected flu-like symptoms from interferon. In addition, a substantial portion of patients did develop transient worsening of underlying neurological symptoms such as seizures, hemiparesis, aphasia, confusion, or depressed level of alertness. All these neurological symptoms resolved spontaneously with discontinuation of interferon, but could become dose limiting in schedules requiring daily or thrice weekly administration. While elevation of aspartate aminotransferase (AST) was a frequent laboratory finding, it was not associated with any clinical manifestations. One patient developed polycythemia vera almost 5 years after initiation of therapy and remains alive without tumor recurrence.

Given the respectable proportion of patients who experienced tumor regression and stabilization, we concluded that the combination of IFN-rα warranted further study in the setting of newly diagnosed high-grade glioma patients.

Phase II Study of Recombinant Interferon-Alpha and Alpha-Difluoromethylornithine in Patients with Recurrent Glioma

While we were studying the combination of IFN-rα with BCNU, as just described, we conducted a separate trial using IFN-rα and α-difluoromethylornithine (DFMO) in patients with recurrent glioma (Buckner et al., unpublished manuscript). Polyamines are involved with normal cellular growth and differentiation [14] and have been found in increased quantities in malignant human brain tumor compared with normal brain tissue or benign brain tumors [15,16]. DFMO blocks polyamine synthesis by irreversible inhibition of the enzyme ornithine decarboxylase and has been shown to inhibit glioma cell growth in vitro [17]. A clinical trial of DFMO with BCNU [18] has suggested potential synergy of these agents in the treatment of patients with glioma. Using renal carcinoma and melanoma cell lines, Kovach and Svingen [10] reported synergistic antiproliferative activity of IFN-rα and DFMO in cell cultures. Subsequently, Edmonson et al. [12] performed a phase I trial, which identified a safe and tolerable schedule of IFN-rα and DFMO. We then performed the following phase II trial to determine the efficacy of IFN-rα and DFMO in patients with recurrent glioma, using the dose and schedule established in the phase I trial.

With the exception that patients may have received prior chemotherapy in this trial, the eligibility criteria and criteria for determining response were identical to the study described previously utilizing IFN-rα and BCNU. In this study, patients received IFN-rα at 36×10^6 units/m^2 s.c. on days 1–7 and DFMO at 2.25 g/m^2 orally four times a day with IFN-rα on days 3–7. Cycles were repeated every 4 weeks until tumor progression or intolerable side effects occurred.

The 29 patients who entered the study included 17 men and 12 women. The median age at study entry was 40 years, ranging from 22 to 70. The Eastern Cooperative Oncology Group (ECOG) performance score was 0 or 1 in 22 patients and 2 or 3 in 7 patients. At initial diagnosis, tumor grade was 1 or 2 in 14 patients, grade 3 or 4 in 14 patients, and unknown in 1 patient. Twenty-two patients had received tumor resection or biopsy at the time of tumor recurrence, providing histological confirmation of tumor; 10 patients had received no prior chemotherapy.

Evidence of toxicity consisted primarily of flu-like symptoms, including fever (82%), chills (76%), lethargy (72%), and myalgias (70%). Nausea occurred commonly (59%) as did vomiting (34%), but was severe in only 10% of patients. Generalized weakness occurred in 41% of patients, and 20% complained of headaches associated with treatment. Neurocortical toxicity, consisting primarily of somnolence and confusion occurred commonly (72%). Fatal toxicity occurred in one patient who became comatose approximately 2 h after the first injection of IFN-rα. At hospitalization, she had evidence of uncal herniation and subsequently died. Hematological toxicity was minimal, consisting of leukocyte nadirs less than 2000/mcl in four patients, none less than 1000/mcl. Similarly, mild thrombocytopenia (platelet nadirs 75 000–100 000/mcl) occurred in five patients.

There was no CT or MRI scan evidence of tumor shrinkage in any patient. Median time to tumor progression was 58 days, and median survival was 213 days. Given that the patients were young and that half had low-grade tumors initially, it is not surprising that the median survival is relatively long in relation to the time to progression. Only one patient remains alive currently. The lack of tumor shrinkage suggests either that the combination of IFN-rα and DFMO is ineffective, or that the doses and schedule used in this protocol were suboptimal. It is possible that lower doses administered on a more frequent basis would be useful.

Pilot Evaluation of Irradiation Combined with Recombinant Interferon-Alpha and BCNU for Primary High-Grade Brain Tumors

Because IFN-rα and BCNU produced durable responses in a reasonable portion of patients with recurrent glioma, and because radiation and BCNU are commonly used to treat patients with high-grade glioma, we performed the following pilot study to determine the appropriate dose and accompanying toxicity in patients with newly diagnosed high-grade glioma [19].

Patients with histological proof of grade 3 or 4 astrocytoma or oligoastrocytoma who were at least 18 years old were eligible to participate in this trial, assuming adequate bone marrow, renal, and hepatic function and the absence of other major medical problems. Initially, patients received radiation therapy consisting of 6480 cGy in 36 fractions along with BCNU, 200 mg/m² intravenously with the first day of radiation. On completion of radiation, patients received IFN-rα at 12×10^6 u/m² s.c. on days 1–3 each week, plus BCNU at 150 mg/m² intravenously on day 3 every 7 weeks. These dosages of IFN-rα and BCNU were repeated for six cycles or until tumor progression or excessive toxicity occurred.

We treated 11 patients with radiation, IFN-rα, and BCNU. Four additional patients, all with grade 4 astrocytoma, enrolled but did not receive IFN-rα. Two patients refused IFN-rα after completing radiation; one patient experienced a major pulmonary embolus that precluded further treatment, and the fourth experienced a fatal myocardial infarction before initiation of IFN-rα. Excessive fatigue occurred with weekly IFN-rα, but treatment was tolerable when IFN-rα was given at weeks 1, 3, and 5 of each 7-week cycle. Myelosuppression was dose limiting with median leukocyte and platelet nadirs being 2000/mcl and 80 000/mcl, respectively. Other toxicities included fever, chills, and myalgias (100%), headache (64%), vomiting (91%), and transient confusion (64%) on the days of IFN-rα administration. Delayed radiotherapy effects included optic atrophy and hemorrhagic infarct (1 patient), radionecrosis (1 patient), and transient hemiparesis and aphasia (1 patient), which resolved with corticosteroids.

All patients who had grade 4 astrocytoma have died. Median and mean survival times were 12.6 and 16.0 months, respectively, including those patients who never received IFN-rα. The four patients with grade 4 astrocytoma who received IFN-rα lived 12.6, 12.7, 29.0, and 44.7 months. In patients with grade 3 astrocytoma or oligoastrocytoma, median and mean survival times were 50.2 and 43.3+ months, respectively, with three patients remaining alive without evidence of tumor progression at 50.2+, 52.4+, and 55.5+ months from study entry. There has been no late neurological toxicity in these long-term survivors. One woman developed galactorrhea and amenorrhea with hyperprolactinemia. Pituitary appearance on CT scan was normal, suggesting hypothalamic damage with loss of suppression of pituitary prolactin production. The symptoms of hyperprolactinemia have been controlled with bromocriptine.

In summary, we identified a safe and tolerable combination of radiation, IFN-rα, and BCNU in this small sample of patients with high-grade glioma. Dose-limiting toxicities are myelosuppression and flu-like symptoms. Transient confusion was common, but mild and reversible. Late neurological sequelae have been minimal. Given the small sample size, we cannot determine the extent to which IFN-rα impacted upon survival. Therefore, we embarked on a phase III trial to determine if there is any survival benefit of adding IFN-rα to radiation and BCNU for patients with high-grade glioma.

Phase III Study of Radiation Therapy plus BCNU with or Without Recombinant Interferon-Alpha in the Treatment of Newly Diagnosed High-Grade Gliomas

In April 1990, the North Central Cancer Treatment Group activated a phase III clinical trial for adult patients with newly diagnosed grade 3 or 4 astrocytoma, oligoastrocytoma, or gliosarcoma. As in the pilot trial discussed earlier, patients must have had satisfactory bone marrow, renal, and hepatic function and no other significant comorbid diseases. Patients were entered into the study within 4 weeks after surgery. Patients were stratified by age, extent of tumor resection, tumor grade, tumor histology, ECOG performance score, and treating institution.

All patients began treatment with radiation (6480 cGy in 36 fractions to the contrast-enhanced tumor plus edema plus a 2-cm margin) and BCNU at 200 mg/m^2 intravenously with the first day of radiation. Patients who remained stable or experienced tumor regression following radiation were then randomized to receive either BCNU alone or IFN-rα plus BCNU. When given alone, BCNU was given at 200 mg/m^2 intravenously every 7 weeks for six additional cycles. When BCNU and IFN-rα were combined, patients received IFN-rα at 12×10^6 u/m² s.c on days 1–3 of weeks 1, 3, and 5 of each 7-week cycle, plus BCNU at 150 mg/m² intravenously on day 3 with IFN-rα every 7 weeks for six cycles. Dose modifications were based on hematological, renal, hepatic, pulmonary, cardiac, and constitutional symptoms Patients received antiemetic, anticonvulsant, and corticosteroid medications based on the judgment of the individual physician.

Between April 1990 and July 1994, 383 patients were registered to the trial. To date, 274 patients have been randomized to the two treatment arms of which 268 patients (134 in each arm) are eligible. Unexpectedly, approximately 28% of patients registered to the trial did not proceed to randomization. The most common reasons for not being randomized were tumor progression, patient refusal, or death. The protocol closed in July 1994 because accrual goals had been met. Treatment of these patients continues, and data are not sufficiently mature to assess the impact of IFN-rα upon survival. However, we can assess the comparative toxicities of the two regimens [20].

As expected, the arm containing IFN-rα experienced more toxic symptoms (Table 2). Flu-like symptoms of fever, chills, lethargy, and myalgia were more common in the IFN-rα group. Similarly, gastrointestinal symptoms of anorexia, nausea, and vomiting were more frequent. Neurological symptoms of headache, neurocortical effects (usually somnolence and confusion), and seizures thought to be related to treatment were all more common with IFN-rα. By contrast, pulmonary toxicity and venous toxicity at the site of chemotherapy administration, although uncommon in both groups, were slightly more common in the BCNU-alone group.

Hematological toxicity was nearly equal in the two groups, with median leukocyte and platelet nadirs in the BCNU-alone group being 2500/mcl and 68 000/mcl, respectively, compared with 2400/mcl and 69 500 mcl, respectively, in the IFN-rα plus BCNU group. Of note, this equitoxic myelosuppression occurred despite a reduction in the dose of BCNU by 25% when IFN-rα was added, confirming pilot data suggesting that BCNU can be safely escalated only to 150 mg/m² when given with IFN-rα.

There have been fatal toxicities in seven patients to date. One patient developed neutropenia and sepsis following the first dose of BCNU before randomization to pastradiation treatment. In the randomized portion of the study, three treatment-

Table 2. Toxicities of patients treated on phase III trial of radiation versus radiation, BCNU, and IFN-rα.

Toxicity	BCNU alone % (n = 124)	IFN-rα + BCNU % (n = 124)
Fever	2	61
Chills	2	55
Lethargy	10	46
Myalgias	1	37
Neurocortical	7	37
Seizures	2	13
Headache	2	23
Anorexia	12	23
Nausea	24	56
Vomiting	15	40
Pulmonary	5	1
IV site toxicity	15	7

BCNU, carmustine; IFN-rα, recombinant inter feron-alpha.

related deaths have occurred in each arm. With BCNU alone, one patient died of each of the following causes: neutropenia with sepsis, intracranial hemorrhage from thrombocytopenia, and radiation necrosis. With IFN-rα plus BCNU, one patient died from neutropenia with sepsis and two died from radiation necrosis.

In summary, considerable toxicity is associated with the combination of radiation, IFN-rα, and BCNU, including flu-like symptoms, gastrointestinal toxicity, and reversible neurocortical toxicity. Myelosuppression is approximately equivalent to that seen with BCNU alone when the dose of BCNU is decreased by 25% in combination with IFN-rα. The proportion of fatal toxicity is low (2%), with either radiation and BCNU or radiation, IFN-rα, and BCNU, but fatal toxicity can occur. The subjective toxicities experienced by the patients will have to be counterbalanced by significant gains in survival to justify adding IFN-rα to radiation and BCNU at the dose and schedule used in this protocol. Survival analysis awaits further patient follow-up.

Conclusion

Interferon-alpha remains an interesting experimental agent in the treatment of primary brain tumors. Preclinical observations suggesting synergy with agents known to be effective in the treatment of gliomas suggest that additional clinical trials are warranted. Our studies have shown that moderately high doses of IFN-rα may be given safely in combination with BCNU and DFMO for recurrent glioma and with radiation and BCNU for newly diagnosed high-grade glioma; however, toxicity including flu-like symptoms, nausea and vomiting, and reversible encephalopathic changes is prominent at the doses used, and further escalation of dose is unlikely to be feasible. On the contrary, smaller doses may be necessary for sustained utilization of the drug in combination with other agents. The 10-month median duration of response with BCNU and IFN-rα in patients with recurrent glioma is encouraging, but the contribution of IFN-rα in producing those results is unknown. While survival in patients with grade 3 and grade 4 gliomas who received radiation, IFN-rα, and BCNU as part of our pilot trial is encouraging, the small sample size does not permit meaningful conclusions regarding the influence of IFN-rα. Results from the recently completed phase III trial comparing radiation and BCNU with radiation, IFN-rα, and BCNU satisfactorily document the safety and toxicity of the regimen and will eventually determine whether IFN-rα improves survival in patients with high-grade glioma.

References

1. Borden EC, Ball LA (1981) Interferon: biochemical, cell growth inhibitory, and immunological effects. Prog Hematol 12:299–339
2. Nakagawa Y, Hirakawa K, Ueda S, Suzuki K, Fukuma S, Kishida T, Imanishi J, Amagai T (1983) Local administration of interferon for malignant brain tumors. Cancer Treat Rep 67:833–835
3. Nagai M, Arai T (1984) Clinical effect of interferon in malignant brain tumours. Neurosurg Rev 7:55–64
4. Mahaley MS Jr, Urso MB, Whaley RA, Blue M, Williams TE, Guaspori A, Selker RG (1985) Immunobiology of primary intracranial tumors. Part 10: Therapeutic efficacy of interferon in the treatment of recurrent gliomas. J Neurosurg 63:719–725
5. Chirigos MA, Pearson JW (1973) Cure of murine leukemia with drug and interferon treatment. JNCI 51:1367–1368, 1973

6. Creagan ET, Kovach JS, Long HJ, Richardson RL (1986) Phase I study of recombinant leukocyte A human interferon combined with BCNU in selected patients with advanced cancer. J Clin Oncol 4:408–413

7. Sunkara PS, Prakash NJ, Mayer GD, Sjoerdsma A (1983) Tumor suppression with a combination of α-difluoromethyl ornithine and interferon. Science 219:851–853

8. Rosenblum MG, Gutterman JU (1984) Synergistic antiproliferative activity of leukocyte interferon in combination with α-difluoromethylornithine against human cells in culture. Cancer Res 44:2339–2340

9. Heston WDW, Fleischmann J, Tackett RE, Ratliff TL (1984) Effects of α-difluoromethylornithine and recombinant interferon-α_2 on the growth of a human renal cell adenocarcinoma xenograft in nude mice. Cancer Res 44:3220–3225

10. Kovach JS, Svingen PA (1985) Enhancement of the antiproliferative activity of human interferon by polyamine depletion. Cancer Treat Rep 69:97–103

11. Talpaz M, Plager C, Quesada J, Benjamin R, Kantarjian H, Gutterman J (1986) Difluoromethylornitihine and leukocyte interferon: a phase I study in cancer patients. Eur J Cancer Clin Oncol 22:685–689

12. Edmonson J, Kovach J, Buckner J, Kvols L, Hahn R (1988) Phase I study of difluoromethylornithine (DFMO) in combination with recombinant alpha-2a-interferon. Cancer Res 48:6584–6586

13. Buckner JC, Brown LD, Cascino TL, O'Fallon JR, Scheithauer BW (1995) Phase II Evaluation of recombinant interferon alpha and BCNU in recurrent glioma. J Neurosurg 82:430–435

14. Pegg AE, McCann PP (1982) Polyamine metabolism and function. Am J Physiol 243: (Cell Physiol 12:)C212–C221

15. Harik SI, Sutton CH (1979) Putrescine as a biochemical marker of malignant brain tumors. Cancer Res 39:5010–5015

16. Yamakazi H, Tsukahara T, Uki J, Matsuzaki S (1986) Elevated levels of free putrescine and N^1-acetylspermidine in cyst fluids of malignant brain tumours. J Neurol Neurosurg Psychiatry 49:209–210

17. Barranco SC, Ford PJ, Townsend CM Jr (1989) Heterogeneous survival and cell kinetics responses of human astrocytoma clones to α-difluoromethylornithine in vitro. Invest New Drugs 7:155–161

18. Prados M, Rodriguez L, Chamberlain M, Silver P, Levin V (1989) Treatment of recurrent gliomas with 1,3-bis (2-chloroethyl)-1-nitrosourea and α-difluoromethylornithine. Neurosurgery 24:806–809

19. Buckner JC, Schomberg PJ, Cascino TL, Burch PA, Shaw EG, Dinapoli RP (1992) Pilot evaluation of radiation, BCNU, and interferon-alpha in patients with high-grade astrocytoma. Proc Am Assoc Cancer Res Annu Meet 33:212 (A1269)

20. Buckner JC, Cascino TL, Schomberg PS, O'Fallon JR, Dinapoli RP, Burch PA, Shaw EG (1993) Toxicity of interferon-alpha (IFN-α), BCNU, and radiation (RT) in high-grade glioma patients. J Neurol Oncol 15:S6

Evaluation of Interferon Therapy on Malignant Gliomas

Masakatsu Nagai, Sousi Okuhata, Kunihiko Watanabe, Jun-ichi Narita, Chikayuki Ochiai, and Toshimoto Arai

Abstract. A phase II, multicenter study was conducted by 34 institutions to evaluate the effectiveness of human fibroblast interferon (IFN) in the treatment of patients with malignant gliomas. The response rates to IFN in glioma patients (evaluable cases, $n = 120$), were 14.0% for malignant glioma, 24.0% for low-grade astrocytoma, and 19.2% overall. No significant difference was observed between systemic administration and local administration. There were only mild adverse reactions.

A randomized trial of combination therapy conducted by 20 institutions indicated a significant difference in response rate between IFN + radiation therapy (19.6%; $n = 51$) and IFN + (1,4-amino-2-methyl-5-pyrimidinyl)-methyl-3-(2-chloroethyl)-3-nitrosourea (ACNU) + radiation therapy (IAR) (41.2%; $n = 51$). A prospective study on long-term maintenance therapy using IFN after IAR therapy obtained high survival rates. From the point of view of survival, 72 evaluable cases of malignant glioma (41 glioblastoma [GB] and 31 malignant astrocytoma [MA]) analyzed in our institution showed a distinct difference in survival rates ($P < .001$). There were no significant differences of survival rates of GB and MA when compared with the results of the Brain Tumor Registry in Japan, although high response rates were obtained as an effect of postoperative remission induction therapy (24.4% for GB, 45.5% for MA). There was a significant relationship between tumor size reduction effect and survival rate in the second and third years. Specifically, IAR therapy was effective for prolongation of the survival period of GB.

With regard to age of GB, a group younger than 54 years showed longer survival compared with an older age group (>55 years). In a comparison of cases that underwent subtotal resection and those who received biopsy, the former group had a longer mean survival time, although this was not statistically significant. Maintenance therapy is another important factor for long survival in which IFN also seemed to be beneficial.

Key words. Interferon—Combination therapy—Maintenance therapy—Survival rate—Response rate

Department of Neurosurgery, Dokkyo University School of Medicine, Mibu, Tochigi 321-02, Japan

Introduction

More than 15 years have passed since interferon (IFN) was first put to clinical use for the treatment of malignant gliomas. In 1979, the special study group on the clinical application of IFN of the Japanese Ministry of Health and Welfare was inaugurated in which the authors participated as members of the sectional meeting on tumors. In April 1981, the brain tumor subcommittee started with members from 15 neurosurgical institutions in Japan. In April 1985, the clinical use of human fibroblast IFN for glioblastoma was approved and registered in the Japanese National Health Insurance System.

In January 1986, a multicenter study of combination therapy started as a prospective phase III study by 20 institutions. In May of the same year, a multicenter study on new indications of IFN was also organized. In December 1990, astrocytoma and medulloblastoma were approved as new indications for IFN therapy by the Ministry of Health and Welfare. Meanwhile, in January 1989 a multicenter study by 92 institutions on maintenance therapy using IFN started; it is still going on.

The authors have organized these studies either as chairmen or as members of the organizing committee, and reported the results of the study [1–6]. In this chapter, the evaluation of IFN therapy on glioma from the results of multicenter studies are reported in Part I; the results of cases in our own institution are described in Part II, especially regarding survival rate.

Part I. Results of Multicenter Studies in Japan on Interferon Therapy for Malignant Glioma

Therapy with IFN Alone

Subjects and Methods

Indications and Patient Selection Eligibility Criteria for IFN Therapy

1. The target tumor was glioma including medulloblastoma
2. Indication of the therapy was decided as follows:
    i. Histologically proven patients
    ii. Patients with measurable tumor lesions on computed tomography (CT) scan images
    iii. A 4-week or longer interval before starting the IFN therapy, if the patient was treated with another therapy previously
    iv. Patients who are expected to be alive at least 2 months after the initiation of IFN therapy
    v. Patients whose performance status is 0–3
    vi. Patients without serious complications

Subjects

The evaluable subjects of the study were 57 cases of malignant glioma (46 glioblastoma [GB] and 11 malignant astrocytoma [MA]; mean age was 40.6 years, ranging from 5 to 67 years; 32 men, 25 women), and 63 other cases of gliomas including low-grade astrocytoma, oligodendroglioma, ependymoma, and medulloblastoma. Thirty-four institutions participated in the study.

IFN Preparation Used

Human fibroblast IFN (natural beta type) produced by Toray (Tokyo, Japan) was used in the study. Specific activity of the preparation was greater than 10^7 IU/mg protein.

Dosage and Administration

1. Routes of administration
    i. Intravenous (i.v.) drip infusion: dissolve in 100–250 ml of physiological saline and administer by i.v. drip infusion
    ii. Local injection: dissolve in an appropriate volume of physiological saline (average, 2 ml) and inject into the medullary space (including intratumor injection)
2. Dosage
    i. Usual adult dose is 3×10^6 IU/body/day
    ii. Dosage should be adjusted for children
    iii. IFN should not be used concomitantly with chemotherapy
3. Administration period
    i. An 8-week period is a guideline; administer every day, if possible
    ii. Administration should be continued for at least 6 weeks, even when the tumor size is stable

Assessment of Therapeutic Response

Every patient was assessed as to clinical response to IFN therapy at 8 weeks after starting, by measurement of the size of mass estimated from the tumor shadow on CT scan and employing criteria as follow:

1. Markedly effective (complete remission, CR): disapperance of a measurable or assessable lesion
2. Effective (partial remission, PR): more than 50% tumor reduction or improvement
3. Unchanged (no change, NC): less than 50% tumor reduction or less than 25% exacerbation
4. Progressive disease (PD): more than 25% tumor enlargement

Results

Response Rate

The response rate to the therapy in 120 evaluable cases is given in Table 1. The response rate of malignant glioma (described as glioblastoma in the table) was 14.0%, that for astrocytoma (low grade) was 24.0%, and the overall response rate was 19.2%.

In the group of systemic administration, the response rate was 19.0%, compared to 19.5% with local administration, the difference being not statistically significant.

Side Effects

As reported before [3–5], the main reactions were fever, leukopenia, and hepatic dysfunction, and these reactions were mild enough to reverse in 3–14 days of the rest of the treatment. Such adverse side effects tended to be less frequent with local than with systemic administration of IFN.

Table 1. Response rate of gliomas to human fibroblast interferon.

Route of administration	Pathological Diagnosis	CR	PR	NC	PD	Total	Response rate (%)
i.v. drip infusion	Glioblastoma[a]		3	12	9	24	12.5
	Astrocytoma	1	4	12	6	23	21.7
	Medulloblastoma	3		14		17	17.6
	Others	2	2	7	4	15	26.7
	Subtotal	6	9	45	19	79	19.0
Intrathecal injection	Glioblastoma	1	4	18	10	33	15.2
	Astrocytoma		1	1		2	50.0
	Medulloblastoma		1	2		3	33.3
	Others		1	2		3	33.3
	Subtotal	1	7	23	10	41	19.5
Total	Glioblastoma	1	7	30	19	57	14.0
	Astrocytoma	1	5	13	6	25	24.0
	Medulloblastoma	3	1	16		20	20.0
	Others	2	3	9	4	18	27.8
	Total	7	16	68	29	120	19.2

CR, Complete remission; PR, partial remission; NC, no change (unchanged); PD, progressive disease.
[a] Includes malignant astrocytoma.
$n = 120$.

Combination Therapy with IFN, ACNU, and Radiation (IAR Therapy)

Subjects and Method

Indications, patient selection, IFN preparation, dosage and administration of IFN, and assessment of the therapy are all the same as with therapy with IFN alone.

Regimen of the Therapy

The regimen of phase III trial of comparing two groups of patients is described in Fig. 1. AR means (1,4-amino-2-methyl-5-pyrimidinyl)-methyl-3-(2-chloroethyl)-3-nitrosourea (ACNU) + radiation, while IAR is IFN, ACNU, and radiation therapy. ACNU ($80 \, mg/m^2$) was given intravenously on day 1 and day 36, and the total dosage of radiation was 50–60 Gy. IFN was administered by the same method as mentioned previously.

Subjects

A total of 102 patients with malignant glioma were randomized into two groups (51 cases each) by means of the envelope method. In the AR group, 22 GB and 29 MA (mean age, 52.8 years; range, 21–74 years; 32 men, 19 women) were admitted; in the IAR group, 27 GB and 16 MA (mean age, 49.7 years; range, 15–75 years; 35 men, 16 women) were registered. There were no significant differences between the background of both groups. Twenty institutions participated in this study.

AR : ACNU + Radiation

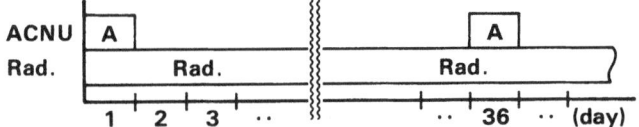

IAR : ACNU + Radiation + Interferon

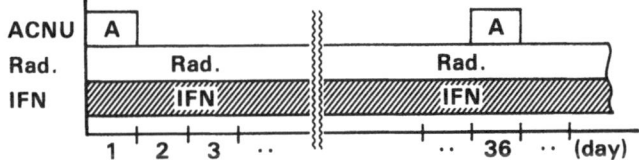

(1) ACNU : 80mg/m², i.v. at day 1 and day 36.
(2) Radiation : total dosis 50–60 Gy.
(3) Interferon-β, (natural type) : 2×10^6 I.U./m², i.v., 5 times/w.
for 8 weeks.

Fig. 1. Regimen of AR therapy and IAR therapy

Table 2. Comparison of response rate in malignant glioma.

Treatment	CR	PR	NC	PD	Response rate, CR + PR (χ^2 test)	
AR ($n = 51$)	3	7	26	15	19.6%	$P < 0.05$
IAR ($n = 51$)	4	17	18	12	41.2%	

AR, ACNU + radiation; IAR, IFN + ACNU + radiation.

Results

Response Rate

Comparison of the response rate of two groups is shown in Table 2. A definite difference is revealed statistically between AR (19.6%) and IAR therapy (41.2%).

Side Effects

Side effects of both AR and IAR therapy tended to be slightly more frequent compared with therapy with IFN alone. There were no significant differences between the side effects of the two groups except for fever in IAR.

Maintenance Therapy

Subjects and Method

A multicenter study on maintenance therapy after the initial remission induction therapy has been conducted since 1991 with the participation of 92 institutions. The patients who were treated by IAR therapy were randomized into two groups. For group A, ACNU was given every 6 weeks, and for group B, the administration of IFN every 1 or 2 weeks was added to ACNU. The doses of ACNU and IFN were same as in the initial therapy. The therapy was continued for as long a period as possible, if there was no tumor progression.

Result

Seventy-eight patients were entered into group A and 81 patients into group B. Up until the present, 1-year and 2-year survival rates of both groups have been analyzed by Kaplan–Meier's method. For group A, the 1-year survival rate was 79.7% and the 2-year rate was 51.1%; for group B, the 1-year rate was 86.3% and the 2-year rate 56.3%. Both groups revealed an extremely high survival rate without a significant difference between them. In both groups, long-surviving cases are increasing in number.

Summary of Part I

1. The response rate to IFN in glioma patients (120 evaluable cases) was 19.2%. No significant difference was observed between systemic administration and local administration.
2. There was only a mild degree of adverse reaction to IFN.
3. In combination therapies, the response rate was 19.6% for AR; it was 41.2% for IAR.
4. IFN was also useful in maintenance therapy of malignant glioma.

Part II. Effect of Interferon Therapy on Malignant Glioma with Survival Analysis of 72 Cases

Subjects and Method

Seventy-two evaluable cases of malignant glioma treated in our institution (Dokkyo University Hospital) from 1980 until the end of 1994 were analyzed, primarily for survival rate.

The subjects of the study were 41 GB (mean age, 48.5 years; range, 6–74 years; 28 men, 13 women) and 31 MA (mean age, 37.8 years; range, 5–65 years; 11 men, 20 women). Indications and patient selection eligibility criteria for IFN therapy are the same as described in Part I.

IFN therapy was performed with radiation as a postoperative adjuvant therapy (IR therapy). Since 1986, the administration of ACNU has been incorporated in the course of therapy (IAR therapy; see Part I). IFN preparation used, dosage, method of administration, and assessment of response are the same as in Part I.

Response rate, survival rate, time to tumor progression (TTP), and the correlation among them were analyzed. Comparisons of those rates between GB and MA, IR and IAR, and age factor were performed. Factors concerning the long-term survival were also analyzed. The survival curve was plotted by Kaplan–Meier's method, and as the statistical analysis, Mann–Whitney's test was used.

Results

Survival Rate, Response Rate, and Correlation Between These Rates

Survival rate is presented in Table 3. Kaplan–Meier plots of survival (Fig. 2) showed a definite statistical difference between GB and MA ($P < .001$). TTP was 11.2 months for

Table 3. Survival rate (%).

Years	1	2	3	4	5
Glioblastoma	41.1	16.2	8.3		
Malignant astrocytoma	74.2	58.2	41.2	17.5	13.6

*P < .01.

Table 4. Response rate (%).

	CR	PR	NC	PD	Total	CR + PR/Total (%)
Glioblastoma	1	9	15	16	41	24.4
Malignant astrocytoma	2	12	12	6	31	45.2

Table 5. Correlation between response rate and survival rate in glioblastoma (%).

Years	1	2	3
CR + PR (10)	66.7	55.6]*	25.2]*
NC (15)	60.0	13.3	6.7
PD (16)	6.3	0	0

*, P < .02.

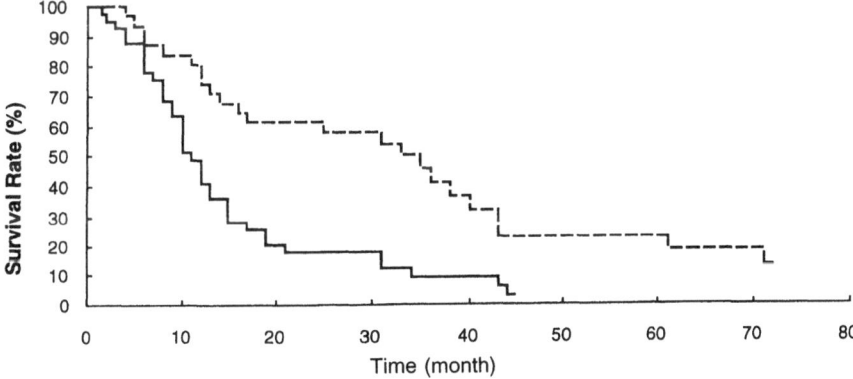

Fig. 2. Kaplan-Meier plots of survival comparing cases of glioblastoma (*solid line, n = 41*) and malignant astrocytoma (*dotted line, n = 31*); P < .001

GB and 21.5 months for MA, and mean survival time was 13.9 months for GB and 34.0 months for MA.

Response rates to the therapy are shown in Table 4; the correlation of these rates with the survival rates of GB and MA are described in Tables 5 and 6, respectively. There was a significant relation between tumor size reduction and survival rate, especially in the second and the third years, for both GB and MA.

Survival Rate Corresponding to Therapy

Survival rates corresponding to each therapy, IR or IAR, are shown in Table 7 (GB) and Table 8 (MA). In cases of GB, the IAR group revealed a significantly longer survival period compared to IR group. In cases of MA, the difference corresponding

Table 6. Correlation between response rate and survival rate in malignant astrocytoma (%).

Years	1	2	3
CR + PR (14)	92.9	83.3	55.6
NC (11)	72.7	45.5	27.3
PD (6)	33.3	33.3	16.7 (%)

*, P < .05.

Table 7. Survival rate corresponding to therapy for glioblastoma (%).

Years	1	2	3
IR (15)	20.0	5.4	2.1
IAR (26)	53.6	21.8	8.8

Kaplan-Meier: **, P < .02; *, P < .05.

Table 8. Survival rate corresponding to therapy for malignant astrocytoma (%).

Years	1	2	3
IR (15)	67.6	54.0	33.3
IAR (16)	75.0	58.6	45.6

N.S., not significant.

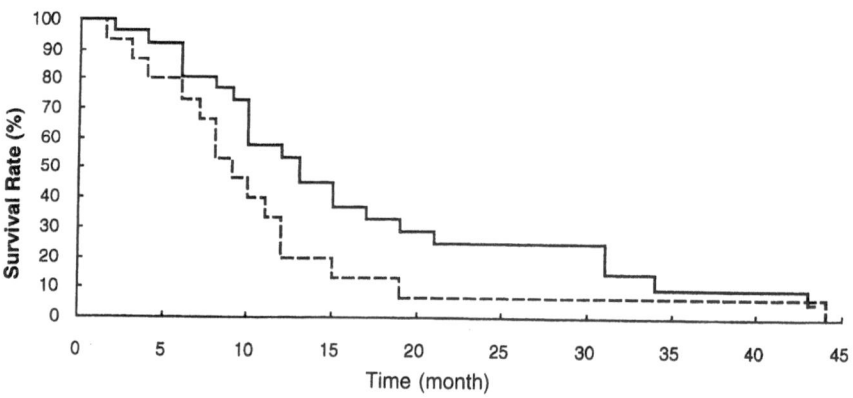

Fig. 3. Kaplan–Meier's plots of survival comparing glioblastoma therapies: IR (IFN [interferon] + radiation), *dotted line* (*n* = 15), IAR (IFN + ACNU + radiation), *solid line* (*n* = 26); P < .01

to each therapy was not seen. Comparison of survival rates of both treatment groups is demonstrated by Kaplan–Meier plots in Fig. 3.

Survival Rate Corresponding to Age

A comparison of survival rates of two age groups was done on the cases of GB. In Kaplan–Meier plots, a longer survival was noticed in the age group of younger than 54 years compared with the age group of older than 55 years, although there was no statistically significant difference (Table 9; Fig. 4).

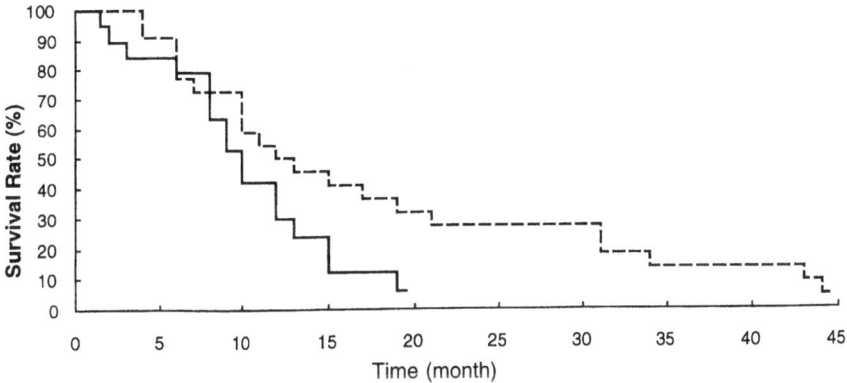

Fig. 4. Kaplan-Meier plots of survival comparing two age groups of age: older than 55 years, *solid line* ($n = 19$); under 54 years, *dotted line* ($n = 22$); $P < .01$

Table 9. Survival rate corresponding to age for glioblastoma (%).

Years	1	2	3
>55 yr. (19)	30.1	5.3	—
<54 yr. (22)	50.0	24.6	12.6

Analysis of Long-Term Survival Cases

Seven cases of GB who survived more than 2 years are listed in Table 10. The patients were relatively young except for one case. Location of the tumor tended to be frontal or in the occipital region, which might be related to the extension of resection. In five cases, more than 95% of the tumor was resected; in the other two cases, 50%. In IAR therapy for six cases, the responses were 1 CR, 4 PR, and 2 NC. In six patients, IFN was also used successfully as a long-term maintenance therapy.

Relation of Survival Time and Resection of Tumor

A comparison of survival time between subtotal resection (>95%) of the tumor and biopsy of the tumor tissue in cases of GB is presented in Table 11. Mean survival time of 12 cases of subtotal resection was 21.8 months, while that of 7 cases of biopsy was 9.7 months. Although the survival period of the subtotal removal group was prolonged, a significant difference was not proven, probably because of the small number of case.

Summary of Part II

1. Survival rates were significantly different between GB and MA ($P < .001$).
2. The tumor size reduction effect of the combination therapy including IFN during remission induction therapy was 24.4% to GB, whereas it was high, 45.5%, to MA.
3. There was a significant relation between tumor size reduction effect and survival rate in the second and the third years for GB and MA.
4. In a comparison between IR and IAR in the remission induction therapy for GB, the IAR survival rate was significantly higher.

Table 10. Long-term survival of glioblastoma patients.

Case	Age(yr)/sex	Location of tumor	Percent resection	Radiation dosage (Gy)	IFN (×10 IU)	Route of IFN	ACNU	Response	Maintenance therapy	Survival (mo)
T.S.	46/M	rF	95	50	555	iv, local	−	NC	IFN	44
A.I.	51/M	rPO	50	50	234	iv, local	+	PR	IFN + MAb	31
Y.S.	24/F	rTO	95	65	267	iv, local	+	PR	IFN + MAb	34
Y.T.	6/F	rF	50	69	108	iv, local	+	NC	IFN	31
M.U.	39/M	rF	95	60	440	iv	+	PR	IFN	63+
F.T.	38/M	IT	95	60	306	iv	+	PR	IFN	43
M.I.	64/F	rO	95	60	45	iv	+	CR	MAb	24+

r, right; l, left; F, frontal; T, temporal; P, parietal; O, occipital; IFN, interferon; mAb, monoclonal antibody; CLN-IgG

Table 11. Comparison of survival time (in months) between subtotal resection (>95%) of tumor and tumor biopsy in cases of glioblastoma.

Subtotal resection (12)	21.8	$* (P < .1)$
Biopsy (7)	9.7	

5. The age group of younger than 54 years showed longer survival than the older group (not significant).
6. In analysis of long-term survival patients, most cases were relatively younger in age, underwent extensive removal of the tumor, and were treated with postoperative IAR therapy followed by long-term maintenance therapy.
7. In a comparison between cases who underwent subtotal resection and those who received biopsy, the survival rate of the former group was higher (not significant).

Discussion

Enthusiastic expectations had been placed on the therapeutic effect of IFN against malignancy early in the 1980s. As to malignant brain tumors, several pioneer works of clinical use of IFN on glioma were also studied in addition to ours. Salford et al. [7] and Boëtius et al. [8] reported on some efficacy of IFN in a small number of malignant glioma patients. They used alpha-type IFN because of the circumstance of production of IFN preparation in Europe. In the United States, the pilot studies were performed with recombinant alpha-IFN by Mahaley et al. [9] in the middle of 1980s, and thereafter recombinant beta-type IFN was also used in several trials [10]. With regard to the type of IFN, we have described the action of the beta type as more superior than the alpha type [3].

Our multicenter group study, inaugurated in 1981 and continued for 5 years, obtained a beneficial effect of IFN on glioma with a response rate of 19.2% [5]. This result, however, disclosed the limitation of the therapy at the same time. To overcome this limitation, several combination therapies had been studied. IAR therapy, which was proposed by Yoshida et al. [11,12] was selected and used in the next muticenter study, which started in 1986. This trial was performed as a prospective phase III study by 20 neurosurgical institutions in Japan. The study revealed a high response rate of about 40% for malignant glioma. In recent years, IAR therapy has been adopted as the first choice of postoperative adjuvant therapy, that is, remission induction therapy, in many institutions or clinics in Japan.

The extremely high survival rates in the multicenter study on maintenance therapy with ACNU and IFN demonstrate the importance of long-term treatment after the initial therapy, although some selection cannot be avoided at the entry of the case. However, a much longer time is needed to analyze the results of long-term survival of so many cases in a multicenter study. For this reason, we performed survival analysis on patients confined to only those treated in our own institution and reported in this chapter.

Comparing the survival rates of 72 patients in our institution with those of the Brain Tumor Registry of Japan [13], no significant differences were recognized between them. In our cases, there was a significant difference between the survival of GB and

MA (P < .001). This fact requires us to reconsider the treatment method for GB. Response rates of IFN therapy as a postoperative remission induction therapy (GB, 24.4%; MA, 45.2%) in our clinic exceeded the results of the multicenter study. It might be said as a natural consequence that those response rates correlated well to the survival rates of 2 years and 3 years.

In comparison of IR and IAR, IAR revealed a significant advantage in 1-year and 2-year survival of GB. There are many reports regarding the combination therapy of anticancer drug and radiation. In 1979, Levin et al. [14] reported that the median time to tumor progression was prolonged to 41 weeks in 46 cases of malignant glioma treated with 1,3-bis (2-chloroethyl)-1-nitrosourea) (BCNU) and radiation. As to ACNU, Matsutani et al. [15] indicated that both response rate and survival rate of 71 cases of GB were raised significantly by combination chemo- and radiotherapies compared with single-therapy treatment. With regard to IAR, Yoshida et al. [16] reported its beneficial results in long-term follow-up in which the survival rates at 3 years was 30% and 18% at 5 years in 60 cases of malignant glioma.

A correlation of survival of GB with age and survival rate of patients older than 55 years was obviously low, although it was not statistically significant. We divided the age groups at 55 years old according to the proposal of von Deimling et al. [17] that the average age of GB type 2 was 56 years, at which age is shown loss of heterozygosity on chromosome 10 (LOH 10) with amplification of the epidermal growth factor (EGFR) gene. Further investigation is needed on this point.

There has been considerable controversy over the concept of treating GB with cytoreductive surgery. Kreth et al. [18] have reported the results of 58 patients treated with stereotactic biopsy followed by radiation therapy and those of surgical resection plus radiation therapy in 57 patients. There was no significant difference between the median survival time for the resection group (39.5 weeks) and for the biopsy group (32 weeks), and the most important factor was the patient's age. In our cases of GB, patients who underwent subtotal resection showed a longer survival time compared with those who received biopsy although there was no significant difference. The study of long-term survival cases in our institution suggests that maintenance therapy is one of the most important factors other than extensive removal of the tumor. These problems remain to be solved in the future.

Conclusions

We can evaluate IFN therapy as follows:

1. IFN therapy is effective in postsurgical remission induction therapy for malignant gliomas.
2. Specifically, IAR therapy is effective for prolongation of the survival period, even for GB.
3. IFN may also be effective in maintenance therapy for long-term survival.

For these reasons, IFN seems to be worthy of much wider application in the future.

References

1. Nagai M, Arai T, Kohno S, Kohase M (1982) Interferon therapy for malignant brain tumors. In: Kono R, Vilcek J (eds) The clinical potential of interferons. University of Tokyo Press, Tokyo, pp 257–273

2. Nagai M, Arai T, Kohno S, Kohase M (1982) Local application of interferon to malignant brain tumors. Texas Rep Biol Med 41:693–698
3. Nagai M, Arai T (1984) Clinical effect of interferon in malignant brain tumours. Neurosurg Rev 7:55–64
4. Nagai M, Arai T, Watanabe K (1988) Treatment of malignant brain tumors with interferon—with special reference to the combination therapy and the maintenance therapy. In: Kawade Y, Kobayashi S (eds) The biology of the interferon system 1988. Kodansha, Tokyo, pp 207–212
5. Nagai M (1989) Clinical effect of human fibroblast interferon (BM532) on malignant brain tumors—with special reference to glioma (in Japanese). J Jpn Soc Cancer Ther 24:638–646
6. Nagai M (1991) Advances of BRM therapy on malignant brain tumors (in Japanese). Jpn J Cancer Chemother 18:188–194
7. Salford LG, Borgstrom S, Brismar J, Brun A, Cronqvist S (1981) Intratumoral and systemic interferon treatment of astrocytoma grade III–IV. Acta Neurochir 56:130–131
8. Boëtius J, Blomgren H, Collins VP, Greitz T, Strander H (1983) The effect of systemic human interferon-alpha administration to patients with glioblastoma. Acta Neurochir 68:239–251
9. Mahaley MS Jr, Urso MB, Whaley RA, Blue M, Williams TE, Guaspari MA (1985) Immunobiology of primary intracranial tumors, part 10: therapeutic efficacy of interferon in the treatment of recurrent gliomas. J Neurosurg 63:719–725
10. Yung W-AK, Castellanos AM, Van Tassel P, Moser RP, Marcus S (1988) Recombinant interferon beta given intravenously in patients with recurrent malignant gliomas. Proc Am Soc Clin Oncol 7:84
11. Yoshida J, Kato K, Wakabayashi T, Enomoto H, Inoue I, Kageyama N (1986) Antitumor activity of interferon-beta against malignant glioma in combination with chemotherapeutic agent of nitrosoureas (ACNU). In: Cantell K, et al (eds) The biology of the interferon system. Nijhoff, Netherlands, pp 399–406
12. Enomoto H, Yoshida J, Kageyama N (1987) The effectiveness of combination therapy with Hu IFN-beta and ACNU against malignant glioma. Neurol Med Chir (Tokyo) 27:6–10
13. The Committee of Brain Tumor Registry of Japan (1992) The brain tumor registry of Japan. Neurol Med Chir (Tokyo) 32 (special issue):478–479
14. Levin VA, Wilson CB, Davis R, Wara WM, Pischer L, Irwin L (1979) A phase III comparison of BCNU, hydroxyurea, and radiation therapy to BCNU and radiation therapy for treatment of primary malignant gliomas. J Neurosurg 51:526–532
15. Matsutani M, Nakamura O, Nagashima T, Asai A, Fujimaki T, Tanaka H, Ueki K, Tanaka Y (1994) Radiation therapy combined with radiosensitizing agents for cerebral glioblastoma in adults. J Neuro-Oncol 19:227–237
16. Yoshida J, Kajita Y, Wakabayashi T, Sugita K (1994) Long-term follow-up results of 175 patients with malignant glioma: importance of radical tumour resection and postoperative adjuvant therapy with interferon, ACNU, and radiation. Acta Neurochir 127:55–59
17. von Deimling A, von Ammon K, Schoenfeld D, Wiestler OD, Seizinger BR, Louis DN (1993) Subsets of glioblastoma multiforme defined by molecular genetic analysis. Brain Pathol 3:19–26
18. Kreth FW, Warnke PC, Scheremet R, Ostertag CB (1993) Surgical resection and radiation therapy versus biopsy and radiation therapy in the treatment of glioblastoma multiforme. J Neurosurg 78:762–766

Clinical Results of Specific Targeting Therapy Against Patients with Malignant Glioma

Makoto Hishii[1], Taizo Nitta[1], Michimasa Ebato[1], Ko Okumura[2], and Kiyoshi Sato[1]

Abstract. Targeting of T or NK cells to tumor cells by bispecific antibodies as a possible way of targeting cancer cells has gained increasing interest in the past few years. We treated 31 patients with malignant glioma by means of local adoptive transfer of lymphokine-activated killer (LAK) cells coupled with bispecific antibodies (anti-CD3Xanti-glioma) as an adjuvant therapy. Approximately 50% of the patients treated with this specific targeting therapy (STT) remain alive at 3-year follow-up, and 40% of the patients are free from recurrence. The effectiveness of this therapy is confirmed by serial computed tomography (CT) scans, which revealed disappearance of remnant tumors in some patients. In addition, histological specimens obtained by the use of CT-guided stereotactic biopsy from the lesions showed marked necrosis and degeneration after STT. However, patients presenting with recurrent glioma were relatively resistant to STT. This is because a hyaline membrane formed on the surface of glioma that may interfere with lymphocyte tracking into the tumor from the operative and histological findings. Five patients developed microbial infection, but 4 cases were treated successfully with the use of antimicrobial drugs. No neurological deterioration was observed after STT. Taken together, STT can produce higher response rates in malignant glioma patients than those achieved with LAK cells only or with other conventional treatments, and might be one of the most promising adjuvant therapies for other types of cancer.

Key words. Malignant glioma—Adoptive immunotherapy—Lymphokine-activated killer cell—Bispecific antibody

Introduction

Intracranial malignant gliomas, especially glioblastoma multiforme, are highly aggressive tumors and associated with very poor prognoses. Significant palliation with good functional recovery cannot yet be achieved. Even with radical surgery followed by radiotherapy and/or chemotherapy, the median time for recurrence is less than 12 months, and the mean survival time is only 2–3 years [1], because the glioma cells are

Department of [1] Neurosurgery and [2] Immunology, Juntendo University School of Medicine, Tokyo 113, Japan

characteristically quite invasive and proliferative. Recently, promising attempts have been made to improve the survival of patients with malignant glioma. One example is adoptive transfer of cytotoxic T lymphocyte (CTL) or lymphokine-activated killer (LAK) cells to patients [2–4]. Adoptive immunotherapy in the neurosurgical field starts with an injection of preactivated autologous lymphocytes via indwelling catheters or directly into the tumors [5,6]. CTL are induced from the patient's peripheral blood lymphocytes (PBL) with antigenic stimulation of autologous tumor cells. To date, many studies have shown difficulties in obtaining specific CTL from glioma patients compared with those of melanoma [7]. On the other hand, LAK cells are a heterogeneous cell population consisting of natural killer (NK) cells, some kinds of T cells, and macrophages, which can lyse NK-resistant tumor or fresh autologous tumor cells without major histocompatibility complex (MHC) restriction [8].

Since 1985, Rosenberg has been using LAK cells to treat malignant melanoma, sarcoma, and renal cell carcinoma. In spite of good in vitro results, the clinical data are not satisfactory [9]. The major problem may be low killer activity and low specificity toward target cells. In view of these problems, there is an urgent need to modify LAK therapy to enhance the affinity, specificity, and lytic potential of killer cells. The bispecific antibody links the target cell directly to CD3 or CD16 on LAK cells, thus enhancing the lytic activity and binding of the T cell to the target cell [10–12]. Both in vitro studies and animal model experiments have shown that specific targeting therapy with this bispecific antibody was effective against various cancers [13,14]. This strategy can be used to target PBL against human glioma cells. Since 1988 we have been developing a specific targeting therapy (STT) in which LAK cells are targeted with bispecific antibodies against malignant glioma patients. Preliminary results of a 1-year follow-up showed that STT is more effective than other treatments in prolonging the time to recurrence for malignant glioma [13]. In this study we evaluated the current results of STT based on the mean recurrence time, median survival time, and side effects.

Materials and Methods

Patients

Thirty-one patients with malignant glioma including 5 recurrent glioma cases were entered into the clinical trial of STT (Table 1). The patients had a mean age of 46 years and included 17 cases of glioblastoma multiforme (grade IV) and 14 cases of

Table 1. Profiles of glioma patients treated with specific targeting therapy (1988–1992).

Cases of malignant glioma: 31 (M:F = 22:9)
Age: 5–71 years (mean, 46.0 yr)
Diagnosis: Glioblastoma multiforme, 17
            Anaplastic astrocytoma, 14
Therapy: Op/Rad/Chem/STT 20
            Op/Rad/STT 9
            Op/STT 2

Op, Operation; Rad, external irradiation; Chem, chemotherapy.

anaplastic astrocytoma (grade III), according to the WHO classification. All cases underwent surgery; 20 cases received whole brain irradiation (50–60 Gy) in addition to a single intracarotid injection of (1,4-amino-2-methyl-5-pyrimidinyl)-methyl-3-(2-chloroethyl)-3-nitrosourea (ACNU, 100 mg), 9 cases received only radiation, and 2 cases lacked any supportive therapies. To qualify for the adoptive immunotherapy, patients had to meet the following criteria: (1) histological evidence of malignant glioma after surgical resection, (2) complete recovery from any apparent toxic side effects of prior radiotherapy or chemotherapy, (3) an adequate hematological status (no leukopenia, thrombocytopenia, or anemia), and (4) no antitumor therapy for at least 4 weeks before entering the trial.

Treatment Schedule

All patients with malignant glioma receiving STT had an indwelling catheter and Ommaya reservoir placed at the edge of the bone flap after tumor debulking. To obtain LAK cells, 100 ml of venous blood was withdrawn from the patients and separated PBL were cultured with 100 U/ml of rIL-2 (Shionogi, Osaka, Japan). After 7 days, half the LAK cells were infused into the patient while the remaining half were infused on day 10 (Fig. 1). Cell numbers ranged from 1 to 1.5 × 10^8 cells/infusion, and cells were preincubated with 100 µg of bispecific antibodies for 30 min before administration. After sterilizing the scalp over the reservoir, we infused bispecific antibody-coated LAK cells at the patient's bedside with a 23-gauge needle. Treatment schedule was six injections over 3 weeks. The bispecific antibodies used in this study were F(ab')2 monomers composed of anti-CD3 monoclonal antibodies (mAb) (OKT3, American Type Culture Collection) chemically conjugated with antiglioma mAb (NE 150) by use of a thiol activating agent 5.5′-dithiobis-(2-nitrobenzoic acid) (DTNB), as described previously [10,14]. To confirm the reactivity of NE 150 with each glioma specimen, surgical specimens were stored at −70°C and were stained with fluorescen isothiocyanate (FITC)-conjugated NE 150 by an immunohistochemical method.

Clinical Evaluation

To compare tumor sizes, all treated patients underwent serial computed tomography (CT) scans using 100 ml of contrast medium. CT scans were performed before surgery, after surgery, and after STT. Neurological status and complications were monitored in all cases. We took histological specimens from the lesion after treatment by a CT-guided stereotactic biopsy in three cases.

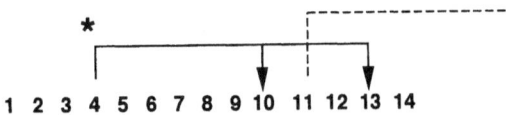

Fig. 1. Treatment schedule of specific targeting therapy. *Asterisk,* blood with drawal; *arrows,* injection of lymphokine-activated killer (LAK) cells

Results

Survival Period

All patients were subjected to a statistical study to investigate the effectiveness of STT, and the data were compared with the Brain Tumor Registry (BTR) in Japan [15]. The survival curve for all malignant glioma patients is shown in Fig. 2. About 50% of the patients treated with STT remained alive more than 3 years from the time of initial diagnosis and treatment. In contrast, all patients treated with LAK therapy died in less than 2.5 years. This difference was statistically significant ($P < .05$). Thereafter, we classified patients into two groups: those suffering from glioblastoma multiforme and those with anaplastic astrocytoma, according to the histological grading. The relative survival rate of each group was calculated yearly up to 3 years. As Table 1 shows, it is evident that STT is more effective in treating malignant glioma than other conventional treatments. For example, according to all studies in Japan (BTR in Japan), fewer than 15% of patients harboring glioblastoma multiforme (GM) are alive after 3 years of initial diagnosis and treatment, but 45% of patients in the STT group are alive. This tendency is more prominent in patients with anaplastic astrocytoma (AA); that is, about two-thirds of the patients with STT are alive after 3 years but fewer than 30% in BTR. No neurological change was noticed before and after treatment.

Table 2. Relative survival rate of patients with malignant glioma after 1, 2, or 3 years.

Type	Therapy	1 yr	2 yr	3 yr
Glioblastoma multiforme	STT	60.5%	45.3%	45.1%
(17 cases)	BTR	47.4%	21.8%	14.8%
Anaplastic astrocytoma	STT	66.9%	66.9%	66.9%
(14 cases)	BTR	64.5%	39.1%	30.3%

STT, Specific targeting therapy; BTR, Brain Tumor Registry in Japan.

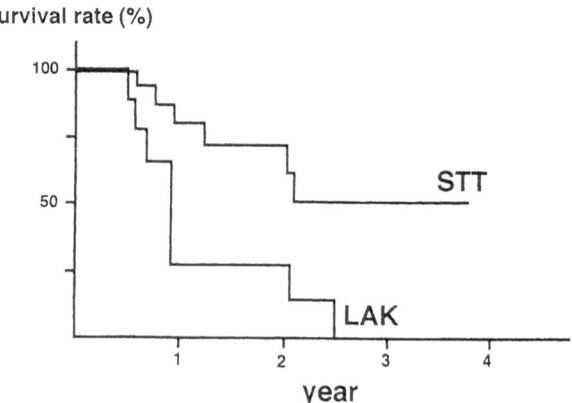

Fig. 2. Data were analyzed using the Kaplan-Meier method; specific targeting therapy (STT) treated patients were found to have a statistically higher survival time than patients treated with LAK cells alone ($P < .05$)

Time to Recurrence

One of the biological characteristics in malignant glioma is recurrence [16]. Even though they may be radically removed, tumors usually recur within 1 year. Of 31 cases in this study, 25 cases, 13 GM and 12 AA, were treated at the time of initial diagnosis. Our study shows that 4 of 13 GM (30.8%) and 6 of 12 AA (50%) are free from recurrence up to 3 years after STT.

Tumor Imaging

In all glioma patients treated with STT, CT scans were serially obtained before and after treatment. The goal of aggressive surgery in malignant glioma is to remove as much tumor as possible. At the initial diagnosis of malignant glioma, a tumor seen as high-density areas by enhanced CT scan was radically resected. Serial CT scans revealed no progression of tumors in about half the patients. In a few cases in which a tumor was located at a surgically inaccessible region, such as the basal ganglia, motor cortex, or brainstem, these remnant high-density lesions disappeared after STT in case 1. In addition, almost all patients demonstrated a distinct thin-ring area of contrast enhancement about the lesion within 2 weeks after STT. Most of the enhancing effects resolved within 1 month. Clinical and neurological evaluation did not reveal any correlation between the development of contrast enhancement and symptoms.

Pathological Examination

After receiving STT, tissue specimens of the above-mentioned thin rings on enhanced CT were obtained by CT-guided stereotactic biopsy in three cases. The biopsied specimens revealed severe necrosis and degenerative change of tumor cells, with no viable cells remaining.

Recurrent Glioma

Five cases of recurrent malignant glioma were also included in this trial. These patients had not received prior immunotherapy. We explored the effect of STT on these recurrent glioma patients. The results showed that three of five patients were refractory to STT. In this patient, reoperation was done to remove the remnant glioma. Intraoperative findings showed that a dense hyaline membrane was formed and extended along the entire surface of recurrent glioma. Histological examination of this membrane revealed multilayer, fibrous connective tissues.

Side Effects

STT was well tolerated. The most prominent side effect was a mild transient fever up to 38.5°C, and this could be controlled by the oral administration of aspirin. Hematological examination showed a mild leukocytosis in about one-third of the patients. Five of 31 cases developed a high fever, and microbial infection was suspected. Acute bacterial (2/5) and fungal (3/5) infection was confirmed by positive microbial culture from the indwelling catheter. Four of 5 cases were successfully treated by intravenous infusion of antibiotics, but 1 patient deteriorated and died of meningitis.

Discussion

Recent advances in cancer research have increased the treatment options available for patients with high-grade astrocytoma. Despite aggressive treatment, approximately 25%–50% of patients with glioblastoma multiforme undergoing surgery and conventional radiation survive 1 year, 10% survive 2 years, and only 1% survive 5 years or longer. Results for patients harboring anaplastic astrocytoma are a little more encouraging, but fewer than 30% survive 3 years [16]. Targeting of cytotoxic T cells to tumor cells by bispecific antibodies as a tool of targeting cancer has gained increasing interest in the past few years [17,18]. CD3 molecules are tightly associated with T-cell antigen receptor and play a key role in transduction of signals by antigen binding to the intracellular enivronment. Anti-CD3 monoclonal antibodies behave similarly to anigen; their binding to CD3 results in modulation of the entire complex from the cell surface [11,19]. Bispecific hybrid antibodies composed of anti-CD3 and antitumor Ab were used to link cloned CTL or PBL with tumor cells, rendering the tumor cells more sensitive to attack by lymphocytes [14]. Therefore, these Abs were considered suitable for cancer immunotherapy due to their specificity toward the target cells. In patients harboring malignant tumors, LAK activity of PBL has been shown to be impaired because of tumor cell-derived suppressive factors [7,20], like TGF-β2 or IL-10, or increase in the population of suppressive macrophages or T lymphocytes.

However, our previous studies showed that impaired LAK activity in glioma patients could be enhanced with the use of bispecific antibodies in vitro. The preliminary clinical study showed that 4 of the 10 patients given STT showed regression of tumor, and in another 4 patients CT scan and histology suggested eradication of the glioma cells left behind after surgery [13]. We presented the current data on 31 patients with malignant glioma treated with the combined administration of LAK cells and bispecific antibodies. By use of this STT, the survival times of malignant glioma patients were increased, and about half the patients treated with STT remained alive more than 3 years from the time of initial treatment. In addition, 10 of 25 patients treated at time of initial diagnosis are still free from recurrence. These results were confirmed by serial CT scans, that is, the remnant glioma disappeared in some patients. Our early findings suggest that STT may be more effective than other treatments, because the survival rate is longer and the recurrence rate is lower.

STT has been ineffective, however, in patients with recurrent malignant glioma. This may be because a fibrous membrane forms between cerebrospinal fluid and tumor cells that may hinder the lymphocytes from attacking glioma cells. Therefore, it is suggested that this hyaline membrane should be resected surgically before STT. Another possibility may be loss of antigenic specificity on glioma cells by prior radiotherapy or chemotherapy, which causes glioma cells to escape from the bispecific antibodies. The pathological findings also confirm the effectiveness of STT in that active remnant glioma cells were replaced by degenerative necrotic tissue after STT. The major complication of infection must be seriously investigated, because fungal infections had been already reported from LAK therapy by Rosenberg et al. [9]. This is not simply caused by technical problems of contamination, but is more likely the result of "immunological paralysis" of the host after receiving killer cells, which may cause opportunistic bacterial or fungal infections.

In conclusion, although further studies will be required, STT appears to offer a promising approach for treating cancer [21,22].

References

1. Quigley MR, Maroon JC (1991) The relationship between survival and the extent of the resection in patients with supratentorial malignant gliomas. Neurosurgery 29:385–389
2. Jacobs SK, Wilson DJ, Kornblith PL (1986) Interleukin-2 and autologous lymphokine-activated killer cells in the treatment of malignant glioma. J Neurosurg 64:743–749
3. Merchant RE, Merchant LE, Cook SHS (1989) Intralesional infusion of lymphokine-activated killer (LAK) cells and recombinant interleukin-2 (rIL-2) for the treatment of patients with malignant brain tumor. Neurosurgery 23:725–732
4. Rosenberg SA, Lotze MT (1986) Cancer Immunotherapy using interleukin-2 and interleukin-2-activated lymphocytes. Annu Rev Immunol 4:681–709
5. Neuwelt EA, Clark K, Kirkpatrick JB (1978) Clinical studies of intrathecal autologous lymphocyte infusions in patients with malignant glioma: a toxicity study. Ann Neurol 4:307–312
6. Young H, Kaplan A, Regelson W (1977) Immunotherapy with autologous white cell infusions ("lymphocytes") in the treatment of recurrent glioblastoma multiforme. A preliminary report. Cancer 40:1037–1044
7. Fontana A, Hengertner H, de Tribolet (1984) Glioblastoma cells release interleukin-1 and factors inhibiting interleukin-2-mediated effect. J Immunol 132:1837–1844
8. Grimm EA, Ramsey KM, Mazumder A (1983) Lymphokine activated killer cell phenomenon. J Exp Med 157:884–897
9. Barba D, Saris CS, Holder C (1989) Intratumoral LAK cell and interleukin-2 therapy of human gliomas. J Neurosurg 70:175–182
10. Nitta T, Sato K, Okumura K (1990) Induction of cytotoxicity in human T cells coated with anti-gliomaXanti-CD3 bispecific antibody against human glioma cells. J Neurosurg 72:476–481
11. Perez P, Hoffman RW, Shaw S (1985) Specific targeting of cytotoxic T cells by anti-T3 linked to anti target cell antibody. Nature 316:354–356
12. Van Lier RAW, Boot JHA, de Groot ER (1987) Induction of T cell proliferation with anti-CD3 switch variant monoclonal antibodies. Eur J Immunol 17:1599–1604
13. Nitta T, Yagita H, Azuma T (1989) Bispecific F(ab') 2 monomer prepared with anti-CD3 and anti-tumor monoclonal antibodies is most potent in induction of cytolysis of human T cells. Eur J Immunol 19:1437–1441
14. Nitta T, Sato K, Yagita H (1990) Preliminary trial of specific targeting therapy against malignant glioma. Lancet 1:368–376
15. The Committee of Brain Tumor Registry of Japan (1992) Brain Tumor Registry of Japan. Neurol Med Chir (Tokyo) 32:385–547
16. Van Dijk JS, Warnaar SO, Van Eedenburg JDH (1989) Induction of tumor-cell lysis by bi-specific monoclonal antibodies recognizing renal-cell carcinoma and CD3 antigen. Int J Cancer 43:344–349
17. Nitta T, Nakata M, Yagita H (1991) Interleukin-2 activated T cells express CD16 and are triggered to target cell lysis by anti-CD16 linked to anti-target heteroantibody. Immunol Lett 28:31–38
18. Titus JA, Garrido MA, Hecht TT (1987) Human T cells targeted with anti-T3 cross-linked to anti-tumor antibody prevent tumor growth in nude mice. J Immunol 138:4018–4022
19. Staerz UD, Kanagawa O, Bevan MJ (1985) Hybrid antibodies can target sites for attack by T cells. Nature 314:628–631
20. Jacobs SK, Wilson DJ, Kornblith PL (1986) In vitro killing of human glioblastoma by interleukin-2-activated autologous lymphocytes. J Neurosurg 64:114–117

21. Pupa SM, Canevari S, Fontanelli R (1988) Activation of mononuclear cells to be used for hybrid monoclonal antibody-induced lysis of human ovarian carcinoma cells. Int J Cancer 42:455–459
22. Watne K, Hannisdal E, Nome O (1992) Combined intra-arterial an systemic chemotherapy for recurrent malignant brain tumors. Neurosurgery 30:223–227

Structural Analysis of Anti-cancer Antibody, CLN-IgG, and Anti-Idiotypic Antibody, Idio-No. 3, for the Study of Idiotope Image Transmission: An Insight into Antigen-Specific Human Monoclonal Antibody Therapy

Hideaki Hagiwara and Yasuyuki Aotsuka

Abstract. The clinical value of a human monoclonal antibody, CLN-IgG, as an antitumor antibody has been studied at the molecular level. By use of computer-aided graphic design, an anti-idiotypic antibody to CLN-IgG termed idio-No. 3 was evaluated as having an epitope image of a tumor-associated antigen TA226; on the other hand, the combining site of CLN-IgG was seen to be in conformity with a counterimage of the epitope of TA226 and presumed to be part of the ligand image to TA226. An anti-paratactic antibody, idio-No. 3 behaves as a mimic antigen on TA226 and binds to p34 antigen that is expressed on glioma cells. Idio-No. 3 was used for monitoring anti anti-idiotypic antibody intensification in the sera of glioma patients to whom CLN-IgG had been administered.

Key words. Tumor-associated antigen—Human monoclonal antibody—Idiotypic antibody—Internal image—Immune network

Introduction

A human monoclonal antibody (HuMoAb) termed CLN-IgG that recognizes the TA226 malignant-associated antigen has been introduced in clinical trials for brain tumor patients in this decade [1,2]. Tumor antigen-specific antibody therapy using a human monoclonal antibody has revealed clinically a number of advantages: no adverse reaction, long serum half-life, accessibility of the antibody to the tumor region, no severe host versus foreign antigen reaction, and the feasibility of long-term repetitive administration.

To delineate the antitumor activity of CLN-IgG, we focused on idiotype network [3,4] occurrence in brain tumor patients who were treated with CLN-IgG. Several attempts have been applied to cancer therapy as to idiotype-specific therapy by using murine antibodies [5,6]. In human cancer patients, however, whether anti-idiotypic antibody and anti anti-idiotypic antibody could be caused by an initial idiotypic HuMoAb has remained obscure. To study the behavior of idiotypic antibody occurrence during the course of antigen-specific HuMoAb therapy, we generated a murine

Hagiwara Institute of Health, Kasai, Hyogo 679-01, Japan

anti-paratactic antibody to CLN-IgG, then verified its idiotope image by computer modeling of the antibody molecule.

Materials and Methods

Generation of Anti-idiotypic Antibodies to CLN-IgG

Newborn mice (Balb/c) were treated to induce tolerance by 100 μg of human IgG at 1 day after birth. After growth, the mice were immunized with Fab fragment of CLN-IgG intraperitoneally. Several murine hybridoma clones were generated by the method of cell fusion with immunized mouse spleen cells and parental cells NS1 [7]. The clone that secretes murine IgG capable of reacting to CLN-IgG but not to irrelevant human IgG was selected as an anti-idiotypic antibody to CLN-IgG. The hybridoma producing anti-idiotypic antibody, idio-No. 3, was propagated in athymic mice and their ascites were used as idio-No. 3 preparation.

Sequencing of CLN-IgG and Idio-No. 3

Heavy- and light-chain genes of CLN-IgG were cloned from λgt10 CLNH11 library using DNA probes encoding partial amino acid sequences of CLN-IgG. DNA sequences of heavy and light chains of idio-No. 3 were determined from DNA fragments amplified by reverse transcriptase-polymerase chain reaction (RT-PCR) using PCR primers corresponding to the leader and constant regions of mouse γ1 and κ. Amino acid sequences of the variable region of the two antibodies were deduced from the DNA sequences.

Three-Dimensional Analysis of the Antibodies

We constructed three-dimensional molecular models of CLN-IgG and idio-No. 3 using program BIOCES as follows: as the first step, we searched the Protein Data Bank (PDB) for the homologous proteins in the amino acid sequence of the antibodies. We then selected the human anti-HIV gp41 antibody 3D6 Fab fragment and the mouse anti-hen lysozyme antibody D11.15 Fv fragment as the reference proteins for modeling CLN-IgG and idio-No. 3, respectively. After an alignment of the amino acid sequences was made using hydrophobic core scores, the amino acid sequence of the reference protein was replaced with that of the antibody to be modeled. The prototype of the models was generated by referring to information about the structure of well-known proteins and by generating main and side chains of the replaced region. The model was then refined by calculations using the Monte Carlo method and molecular mechanics.

Identification of Antigens Recognized by CLN-IgG and Idio-No. 3

The crude membrane fraction of U-251MG human glioma cells was prepared and the proteins were analyzed by sodium dodecyl sulfate-polyacrylamide gel electrophoresis (SDS-PAGE). The proteins were electroblotted onto nitrocellulose membrane and the purified antibody was then reacted at room temperature for 1 h.

The reaction sites with peroxidase-conjugated anti-human/mouse antibody were detected by the method of enhanced chemiluminescent assay (Amersham, Buckinghamshire, UK). The x-ray film was exposed for 1 min and developed to visualize the sensitized bands.

Results

Characterization of CLN-IgG

CLN-IgG is a human monoclonal antibody secreted from a human-human hybridoma termed CLNH11 [8]. CLNH11 cell stably produces IgG in serum-free media at a concentration of 10 μg/ml. Amino acid sequences in the heavy chains and light chains of CLN-IgG were completely determined, identifying an antibody having an γ1 and ϰ isotype. CLN-IgG bound various tumor cells and showed antibody-dependent cell cytotoxicity (ADCC) and complement-dependent cytotoxicity (CDC) [9–11]. Growth inhibition activity of CLN-IgG was assessed by the athymic mice system.

Characterization of Anti-idiotypic Antibody Idio-No. 3

By means of cell fusion we obtained murine hybridoma clones producing anti-CLN-IgG. By nature of inhibitory activity of CLN-IgG binding to target cells and no reactivity to irrelevant human IgG with isotype match, we selected a clone termed idio-No. 3 producing IgG1.

Idio-No. 3 could only bind to the complete configuration of CLN-IgG and caused delayed-type hypersensitivity in the animal model. Taking these characteristics into consideration, we confirmed that idio-No. 3 must have a counterimage of the CLN-IgG antigen-combining site. That is to say, idio-No. 3 should have a tumor antigen epitope image in its paratope. To confirm this model, we designed tertiary structures of each antibody on the basis of visible verification.

Three-Dimensional Structure of CLN-IgG Fab

We designed a space-filling model of CLN-IgG using computer graphics by referring to the structure of human anti-HIV gp41 antibody (Fig. 1a). The complete mode of the paratope was delineated with six complementary determining regions (CDRs), which strikingly contribute to the antigen-combining site of CLN-IgG (colored yellow). The distinctive feature of the CDR conformation is that a positively charged arginine (Arg) residue of heavy-chain CDR3 protrudes from the middle of the CDR regions.

Paratope Structure of Idio-No. 3 Fv

By means of three-dimensional molecular modeling of idio-No. 3 assisted by computer graphics, we designed a space-filling model of the idio-No. 3 Fv fragment based on the structure of murine anti-hen lysozyme antibody; its paratope, composed of six CDRs, is colored red in Fig. 1b. A prominent feature of this CDR region was a shallow

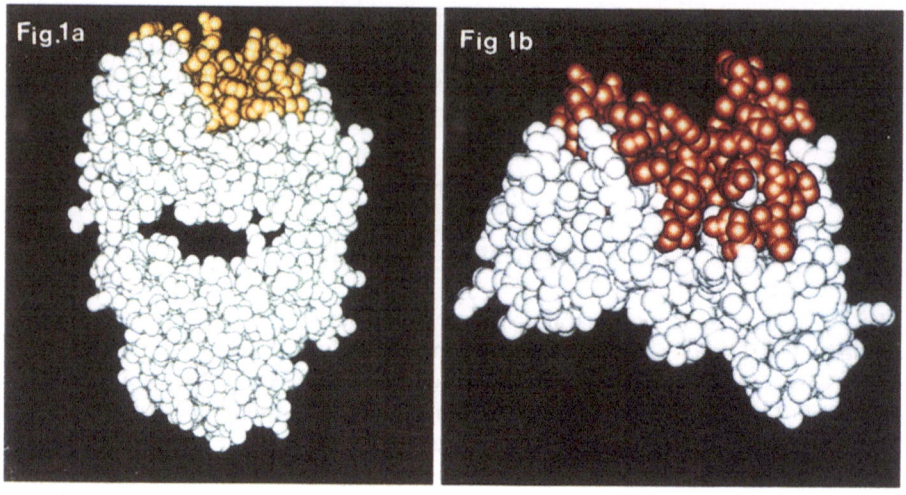

Fig. 1a,b. Space-filling models of CLN-IgG Fab and idio-No. 3 Fv. Complementary determining regions (CDRs) of CLN-IgG (a) and idio-No. 3 (b) were colored yellow and red, respectively

groove formed by negatively charged glutamates (Glu) and aspartates (Asp), which are located in the heavy-chain CDR3. As CLN-IgG was shown to recognize the antigen TA226 even under denaturing conditions, we suppose that the epitope should ride on a linear polypeptide of TA226, and it could be accessible to CLN-IgG under stressed conditions. An idiotope of idio-No. 3, which can mimic TA226 epitope, could also present a linear epitope.

Docking Model of Two Paratopes

We tried to dock the two models, with paratope-to-paratope interaction of CLN-IgG and idio-No. 3, on a computer monitor using a protein–protein docking program (BIOCES/DK). The paratope models we obtained, as mentioned previously, suggest that binding of CLN-IgG and idio-No. 3 might be mediated by electrostatic interaction. Thus, the docking was first carried out so that the protruding Arg residue of CLN-IgG CDRs interacted with the acidic region of idio-No. 3 CDRs; in the second attempt, collisions between atoms forming CDRs were avoided (Fig. 2). Features of recognition sites of two antibodies were comprehensible as a typical concave/convex model of proteins. However, possible recognition patterns had more variations because of delicate deviations in inter-molecular positioning.

Identification of Antigens Recognized by CLN-IgG and Idio-No. 3

The antigen recognized by CLN-IgG was identified from the human glioma cell line U-251MG as a malignant cell-associated common antigen TA226 that includes two different moieties having molecular weights of 60k and 53k in SDS-PAGE [12] (Fig. 3). The antigen recognized by idio-No. 3 was also identified from U-251MG and found to be a single polypeptide having a molecular weight of 34k (p34) (Fig. 3).

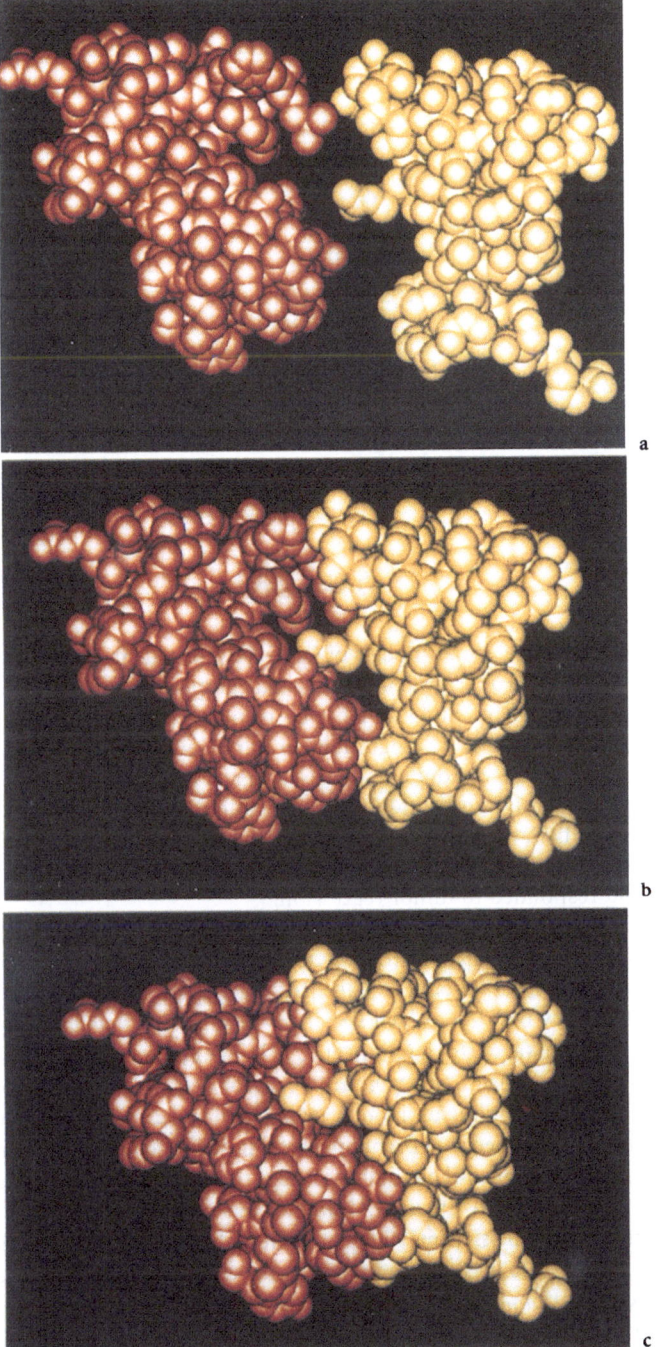

Fig. 2a–c. Docking of CLN-IgG and idio-No. 3 was performed (a–c) using BIOCES/DK docking program. CDRs of CLN-IgG and idio-No. 3 are colored yellow and red, respectively

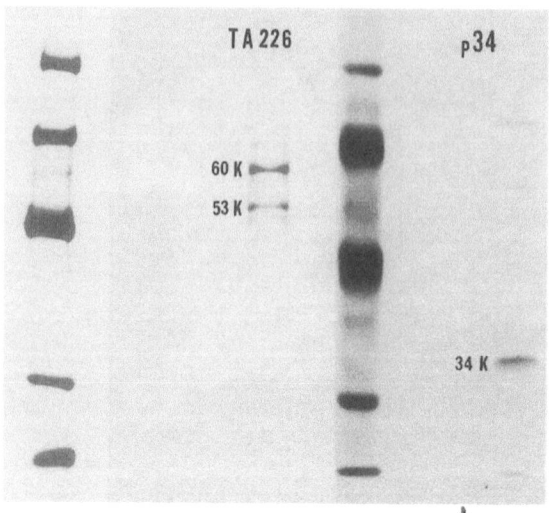

Fig. 3. Identification of antigens recognized by CLN-IgG and idio-No. 3. CLN-IgG recognizes TA226 (60K/53K, *left*); idio-No. 3 recognizes p34 (*right*)

Discussion

Three-dimensional molecular models of CLN-IgG and anti-paratactic antibody idio-No. 3 were constructed using computer-aided graphics design. The mode of the combining site of CLN-IgG and idio-No. 3 corresponds to the feature of paratope and epitope in antigen–antibody recognition. In particular, the paratope of idio-No. 3 shared a feature of the epitope on TA226 antigen. Thus, when antigen-mimicking anti-idiotypic antibody can be induced in the patient, it can elicit anti anti-idiotypic antibody, which behaves like CLN-IgG. In the clinical trials, the unfamiliar anti anti-idiotypic antibody induction was found in glioma patients who were treated with CLN-IgG and responded to tumor regression.

Repetitive administration of CLN-IgG augmented CLN-IgG-like antibody in good responders during the course of treatment (Fig. 4) [13]. Further, anti anti-idiotypic antibody production in the patient was intensified aperiodically in accordance with duration of efficacy besides antigen specificity (Fig. 5). This phenomenon has been called the "idiotope wave" by Hagiwara et al. [13]. We cannot explain precisely why an aperiodical wave response of idiotypic antibody was observed in the good responders. At least, numerous idiotypic antibodies evoked by an paratactic antibody CLN-IgG may participate the sequence of event on idiotypic antibody induction. Open network theory permits us to transmit an idiotope image to successive idiotopes whether they are constituents or nonconstituents of immune networks. From this point of view, the paratope image transmission may have considerable influence on the other immune systems, such as cytotoxic T-cell induction to the antigen-presenting cells, leading to tumor cell elimination. Hence, modeling of the idiotope image provides a new insight regarding tumor immunity by anti-tumor antibody.

In practice, it is useful to measure the specific idiotypic antibody occurrence in patients who are responding to antigen-specific HuMoAb therapy. Clinically, intensification of anti anti-idiotypic antibody means that patients who received antigen-specific HuMoAb therapy could rebuild intrinsic anti-tumor competence to malignancy. In this sense, studying epitope–paratope image recognition will relate

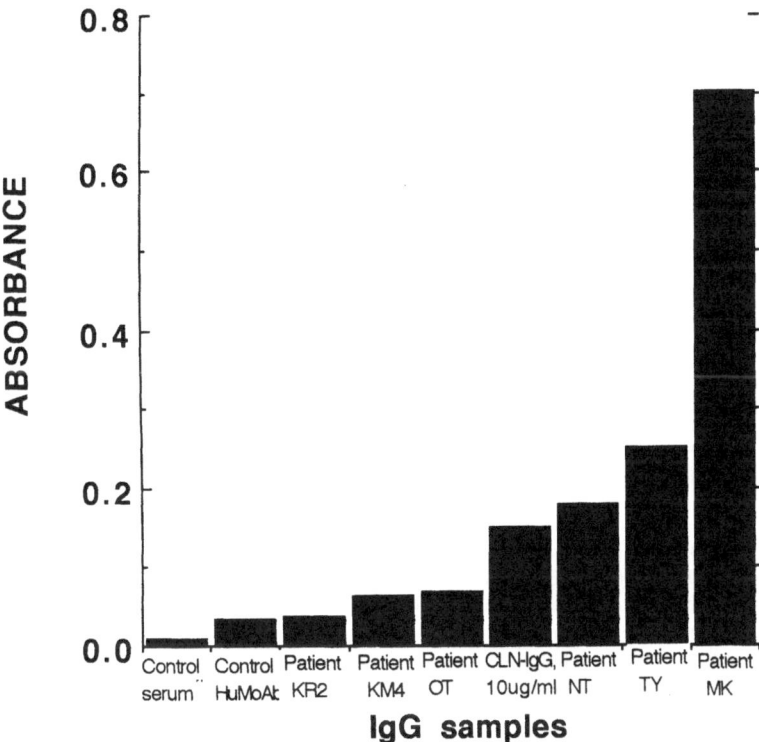

Fig. 4. Reactivity of serum IgG of glioma patients who were treated with CLN-IgG to live glioma cells. U-251MG cells were synchronously cultured overnight in Dulbecco's Modified Eagle medium plus Ham's F-12 medium (DF) +10% fetal bovine serum (FBS) in the presence of Nocodazole (SIGMA). The cells were harvested by shaking without trypsinization and inoculated into a 96-well plate. The purified antibody or serum of the patients was added to the cells in the well, in an amount stoichiometrically corresponding to 1 µg/ml CLN-IgG and incubated at 37°C for 1 h. The first antibody was removed and the wells were washed with gelatin buffer. The first antibody reaction was assessed by enzyme-linked immunosorbentassay (ELISA) using the ABC (avidin–Biotin complex) method. Equivalency of concentration was achieved at 1:245, 1:62, and 1:84 dilutions of sera from patients NT, TY, and MK (who were good responders), respectively. KR2, KM4, and OT are patient sera diluted 1:1. Human monoclonal antibody (HuMoAb) was irrelevant human monoclonal antibody TOH/D5 with the same isotype of CLN-IgG.

closely to a mechanism of tumorigenicity and immunity through antigen and its ligand interaction. CLN-IgG recognized TA226, and idio-No. 3 recognized p34 antigen; taking the counterimaginable relationship of these antibodies into consideration, p34 may behave as a ligand to TA226.

We have presented portraits of idiotope images of anti-cancer antibodies derived by computer-aided graphics in this chapter. Comprehending the host immune response that might allow patient respite from the tumorous stage in antigen-specific HuMoAb therapy.

Acknowledgments. We thank Mr. Y. Yamamoto and Mr. H. Yuasa for their skillful assistance regarding antibody and antigen preparation. This work was partially supported by Japan Pharmaceutical Development Co. in Osaka.

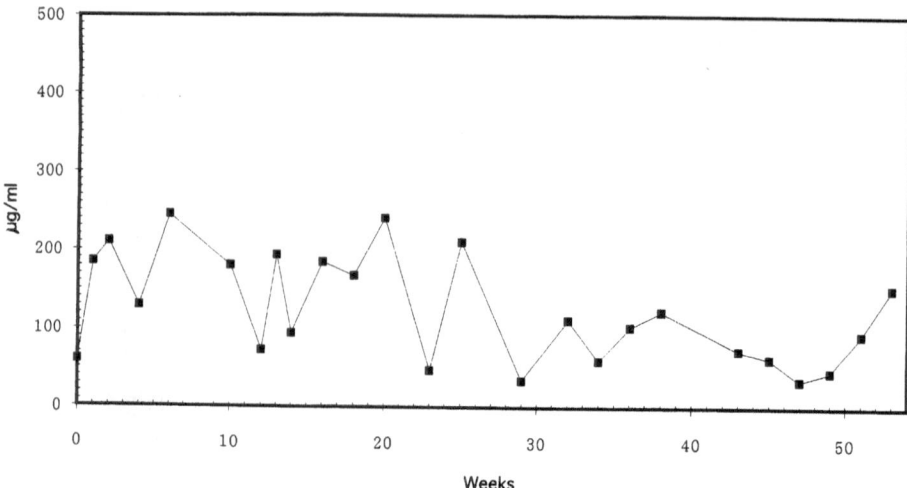

Fig. 5. Aperiodic intensification of the paratope image of anti anti-idiotypic antibody by CLN-IgG administration in malignant astrocytoma patient. The patient (NT) received a 1-mg dose of CLN-IgG twice weekly. The content of CLN-IgG paratope-carrying IgG in the serum was measured intermittently using anti-paratactic antibody in $2M$ NaCl + $5M$ urea. The concentration of anti anti-idiotypic antibody was measured as the amount of IgG corresponding to that of CLN-IgG calculated from a dose-dependent curve. Each point represents the content of CLN-IgG equivalent in the serum, indicated by the mean value of triplicate trials

References

1. Taomoto K, Ijichi A, Matsumoto S, Hagiwara H (1991) Antitumor effects of human monoclonal antibodies on human malignant glioma xenografts and their clinical application. In: Tabuchi K (ed) Biological aspects of brain tumors. Springer, Berlin Heidelberg Tokyo, pp 452–463
2. Nagai M, Arai T, Watanabe K, et al (1991) Clinical application of rediolabeled human x human monoclonal antibody with interferon in the treatment of malignant glioma—preliminary report. In: Paoletti P et al (eds) Neuro-oncology. Kluwer, Dordrecht, pp 153–159
3. Jerne NK, Roland J, Cazenave P-A (1982) Recurrent idiotopes and internal images. EMBO J 1:243–247
4. Lundvkvist I, Coutinho A, Varela F, Holmberg D (1989) Evidence for a functional idiotypic network among natural antibodies in normal mice. Proc Natl Acad Sci USA 86:5074–5078
5. Herlyn D, Linnenbach A, Koprowski H, Herlyn M (1991) Epitope- and antigen-specific cancer vaccines. Int Rev Immunol 7:245–257
6. Bhattacharya-chatterjee M, Foon KA, Köhler H (1991) Antiidiotype monoclonal antibodies as vaccines for human cancer. Int Rev Immunol 7:289–302
7. Köler G, Milstein C (1975) Continuous culture of fused cells secreting antibody of predefined specificity. Nature 256:495–497
8. Hagiwara H, Sato HG (1983) Human × human hybridoma producing monoclonal antibody against autologous cervical carcinoma. Mol Biol Med 1:245–252
9. Kokunai T, Tamaki N, Matsumoto S (1990) Antigen related to cell proliferation in malignant gliomas recognized by a human monoclonal antibody. J Neurosurg 73:901–908
10. Osumi K, Nagao J, Yuasa H, et al (1992) Antibody-dependent cell-mediated cytotoxicity on human cervical carcinoma cell line, ME-180, with human monoclonal antibody. Cancer Lett 62:179–183

11. Umesaki N, Kawabata M, Kanaoka Y, et al (1991) Reactivity and cytotoxicity of human monoclonal antibody (CLN-IgG) to the gynecological malignancies. J Jpn Soc Cancer Ther 26(1):14–20
12. Aotsuka Y, Hagiwara H (1988) Identification of a malignant cell associated antigen recognized by a human monoclonal antibody. Eur J Cancer Clin Oncol 24:829–837
13. Hagiwara H, Nagao J, Yamamoto Y, et al (1993) Concentrated induction of tumor antigen-specific anti-anti-idiotypic antibody in the serum of brain tumor patient treated with human monoclonal antibody CLN-IgG. In: Proceedings of the Japanese Cancer Association, 52nd Annual Meeting Oct. 7, Sendai, p 429

Clinical Effect of CLN-IgG on Glioma and Its Correlation with the Induction of Antianti-Idiotypic Antibody in the Serum

Masakatsu Nagai[1], Jun-ichi Narita[1], Kunihiko Watanabe[1],
Masaru Endoh[1], Chikayuki Ochiai[1], and Hideaki Hagiwara[2]

Abstract. CLN-IgG is a monoclonal antibody (Ab) produced from a human–human hybridoma recognizing the tumor common antigen (Ag) TA226. In a clinical trial of CLN-IgG treatment conducted in 16 cases of glioma, 1 mg of the Ab was administered to patients twice a week for more than 8 weeks. The induction of antianti-idiotypic Ab (Ab3) in the serum of patient was measured using anti-CLN-IgG idiotype Ab (idiono.33). In 2 cases of complete remission and 3 cases of partial remission treated with CLN-IgG, high levels of Ab3 were detected. The induction of Ab3 was correlated to the clinical effect of the treatment. CLN-IgG is beneficial for the long-term maintenance therapy of glioma without an adverse side effect.

Key words: Glioma—Monoclonal antibody—CLN-IgG—Maintenance therapy

Introduction

CLN-IgG is a monoclonal antibody (MoAb) produced from a human–human hybridoma by Hagiwara et al. in 1983 [1,2]. This MoAb recognizes the tumor common antigen (Ag) TA226 and shows affinity for glioma cells [3]. A phase II clinical trial of CLN-IgG for the treatment of glioma has been conducted since 1990 in several institutions in Japan. At the same time, the correlation of induction of antianti-idiotypic antibody (Ab3) in the sera of patient with clinical effectiveness was also studied.

Clinical Material and Methods

Patient Selection

We submitted 16 cases of glioma (9 glioblastoma [GB], 5 malignant astrocytoma [MA], and 2 low-grade astrocytoma [A]) to the CLN-IgG treatment for the purpose of long-term maintenance therapy. The mean age of the patients was 45.8 years (range, 12–66 years); 7 were male and 9 were female. In 14 primary cases, CLN-IgG treatment was inaugurated 4 weeks after postoperative adjuvant therapy (interferon-

---

[1] Department of Neurosurgery, Dokkyo University School of Medicine, Mibu, Tochigi 321-02, Japan
[2] Hagiwara Institute of Health, Kasai, Hyogo 679-01, Japan

1-(4-amino-2-methyl-5-pyrimidynl-3-(2-chloroethyl)-3-nitrosoured hydrochloride (ACNU)–radiation therapy), and in 2 recurrent cases, a wash-out interval of 4 weeks was made between the end of previous therapy and the start of CLN-IgG treatment.

Monoclonal Antibody Used

MoAb used in this study was produced by Hagiwara et al. [1,2] by means of the fusion of the human lymphoblastoid B-cell line UC729-6 and lymphocytes from the metastatic lymph node of human squamous cell carcinoma of the uterine cervix. The fused cells were cloned and produced a MoAb named CLN-IgG. This MoAb possesses gamma-1 and kappa chains; its molecular weight is 150000. It was prepared as a freeze-dried powder passed through a 0.22-μm-pore filter supplied by the Hagiwara Health Institute.

Method of Administration

Intravenously, 1 mg of CLN-IgG dissolved in 2 ml of distilled water was given twice a week for more than 8 weeks for as long as possible.

Measurement of Ab3

The titer of Ab3 induced in the serum of each patient was measured once every 2 weeks using Ab2 (idio-No.33), an anti-paratope antibody against CLN-IgG (see the chapter by H. Hagiwara and Y. Aotsuka, this volume). The grade of induction of Ab3 was assessed as follows: greater than 200 μg/ml, 3+; greater than 100 μg/ml, 2+; and less than 100 μg/ml, 1+.

Evaluation of Efficacy of the Therapy

The efficacy of the therapy was assessed according to the criteria of the Ministry of Health and Welfare in Japan for the evaluation of the clinical effect of cancer chemotherapy on solid tumors measured by computed tomography (CT) scan or magnetic resonance imaging (MRI): complete remission (CR) is disappearance of a measurable or assessible lesion; partial remission (PR) is more than 50% tumor reduction; no change (NC) is less than 50% of tumor reduction plus progressive disease (PD).

Results

As shown in the list of cases treated with CLN-IgG (Table 1), Ab3 was induced and detected in nine cases (2 GB, 5 MA, and 2 A). Reduction of the tumor size was noticed in six cases (2 CR, 4 PR) of these nine, which indicates obvious correlation to the Ab3 induction. Regarding the grade of Ab3 induction in CR cases, one case of GB was 2+, one case of MA was 1+, and in PR cases (all MA), one case was 3+ and two cases were 2+. Thus, there was no relation between the grade of Ab3 induction and the reduction rate of tumor size. Another Ab3-positive case of MA was assessed as NC, but this patient has survived for a long period (more than 2 years). In four cases of NC and four cases of PD, the induction of Ab3 was not detected in the sera at all.

Table 1. Cases of glioma patients treated with CLN-IgG.

Case	Age	Sex	Pathology	Operation	Adjuvant therapy	PS	CLN Start dose (mg)	Total	Response	Survival time (mo)	Detection of Ab-3	Outcome (PS)
1 N.T.	28	F	MA	91.8.	IAR-JET	1	92.3.	138+	PR	>30	3+	Alive (1)
2 K.M.	40	F	GB	91.3.	AR-JET	4a	92.4.	53	PD	5	—	Died
3 K.R.	66	M	GB	91.11.	IAR-A	4a	92.4.	37	NC	6	—	Died
4 U.T.	12	M	MA	91.1.	IAR-A	0	92.7.	113+	NC	>26	2+	Alive (0)
5 I.M.	66	F	GB	92.7.	IAR	0	92.10.	188+	CR	>23	2+	Alive (0)
6 H.K.	41	M	GB	92.7.	IAR	0	92.10.	21	PD	3	—	Died
7 H.H.	26	F	MA	92.1.	IAR	1	93.2.	166+	CR	>19	3+	Alive (0)
8 S.K.	42	F	MA	92.1.	IAR	0	93.3.	77+	PR	>18	2+	Alive (1)
9 I.H.	46	M	MA	93.2.	IAR	0	93.5.	72+	PR	>16	2+	Alive (0)
10 S.Y.	35	F	GB	93.1.	IAR	1	93.5.	24	PD	3	—	Died
11 S.J.	47	M	GB	93.2.	IAR-I	3	93.5.	32	NC	3	—	Died
12 T.T.	60	F	GB	93.1.	IAR	1	93.6.	42	NC	8	—	Died
13 T.T.	57	F	GB	93.3.	AR	4	93.7.	37	PD	4	—	Died
14 A.S.	47	F	A	93.5.	IAR	2	93.8.	79+	PR	>13	2+	Alive (0)
15 F.M.	63	M	GB	93.8.	IAR	3	93.11.	35	PD	10	1+	Alive (4)
16 S.M.	56	M	A	90.11.	IAR	2	94.1.	60+	NC	>8	2+	Alive (1)

F, female; M, male; A, astrocytoma; MA, malignant astrocytoma; GB, glioblastoma; I, interferon; A, ACNU; R, radiation; J, carboplatin (JM-8); ET, etoposide; CR, complete remission; PR, partial remission; NC, no change; PD, progressive disease; PS, performance state.
a Recurrent case.

An adverse side effect from CLN-IgG has never been observed, which allows long-term treatment with this MoAb even for nearly 3 years.

Titer of Ab3 in the serum became detectable after the administration of 5–10 mg in most cases, reached the peak value about 10–30 mg, and revealed an aperiodic wave-like curve thereafter. In cases that responded after the long-term treatment, the elevation of Ab3 titer was also slow but the higher level of titer had been maintained for a long period.

Serial pictures of MRI and Ab3 curves of two cases of CR are seen in Figs. 1 and 2.

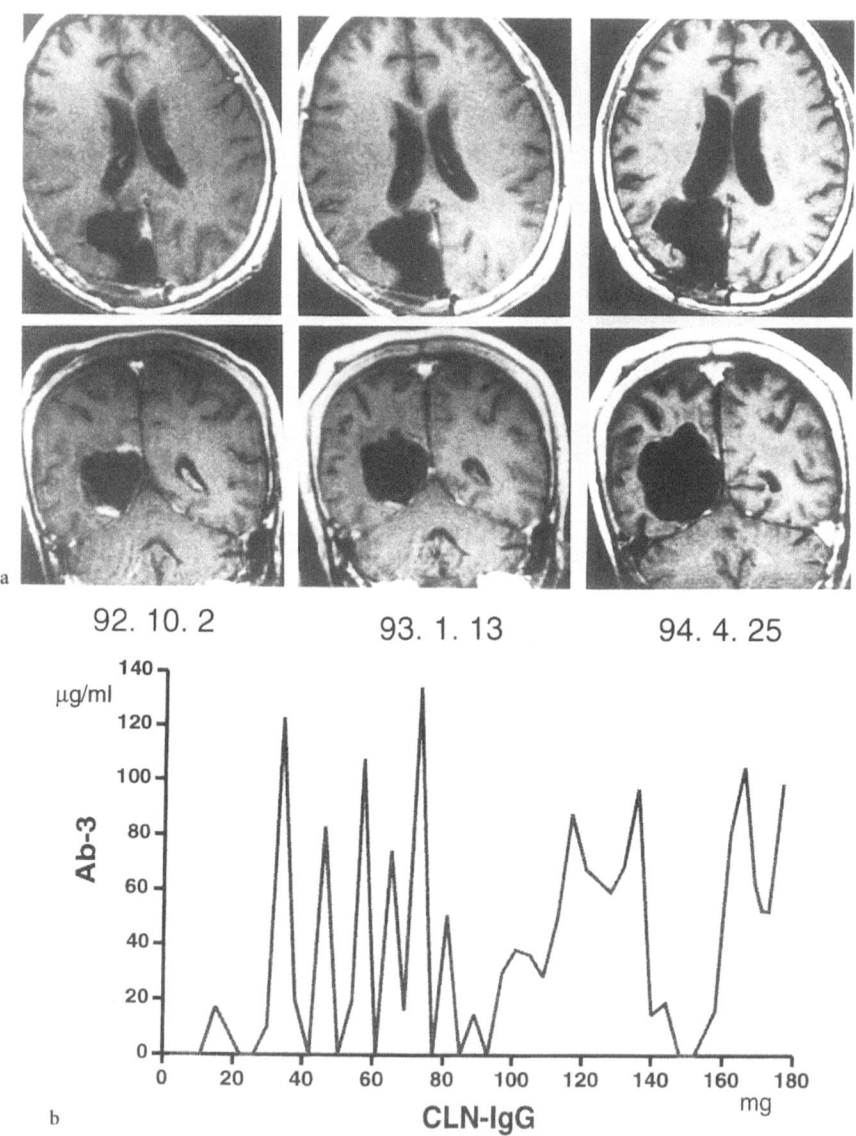

Fig. 1. a Serial computed tomography (CT) scan of case 5 (66-year-old woman, right-occipital glioblastoma) evaluated as complete remission. **b** The titer of Ab3 in the serum of case 5. An aperiodic rhythmic curve is plotted

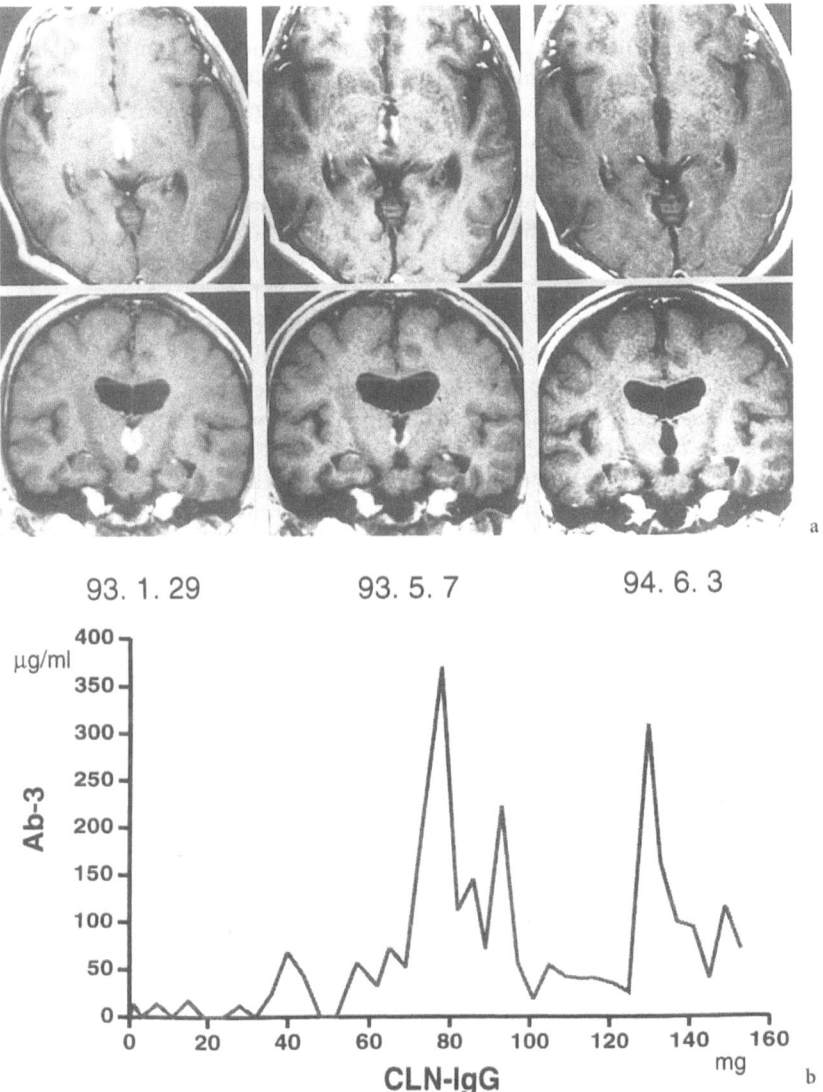

Fig. 2. a Serial CT scan of case 7 (24-year-old woman, malignant astrocytoma in the hypothalamus) evaluated as complete remission. **b** The titer of Ab3 in the serum of case 7. The higher titers are induced corresponding to the increasing dosage of monoclonal antibody (MoAb)

Discussion

The affinity of CLN-IgG for glioma cells with growth control has been demonstrated by Kokunai et al. [3] and Taomoto et al. [4] by in vitro and in vivo studies. Regarding the mechanism, the antitumor action of MoAb is attributed to ADCC and/or CDC [5,6]. The action of CLN-IgG is also proven as a mechanism through the recognition of a tumor common antigen TA226 (60k/53k) [7]. Recently, Jerne's idiotype network theory [8] has been considered as one of the antitumor mechanism, although its evidence has remained obscure. The concept of an idiotypic network has been confirmed remarkably, because the measurement of Ab3 in the serum became possible using an antiparatope antibody against CLN-IgG (Ab2, idio-No.33 and -No.3) that was produced from Balb/c hybridoma (see the chapter by H. Hagiwara and Y. Aotsuka, this volume). It might be said that the correlation between induction of Ab3 in the serum and effectiveness on the tumor reduction was elucidated in our clinical study.

The cause of aperiodic wavelike induction of Ab3 is supposed to be a cyclic course of production and consumption of internal images—Ab1–Ab2–Ab3–Ab2—and so on. Ab2 is the internal image of the antigen (Ag) itself and shows the functions of enhancement and retention of Ag presentation. For this reason, Herlyn et al. [9] reported the clinical use of Ab2 for the postoperative treatment of colorectal cancer. Further extensive investigation is needed to clarify the connection of an idiotype network with the killing mechanism by the killer T cell.

MoAb produced from a human–human hybridoma has an advantage compared to a mouse-human hybridoma in that it can be easily transferred to the clinical application. In fact, the clinical trial with human MoAb CLN-IgG has been carried out smoothly and safely without any adverse effect. Taomoto et al. [10] reported the beneficial clinical effect of CLN-IgG therapy in 38 cases of glioma, in 11 cases of which Ab3 were detected in the sera. In our clinical trial, cases of MA responded to the CLN-IgG therapy; 3 of 5 cases showed remission (CR or PR) in reduction of tumor size; furthermore, in most cases the prolongation of survival period was observed. In cases of GB, however, the responsiveness was poor except for 1 case in which subtotal resection of the tumor could be achieved. From these results, we can say that CLN-IgG therapy is useful for the long-term maintenance therapy for MA, while it does not show efficacy for GB so that more extensive chemotherapy is required.

The synthesis of Ab2 (idio-no.33) enabled us to measure the titer of Ab3 in the serum of patients. In the nonresponding cases, Ab3 was never detected in the sera after the administration of 5–10mg of CLN-IgG. Thus, the correlation between the clinical effect and the induction of Ab3 was also indicated from this point of view. Moreover, this fact may be utilized as a sensitivity test to determine the indication for therapy.

To overcome the limitation of a single use of MoAb, several clinical trials of targeting therapy using MoAb combined with a radioisotope or anticancer drug have been conducted. We have reported on the good clinical effect of radioimmunotherapy using I-131-labeled CLN-IgG administered locally for the treatment of glioma including GB [11]. However, it became clear in this study that even a single use of CLN-IgG revealed clinical effects, at least on MA, and thus the therapy seems to be worthy of further investigations.

Conclusion

A phase II clinical trial of human MoAb CLN-IgG for the treatment of glioma can be conducted safely for a long time period. Beneficial results were obtained, especially in the case of MA, corresponding to the induction of Ab3 in the serum of patients. CLN-IgG treatment holds future promise as a long-term maintenance therapy for glioma.

References

1. Hagiwara H, Sato G (1983) Human × human hybridoma producing monoclonal antibody against autologous cervical carcinoma. Mol Biol Med 1:245–252
2. Glassy MC, Handley HH, Hagiwara H, Hoyston I (1983) UC729-6, a human lymphoblastoid B-cell line useful for generating antibody-secreting human-human hybridomas. Proc Natl Acad Sci USA 80:6327–6331
3. Kokunai T, Tamaki N, Matsumoto S (1990) Antigen related to cell proliferation in malignant gliomas recognized by a human monoclonal antibody. J Neurosurg 73:901–908
4. Taomoto K, Ijichi A, Matsumoto S, Hagiwara H (1991) Anti-tumor effect of human monoclonal antibodies on human malignant glioma xenografts and their clinical application. In: Tabuchi K (ed) Biological aspects of brain tumors. Springer, Berlin Heidelberg Tokyo, pp 452–463
5. Hagiwara H, Aotsuka Y (1987) Cytotoxicity of mixed human monoclonal antibodies reacting to tumor antigens. Acta Paediatr Jpn 29:552–556
6. Takahashi H, Belser PH, Atkinson BF, Sela BA, Ross AH, Biegel J, Emanuel B, Sutton L, Koprowski H, Herlyn D (1990) Monoclonal antibody-dependent, cell-mediated cytotoxicity angainst human malignant gliomas. Neurosurgery (Baltimore) 27:97–102
7. Aotsuka Y, Hagiwara H (1988) Identification of a malignant cell-associated antigen recognized by a human monoclonal antibody. Eur J Cancer Clin Oncol 24:829–838
8. Jerne NK (1974) Towards a network theory of the immune system. Ann Immunol (Inst Pasteur) 125C:373–389
9. Herlyn D, Weetndorf M, Schmoll E, Iliopoulos D, Schedel I, Dreikhausen U, Raab R, Ross AH, Jakshe H, Scriba M, Koprowski H (1987) Anti-idiotype immunization of cancer patients: modulation of the immune response. Proc Natl Acad Sci USA 84:8055–8059
10. Taomoto K (1994) Cytokine therapy on glioma—monoclonal antibody (in Japanese). Clin Neurosci (Jpn) 12:672–675
11. Nagai M, Arai T, Watanabe K, Ichikawa K, Watari T (1991) Clinical application of radiolabeled human × human monoclonal antibody with interferon in the treatment of malignant glioma. In: Paoletti P, Takakura K, Walker MD, Butti G, Pezzota S (eds) Neuro-oncology. Kluwer, Dordrecht, pp 153–159

Section 2. Gene Therapy (Basic Studies)

Gene Therapy for Central Nervous System Tumors

Suzanne Dee, James Fick, and Mark A. Israel

Abstract. Molecular oncology and recombinant DNA technologies have greatly increased our understanding of molecular mechanisms that are altered during malignant transformation, facilitating the development of new approaches to cancer treatment. Rapid progress in the development of gene therapy for the treatment of nervous system tumors could impact greatly on the practice of neuro-oncology. In this report, we describe potential strategies and review recent advances for the use of gene therapy to treat these tumors.

Key words. Gene therapy—Brain tumors—Immunotherapy—Viral-directed enzyme/Prodrug therapy—Drug resistance

Introduction

Recombinant DNA technology has ushered in an era of molecular oncology in which the genetic basis for malignant transformation is now recognized and is being intensely examined. Knowledge of the genetic alterations associated with the development of tumors has provided key insights into the molecular basis of neoplastic disease. This has important implications for the fields of neuropathology and neuro-oncology. The development of new diagnostic methods that use recombinant DNA techniques to screen tumors for mutated genes will undoubtedly contribute to our understanding of the actual molecular disorders that underlie tumor development. It is possible that such tests will one day predict the biological behavior of a specific tumor, thus enabling physicians to prescribe individualized therapy for patients with a specific oncogenetic diagnosis.

Current treatments for brain tumors are not usually potent, durable, or tumor selective. Gene therapy distinguishes itself from conventional approaches to therapy because advances in molecular genetics have made it possible to selectively express gene products in either normal or tumor cells. This provides an opportunity to test new therapeutic approaches to cancer based on the transfer of genetic material. Such novel therapeutic initiatives include enzyme-prodrug strategies, attempts to induce antitumor immunity with molecular approaches designed to increase tumor

Preuss Laboratory for Molecular Neuro-oncology, Brain Tumor Research Center, Department of Neurological Surgery, School of Medicine, University of California, San Francisco, San Francisco, CA 94143-0520, USA

389

antigenicity and augment host response mechanisms, and the modulation of molecular pathways mediating the malignant phenotype. To date, gene transfer approaches have been used in human patients to answer fundamental questions of tumor biology as well as to correct congenital enzymatic deficiencies. Undoubtedly, gene therapies will play an important role in the design of investigational treatment approaches for cancer in the future (for review, see [1–10]).

Gene Therapy Strategies and Techniques

Gene therapy strategies for the treatment of central nervous system tumors can be conveniently divided into three categories (Table 1): (1) those that involve the downregulation or inactivation of oncogenes, (2) those leading to the replacement of tumor suppressor genes, and (3) those strategies that result in the addition of new genetic material (transgenes) to normal or malignant cells. The downregulation of gene products contributing to the malignant features of a tumor is the goal of "antisense" strategies. The overexpression of an oncogene can promote the clonal expansion of a mutant cell leading to tumor formation. This predicts that the downregulation of inappropriately activated gene sequences would inhibit the growth of tumor cells [11–16]. Using antisense technologies targeted against the c-*sis* oncogene product [17] or the product of the bFGF gene [18], investigators have been able to inhibit the growth of astrocytic tumor cell lines. Gene therapy strategies that would target the transfer of antisense molecules, ribozymes, or specific proteases within tumor cells are being explored in animal models.

Other therapeutic strategies have focused on the transfer of genetic material to tumor cells with the intent of altering various cellular activities. This type of approach includes the selective expression of a transgene to enhance tumor susceptibility to a particular therapy or to protect normal cells from the toxicity associated with irradiation or chemotherapy. The most widely evaluated of such strategies has involved the transfer of drug resistance genes to bone marrow stem cells [19–22]. Such strategies have involved genes that are of central importance for the treatment of central nervous system malignancies, such as *mdr* or other genes encoding proteins which confer specific resistance to the nitrosoureas [23–26]. It is anticipated that higher doses of chemotherapy would be tolerated after such autologous cells were returned to the patient, enhancing the efficacy of currently available chemotherapeutic agents.

One novel gene therapy approach employs autologous tumor cells as a vaccine. Current strategies for the development of tumor vaccines typically involve the transduction of a cytokine gene into primary cultures of tumor cells obtained at the time of surgery. The cells are expanded in culture and then inoculated intradermally or subcutaneously following irradiation to prevent their replication [10, 27–29]. Preliminary results from studies performed in murine tumor models suggest that granulocyte-macrophage colony-stimulating factor (GM-CSF) is particularly effective in inducing potent antitumor immunity [30]. The local rejection of tumor cells ex-

Table 1. Conceptual gene therapy strategies for central nervous system tumors.

Gene inactivation or downregulation
Gene addition
Gene replacement

pressing GM-CSF has been shown to result in the elimination of established primary and metastatic tumors as well as to protect against rechallenges with unmodified tumor. This suggests that tumor vaccines could play a role in therapies directed against known tumor sites, undetected microscopic tumor deposits, and recurrent disease [31–34]. Presumably, GM-CSF facilitates the functioning of antigen-presenting cells, which play a critical role in the recognition of the tumor antigens by the host immune system. Other genes that are being transferred into tumor cells in an attempt to increase tumor antigenicity include costimulatory molecules such as B7 [35, 36] and specific major histocompatibility complex (MHC) genes. The identification of tumor-specific antigens, such as the melanoma antigen (MAGE) expressed by melanomas [37–41], might improve the antitumor specificity of immunotherapy. Candidate molecules for the development of such vaccines include products of mutated oncogenes, oncofetal antigens, and viral proteins produced by neoplastic cells in viral-induced tumors.

Other strategies are being pursued to enhance the sensitivity of tumor cells to drugs that are otherwise innocuous or have a low cytotoxic potential. One such approach involves the transduction of tumor cells with enzymes not otherwise present in the body that can convert an inactive prodrug to a cytotoxic drug. Best studied among these approaches is a gene therapy strategy known as viral directed enzyme prodrug therapy (VDEPT) [42]. VDEPT utilizes retroviral vectors and has proven to be effective in eliminating some types of experimental brain tumors in rodent models [43–49]. The basis of this approach is straightforward: a viral gene encoding an enzyme that converts an inactive prodrug into a therapeutically active metabolite is transferred selectively into tumor cells. This enzyme can then mediate a cytotoxic effect in the infected cell. A key feature of this therapy for brain tumors is that the targets for retroviral vector-mediated gene transfer are dividing cells [50–52], such as tumor cells, and in the mature nervous system most normal cells are postmitotic. Therefore, tumor cells are targeted by the retroviral vectors and expression of the transduced gene is limited to tumor cells.

The most extensively studied VDEPT strategy for the treatment of brain tumors has used a recombinant retroviral vector containing the thymidine kinase gene from herpes simplex virus type 1 (HSV-tk). Following recombinant retroviral vector infection of a tumor cell, the HSV-tk gene is stably integrated into the host cell genome. The thymidine kinase enzyme encoded by mammalian cells does not have high affinity for guanine analogs such as ganciclovir (GCV), which HSV-tk will avidly phosphorylate. The phosphorylated GCV metabolites are suitable substrates for mammalian DNA polymerases, and the incorporation of these nucleotide analogs into the cellular genome during DNA replication leads to tumor cell death. Because GCV is not a substrate for mammalian thymidine kinase, this drug does not harm normal cells when given in therapeutic doses.

Following the direct inoculation of retroviral vectors into established intracerebral tumors in rodents, the transduction efficiency of tumor cells is rarely greater than 1%. However, when xenografted tumors are injected with a murine fibroblast packaging cell line engineered to produce recombinant retroviral vectors containing a marker gene, the percentage of tumor cells expressing the marker gene can be increased to 10% [53]. While this suggests that only 10% of a tumor can be expected to respond to GCV therapy, it has been shown that in some brain tumor models infection with the HSV-tk-containing retrovirus and treatment with GCV leads to a degree of cell death that far exceeds the number of cells expressing the transduced HSV-tk gene. Such experiments indicate that the 9L rat brain tumor could be eliminated after treatment with GCV when as few as 10% of the cells expressed the HSV-tk gene [44]. This is referred to as the "bystander effect," but the mechanism of this phenomenom is not known [54–56].

To date, no evidence of toxicity to the normal brain in animals treated with this gene therapy strategy has been reported, and this suggests that the bystander cytotoxic effect is tumor specific. Also, toxicity to organs outside the nervous system has not been detected, and no retroviral vector-induced secondary malignancies have occurred [48]. Evidence for the bystander effect has also been observed by several groups using the HSV-tk/GCV gene therapy strategy to treat a variety of tumor types in animal models [57–61]. The VDEPT gene therapy approach for experimental brain tumors appears to offer several potential advantages over conventional therapies used to treat brain tumors in human patients. Retroviral-mediated gene transfer is selective for tumor cells in animal models, and there is no systemic toxicity associated with the administration of therapeutic doses of the prodrug GCV. While the bystander effect results in the death of a greater number of tumor cells than would be predicted by the number of cells that express the HSV-tk gene, this toxicity appears to remain tumor specific. Investigational trials evaluating the safety of HSV-tk/GCV treatment strategies in human patients with recurrent malignant gliomas are currently underway. Whether the successes of this approach in animals can be duplicated in patients remains an open question. Other therapeutic strategies incorporating the major conceptual features of the VDEPT approach to the management of tumors are listed in Table 2.

Gene therapy strategies that involve the in vivo transfer of genetic material or the transfer of genes to all or most of the tumor cells are problematic in that the currently available gene transfer systems are unlikely to successfully provide for such demanding requirements. The specific choice of a gene transfer technique will depend on the demands for accuracy, efficiency, and stable gene expression of any particular gene therapy strategy. For example, a tumor vaccine gene therapy approach has only limited requirements for the efficiency and accuracy of gene transfer. Furthermore, even if the expression of the transferred gene is not stable for a prolonged period of time, it is possible that only a very short period of cytokine production would be necessary for the development of a sustainable host immune response.

On the other hand, the VDEPT strategy may require that the prodrug-activating gene be transferred to all or almost all the tumor cells and that this transfer (or at least gene expression) must be accurately targeted to the tumor cell or unwanted toxicity to normal tissue can be expected. The gene transfer techniques that are currently available (Table 3) vary dramatically, not only in their practicality for use in vitro and in vivo but also in other characteristics. The transfer technologies currently being used for human gene therapy trials are limited. Only liposome-mediated transfer is being

Table 2. Viral-directed enzyme prodrug therapy (VDEPT).

Prodrug	Enzyme	Cytotoxic metabolite
Adenine arabinoside	HSV-tk	Ara-ATP
5-Fluorocytosine	Cytosine deaminase	5-Fluorouracil
Ganciclovir	HSV-tk	GCV-P

HSV-tk, herpes simplex virus type 1; ATP, adenosine triphosphate; GCV-P, ganciclovir phosphate.

Table 3. Gene delivery systems.

Physical methods
    Calcium phosphate precipitation
    Electroporation
    Microinjection
    Protoplast fusion
    Liposomal transfer
    Receptor-mediated delivery
    Tissue injection
Viral vectors
    Retroviruses
    Herpesviruses
    Adenoviruses

used from among the various physical gene transfer systems, and in the case of cancer studies, retroviral vectors are also being utilized. These systems, although the most efficient of those currently available, are still very inefficient in vivo and it is likely that greatly enhanced gene transfer systems will be needed if gene therapy strategies targeting tumor cells dispersed throughout the body are to be pursued.

Summary and Conclusions

We should anticipate that gene therapy protocols for the treatment of central nervous system tumors will initially be designed to augment conventional therapies of proven efficacy. This will certainly be the case for brain tumors in which multimodality approaches to therapy already predominate. Among the gene therapy approaches currently being investigated, some may prove to be superior to standard therapy, while others may provide insights into mechanisms that could be exploited in the design of new therapies. The VDEPT gene therapy strategy has been shown to eliminate experimental brain tumors in animal models and is currently being evaluated for the treatment of human brain tumors in several different clinical protocols. It seems likely that interest in this field will continue to grow and will lead to the emergence of a more recognizable role for gene therapy in the management of central nervous system tumors.

References

1. Friedmann T (1992) A brief history of gene therapy. Nature Genet 2:93–98
2. Miller AD (1992) Human gene therapy comes of age. Nature 357:455–460
3. Kennedy PGE, Steiner I (1993) The use of herpes simplex virus vectors for gene therapy in neurological diseases. Q J Med 86:697–702
4. Morgan RA, Anderson WF (1993) Human gene therapy. Annu Rev Biochem 62:191–217
5. Tolstoshev P (1993) Gene therapy, concepts, current trials and future directions. Annu Rev Pharmacol Toxicol 33:573–596
6. Culver KW, Blaese RM (1994) Gene therapy for cancer. Trends Genet 10:174–178
7. Friedmann T (1994) Gene therapy for neurological disorders. Trends Genet 10:210–214
8. Uckert W, Walther W (1994) Retrovirus-mediated gene transfer in cancer therapy. Pharmacol Ther 63:323–347
9. Kerr WG, Mule JJ (1994) Gene therapy—current status and future prospects. J Leukocyte Biol 56:210–214

10. Miller AR, McBride WH, Hunt K, Economou JS (1994) Cytokine-mediated gene therapy for cancer. Ann Surg Oncol 1:436–450
11. Zon G (1990) Innovations in the use of antisense oligonucleotides. Ann NY Acad Sci 616:161–172
12. Calabretta B (1991) Inhibition of protooncogene expression by antisense oligodeoxynucleotides: biological and therapeutic implications. Cancer Res 51:4505–4510
13. Calabretta B, Skorski T, Szczylik C, Zon G (1993) Prospects for gene-directed therapy with antisense oligodeoxynucleotides. Cancer Treat Rev 19:169–179
14. Carter G, Lemoine NR (1993) Antisense technology for cancer therapy: does it make sense? Br J Cancer 67:869–876
15. Milligan JF, Jones RJ, Froehler BC, Matteucci MD (1994) Development of antisense therapeutics. Implications for cancer gene therapy. Ann NY Acad Sci 716:228–241
16. Yung WK (1994) New approaches in brain tumor therapy using gene transfer and antisense oligonucleotides. Curr Opin Oncol 6:235–239
17. Nitta T, Sato K (1994) Specific inhibition of c-*sis* protein synthesis and cell proliferation with antisense oligodeoxynucleotides in human glioma cells. Neurosurgery (Baltimore) 34:309–314
18. Morrison RS, Giordano S, Yamaguchi F, Hendrickson S, Berger MS, Palczewski K (1993) Basic fibroblast growth factor expression is required for clonogenic growth of human glioma cells. J Neurosci Res 34:502–509
19. Mickisch GH, Aksentijevich I, Schoenlein PV, Goldstein LJ, Galski H, Stahle C, Sachs DH, Pastan I, Gottesman MM (1992) Transplantation of bone marrow cells from transgenic mice expressing the human MDR1 gene results in long-term protection against the myelosuppressive effect of chemotherapy in mice. Blood 79:1087–1093
20. Sorrentino BP, Brandt SJ, Bodine D, Gottesman M, Pastan I, Cline A, Nienhuis AW (1992) Selection of drug-resistant bone marrow cells in vivo after retroviral transfer of human MDR1. Science 257:99–103
21. Deisseroth AB, Zu Z, Claxton D, Hanania EG, Fu S, Ellerson D, Goldberg L, Thomas M, Janicek K, Anderson WF, et al (1994) Genetic marking shows that Ph+ cells present in autologous transplants of chronic myelogenous leukemia (CML) contribute to relapse after autologous bone marrow in CML. Blood 83:3068–3076
22. Gottesman MM, Germann UA, Aksentijevich I, Sugimoto Y, Cardarelli CO, Pastan I (1994) Gene transfer of drug resistance genes. Implications for cancer therapy. Ann NY Acad Sci 716:126–138
23. Berhane K, Hao XY, Egyhazi S, Hansson J, Ringborg U, Mannervik B (1993) Contribution of glutathione transferase M3-3 to 1,3-bis(2-chloroethyl)-1-nitrosourea resistance in a human non-small cell lung cancer line. Cancer Res 53:4257–4261
24. Marathi UK, Kroes RA, Dolan ME, Erickson LC (1993) Prolonged depletion of 06-methylguanine DNA methyltransferase activity following exposure to 06-benzylguanine with or without streptozotocin enhances 1,3-bis(2-chloroethyl)-1-nitrosourea sensitivity in vitro. Cancer Res 53:4281–4286
25. Marathi UK, Dolan ME, Erickson LC (1994) Extended depletion of 06-methylguanine-DNA methyltransferase activity following 06-benzyl-2'-deoxyguanosine or 06-benzylguanine combined with streptozotocin treatment enhances 1,3-bis(2-chloroethyl)-1-nitrosourea cytotoxicity. Cancer Res 54:4371–4375
26. Gerson SL, Berger SJ, Varnes ME, Donovan C (1994) Combined depletion of 06-alkylguanine-DNA alkyltransferase and glutathione to modulate nitrosourea resistance in breast cancer. Biochem Pharmacol 48:543–548
27. Pardoll D (1992) New strategies for active immunotherapy with genetically engineered tumor cells. Curr Opin Immunol 4:619–623
28. Pardoll D (1992) Immunotherapy with cytokine gene-transduced tumor cells: the next wave in gene therapy for cancer. Curr Opin Oncol 4:1124–1129
29. Forni G, Giovarelli M, Cavallo F, Consalvo M, Allione A, Modesti A, Musiani P, Colombo MP (1993) Cytokine-induced tumor immunogenicity: from exogenous cytokines to gene therapy. J Immunother 14:253–257

30. Dranoff G, Jaffee E, Lazenby A, Golumbek P, Levitsky H, Brose K, Jackson V, Hamada H, Pardoll D, Mulligan RC (1993) Vaccination with irradiated tumor cells engineered to secrete murine granulocyte-macrophage colony-stimulating factor stimulates potent, specific, and long-lasting anti-tumor immunity. Proc Natl Acad Sci USA 90:3539–3543

31. McCabe ER (1993) Clinical application of gene therapy: emerging opportunities and current limitations. Biochem Med Metab Biol 50:241–253

32. Ogasawara M, Rosenberg SA (1993) Enhanced expression of HLA molecules and stimulation of autologous tumor infiltrating lymphocytes following transduction of melanoma cells with gamma-interferon genes. Cancer Res 53:3561–3568

33. Zatloukal K, Schmidt W, Cotten M, Wagner E, Stingl G, Birnstiel ML (1993) Somatic gene therapy for cancer: the utility of transferrinfection in generating "tumor vaccines." Gene 135:199–207

34. Celis E, Tsai V, Crimi C, DeMars R, Wentworth PA, Chesnut RW, Grey HM, Sette A, Serra HM (1994) Induction of anti-tumor cytotoxic T lymphocytes in normal humans using primary cultures and synthetic peptide epitopes. Proc Natl Acad Sci USA 91:2105–2109

35. Li Y, McGowan P, Hellstrom I, Hellstrom KE, Chen L (1994) Costimulation of tumor-reactive CD4+ and CD8+ T lymphocytes by B7, a natural ligand for CD28, can be used to treat established mouse melanoma. J Immunol 153:421–428

36. Janeway CA Jr, Bottomly K (1994) Signals and signs for lymphocyte responses. Cell 76:275–285

37. Platsoucas CD (1991) Human autologous tumor-specific T cells in malignant melanoma. Cancer Metastasis Rev 10:151–176

38. Topalian SL, Hom SS, Kawakami Y, Mancini M, Schwartzentruber DJ, Zakut R, Rosenberg SA (1992) Recognition of shared melanoma antigens by human tumor-infiltrating lymphocytes. J Immunother 12:203–206

39. Uchiyama A, Hoon DS, Morisaki T, Kaneda Y, Yuzuki DH, Morton DL (1993) Transfection of interleukin 2 gene into human melanoma cells augments cellular immune response. Cancer Res 53:949–952

40. Kawakami Y, Eliyahu S, Delgado CH, Robbins PF, Sakaguchi K, Appella E, Yannelli JR, Adema GJ, Miki T, Rosenberg SA (1994) Identification of a human melanoma antigen recognized by tumor-infiltrating lymphocytes associated with in vivo tumor rejection. Proc Natl Acad Sci USA 91:6458–6462

41. Oaks MK, Hanson JP Jr, O'Malley DP (1994) Molecular cytogenetic mapping of the human melanoma antigen (MAGE) gene family to chromosome region Xq27-qter: implications for MAGE immunotherapy. Cancer Res 54:1627–1629

42. Huber BE, Richards CA, Austin EA (1994) Virus-directed enzyme/prodrug therapy (VDEPT). Selectively engineering drug sensitivity into tumors. Ann NY Acad Sci 716:104–114

43. Ezzerdine ZD, Martuza RL, Platika D, et al (1991) Selective killing of glioma cells in culture and in vivo by retrovirus transfer of the herpes simplex thymidine kinase gene. New Biol 3:608–614

44. Culver KW, Ram Z, Walbridge S, et al (1992) In vivo gene transfer with retroviral vector-producer cells for treatment of experimental brain tumors. Science 256:1550–1552

45. Takamiya Y, Short MP, Ezzerdine ZD, et al (1992) Gene therapy of malignant brain tumors: a rat glioma line bearing the herpes simplex virus type 1-thymidine kinase gene and wild type retrovirus kills other tumor cells. J Neurosci Res 33:493–503

46. Ram Z, Culver KW, Walbridge S, et al (1993) In situ retroviral-mediated gene transfer for the treatment of brain tumors in rats. Cancer Res 53:83–88

47. Takamiya Y, Short MP, Moolten FL, et al (1993) An experimental model of retrovirus gene therapy for malignant brain tumors. J Neurosurg 79:104–110

48. Ram Z, Culver KW, Walbridge S, et al (1993) Toxicity studies of retroviral-mediated gene transfer for treatment of brain tumors. J Neurosurg 79:400–407

49. Barba D, Hardin J, Ray J, et al (1993) Thymidine kinase-mediated killing of rat brain tumors. J Neurosurg 79:729–735

50. Springett GM, Moen RC, Anderson S, et al (1993) Infection efficiency of T lymphocytes with amphotropic retroviral vectors is cell cycle dependent. J Virol 63:3865–3869

51. Miller DG, Adam MA, Miller AD (1990) Gene transfer by retrovirus vectors occurs only in cells that are actively replicating at the time of infection. Mol Cell Biol 10:4239–4242

52. Roe T, Reynolds TC, Yu G, et al (1993) Integration of murine leukemia virus DNA depends on mitosis. EMBO J 12:2099–2108

53. Short MP, Choi BC, Lee JK, et al (1990) Gene delivery to glioma cells in rat brain by grafting of a retrovirus packaging cell line. J Neurosci Res 27:427–433

54. Kolberg R (1994) The bystander effect in gene therapy: great, but how does it work? J NIH Res 6:62–64

55. Bi WL, Parysek LM, Warnick R, et al (1993) In vitro evidence that metabolic cooperation is responsible for the bystander effect observed with HSV tk retroviral gene therapy. Hum Gene Ther 4:725–731

56. Moolten FL (1986) Tumor chemosensitivity conferred by inserted herpes thymidine kinase genes: paradigm for a prospective cancer control strategy. Cancer Res 46:5276–5281

57. Moolten FL, Wells JM (1990) Curability of tumors bearing herpes thymidine kinase genes transferred by retroviral vectors. J Natl Cancer Inst 82:297–300

58. Vile RG, Hart IR (1993) Use of tissue-specific expression of the herpes simplex virus thymidine kinase gene to inhibit growth of established murine melanomas following direct intratumoral injection of DNA. Cancer Res 53:3860–3864

59. Caruso M, Panis Y, Gagandeep S, et al (1993) Regression of established macroscopic liver metastasis after in situ transduction of a suicide gene. Proc Natl Acad Sci USA 90:7024–7028

60. Freeman SM, Abboud CN, Whartenby KA, et al (1993) The "bystander effect": tumor regression when a fraction of the tumor mass is genetically modified. Cancer Res 53:5274–5283

61. Banerjee D, Zhao SC, Li MX, Schweitzer BI, et al (1994) Gene therapy utilizing drug resistance genes—a review. Stem Cells 12:378–385

Application of the Apoptotic Gene to Gene Therapy of Malignant Gliomas

Akio Asai, Chifumi Kitanaka, Akinori Sugiyama, Kazuhiko Mishima, and Yoshiyuki Kuchino

Abstract. The s-*myc* gene is a unique *myc* family gene without introns that was isolated from a rat genomic library using the v-*myc* exon 3 region as a probe. Significant expression of the s-*myc* gene was detected in rat embryo chondrocytes committed to programmed cell death. Gene transfection experiments showed that s-*myc* expression in rat and human glioma cells killed the cells by apoptosis induction. These observations, indicating that s-Myc can act as an apoptosis inducer in vivo and in vitro, suggest that the s-*myc* gene might be useful for gene therapy of gliomas. To test this possibility, we introduced the s-*myc* gene (pCEP4smyc), linked to the cytomegalovirus promoter, into glioma-bearing rats. Surprisingly, injection of pCEP4smyc plasmid DNA together with rat 9L or C6 glioma cells completely prevented 9L- or C6-derived tumor formation in the brain or the hind leg of rats. A similar dramatic antitumor effect induced by s-*myc* gene expression was observed at a site distant from the original site at which the s-*myc* gene and glioma cells were coinjected. These results indicated that s-*myc* expression has the potential to elicit a host antitiumor immune response.

Key words. s-*myc*—c-*myc*—wt-*p53*—Gliogblastoma—Gliosarcoma

Introduction

The immune system has been shown to play a protective role in malignancy. However, tumors generally lack the ability to present antigen-specific signals to T lymphocytes effectively and so escape the normal host immune defense system. Plautz et al. [1] recently demonstrated that stimulation of the immune system by introduction of a recombinant gene encoding major histocompatibility complex (MHC) proteins caused sensitization to unrecognized tumor antigens and had a therapeutic effect on established tumors in vivo. In addition, Townsend and Allison [2] showed that introduction of cDNA encoding B7 into melanoma cells induced rejection of a melanoma in vivo. B7 is a costimulatory ligand expressed on the surface of antigen-presenting cells and is required for effective interaction with the CD28 molecule on the T-cell

Biophysics Division, National Cancer Center Research Institute, Tsukiji 5-1-1, Chuo-ku, Tokyo 104, Japan

surface. These findings indicate that tumors may be intrinsically capable of presenting antigen-specific signals to T cells, but that the magnitude of the signals is not enough for full activation of T cells.

The intracellular roles of *myc* family gene products in cell proliferation, differentiation, and transformation have been studied extensively, mainly in vitro systems, but their roles in the development of immunogenic phenotypes have not been examined except that of N-Myc, which has been shown to have a role in repression of expression of MHC class I antigen [3,4]. In this study, we demonstrate that one of the Myc family proteins, s-Myc, modulates the immunogenicity of rat glioma cells and elicits an effective antitumor immune response in tumor-bearing animals. This is the first demonstration that a Myc family protein has a potential to eradicate, through the immune system, gliomas formed in rats. We also show the efficiency of tumor regression by transfer and expression of the s-*myc* gene, and discuss the specificity of the host antitumor immune response mediated by s-*myc* expression.

Results and Discussion

The s-*myc* gene isolated from a rat genomic library retains approximately 60% nucleotide sequence homology with the coding sequence of the rat N-*myc* gene, but has no introns in the coding region [5]. It encodes a protein consisting of 429 amino acids and contains all the functional domains conserved in the Myc family proteins except for the sequence context required for phosphorylation by casein kinase II (CKII) in the internal acidic domain (domain IV). However, in contrast to c-Myc and N-Myc, which have been implicated in cell proliferation, differentiation, and transformation, constitutive expression of the s-*myc* gene linked to the SV40 promoter suppressed not only the growth activity of neural tumor cells, but also their tumorigenicity in nude mice [5,6].

We previously demonstrated weak expression of s-*myc* mRNA in the head and neck of rat embryos by Northern blot analysis probed by the cloned s-*myc* gene [7]. However, more precise analysis showed that s-*myc* mRNA was not expressed in the rat embryo brain, including the cerebrum and cerebellum, but was expressed in rat embryo tissues such as the cartilage of the skull base and the sternum. In situ hybridization and RNase protection analysis using an antisense riboprobe confirmed the synthesis of s-*myc* mRNA in rat embryo cartilage, not only that of the head and neck but also that of ventral and dorsal parts of the body including the vertebral and sternal bones [7]. For instance, as shown in Fig. 1, a 208-nucleotide (nt) band containing the sequence encoding the internal acidic domain (domain IV) was detected with antisense s-*myc* riboprobe in rat embryos in the head, neck, spine, and ribs, but not in the distal extremities. Moreover, immunohistochemical analysis with s-Myc polyclonal antibody demonstrated staining in the peripheral regions of the vertebral bones and the sternal bones. These observations showed that the s-*myc* gene is an active gene expressed in rat embryo cartilage despite its intronless structure. In the peripheral region of rat embryo cartilage, some cells are being committed to differentiation into hypertrophic chondrocytes that undergo programmed cell death. Based on these findings, we concluded that s-Myc may have a crucial role in induction of programmed cell death of rat embryo chondrocytes.

To support this conclusion, we transfected the s-*myc* gene linked with the human metallothionein promoter into rat glioma and fibroblast cells by the lipofectin-medi-

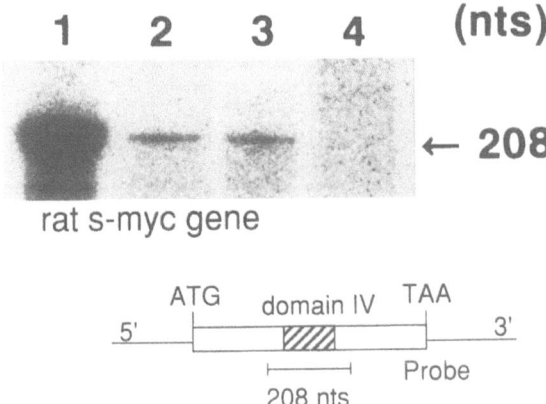

Fig. 1. Expression of s-*myc* mRNA in rat embryo cartilage of bones: RNase protection analysis of s-myc mRNA. Total poly (A⁺)RNA was prepared from various tissues of rat embryos on day 16 of gestation as described previously [17] and subjected to RNase protection analysis. For RNase protection analysis, a DNA fragment corresponding to nucleotides 4763 to 4970 of the s-Myc protein coding region [5], which contains the sequence encoding the s-Myc-specific unique peptide with the sequence context for phosphorylation by CKII, was subcloned into a plasmid vector pTZ18R. ^{32}P-Labeled antisense s-*myc* riboprobe of 281 nucleotides (nt) was synthesized using a commercial transcription kit (Promega, Madison, WI, USA) with T7 RNA polymerase (Boehringer Mannheim, Germany) and α-^{32}P-uridine triphosphate (-UTP) (800 Ci/mmol, Dupont/NEN, [Boston, MA, USA]). Total poly(A⁺)RNA (30 μg) was hybridized for 18 h to 8×10^4 dpm of antisense riboprobe and then digested with RNase A and T_1 as recommended by the manufacturer (Promega). Products were then separated by sodium dodecyl sulfate-(SDS)-polyacrylamide gel electrophoresis containing 8% urea. *Lane 1*, s-*myc* transfectant; *lane 2*, rat embryonal head and neck; *lane 3*, spine and ribs; *lane 4*, embryonal extremities

ated transfection method. In s-*myc* transfectants isolated by selection with the neomycin analog G418, s-*myc* gene expression was induced by addition of zinc sulfate in a dose-dependent manner. For example, as shown in Fig. 2a, s-*myc* expression in the s-*myc* transfectant U251smyc10 from human glioma U251 cells was not detectable without zinc sulfate treatment, but was induced by addition of 200 μM zinc sulfate. The level of s-*myc* expression in the cells reached a maximum at 4 h after induction and then gradually decreased. In contrast, the levels of c-*myc* and β-actin mRNAs remained unchanged after induction of s-Myc synthesis or addition of zinc sulfate (data not shown). Synthesis of the s-Myc protein in U251smyc10 cells was also verified by Western blot analysis with anti-s-Myc antibody (Fig. 2b). Similar induction of the s-*myc* gene product was observed in other s-*myc* transfectants, 9Lsmyc7 from rat 9L glioma cells and C6smyc4 from rat C6 glioma cells, on addition of 160 μM zinc sulfate (data not shown).

Microscopic analysis indicated that glioma cells started to detach from the plastic dishes within 6 h after s-Myc induction (Fig. 3). Three days after s-Myc induction, almost all U251smyc10 cells died and became floating. These floating cells showed typical morphological changes of apoptosis, such as condensation of the nucleus, chromatin localization in the periphery of the nucleus, and formation of translucent cytoplasmic vacuoles on electron microscopic examination. Progressive degradation of chromosomal DNA with a ladder of DNA fragments, which is also typical of

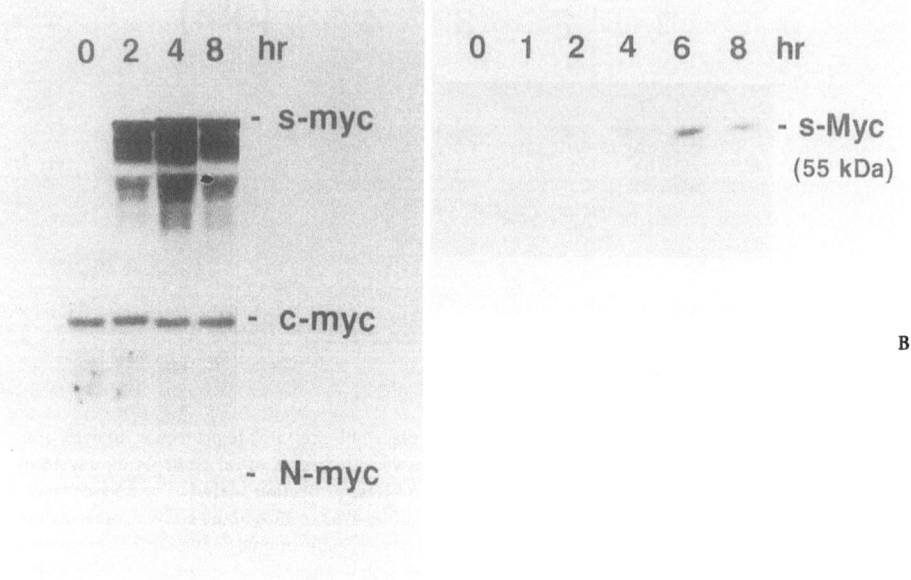

A

B

Fig. 2 A,B. Expression of the s-*myc* gene product in s-*myc* transfectants by addition of zinc sulfate. **A** Northern blot analysis of s-myc mRNA with the 2.9-kbp fragment of the s-*myc* gene. Poly(A⁺)RNA (2 mg) from U251smyc10 cells collected at the indicated time after addition of 200 μM zinc sulfate was hybridized with a nick-translated ³²P-labeled s-*myc* probe. The same filter was subsequently hybridized with ³²P-labeled c-*myc* and N-*myc* probes. Poly(A⁺)RNA prepared from various rat tissues and exponentially growing cultured cells was subjected to Northern blot analysis in formaldehyde-agarose gel [17] and probed with a ³²P-labeled *Eco*RI-*Bst*BI fragment (2.9 kbp) of the rat s-*myc* gene, the *Bgl*II-*Hpa*I fragment (823 bp) of the rat c-*myc* exon 3 region [18], and the *Hinc*II-*Pst*I fragment (590 bp) of the rat N-*myc* exon 3 region [19]. **B** Western blot analysis of the s-Myc protein synthesized in s-*myc* transfectants with s-Myc polyclonal antibody. Crude lysates (10 mg) were prepared from U251smyc10 cells as described by Blackwood et al. [20] at the indicated times after induction by 200 μM zinc sulfate and separated by electrophoresis using a 10% polyacrylamide gel with 0.1% SDS. Proteins were transferred electrophoretically to a nitrocellulose membrane, which was subjceted to Western blot analysis using s-Myc polyclonal antibody against the synthetic peptide consisting of 13 amino acids from position 224 to 238 of the s-Myc protein [7] as probe. After washing with phosphate-buffered saline (PBS), the filter was incubated with biotinylated goat antirabbit IgG. The filter was further incubated in avidin–biotin complex (ABC) solution containing alkaline phosphatase conjugated streptoavidin–biotin complex (Vector, Burlingame, CA, USA) and subsequently in substrate solution (Bio-Rad, Hercules, CA, USA)

apoptosis, was also observed in the glioma cells after s-Myc induction. Similar characteristics of apoptosis were observed in 9Lsmyc7 and C6smyc4 cells [7]. Zinc sulfate-inducible s-Myc expression was observed in s-*myc* transfectants from Rat-1, NIH3T3, and rat hepatoma dRLh84 cells. However, in Rat-1, NIH3T3, and rat hepatoma dRLh84 cells, induction of s-Myc by zinc sulfate did not affect cell viability. Zinc ion is known to be toxic to mammalian cells. Thus, to rule out the possibility that cell death was induced in glioma cells by the toxicity of zinc sulfate, we carried out colony formation assay using the s-*myc* gene subcloned into a constitutive expression vector. The analytical data demonstrated that glioma cells transfected with the s-*myc* gene linked to either the cytomegalovirus promoter or the SV40 promoter did not form grossly visible colonies expressing s-Myc in culture medium without zinc sulfate (data not shown). These results indicated that the s-Myc protein itself acts as a cell-type-specific apoptosis inducer even in the presence of serum growth factors.

Although the physiological functions of s-Myc and the molecular mechanism of apoptosis induction by s-Myc expression are still unclear, we examined whether s-Myc as an apoptosis inducer can suppress the development of gliomas in vivo. To test this possibility, we introduced the s-*myc* gene into glioma-bearing rats. For transfection of the s-*myc* gene, the 2.2-kilo base pair (kbp) *Dra*I fragment containing the entire open reading frame of the s-*myc* gene was subcloned into the *Pvu*II site of an episomal expression vector pCEP4 (Invitrogen, San Diego, CA, USA) containing the promoter sequence of cytomegalovirus to obtain pCEP4smyc. A suspension of rat 9L gliosarcoma cells (4×10^4) with lipofectin-treated pCEP4smyc plasmid DNA was injected stereotactically into the basal ganglia of the brain of syngeneic Fischer F344 rats without prior cloning of s-*myc* transfectants. The efficiency of gene transfection in an in vitro system by the lipofectin-mediated gene transfection method is generally less than 3% [8], so we expected that in situ transfection of the lipofectin-treated s-*myc* gene into glioma cells would produce very low numbers of s-*myc* transfected cells. However, unexpectedly, after stereotactic injection of 9L cells together with the s-*myc* gene, no tumors formed in the brain of six rats within 2 months (Table 1). In particular, one of the rats injected with 9L cells together with pCEP4smyc DNA developed signs of intracranial hypertension, such as cerebrospinal fluid (CSF) rhinorrhea, drowsiness, and left-sided hemiparesis 16 days after the injection, implying that a tumor large enough to impair the nervous system was formed in the brain; however, the next week the neurological status of this rat was stabilized and even improved, and the rat fully recovered 50 days after the injection, suggesting that the tumor regressed completely in vivo. On autopsy of the brain of this rat to observe morphological changes of the brain tissues around the injection site, no tumor cells were observed but massive lymphocyte and macrophage infiltration was seen around the putative tumor bed [9]. These findings strongly suggested that the host immune system may have contributed to the regression of gliomas in vivo.

Contrary to the antitumor effect of s-Myc, injection of either 9L cells with plasmid DNA carrying the c-*myc* gene (pCEPcmyc) or the wt-*p53* gene (pCEPp53) failed to inhibit the formation of brain tumors (see Table 1), although wt-*p53* expression induced apoptotic cell death of glioma cells with higher efficiency than s-Myc in an in vitro system. Injection of the parental 9L cells alone and cells with the pCEP4 vector DNA itself as controls formed brain tumors large enough to kill the animals within 4 weeks.

Table 1. Survival rate of rats after intracerebral injection of 9L glioma cells.

Protocol	Survival rate	Survival time (days)
9L	0/6 (0%)	18.2 ± 1.0 (18, 17, 20, 18, 19, 17)
9L + Lipo	0/6 (0%)	21.0 ± 1.7 (19, 19, 22, 23, 21, 22)
9L + Lipo + pCEP4	0/6 (0%)	21.2 ± 1.4 (21, 22, 19, 20, 23, 22)
9L + Lipo + pCEP4p53	0/6 (0%)	26.2 ± 5.4 (27, 27, 29, 20, 27, 27)
9L + Lipo + pCEP4cmyc	0/6 (0%)	21.0 ± 2.1 (20, 24, 20, 23, 21, 19)
9L + Lipo + pCEP4smyc	6/6 (100%)	All alive

9L cells (4×10^4) together with lipofectin (Lipo) or lipofectin-treated plasmid DNA (300 ng) were injected stereotactically into the basal ganglia of the brain. Tumor formation was confirmed at autopsy.

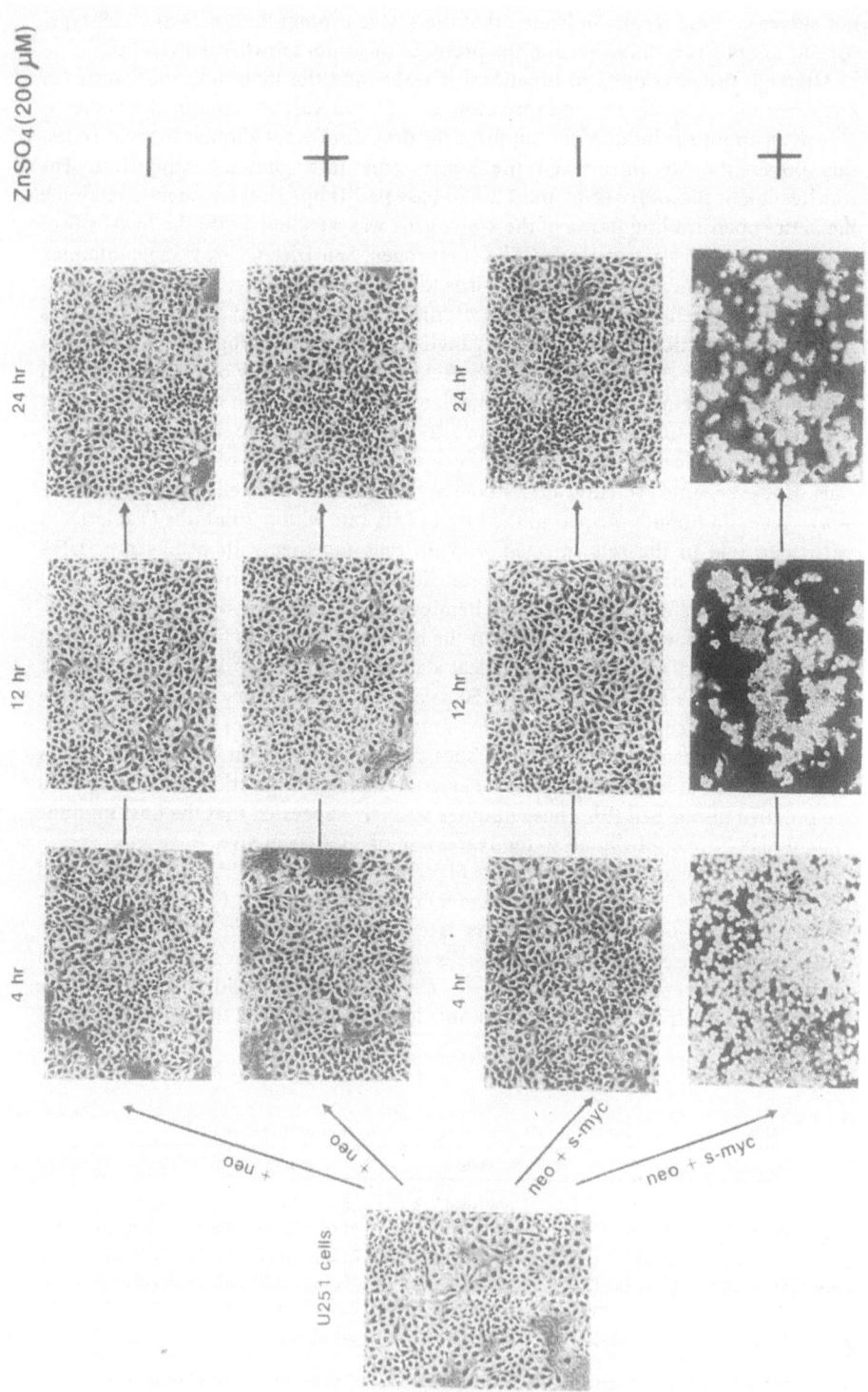

Considering the efficiency of gene transfection in situ, we speculated that a host antitumor immune response might be elicited by coinjection of glioma cells and the s-*myc* gene. To support this speculation, we reinjected 4×10^6 parental 9L cells alone into the hind legs of rats that survived the first injection of 9L cells with the s-*myc* gene. Surprisingly, no tumors developed in these rats at the two sites of injection within the next 60 days. To confirm this finding, we injected 4×10^6 9L cells with pCEP4smyc DNA subcutaneously into the right hind leg of six normal rats, and at the same time, the same number of parental tumor cells alone into their left hind leg. Sixty days later, all the animals injected with 9L cells and the s-*myc* gene were free from tumors in both the right and left leg [9]. However, after injection of 9L cells alone or with the pCEP4 vector itself, tumors formed in both legs of the rats. Similarly, injection of pCEP4cmyc or pCEP4p53 plasmid DNA together with 9L glioma cells (4×10^6) into the hind legs formed subcutaneous tumors in both hind legs of the rats within 30 days after the injections. These results strongly suggested that s-Myc expression can modulate tumor immunogenicity and provoke host antitumor effects, but that c-*myc* and wt-*p53* gene transfection cannot.

To ensure that expression of the s-Myc protein was really required for elicitation of the host antitumor immune response, we injected into rats an s-*myc* transfectant, 9Lsmyc7, derived from 9L cells. This transfectant contained two copies of the exogenous s-*myc* gene and produced a low level of the intact s-Myc protein constitutively. As expected, all six rats in which 4×10^6 9Lsmyc7 cells were injected subcutaneously into a hind leg remained tumor free for 2 months after the injection. Intracranial or subcutaneous injection of 9Lsmyc7 cells also prevented the formation of gliosarcomas at distant sites. To confirm that the host antitumor phenomenon is specifically associated with s-*myc* gene expression, we injected 9Lsmyc7 cells rendered nonviable by 5000 rads of ^{60}Co irradiation subcutaneously into rats. All six rats injected with irradiated 9Lsmyc7 cells were tumor free for 2 months, indicating that the antitumor effect of s-*myc* transfection was not lost after irradiation. However, injection of parental 9L cells rendered nonviable by ^{60}Co irradiation with or without the s-*myc* gene allowed the formation of large subcutaneous tumors in the contralateral side in rats within 30 days after injection. From these results, we concluded that the remote antitumor phenomenon was induced equally by intracranial and subcutaneous injections of the s-*myc* transfectant and that elicitation of the host

---

Fig. 3. Microscopic analysis of induction of s-Myc expression in glioma cells. Several lines of human glioma cells transfected with either pSVneoHMTter plasmid DNA or pSVneoHMTtersmyc plasmid DNA carrying the s-*myc* gene were established as described previously. Each clone was cultivated in Dulbecco's modified essential medium supplemented by 10% fetal calf serum (FCS) and 600 μg/ml of glutamine. Expression of the s-*myc* gene in transfectants was induced by addition of 200 μM zinc sulfate. After addition of zinc sulfate, morphological changes of glioma cells were examined by microscopy at the indicated times. Gene transfection: an expression plasmid vector (pSVneoHMTter) with a human metallothionein promoter and the neomycin-resistant gene was used for induction of s-Myc-dependent apoptosis. The *Dra*I fragment (2.1 kbp) of the s-*myc* gene containing the entire protein coding region was subcloned into the blunted *Bam*HI site of the vector to obtain pSVneoHMTtersmyc. The pSVneoHMTter or pSVneoHMTtersmyc plasimd DNA was transfected into human glioma U251 cells by the lipofectin-mediated transfection method [8]. After initial screening with G418, several drug-resistant clones were subcloned, and s-*myc* expression-positive clones were then selected by Northern blot analysis using the *Eco*RI-*Bst*BI fragment of the s-*myc* gene as probe

antitumor immune response depended entirely on s-*myc* gene expression in the tumor cells.

The specificity of the host antitumor immune response mediated by s-Myc expression was examined by transplantation experiments using two other types of tumor cells that did not express the s-*myc* gene endogenously, C6 glioblastoma cells and B104 neuroblastoma cells. As with 9L cells, injection of the C6 cells together with the s-*myc* gene completely prevented C6- and 9L-derived tumor formation at a distant site in all six rats tested. However, injection of B104 cells, even together with the s-*myc* gene, did not inhibit the development of B104- or 9L-derived tumors at either the original injection site or on the contralateral side [9]. Moreover, introduction of c-Myc had no ability to alter the immunogenic phenotype of either glioma or neuroblastoma cells. These findings clearly demonstrated that the host antitumor immune response was specifically elicited by expression of the s-*myc* gene and that it could distinguish between glioma and neuroblastoma cells, but not between 9L and C6 cells. In addition, these observations suggested that 9L and C6 cells may have a common tumor antigen distinct from that of B104 cells.

Finally, it should be noted that the host antitumor immune response elicited by s-Myc expression eradicated gliomas already established in rats. Two weeks after injection of 4×10^6 9L cells alone into the right hind leg of six rats, we injected the same number of 9L cells together with pCEP4smyc plasmid DNA in their left hind legs. After the second injection, the tumors in the original injection site continued to grow for 2–3 weeks; at about 4 weeks, however, the tumors gradually began to decrease in size, and massive mononuclear cell infiltration consisting mainly of CD8+ T cells was induced around the tumors. These observations support the foregoing conclusion that glioma eradication in rats resulted from an immune phenomenon involving alteration of glioma cell immunogenicity and consequent provocation of a host immune response.

Establishment of a cell line from surgical tumor materials has proved very difficult, and this has been one of the major obstacles to success in gene therapy. To overcome this problem, we injected glioma cells mixed with lipofectin-treated recombinant plasmid DNA without prior cloning of gene transfectants. Although the transfection efficiency of the gene into tumor cells is 3% or less, this treatment may have a marked antitumor effect in patients. Indeed, a limited number of glioma cells transfected with the s-*myc* gene in situ eradicated gliomas established in rat brain. This finding indicated that it is not necessary to clone a tumor cell line transfected with a desired gene for gene therapy. Thus, the present protocol not requiring cloning of s-*myc* transfectants provides a possible procedure for use in clinical trials of gene therapy on brain tumors.

Selection of a vector system for potent and cell-type-specific expression of an introduced gene in vivo is another difficulty. In this study, we adopted the lipofection method to introduce a recombinant DNA into glioma cells in vivo and an expression vector pCEP4 containing the cytomegalovirus promoter to obtain active expression of the gene desired for gene therapy. Although we fortunately obtained sufficient expression to inhibit glioma formation in vivo using this system, further experiments are required before concluding that this system for gene transfection using the pCEP4 vector and the lipofection method is best for clinical trials.

The most notable finding in this study was that s-Myc expression in glioma cells alters the tumor immunogenicity and results in cell-type-specific elicitation of the host immune response against gliomas. This is the first demonstration that a Myc family protein has a potential to elicit an effective antitumor immune response in tumor-bearing rats. Although the molecular mechanism of the alteration of tumor immunogenicity by s-Myc expression is unknown, we recently found that s-Myc acts as a transcription factor through binding to the E-box sequence. Therefore, s-Myc might play an important role in upregulation of (1) a glioma-specific antigen, (2) MHC proteins or B7 proteins, or (3) some other unknown gene products to render glioma cells capable of effective presentation of the tumor antigen.

The s-Myc protein has approximately 60% amino acid sequence homology with the rat N-Myc protein [5]. Previous reports showed that N-Myc expression causes downregulation of expression of MHC class I antigen [3,4], which is required for effective presentation of a tumor antigen to T cells. Therefore, s-Myc might also be involved in regulation of the expression of MHC class I antigen, and tumor regression in glioma-bearing rats might be caused by upregulation or reversion of MHC class I antigen induced by functional competition between N-Myc and s-Myc. In fact, pre-liminary immunohistochemical analysis using anti-rat MHC class I antigen antibody showed a slight increase in the level of expression of MHC class I antigen in s-*myc*-transfected glioma cells. However, the level was not sufficient to explain elicitation of s-Myc-mediated antitumor immune response (data not show). Huang et al. recently [10] reported that in some cases MHC class I-restricted tumor antigen is transferred to host bone marrow-derived antigen presenting cells and causes priming of an immune response in the cells. Their data suggest that expression of MHC class I antigen in glioma cells may not necessarily be required for effective presentation of a tumor antigen to T cells. If this is so, s-Myc expression might play a crucial role in upregulation of the synthesis of a glioma-specific antigen in the tumor cells. The molecular mechanism of regulation of expression of the glioma-specific antigen by s-Myc expression is unknown, but some cell-type-specific function might be important to eliminate side effects of introduction of a recombinant plasmid DNA in gene therapy.

The s-Myc protein is distinct from other Myc family proteins in that it does not have CKII sites in the internal acidic domain. Therefore, expression of its cell-type-specific function may be the result of this unique structural feature. The Myc protein has been reported to associate with at least two transcription factors, TFII-I and YY-1 and to alter the transcription efficiency of genes having the Inr promoter [11,12]. Moreover, the Myc protein has been demonstrated to interact with the retinoblastoma protein and Rb-related p107 protein, resulting in suppression of Myc function [13,14]. The s-Myc protein has all the highly conserved domain structures common to Myc family proteins except the sequence context required for phosphorylation by CKII in the internal acidic domain. Like c-Myc, the transcription activity of c-Jun as a tran-scription factor is known to be regulated by phosphorylation. Lin et al. [15] have reported that phosphorylation of c-Jun at Thr 231, Ser 243, and Ser 249 by CKII specifically inhibits its DNA binding activity without modulating its transactivation potential. In addition, Arias et al. [16] demonstrated that CKII-phosphorylated c-Jun could not bind to cyclic AMP-responsive element-binding protein (CBP). Taken to-gether, these findings suggest that s-Myc lacking CKII sites in domain IV might have different association constants with proteins such as TFII-1 and YY1 from those of c-Myc. These differences might be required for expression of s-Myc-specific unique biological functions. Another possible explanation for prescription of the cell-type specificity is that s-Myc may have the potential to associate with a factor specifically present in glioma cells that does not associate with other Myc proteins, resulting in expression of glioma-specific s-Myc function. If this is so, isolation and characterization of this protein as well as a glioma-specific antigen could be very important and interesting for understanding the molecular mechanism of the development of the immunogenic phenotype in glioma cells.

Finally, it should be noted that the s-Myc-mediated anti-tumor effect is not lost in glioma cells rendered nonviable by ^{60}Co irradiation. This finding indicates the possibility of developing a new system for cancer therapy using killed glioma cells that have been expressing exogenously incorporated s-*myc* gene as a vaccine. Thus, identification of the genes encoding glioma-specific tumor-rejection antigens may facilitate the development of vaccination therapy for gliomas.

References

1. Plautz GE, Yang ZY, Wu BY, Gao X, Huang L, Nabel GJ (1993) Immunotherapy of malignancy by in vivo gene transfer into tumors. Proc Natl Acad Sci USA 90:4645–4649
2. Townsend SE, Allison JP (1993) Tumor rejection after direct co-stimulation of CD8+ T cells by B7-transfected melanoma cells. Science 259:368–370
3. Bernards R, Dessain SK, Weinberg RA (1986) N-*myc* amplification causes down-modulation of MHC class I antigen expression in neuroblastoma. Cell 47:667–674
4. Van't Veer LJ, Beijersbergen RL, Bernards R (1993) N-myc suppresses major histocompatibility complex class I gene expression through down-regulation of the p50 subunit of NF-𝜘B. EMBO J 12:195–200
5. Sugiyama A, Kume A, Nemoto K, Lee SY, Asami Y, Nemoto F, Nishimura S, Kuchino Y (1989) Isolation and characterization of s-*myc*, a member of the rat *myc* gene family. Proc Natl Acad Sci USA 86:9144–9148
6. Asai A, Miyagi Y, Sugiyama A, Gamanuma M, Hong SI, Takamoto S, Nomura K, Matsutani M, Takakura K, Kuchino Y (1994) Negative effects of wild-type p53 and s-Myc on cellular growth and tumorigenicity of glioma cells: implication of the tumor suppressor genes for gene therapy. J Neurooncol 19:259–268
7. Asai A, Miyagi Y, Sugiyama A, Nagashima Y, Kanemitsu H, Obinata M, Mishima K, Kuchino Y (1994) The s-Myc protein having the ability to induce apoptosis is selectively expressed in rat embryo chondrocytes. Oncogene 9:2345–2352
8. Felgner PL, Gadek TR, Holm M, Roman R, Chan HW, Wenz M, Northrop JP, Ringold GM, Danielsen M (1987) Lipofection: a highly efficient, lipid-mediated DNA-transfection procedure. Proc Natl Acad Sci USA 84:7413–7417
9. Asai A, Miyagi Y, Hashimoto H, Lee SH, Mishima K, Sugiyama A, Tanaka H, Mochizuki T, Yasuda T, Kuchino Y (1994) Modulation of tumor immunogenicity of rat glioma cells by s-Myc expression: eradication of rat gliomas in vivo. Cell Growth & Differ 5:1153–1158
10. Huang AYC, Golumbek P, Ahmadzadeh M, Jaffee E, Pardoll D, Levitsky H (1994) Role of bone marrow-derived cells in presenting MHC Class I-restricted tumor antigens. Science 264:961–965
11. Roy AL, Carruther C, Gutjahr T, Roeder RG (1993) Direct role for Myc in transcription initiation mediated by interactions with TFII-I. Nature 365:359–361
12. Shrivastava A, Saleque S, Kalpana GV, Artandi S, Goff SP, Calame, K (1993) Inhibition of transcriptional regulation Yin-Yang-1 by association with c-Myc. Science 262:1889–1892
13. Rustgi AK, Dyson N, Bernards R (1991) Amino-terminal domains of c-myc and N-myc proteins mediate binding to the retinoblastoma gene product. Nature 352:541–544
14. Gu W, Bhatia K, Magrath IT, Dang CV, Dalla-Favera R (1994) Binding and suppression of the Myc transcriptional activation domain by p107. Science 264:251–254
15. Lin A, Frost J, Deng T, Smeal T, Al-Alawi N, Kikkawa U, Hunter T, Brenner D, Karin M (1992) Casein kinase II is a negative regulator of c-Jun DNA binding and AP-1 activity. Cell 70:777–789

16. Arias J, Alberts AS, Brindle P, Claret FX, Smeal T, Karin M, Feramisco J, Montiminy M (1994) Activation of cAMP and mitogen responsive genes relies on a common nuclear factor. Nature 370:226–229

17. Nagane M, Asai A, Shibui S, Nomura K, Matsutani M, Kuchino Y (1992) Expression of O^6-methylguanine-DNA methyltransferase and chloroethylnitrosourea resistance of human brain tumors. Jpn J Clin Oncol 22:143–149

18. Hayashi K, Makino R, Kawamura H, Arisawa A, Yoneda K (1987) Characterization of rat c-*myc* and adjacent regions. Nucleic Acids Res 15:6419–6436

19. Sugiyama A, Miyagi Y, Shirasawa Y, Kuchino Y (1991) Different usage of two polyadenylation signals in transcription of the N-*myc* gene in rat tumor cells. Oncogene 6:2027–2032

20. Blackwood EM, Lüscher B, Eisenman RN (1992) Myc and Max associate in vivo. Genes & Dev 6:71–80

Experimental Therapy for Malignant Brain Tumors Using Genetically Engineered Herpes Simplex Virus Type 1

Toshihiro Mineta[1,2], Samuel D. Rabkin[2], and Robert L. Martuza[2]

Abstract. We are exploring a novel experimental treatment for malignant brain tumors utilizing a genetically engineered, attenuated, replication-competent herpes simplex virus type 1 (HSV-1). Our previous studies demonstrated that a thymidine kinase-deficient HSV-1 mutant (*dl*sptk) could destroy human glioma cells in an animal brain tumor model. This HSV-1 mutant has a 360-base pair deletion in the thymidine kinase gene, allowing for replication in dividing tumor cells but not in nondividing cells. We hypothesized that such HSV-1 mutants might replicate in actively growing tumor cells and effectively kill malignant brain tumors while sparing normal brain cells. So that this therapy could become an effective clinical choice, we have examined different HSV-1 mutants. We tested a ribonucleotide reductase-deficient mutant as an experimental treatment for malignant brain tumors. The HSV-1 mutant *hr*R3, containing *Escherichia coli lacZ* gene in the ICP6 gene that encodes the large subunit of ribonucleotide reductase, is hypersensitive to antiherpetic agents acyclovir and ganciclovir while *dl*sptk is resistant. We have demonstrated that *hr*R3 destroyed human glioblastoma cells in vitro and in vivo as well as *dl*sptk. These results have stimulated interest in the possible clinical trial of *hr*R3 for the treatment of malignant brain tumors.

Key words. Glioma—Viral therapy—Herpes simplex virus type 1—Antitumor agent—Neurovirulence

Introduction

Malignant gliomas remain one of the most deadly forms of cancer in humans. Despite many recent advances in neurosurgical techniques, radiation therapy, and chemotherapy, the prognosis for patients with malignant brain tumors has not improved dramatically. The 5-year survival rate for glioblastoma multiforme is 5.5% or less [1–4]. This led us to examine novel therapeutic approaches using genetically engineered viruses. In the past, viruses have been suggested as potentially useful antineoplastic agents. Several viruses have been tested for their ability to treat various types of

[1] Departments of Neurosurgery and Immunology, Saga Medical School, Nabeshima, Saga 849, Japan
[2] Georgetown Brain Tumor Center and Department of Neurosurgery, Georgetown University Medical Center, Washington, DC 20007, USA

tumors in animals and shown to be capable of inducing some degree of tumor regression [5–7].

The proposed therapeutic mechanisms of viral cancer therapy include (i) direct cell killing by the virus, called oncolysis, and (ii) producing new antigens on the tumor cell surface to induce immunological rejection, a phenomenon called xenogenization [6]. Several animal tumor models have been used to study oncolysis with wild-type viruses, passage-attenuated viruses, or infected preparations. A major drawback in these early animal studies, however, was systemic infection by the virus. The disadvantage is that they do not necessarily distinguish between dividing cells and nondividing cells. To avoid systemic infection, the genetic engineerings of viruses for use as antineoplastic agents has focused on generating altered viruses that are not capable of replication in nondividing cells.

Recent studies indicate that genetically engineered viruses, derived from a retrovirus or herpes simplex virus type 1 (HSV-1) may have therapeutic potential for the treatment of malignant gliomas. In one approach, replication-defective retroviruses bearing the HSV-thymidine kinase gene carried this gene into the brain tumor cells, which conferred sensitivity of the tumor cells to the antiherpetic drug ganciclovir, while nondividing cells in the brain do not integrate this gene and were resistant to the drug [8–12]. However, the use of replication-defective retroviruses for treating malignant gliomas requires producer cells and might be limited because each replication-defective retrovirus particle can enter only a single cell and cannot productively infect others thereafter.

In another scheme, replication-competent HSV-1 mutants with a deletion in the thymidine kinase or ribonucleotide reductase gene replicate in and thereby destroy tumor cells, but cannot replicate in nondividing cells in the adult central nervous system [13–15]. These HSV-1 mutants have the advantage of being able to enter one tumor cell, make multiple copies, lyse the cell, and spread to additional tumor cells. This strategy is based on the previously noted fact that a malignant glioma is a dividing population within a relatively nondividing population of normal nervous system cells. In the dividing tumor cell populations, it is therefore expected that relatively high levels of enzymes necessary for DNA synthesis will be present, such as thymidine kinase (TK), DNA polymerase, and ribonucleotide reductase (RR). We therefore hypothesized that a HSV-1 mutant lacking the key enzyme for DNA synthesis might be able to divide and replicate within the tumor cells and effectively treat tumors while sparing normal brain cells.

Experimental Glioma Therapy with TK-Deficient HSV-1 Mutant

We initially used the thymidine kinase gene-deficient (TK$^-$) HSV-1 mutant *dl*sptk for the experimental glioma therapy. The HSV-1 mutant *dl*sptk is derived from the wild-type strain KOS and has a 360-base pair (bp) deletion in the TK gene (Fig. 1a) [16]. HSV-TK is an enzyme involved in pyrimidine metabolism, where it catalyzes the phosphorylation of thymidine that is incorporated into viral DNA. HSV-TK$^-$ mutants replicate poorly in nervous tissue and exhibit reduced neurovirulence [17,18]. We demonstrated previously that *dl*sptk treatment was effective in killing human malignant glioma monolayers in culture as well as in slowing subcutaneous glioma tumor growth in athymic mice [13]. Additionally, *dl*sptk treatment prolonged overall survival in athymic mice with intracerebral human glioma xenografts. These results

a. *dl*sptk: thymidine kinase negative HSV-1 mutant

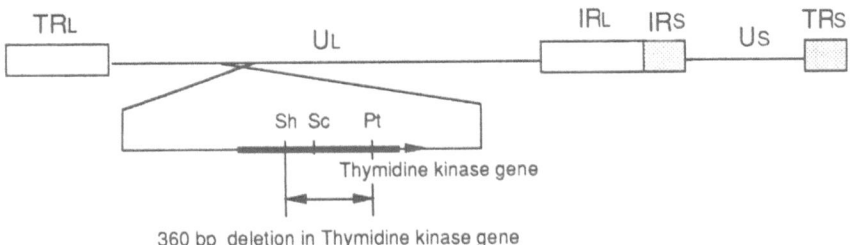

b. *hr*R3: *lacZ* gene insertion HSV-1 mutant in ICP6 gene

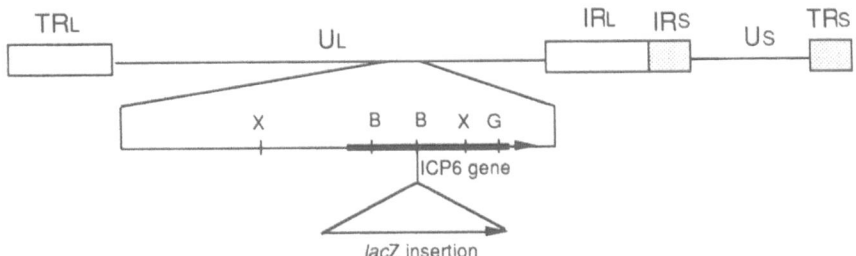

Fig. 1a,b. Schematic representation of the genome structure of *dl*sptk and *hr*R3. **a** *dl*sptk, thymidine kinase-deficient herpes simplex virus type 1 (HSV-1) mutant. The HSV-1 genome is depicted conventionally with unique sequences U_L and U_S (as *solid lines*) and major repeat elements (TR$_L$ and IR$_L$, *open boxes*; TR$_S$ and IR$_S$, *shaded boxes*). *Diagonal lines* connect to an expanded view of the thymidine kinase gene region. Selected restriction endonuclease restriction sites are indicated above the line. Location of the deletion mutation of the *dl*sptk mutant is shown. *Sph* I, Sh-; *Sac* I, Sc-; *Pst* I, Pt-. (Modified with permission from [16]). **b** *hr*R3, *lacZ* gene insertion HSV-1 mutant in ICP6 gene. The expanded domain of the U_L region shows the location of the ICP6 gene that encodes the large subunit of ribonucleotide reductase. Mutant *hr*R3 contains the structural gene of *lacZ* inserted in this gene. *Bam* HI, B-; *Bgl* II, G-; *Xho* I, X-. (Modified from [22])

suggest that genetically engineered HSV-1 mutants have therapeutic potential for malignant gliomas.

Since this initial study of *dl*sptk, we have examined the effects of *dl*sptk on medulloblastoma, malignant meningioma, and neurofibrosarcoma cells to expand this therapy to other nervous system tumors that do not respond to conventional treatment. In cell culture, we demonstrated that *dl*sptk could cause a spreading and destructive infection in these cells. Further, *dl*sptk could inhibit the in vivo tumor growth of medulloblastoma and malignant meningioma in subcutaneous or subrenal capsule tumor models [14]. These results demonstrate that HSV-1 mutants can kill a wide variety of nervous system tumors and can be used for further investigation of this potential modality for tumor therapy.

Experimental Glioma Therapy with RR-Deficient HSV-1 Mutant

While our initial studies focused on HSV-TK$^-$ mutant, we have also explored other mutant viruses with attenuated neurovirulence. In considering clinical trials of this therapeutic approach, an important issue is the resistance of the HSV-TK⁻ mutant to commonly used antiherpetic agents such as acyclovir and ganciclovir. The possible side effect of using replication-competent HSV-1 mutants for malignant brain tumor therapy is the production of encephalitis. Therefore, although *dl*sptk is sensitive to foscarnet and vidarabine, it would be beneficial to use a HSV-1 mutant that is sensitive or hypersensitive to the favored antiherpetic agents acyclovir and ganciclovir.

HSV-1 encodes a ribonucleotide reductase (RR) consisting of two nonidentical subunits. The large subunit (mol wt, 140 000), designated RR1 or ICP6 (ICP, infected cell protein), is tightly associated to the small subunit (mol wt, 38 000) [19]. The enzyme RR plays an essential role in the de novo DNA synthesis catalyzing the reduction of ribonucleoside diphosphate [20]. HSV-RR is required for efficient viral growth in nondividing cells but not in many dividing cells [21–24]. In mice, RR-deficient (RR⁻) HSV-1 mutants have been shown to have reduced neurovirulence [25]. Cellular RR is present only in actively dividing cells. Postmitotic neurons should have little or no RR activity. Furthermore, previous studies have demonstrated that the HSV-RR⁻ mutant is hypersensitive to acyclovir [26]. We would predict, therefore, that the HSV-RR⁻ mutant might effectively treat malignant gliomas as well as possessing the antiherpetic drug hypersensitivity.

We have studied the efficacy of the HSV-RR⁻ mutant *hr*R3, which possess the structural gene of *Escherichia coli lacZ* gene inserted into the ICP6 gene of wild-type HSV-1 KOS (Fig. 1b) [20]. The presence of the *lacZ* gene in the HSV-1 genome allows identification of virally infected tumor cells using β-galactosidase histochemistry. To determine whether a HSV-RR⁻ mutant can destroy malignant glioma cells, subconfluent monolayers of U-87MG human glioblastoma cells were infected with *hr*R3 [multiplicity of infection (MOI), 0.1 plaque-forming unit (pfu) per cell]. The cytopathic efficacy of *hr*R3 to U-87MG cells was almost the same as that of *dl*sptk. Additionally, we studied β-galactosidase expression in *hr*R3-infected U-87MG cells. Scattered positive X-gal (5-bromo-4-chloro-3-indolyl-β-D-galactopyranoside) staining cells were seen on day 1 postinfection, indicative of infected cells. Spread was seen at day 2 with multiple foci of infected cells. By day 3, the entire monolayer of cells was destroyed. X-gal-stained cells became round, lost normal morphological features, and lifted off the plate (Fig. 2).

We next studied the effect of *hr*R3 on subcutaneous U-87MG human glioblastoma xenografts in athymic mice and demonstrated that *hr*R3 significantly inhibited tumor growth compared with medium-treated controls in this situation as well. To assess the spread of virus in U-87MG tumors in vivo, we stained these *hr*R3-treated subcutaneous tumors with X-gal to examine the extent of β-galactosidase expression. On day 3 posttreatment, we observed positive X-gal-staining cells at injection sites. Further, the area of positive X-gal-staining within the tumor was expanded on days 7 and 14, which suggests spread of the virus [15]. These results demonstrate that the presence of the *lacZ* gene in the genomic DNA of HSV-1 mutants provides a sensitive mean to track viral infection within the tumor tissues.

In this study, we have demonstrated that HSV-RR⁻ mutant *hr*R3, as well as the HSV-TK⁻ mutant *dl*sptk, destroyed human U-87MG cells in vitro and in vivo. An important difference between these HSV-1 mutants is that *hr*R3 is hypersensitive to acyclovir while *dl*sptk is resistant. Relative to viral replication outside the tumor, HSV-TK⁻ mutants are resistant to the most commonly used antiherpetic nucleoside analog and are therefore currently difficult to treat, whereas HSV-RR⁻ mutants are hypersensitive to this treatment. We have also demonstrated that *hr*R3 is approxi-

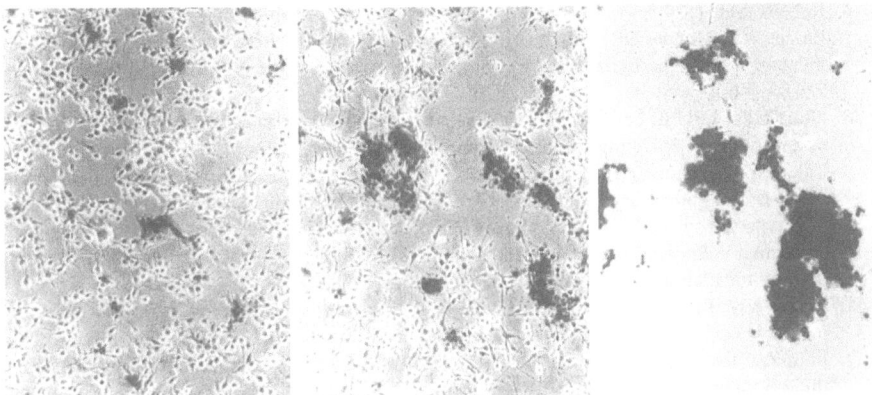

Fig. 2. β-Galactosidase expression in *hr*R3-infected U-87MG cells on day 1 (*left*), day 2 (*center*), and day 3 (*right*) postinfection. Cells were infected with *hr*R3 at an MOI multiplicity of infection of 0.1 and histochemically stained for the presence of β-galactosidase activity on the days indicated

mately tenfold more sensitive to ganciclovir than is the wild-type HSV-1 strain KOS; the median effective dose for *hr*R3 is 4–5 ng/ml while the median effective dose for KOS is 40–50 ng/ml [15]. These data suggest that HSV-RR⁻ mutants have an additional safety advantage over HSV-TK⁻ mutants, the drug of choice for treating HSV-1.

In this brief review, we have outlined our experimental treatment of malignant brain tumors using HSV-TK⁻ and HSV-RR⁻ mutants. To optimize this therapy for clinical trial, it is important to examine different attenuated HSV-1 strains or mutants. Further studies are needed to explore the effects of viruses engineered to contain multiple mutations, which may reduce the possibility of wild-type reversion and confer several important safety advantages for possible use in clinical trials.

Acknowledgments. We thank Dr. Donald M. Coen (Harvard Medical School, Boston, MA) for providing *dl*sptk, and Dr. Sandra K. Weller (University of Connecticut Health Center, Framington, CT) for providing *hr*R3. This study was supported in part by grants from the National Institute of Health (CA60176 and NS323677) to R. L. M.

References

1. Walker MD, Green SB, Byar DP (1980) Randomized comparisons of radiotherapy and nitrosoureas for the treatment of malignant glioma after surgery. N Engl J Med 303:1323–1329
2. Mahaley MS, Mettlin C, Natarajan N, et al (1989) National survey of patterns of care for brain-tumor patients. J Neurosurg 71:826–836
3. Kim TS, Halliday AL, Headley-Whyte ET, et al (1991) Correlates of survival and the Daumas-Duport grading system for astrocytomas. J Neurosurg 74:27–37
4. Schoenberg BS (1983) The epidemiology of central nervous system tumors. In: Wlaker MD (ed) Oncology of the nervous system. Nijhoff, Boston, pp 1–30
5. Taylor MW, Cordell B, Souhrada M, et al (1971) Viruses as an aid to cancer therapy: regression of solid and ascites tumors in rodents after treatment with bovine enterovirus. Proc Natl Acad Sci USA 68:836–840

6. Kobayashi H (1979) Viral xenogenization of intact tumor cells. Adv Cancer Res 30:279–299
7. Cassel WA, Murray DR, Phillips HS (1983) A phase II study on the postsurgical manage-ment of stage II malignant melanoma with a newcastle disease virus oncolysate. Cancer 52:856–860
8. Short MP, Choi BC, Lee JK, et al (1990) Gene delivery to glioma cells in rat brain by grafting of a retrovirus packaging cell line. J Neurosci Res 27:427–439
9. Takamiya Y, Short MP, Ezzenddine ZD, et al (1992) Gene therapy of malignant brain tumors: a rat glioma line bearing the herpes simplex virus type 1-thymidine kinase gene and wild type retrovirus kills other tumor cells. J Neurosci Res 33:493–503
10. Takamiya Y, Short MP, Moolten FL, et al (1993) An experimental model of retrovirus gene therapy for malignant brain tumors. J Neurosurg 79:104–110
11. Culver KW, Ram Z, Walbridge S, et al (1992) In vivo gene transfer with retroviral vector-producer cells for treatment of experimental brain tumors. Science 256:1550–1552
12. Ram Z, Culver KW, Walbridge S, et al (1993) In situ retroviral-mediated gene transfer for the treatment of brain tumors in rats. Cancer Res 53:83–88
13. Martuza RL, Malick A, Markert JM, et al (1991) Experimental therapy of human glioma by means of a genetically engineered virus mutant. Science 252:854–856
14. Markert JM, Coen DM, Malick A, et al (1992) Expanded spectrum of viral therapy in the treatment of nervous system tumors. J Neurosurg 77:590–594
15. Mineta T, Rabkin SD, Martuza RL (1994) Treatment of malignant glioma using ganciclovir-hypersensitive, ribonucleotide reductase-deficient herpes simplex viral mutant. Cancer Res 54:3963–3966
16. Coen DM, Kosz-Vnenchak M, Jacobson JG, et al (1989) Thymidine kinase-negative herpes simplex virus mutants establish latency in mouse trigeminal ganglia but do not reactivate. Proc Natl Acad Sci USA 86:4736–4740
17. Field HJ, Wildy P (1978) The pathogenicity of thymidine kinase-deficient mutants of herpes simplex virus in mice. J Hyg Camb (Lond) 81:267–277
18. Field HJ, Darby G (1980) Pathogenicity in mice of strains of herpes simplex virus which are resistant to acyclovir in vitro and in vivo. Antimicrob Agents Chemother 17:209–216
19. Duita BM (1983) Ribonucleotide reductase induced by herpes simplex virus has a virus-specific constituent. J Gen Virol 64:513–521
20. Thelander L, Reichard P (1979) Reduction of ribonucleotide. Annu Rev Biochem 48:133–158
21. Preston VG, Palfreyman JW, Duita BM (1984) Identification of a herpes simplex virus type 1 polypeptide which is a component of the virus-induced ribonucleotide reductase. J Gen Virol 65:1457–1466
22. Goldstein DJ, Weller SK (1988) Herpes simplex virus type 1-induced ribonucleotide reductase activity is dispensable for virus growth and DNA synthesis: isolation and charac-terization of an ICP6 *lacZ* insertion mutant. J Virol 62:196–205
23. Goldstein DJ, Weller SK (1988) Factor(s) present in herpes simplex virus type 1-infected cells can compensate for the loss of the large subunit of the viral ribonucleotide reductase: characterization of an ICP6 deletion mutant. Virology 166:41–51
24. Jacobson JG, Leib DA, Goldstein DJ, et al (1989) A herpes simplex virus ribonucleotide reductase deletion mutant is defective for productive acute and reactivable latent infections of mice and for replication in mouse cells. Virology 173:276–283
25. Cameron JM, McDougall I, Marsden HS, et al (1988) Ribonucleotide reductase encoded by herpes simplex virus is a determinant of the pathogenicity of the virus in mice and a valid antiviral target. J Gen Virol 69:2607–2612
26. Coen DM, Goldstein DJ, Weller SK (1989) Herpes simplex virus ribonucleotide reductase mutants are hypersensitive to acyclovir. Antimicrob Agents Chemother 33:1395–1399

Investigations of Retroviral-Mediated Gene Therapy for Malignant Glioma: Transduction with HTK-Bearing Retroviruses Sensitizes Glioma Cells to Ganciclovir

Yasuyoshi Miyao[1], Keiji Shimizu[1], Masakazu Tamura[1,3],
Masanobu Yamada[2], Kazuyoshi Tamura[1], Haruhiko Kishima[1],
Kensuke Nakahira[3], Tadanori Yoshimatsu[3], Katsuhiko Mikoshiba[4],
Kazuhiro Ikenaka[3], and Toru Hayakawa[1]

Abstract. We have demonstrated that retrovirus-mediated herpes simplex virus type I (HTK) genes transferred to mouse glioma cells caused those glioma cells to be selectively sensitive to ganciclovir (GCV) in which myelin basic protein (MBP) promoter controlled these killer genes (MBP1.3/pNT230) in vitro. For this study, to know what percentage of retrovirus-transduced glioma cells is sufficient to kill most other wild glioma cells in vivo, we made an in vivo glioma model that contained several percentages (0%, 10%, 25%, 50%, and 100%) of retrovirus-transduced glioma cells. Mouse glioma models with 1×10^5 wild-type Rous sarcoma virus (RSV-M) glioma cells developed a large tumor mass in their brain even with the GCV treatment. However, the tumor mass was much smaller in a model containing 25% HTK-transduced cells, and the glioma model containing 50% HTK-transduced cells caused small tumor mass formation only in half of this group. Control mice that received only HTK-transduced glioma cells without GCV treatment suffered large tumor masses in the same way as did mice that received totally wild-type RSV-M glioma cells with GCV treatment. Therefore, glioma-affected mice may be rescued if one-fourth of the glioma cells are transduced with the MBP1.3/pNT230 retroviruses. We will investigate mechanisms of this phenomenon (bystander effect).

Key words. Malignant glioma—Gene therapy—MBP promoter—Bystander effect

Introduction

We have demonstrated that retrovirus-mediated herpes simplex virus type I (HTK) genes were transferred to mouse glioma cells and that these glioma cells were selectively sensitive to ganciclovir (GCV) in which myelin basic protein (MBP) promoter controlled these killer genes (MBP1.3/pNT230) in vitro [1]. If the MBP promoter is used as a regulator of HTK gene expression, gene therapy of malignant gliomas using

[1] Department of Neurosurgery, Osaka University Medical School, Osaka 565, Japan
[2] Department of Neurosurgery, The Center for Adult Diseases, Osaka 537, Japan
[3] National Institute for Physiological Sciences, Okazaki National Research Institutes, Okazaki, Aichi 444, Japan
[4] Institute of Medical Science, University of Tokyo, Tokyo 108, Japan

a retrovirus vector should cause few of the side effects, such as bone marrow suppression, that always accompany cancer chemotherapy.

Clinical trials of gene therapy have begun in the United States, not only for genetic diseases such as adenosine deaminase deficiency [2,3] but also for diverse diseases ranging from cancer to acquired immunodeficiency syndrome (AIDS). Among the methods available for delivering genes into mammalian cells, recombinant retroviruses are one of the most useful vehicles for targeting dividing cells, including malignant cells, because of broad host range and the stability inherent in chromosomal integration [4]. Although one of the limitations of retrovirus vectors is a low infectious viral titer, it is not necessary to transduce the HTK gene into every glioma cell. Glioma cells that are not transduced with the HTK gene-bearing retrovirus are also sensitive to GCV because of the sensitivity of surrounding glioma cells that were transduced with HTK gene-bearing retroviruses [5]. This phenomenon has been called the bystander effect [5], and it may occur partly because of the movement of ganciclovir triphosphate from transduced cells to non transduced cells [6] or partly because of host immunity to the viral-infected cells, or vice versa. Although it is important to investigate the mechanisms of the bystander effect, it is more important clinically to know what percentage of retrovirus-transduced glioma cells is sufficient to kill most wild-type glioma cells. In this chapter, we report our in vivo glioma model, which contained several percentages (0%, 10%, 25%, 50%, and 100%) of retrovirus-transduced glioma cells. After treatment with GCV, the mice were killed and the diameter of their tumors was measured.

Materials and Methods

Transduction of HTK-Bearing Retrovirus to Rous Sarcoma Virus Glioma Cells

Rous sarcoma virus (RSV-M) glioma (an anaplastic astrocytoma line derived from C3H/HeN mice) [7] was grown in Dulbecco's modified Eagle's medium (DMEM) containing 10% fetal bovine serum (FBS) (DMEM10). Ecotropic Psi-2 cells (kindly provided by Dr. Mulligan [8]) were also grown in DMEM10.

The MBP1.3/pNT230 (Fig. 1b) was transferred to Psi-2 cells by the calcium phosphate method as described previously [1]. After 48h transfection, G418 selection (1.0mg/ml) was performed, and high-titer virus-producing cells were selected by a simplified HTK gene product-amplification method [9]. The supernatant of Psi-2 cells, which produce the MBP1.3/pNT230 retroviruses, was added to the culture medium of RSV-M glioma cells with 8µg/ml polybrene (Aldrich, Milwaukee, WI, USA) and cultured for 5h at 37°C. The medium was then replaced by fresh virus-free medium, the cells were cultured for 48h at 37°C, and G418 (final concentration, 0.2mg/ml) was added to the RSV-M glioma cells. Glioma cells resistant to G418 were then harvested and used as recombinant retrovirus-transduced glioma cells.

In Vitro Sensitivity of Retrovirus-Transduced Cells to Ganciclovir

Retrovirus-transduced cells (2×10^4/well) were seeded in triplicate in flat-bottomed 96-well plates, and GCV was added at a final concentration of 0–1000nM (0, 15, 30, 60, 125, 250, 500, or 1000nM). Following incubation for 48–72h, cells were fixed with methanol for 1min at room temperature and stained for 5min with 100µl of 0.2%

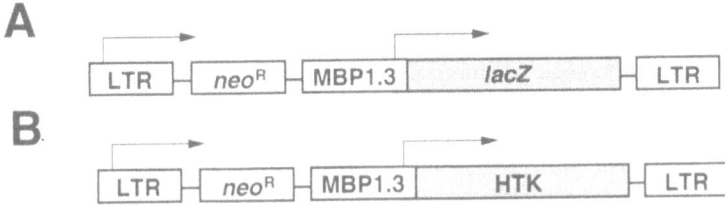

Fig. 1A,B. Construction of MBP1.3/pIP200 (**A**) and MBP1.3/pNT230 (**B**). MBP1.3/pIP200 contains the neomycin phosphotransferase (*neo*^R) gene and the *E. coli lacZ* gene within two Moloney murine leukemia virus long terminal repeats (LTRs). Myelin basic protein (MBP) promoter (MBP1.3) was inserted between the *neo*^R and the *lacZ* genes (**A**). The MBP1.3/pNT230 contains the *neoR* gene and the 2.8-kb herpes simplex virus type I (HTK) gene, whose expression was directed by MBP promoter (**B**)

crystal violet in 2% aqueous methanol. After washing the plates with running water for 10 min and drying them at room temperature, 200 μl of 1% laurylsarkosine was added and the plates were agitated gently for 20 min. The degree of violet staining was analyzed at a wavelength of 540 nm using an immunoreader (ImmunoReader NJ-2000, InterMed, Tokyo, Japan). Then the viability rate was calculated by the following formula: percent cell survival = (mean experimental OD_{540}/mean control OD_{540}) × 100, where control OD_{540} was the absorbance of the well without ganciclovir.

Transplantation of RSV-M Glioma Cells Containing Various Percentages of Cells Transduced with HTK-Bearing Retrovirus into Mouse Brain

Adult C3H/HeN mice were anesthetized by an intraperitoneal injection of pentobarbital and fixed to a stereotactic frame (David Kopf Instrument, Tujunga, CA, USA) as described before [10]. The skin over the head was incised to expose the skull. The right frontal bone was drilled with a dental bur to produce a small burrhole. Suspensions of RSV-M glioma cells at a concentration of 1×10^5 cells/2 μl, which contained 0%, 10%, 25%, 50%, and 100% of HTK-bearing RSV-M glioma cells were stereotaxically inoculated into the right striatum through the burrhole at the following coordinates: 2 mm lateral; 0.2 mm rostral to bregma; 3 mm below the skull. The skin was sutured with 4-0 nylon. After 3 days of tumor inoculation, 25 mg/kg of GCV in 250 μl saline was injected intraperitoneally twice a day for 14 days. Body weight of each mouse was measured every day. The mice were killed on the next day of the last ganciclovir treatment, and systemically perfused with 4% paraformaldehyde and then 0.5% glutaradehyde in phosphate buffered saline. After fixation with the same fixative for 24 h, the brain was sliced in 200-μm thickness with a microslicer.

Results and Discussion

Selective Killing by Ganciclovir of Glioma Cells Transduced with Retrovirus Containing the MBP Promoter-HTK Gene

Forty-eight hours after transduction of the MBP1.3/pNT230 into Psi-2 cells by the calcium phosphate coprecipitation method, stable transformants were selected by the addition of G418 at a concentration of 1.0 mg/ml. Infectious retrovirus particles were produced by ecotropic Psi-2 cells, and RSV-M glioma cells were incubated with these particles for 48 h. Transduced glioma cells were also selected using G418 (0.4 mg/ml), and these glioma cells were used for the sensitivity assay to determine the activity of GCV.

RSV-M mouse glioma cells transduced with the MBP1.3/pNT230 retroviruses (Fig. 1b) containing the 1.3-kb MBP promoter and the HTK gene showed increased sensitivity to ganciclovir when compared to both parental cells and those transduced with the MBP1.3/pIP200 (Fig. 1a) containing the MBP promoter directing the *lacZ* gene as a control. Twenty percent of the parental and pIP200/MBP1.3-transduced glioma cells survived at a ganciclovir concentration of 250 μM and 50% cells survived at 50 μM (data not shown). The viability of these cells was not affected by 1 μM ganciclovir, whereas the viability rate of RSV-M glioma cells transduced with retrovirus containing the HTK gene was less than 10% at this concentration, and the ganciclovir concentration producing 50% survival was 100 nM (Fig. 2). Therefore, glioma cells producing HTK were 500 times more sensitive to ganciclovir than parental RSV-M cells or glioma cells transduced with retrovirus without HTK gene.

These data strongly suggest that nucleoside analogs, at a concentration that does not affect the survival of normal dividing cells, can specifically kill glioma cells in which HTK gene expression is driven through the MBP promoter.

Glioma Cells Were Also Sensitive to GCV In Vivo when at Least 25% of Implanted Cells Were Transduced with HTK-Bearing Retroviruses

To know what percentage of retrovirus-transduced glioma cells is sufficient to kill most other wild-type glioma cells, we made a mouse intracranial glioma model that

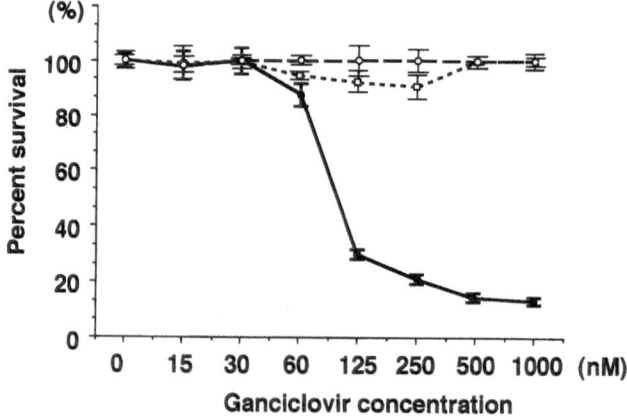

Fig. 2. Percent survival of cultured cells incubated with ganciclovir. Triplicate cultures (2×10^4/well) of RSV-M glioma cells (*open squares, dashed line*), cells transduced with MBP1.3/pIP200 (*open circles, hatched line*), and cells transduced with MBP1.3/pNT230 (*closed circles, solid line*) were incubated with various concentrations of ganciclovir for 72 h and then stained with crystal violet (see Materials and Methods). RSV-M mouse glioma cells were sensitive only when the retrovirus vector containing the HTK gene under control of the MBP promoter was added to a ganciclovir concentration of 125 nM or greater (*closed circles*), but original RSV-M glioma cells (*open squares*) or cells transduced with a nontoxic gene (*lacZ* gene) (*open circles*) were not sensitive to ganciclovir. *Bars*, standard error of mean

contained various percentages of HTK-transduced glioma cells, and then treated by ganciclovir as described in Materials and Methods.

After GCV treatment of mouse intracranial glioma models that contained wild-type RSV-M glioma cells and HTK-transduced glioma cells, tumor masses formed in the brain were measured in their longer diameter and evaluated (Fig. 3). The mouse glioma model with 1×10^5 wild-type RSV-M glioma cells resulted in a large brain tumor mass even with the GCV treatment. However, a glioma model with the same amount of cells but with 10% of HTK-transduced glioma cells developed as tumor mass about half the size by use of GCV treatment. Tumor mass was much smaller in the glioma model containing 25% HTK-transduced cells, and the glioma model containing 50% HTK-transduced cells caused small tumor mass formation only in half this group (Fig. 4). Control mice that received only HTK-transduced glioma cells without GCV treatment suffered with large tumor masses in the same way as mice which received totally wild-type RSV-M glioma cells with GCV treatment (Fig. 3a).

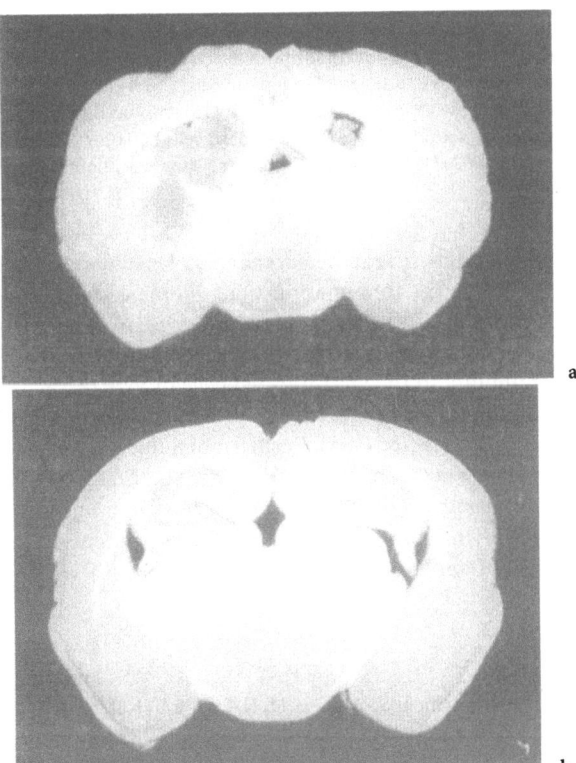

a

b

Fig. 3a,b. Photographs of tumor mass of intracranial glioma models. **a** Huge glioma mass was observed in the brain of in vivo glioma model in which 100% wild-type glioma cells were inoculated. In contrast to **a**, only a small glioma mass was observed in the brain of the model in which 25% HTK gene-transduced glioma cells were inoculated (data not shown). **b** No tumor mass was seen in the brain of the model that was inoculated with 100% HTK-transduced glioma cells with ganciclovir (GCV) treatment. ×10

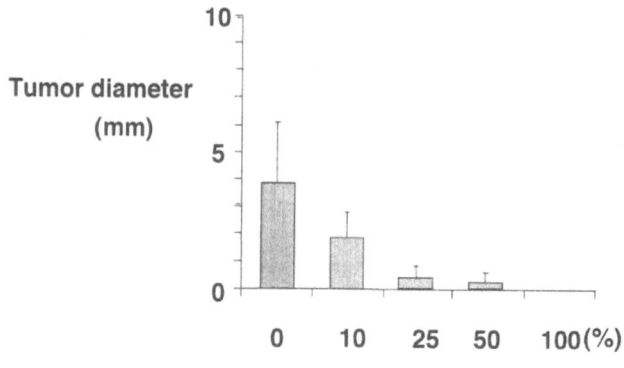

Percentage of HTK-bearing glioma cells

Fig. 4. Tumor diameter of in vivo glioma model inoculated with glioma cells containing various percentages of HTK-transduced cells among wild-type glioma cells (0%, 10%, 25%, 50%, and 100%). After GCV treatment (see Materials and Methods) in mouse intracranial glioma models containing both wild-type RSV-M glioma and HTK-transduced glioma cells, tumor masses formed in the brain were measured in their longer diameter and evaluated (also see Fig. 3). The mouse glioma model with 1×10^5 wild-type RSV-M glioma cells (0% group) developed a 3.7 ± 2.3 mm brain tumor mass even with GCV treatment. However, the glioma model with the same amount of cells but with 10% of HTK-transduced glioma cells resulted in a 1.8 ± 1.1 mm tumor mass with GCV treatment. The tumor mass was much smaller in the glioma model containing 25% HTK-transduced cells (0.3 ± 0.3 mm); further-more, the glioma model containing 50% HTK-transduced cells had only a small tumor mass forma-tion. Every mouse of the 100% HTK-transduced group rejected any glioma cells

These data strongly suggest that the glioma model can be rescued if the retrovirus vector delivers the HTK gene into one-fourth of glioma cells. This phenomenon has been called the bystander effect, and it may occurr partly because of movement of ganciclovir triphosphate from transduced cells to non-transduced cells or partly because of host immunity to the viral-infected cells or vice versa. This phenomenon was also observed in vitro sensitivity assay, but it may be more obvious in vivo than in an in vitro assay (unpublished data). Furthermore, this phenomenon was observed less often in an in vivo assay using nude mice. These data suggest that there are some possibilities this occurred partly because of the host immunity in addition to the movement of ganciclovir triphosphate through the gap junction. We will investigate mechanisms of the bystander effect.

References

1. Miyao Y, Shimizu K, Moriuchi S, Yamada M, Nakahira K, Nakajima K, Nakao J, Kuriyama S, Tsujii T, Mikoshiba K, Hayakawa T, Ikenaka K (1993) Selective expression of foreign genes in glioma cells: use of the mouse myelin basic protein gene promoter to direct toxic gene expression. J Neurosci Res 36:472–479
2. Culver KW, Osborne WRA, Miller AD, Fleisher TA, Berger M, Anderson WF, Blaese RM (1991) Correction of ADA deficiency in human T lymphocytes using retroviral-mediated gene transfer. Transplant Proc 23:170–171
3. Blaese RM, Culver KW, Chang L, Anderson WF, Mullen C, Nienhuis A, Carter C, Dunbar C, Leitman S (1993) Treatment of severe combined immunodeficiency disease (SCID) due to

adenosine deaminase deficiency with autologous lymphocytes transduced with human ADA gene, Hum Gene Ther 4:521–527

4. Cone R, Mulligan RC (1984) High efficiency gene transfer into mammalian cells: generation of helper-free recombinant retrovirus with broad mammalian host range. Proc Natl Acad Sci USA 81:6349–6353

5. Culver KW, Ram Z, Wallbridge S, Ishii H, Oldfield EH, Blaese RM (1992) In vivo gene transfer with retroviral vector-producer cells for treatment of experimental brain tumors. Science 256:1550–1552

6. Freeman SM, Abbound CN, Whartenby KA, Packman CH, Koeplin DS, Moolten FL, Abraham GN (1993) The "bystander effect": tumor regression when a fraction of the tumor mass is genetically modified. Cancer Res 53:5274–5283

7. Kumanishi T, Ikuta F, Yamamoto T (1971) Brain tumors induced by Rous sarcoma virus, Schmidt-Ruppin strain III. Morphology of brain tumors induced in adult mice. J Natl Cancer Inst 46:539–559

8. Mann R, Mulligan RC, Baltimore D (1983) Construction of a retrovirus packaging mutant and its use to produce helper-free defective retrovirus. Cell 33:153–159

9. Miyao Y, Shimizu K, Tamura M, Yamada M, Tamura K, Nakahira K, Kuriyama S, Hayakawa T, Ikenaka K (1995) A simplified general method for determination of recombinant retrovirus titers. Cell Struct Funct 20:177–183

10. Yamada M, Shimizu K, Miyao Y, Hayakawa T, Ikenaka K, Nakahira K, Nakajima K, Kagawa T, Mikoshiba K (1992) Retrovirus-mediated gene transfer targeted to malignant glioma cells in murine brain. Jpn J Cancer Res 83:1244–1247

Cytokine Gene Therapy of Malignant Glioma by Means of DNA/Liposomes

Jun Yoshida[1], Toshihiko Wakabayashi[1], Masaaki Mizuno[1],
Toru Takaoka[1], Sho Okamoto[1], Hideho Okada[1], Kunyu Harada[2],
and Kunio Yagi[3]

Abstract. During the past two decades, there have been major advances in our under-standing of tumor-associated genes that control cell growth and differentiation and in techniques using a variety of viral and nonviral vectors for delivering genes into mammalian cells. These developments have provided us with opportunities of gene therapy for cancer patients, and there is a rapidly growing number of cancer gene therapies worldwide. In this chapter, molecular abnormalities in the evolution of malignant glioma and recent basic experimental studies of gene therapy are reviewed. Our approach to gene therapy for brain tumors is selective in vivo gene transfer by means of immunoliposomes entrapping a plasmid vector. We have demonstrated in our experimental studies that a remarkable antitumor effect could be obtained by intratumoral injection of the liposome-entrapped interferon-β gene or the tumor necrosis factor-α gene.

Key words. Gene therapy—Cytokine—Malignant Glioma

Characteristics of Malignant Glioma

Malignant glioma (anaplastic astrocytoma and glioblastoma) is a parenchymal tumor in the brain of the central nervous system (CNS) that aggressively infiltrates into the surrounding normal brain tissue. Total resection of tumor by surgery is impossible, and even if patients receive extensive surgical resection of tumor and postoperative adjuvant therapy of radiation and immunochemotherapy, average survival time is less than 2 years [1] (Fig. 1). Nevertheless, this malignant glioma has important features as a candidate for gene therapy. The brain is a closed cavity separated from the general circulation system by the blood–brain barrier, and it has been noted to be an immunologically privileged site with no lymphatic system. Normal brain cells of glia and neuron are relatively quiescent compared to the tumor cells. Furthermore, the glioma arising from a glia is a localized tumor in the CNS with no extra-CNS metastasis.

---

[1] Department of Neurosurgery, Nagoya University School of Medicine, Nagoya 466, Japan
[2] Department of Neurosurgery, Hiroshima University, Hiroshima 734, Japan
[3] Institute of Applied Biochemistry, Yagi Memorial Park, Gifu 505-01, Japan

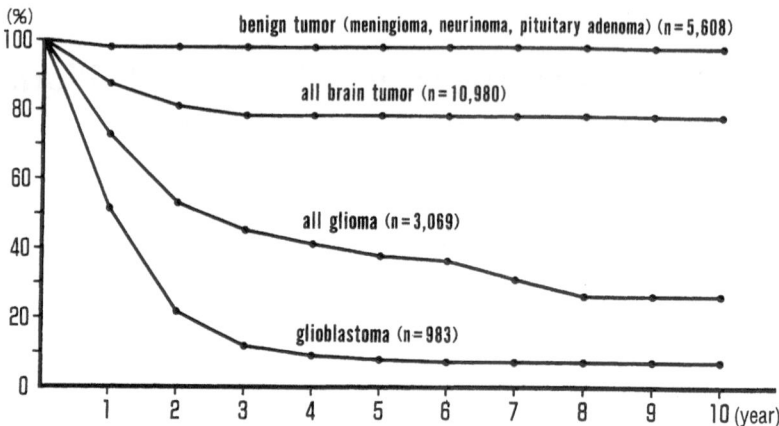

Fig. 1. Relative survival rates of different types of primary brain tumor [37]

Molecular/Genetic Abnormalities of Malignant Glioma

Astrocytic gliomas are the most frequent human brain tumors. They are classified into three malignancy grades on the basis of histopathological parameters. The most commonly encountered genetic alteration in astrocytic gliomas is loss of heterozygosity (LOH) on chromosome 17p [2]. This alteration occurs in approximately half of all grades of malignancy, and most of these are mutations in the conserved region of the p53 genes [3]. Low-grade astrocytomas bear a significant risk of malignant progression. LOH of chromosome 9p21 and chromosome 10 are known for potential involvement in this progression event [4]. Multiple tumor suppressor-1 (MTS-1) gene for a newly identified inhibitor of cell cycle-dependent kinase 4 (CDK-4), a protein that goes by the name p16, has been confirmed to be localized in the area of 9p21 [5]. It was recently reported that deletion of the genes occurs frequently in anaplastic astrocytoma and glioblastoma [6].

Amplification of the epidermal growth factor receptor (EGFR) gene is the most common genetic alteration in glioblastoma [7]. Several cytokines and growth factors are related to the autocrine or paracrine growth of human glioma cells. Platelet-derived growth factor (PDGF) [8], insulin-like growth factor-II (IGF-II) [9], tumor necrosis factor-α (TNF-α), interferon-β (IFN-β) [10,11], and transforming growth factor-β (TGF-β) have been reported to be synthesized from human glioma cells and released constitutively or by various means of induction; they are believed to stimulate or inhibit the growth of glioma cells themselves (Fig. 2).

Gene Therapy for Brain Tumors

Since the first gene therapy was started on 14 September in 1990 in the United States for a patient with severe combined immunodeficiencies [12], various human gene therapies have been proposed and carried out. Target diseases of this therapy are now expanding from congenital metabolic disorders to malignant neoplastic tumors, which cannot be cured by existing treatments [13]. Three approaches of cancer gene

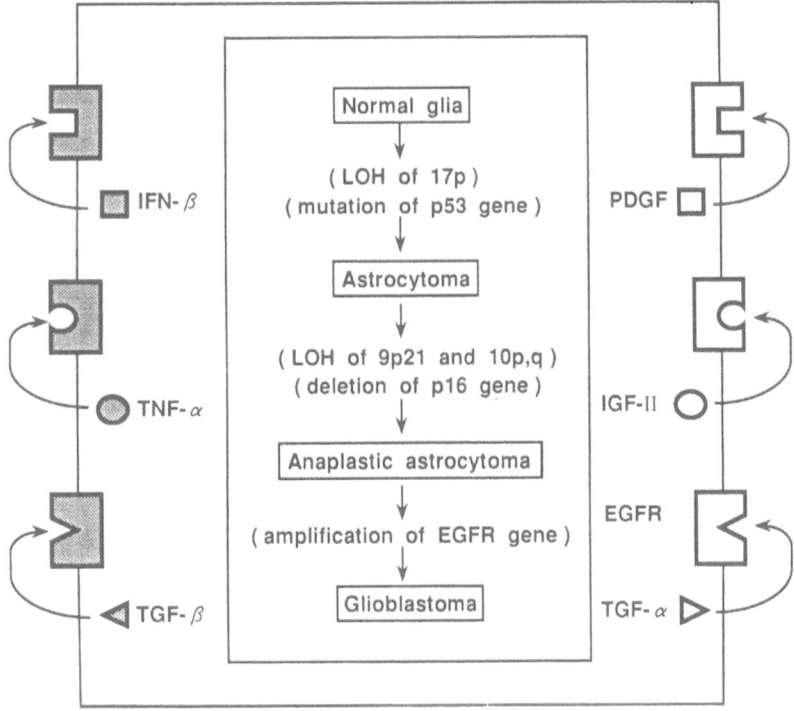

Fig. 2. Molecular/genetic abnormality of malignant glioma from normal glia to glioblastoma. LOH, loss of heterozygosity; IFN-β, interferon-β; TNF-α, tumor necrosis factor-alpha; TGF-β, transforming growth factor-β; PDFG, platelet-derived growth factor; IGF-II, insulin-like growth factor II; EGFR, epidermal growth factor receptor; TGF-α, transforming growth factor-alpha

therapy are proposed: repairing an oncogene or suppressor oncogene, transduction of a toxic gene into tumor cells, and augmentation of a gene that activates tumor immunity.

In 1992, for patients with malignant brain tumor, a team of National Institutes of Health (United States) biologists and neurosurgeons started a remarkable new form of treatment: molecular neurosurgery based on gene therapy [14]. Mouse cells were genetically modified by inserting a retroviral vector carrying a herpes gene coded for thymidine kinase. When the mouse cells were injected directly into a brain tumor, they start pumping out copies of the retroviral vector, which infect nearby tumor cells. The infected tumor cells now produced herpes simplex thymidine kinase (HS-tk), laying themselves open to attack by intravenous injection of the antiviral drug ganciclovir.

In 1994, a team from Howard Hughes Medical Intitute and Baylor College of Medicine (United States) reported the efficacy of adenovirus (ADV) -mediated gene therapy to treat brain tumor [15]. Tumors were generated in syngeneic rats by stereotaxic implantation of 9L gliosarcoma cells into the caudate nucleus. Eight days later, the tumors were injected and transduced in situ with a replication-defective ADV carrying the HS-tk gene, and the rats were treated with ganciclovir. No tumors were detected in animals treated with ADV-tk and with ganciclovir at doses greater than 80 mg/kg, and all animals remained alive longer than 80 days after tumor induction whereas all untreated animals died by 22 days.

DNA/Liposome

Advances in gene therapy depend in large part on the development of delivery systems capable of efficiently introducing DNA into the target cells. There are two delivery systems, viral and nonviral. Viral vectors using retrovirus and adenovirus are most commonly applied for human gene therapy, while nonviral vectors, especially the liposome-entrapped plasmid vector, are known to be much safer because they are noninfectious and nonimmunogenic.

Liposomes, artificially generated lipid vesicles that can entrap drugs within their aqueous compartment or in the lipid bilayer, have been regarded as a useful delivery system [16], including gene transfer [17] (Fig. 3). In 1987, Felgner et al. [18] developed a cationic liposome with N-[1-(2,3-dioleyloxy) propyl]-N,N,N-trimethylammonium chloride (DOTMA). The authors reported that DOTMA interacts spontaneously with DNA to form a DNA–lipid complex and facilitates fusion of the complex with the cell membrane, resulting in both uptake and expression of the DNA. They also reported that the lipofection is from 5- to more than 100 fold more effective than either the calcium phosphate or the diethylaminoethyl (DEAE) dextran transfection technique [18].

Since this pioneer work, cationic liposome-mediated gene transfer has been widely used in the field of basic molecular biology and for gene therapy studies. Several groups have explored more efficient and less toxic cationic liposome compositions using different cationic lipids.

We have developed novel cationic liposomes with high transfection efficiency and low cytotoxicity that permit using these for in vivo gene transfer. Our liposomes are multilamellar vesicles (MLV) prepared by a simple procedure with N-(α-trimethyl ammonioacetyl)-didodecyl-D-glutamate chloride (TMAG), dilauroyl phosphatidylcholine (DLPC), and dioleoyl phosphatidyl ethanolamine (DOPE) in a molar ratio of 1:2:2 [19]. The liposomes entrapped expression vectors of plasmids

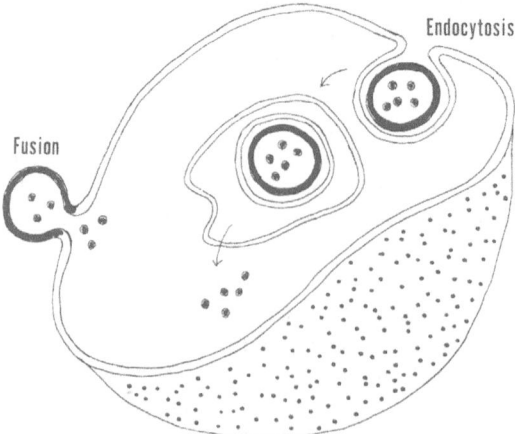

Fig. 3. Interaction of cell and liposome to transfect tumor cells with a toxic gene

and transfected them into the cells. In our system, the gene was transfected mainly by endocytosis of liposomes and expressed predominantly in proliferating cells. The expression rate was generally 10–20% in cultured neoplastic cells in vitro.

Immunoliposomes

To transfer the gene selectively and efficiently into target cells, we coupled a monoclonal antibody (MCA) with the liposomes (immunoliposomes). The G-22 MCA devised by us [20] is noted to be selectively binding with human glioma cells. We utilized its radiolabeled form for radioimaging (Fig. 4) or radioimmunotherapy of malignant glioma [21]. Recently, we identified the G-22 MCA-reactive antigen to be a 85-kDa CD44 overexpressed on the surface of glioma cells [22]. CD44 is an integral membrane glycoprotein expressed by a variety of hematopoietic and non-hematopoietic cells, originally described as a homing receptor of lymphocytes. CD44 belongs to the proteoglycan binding family, with hyaluronate, collagens, and fibronectin as major ligands to confer cell–matrix contacts.

The standard or hematopoietic (CD44H) form of the protein is a transmembrane molecule with a molecular weight of 85 000–90 000, and approximately 20 different CD44 isoforms, ranging in molecular weight from 90 000 to 300 000, are generated by alternative splicing of transcripts of a single gene. On the other hand, although CD44H is expressed by almost all normal human tissues, its overexpression has been reported to be associated with aggressive invasion, dissemination, and metastasis of melanoma and glioma cells. In our experiments, the proportion of the glioma cells that expressed the transferred DNA sequences and the absolute levels of expression obtained were markedly higher when using the immunoliposomes than those achieved with the DNA/liposomes alone [23].

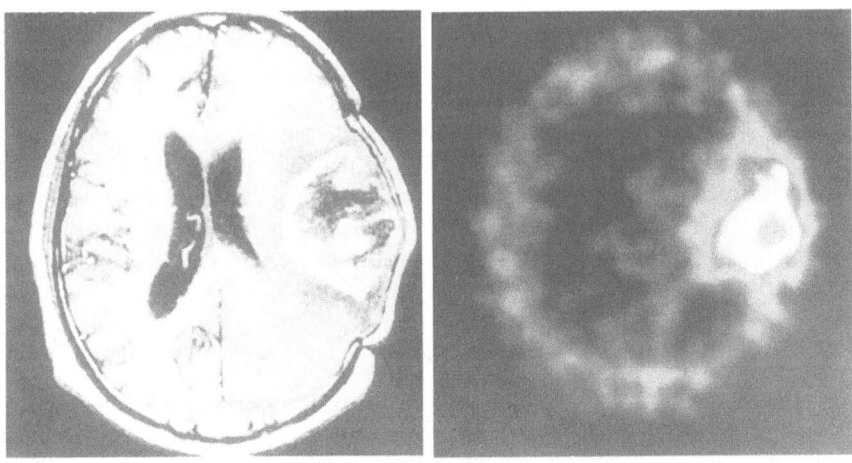

a   b

Fig. 4a,b. Specific binding of G-22 MCA (monoclonal antibody) to malignant glioma cells is shown by (a) magnetic resonance imaging (MRI) and (b) single photon emission computed tomography (SPECT) ([111In] G-22 MCA)

Cytokine Gene

Interferon (IFN) and tumor necrosis factor (TNF) are produced in human glioma cells and known to act a negative growth factor to them; the growth of glioma is suggested to be deeply related to these autocrine or paracrine cytokines [10,11]. Furthermore, these cytokines modulate the expression of the cell-surface antigens, including major histocompatibility complex (MHC) antigens [24] and cell adhesion molecules, thus providing a potential regulatory mechanism for local immune reactivity. In our study, glioma cells transfected IFN-γ or TNF-α genes produced and secreted the cytokines continuously, resulting in the induction of MHC antigens and intercellular adhesion molecule-1 (ICAM-1) on the surface of glioma cells [25,26].

Cytokine Gene Therapy with DNA/Liposome

In Vitro Experiments

IFN-β

Antiproliferative activity of interferons (IFNs) was reported by Parker et al. for the first time in 1962. Gresser et al. confirmed this activity by both in vitro and in vivo studies, and Strander et al. introduced systemic administration of human IFNs for the treatment of patients with malignant tumors. Clinical trials of IFNs for malignant glioma started in 1980 and their effectiveness, especially that of human IFN-β (HuIFN-β), has been noted [27]. However, the result of systemic administration of HuIFN-β was not satisfactory, and thus we have been striving to develop a new interferon therapy using transfection-induced HuIFN-β.

We transfected human glioma cells with an eukaryotic expression vector of the HuIFN-β gene (pSV2IFN-β) by means of our novel cationic liposomes, and found that HuIFN-β produced in the cells had a much stronger inhibitory effect on the growth of the cells than exogenously added HuIFN-β [23]. From results of some other experiments, we considered that the mechanism of the growth-inhibitory effect of transfection-induced HuIFN-β is different from that of an exogenous one (Fig. 5). The former is suggested to be cytocidal to the transfected glioma cells [28], and it seems to be ascribed to HuIFN-β produced in the cells transfected with its gene by the process of apopotosis. The production of HuIFN-β in the cells and its release from the transfected cells were increased by the use of immunoliposomes coupled with G-22 MCA, or by the treatment of cells with TNF-α before the transfection [29]. Correspondingly, the antitumor effect of the transfection-induced HuIFN-β was significantly elevated.

TNF-α

TNF-α was originally discovered in mouse serum by Carswell and colleagues in 1975. It is a cytokine that possesses a wide variety of biological activity and immunomodulatory properties, although the problem of dose-limiting toxicity of TNF-α was reported in its clinical trials [30]. Rosenberg et al. [32] began immunotherapy for cancer patients by gene transfer instead of administration of TNF-α either by adding TNF-α gene to the tumor-infiltrating lymphocytes (TILs) to make them more effective [31] or by adding TNF-α gene to the tumor cells to induce

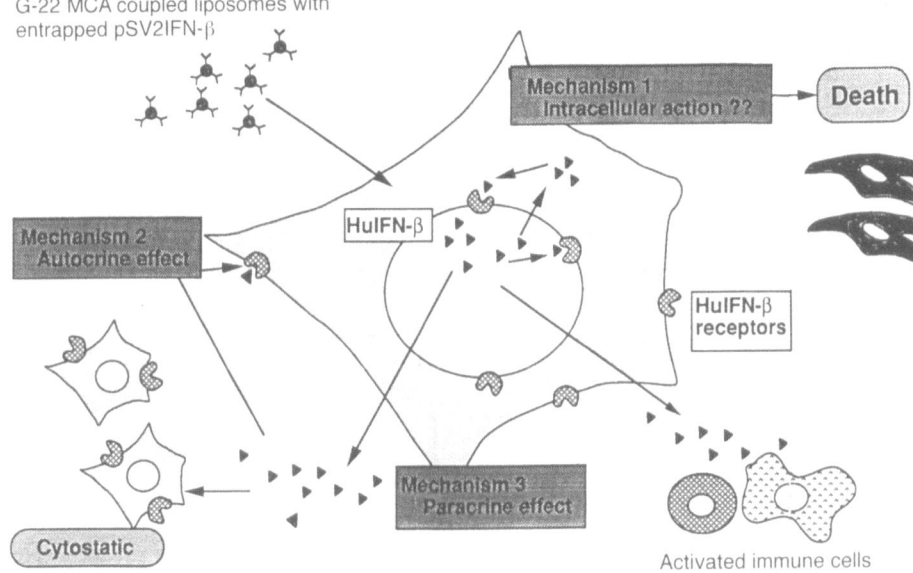

Fig. 5. Mechanisms of antitumor effect of HuIFN-β (human interferon-β): autocrine, paracrine, or intracellular action

the host immune system [32]. In our experimental studies, we found that human TNF-α (HuTNF-α) was produced in the glioma cells transfected with liposomes with entrapped pcDVTNF-α and that the growth-inhibitory effect of transfection-induced HuTNF-α was much stronger than that of exogenously added HuTNF-α.

When we analyzed the mechanism, we found that it was the result of transmembrane-formed TNF-α. TNF-α has a 76-residue-long precursor sequence containing both hydrophobic and hydrophilic regions, and its long precursor sequence serves to anchor the TNF-α precursor polypeptide in the plasma membrane [33]. The transmembrane-formed TNF-α was identified in cytotoxic T lymphocytes (CTLs), macrophages, and activated monocytes, and it has been suggested to play an important role in modulating host immunity. By the transfection of TNF-α gene into human glioma cells, transfected cells secreted soluble TNF-α and also expressed transmembrane-formed TNF-α. We found that the TNF-α gene-transfected cells grew the same as nontransfected ones and obtained protective function against the cytotoxicity of exogenous TNF-α. Further, it has been interestingly demonstrated that the transfected cells have a potentiality of growth inhibition or cytotoxicity toward the adjacent nontransfected glioma cells through the transmembrane-formed TNF-α by cell-to-cell contact (Fig. 6).

In Vivo Experiments

In vivo experiments using transplanted solid tumors of human glioma clearly showed that HuIFN-β or HuTNF-α was expressed in the solid tumor [34,35] and that growth of the tumor was inhibited by intratumoral injection of liposomes with entrapped pSV2IFN-β or pcDVTNF-α, while a high dose of exogenous HuIFN-β or HuTNF-α did

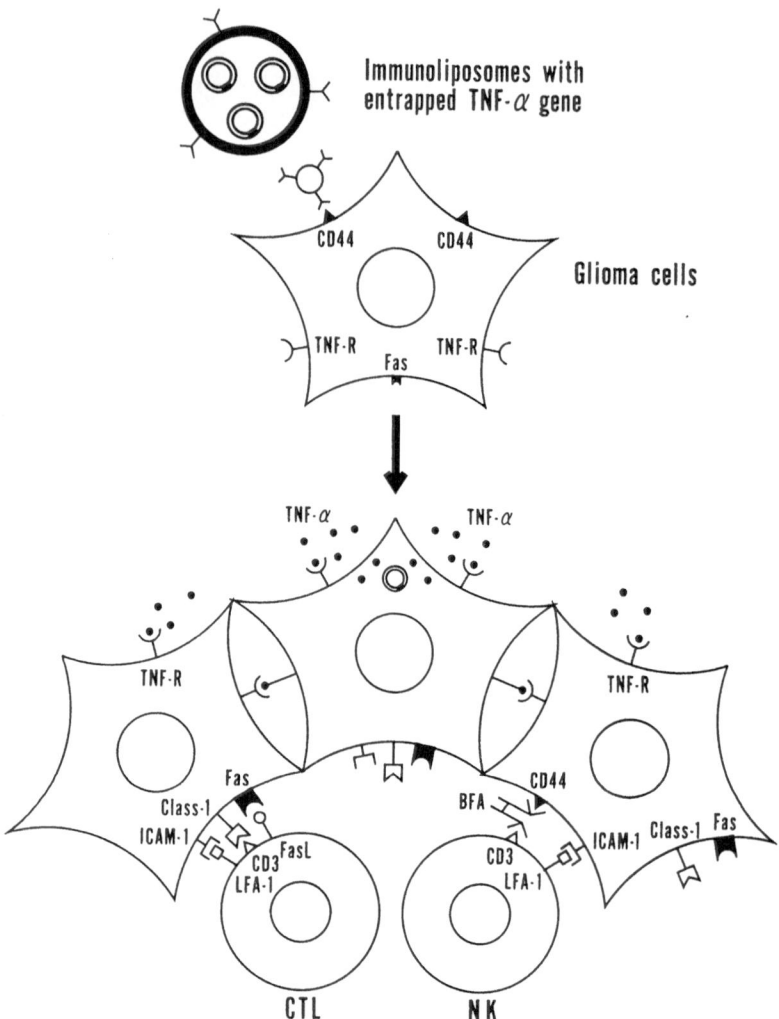

Fig. 6. Mechanism of antitumor effect with TNF-α gene therapy by means of DNA/liposomes on human glioma cells. TNF-R, tumor necrosis factor receptor; FasL, Fas ligand; ICAM-1, intercellular adhesion molecule-1; BFA, bifunctional antibody; LFA-1, lymphocyte function-associated antigen-1; CTL, cytotoxic T lymphocyte; NK, natural killer cell

not significantly inhibit the growth of human glioma [34,35]. When the liposomes were repeatedly injected into the tumor, the number of transfected cells in a tumor was increased and the growth-inhibitory effect to the solid tumor was enhanced. The intraperitoneal injection of a small amount of TNF-α (1000 U) inhibited tumor growth only slightly. On the other hand, prior treatment with TNF-α followed by intratumoral injection of liposomes with entrapped pSV2IFN-β (150 nmol lipids and 3 μg DNA) gave a remarkable effect. The subcutaneous tumors regressed completely in all nude mice tested (Fig. 7); they were tumor free and surviving at the 250th day, the longest time for follow-up [29].

We confirmed the antitumor effect of transfection-induced HuIFN-β by the use of human glioma produced in the brain of nude mice [36]. When we injected human glioma cells of 2×10^5 cells/2 µl into the cerebral hemisphere, the human gliomas grew in the mouse brain and produced a huge brain tumor. For evaluation of the antitumor effect, we injected liposomes with entrapped pSV2IFN-β (30 nmol lipids and 0.6 µg DNA/2 µl) into the tumor growing in the brain once every other day for six times. We started the treatment at different days after the transplantation and killed all animals at the 31st day. The transplanted glioma was checked with naked eye and light microscopic observation, demonstrating that the transplanted glioma disappeared completely when liposomes with entrapped pSV2IFN-β were injected repeatedly into the tumor.

Complete disappearance of the transplanted glioma was seen in 100% of nude mice if the treatment was started 3 days after transplantation; when it was started at 7 days or 9 days, the tumor-free ratio was 5/7 (71%) or 2/7 (29%), respectively. Even when the tumor did not disappear, the residual tumors found in the treated animals were smaller than in animals that were untreated or treated with empty liposomes.

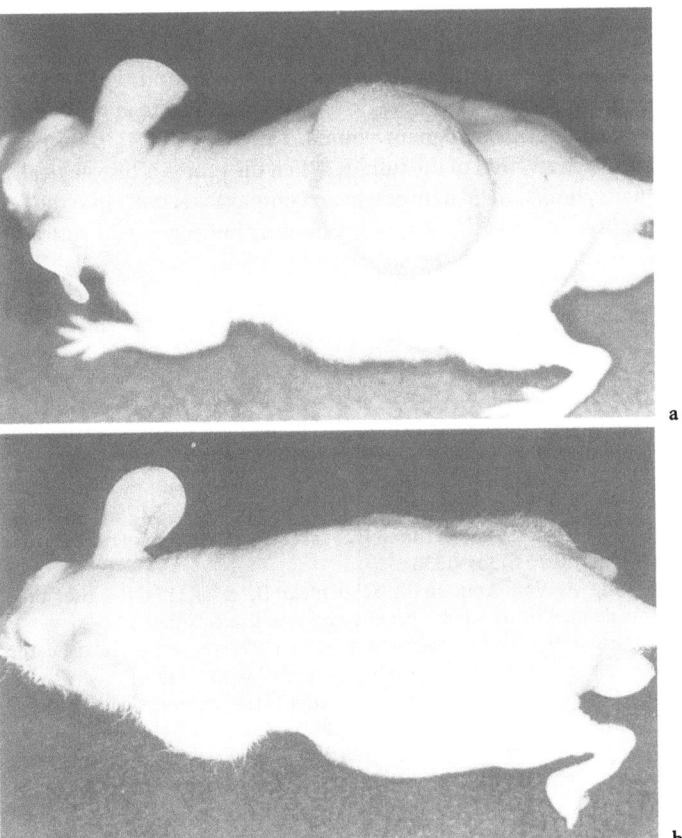

a

b

Fig. 7. Antitumor effect of intratumoral injection of liposomes with entrapped pSV2IFN-β and prior treatment of TNF-α. **a** Control. **b** Two months after treatment

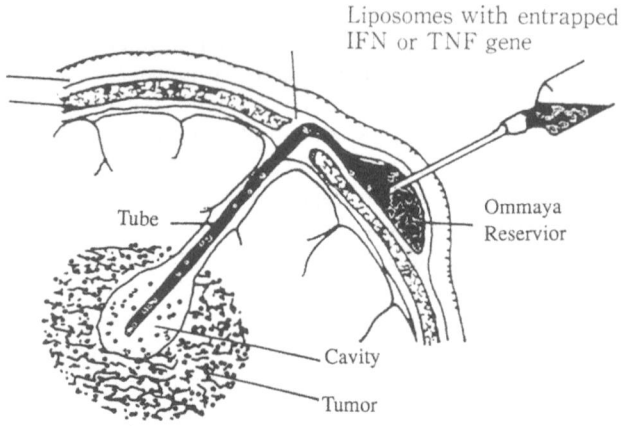

Liposomes with entrapped
IFN or TNF gene

Fig.8. Molecular
neurosurgery for
malignant glioma

Tube

Ommaya
Reservior

Cavity

Tumor

Molecular Neurosurgery

Our in vitro and in vivo experiments have confirmed that cytokine gene transfer by means of DNA/liposomes has promising clinical application (Fig. 8). On approval of the Institutional and National Review Board, we would like to apply our cytokine gene therapy for patients with malignant glioma. Patients with brain tumor will first be treated by surgical resection of the tumor. When the tumor is histologically diagnosed to be malignant glioma, we plan to set up an Ommaya reservoir into the tumor cavity. We will then directly inject the G-22 MCA binding liposomes with entrapped HuIFN-β or HuTNF-α genes through the Ommaya reservoir.

References

1. Yoshida J, Kajita Y, Wakabayashi T, et al (1994) Long-term follow-up results of 175 patients with malignant glioma: importance of radical tumour resection and postoperative adjuvant therapy with interferon, ACNU and radiation. Acta Neurochir (Wien) 127:55–59
2. Von Deimling A, Eibl RH, Ohgaki H, et al (1992) p53 mutations are associated with 17p allelic loss in grade II and grade III astrocytoma. Cancer Res 52:2987–2990
3. Rasheed BKA, Mclendon RE, Herndon JE, et al (1994) Alteration of the TP53 gene in human gliomas. Cancer Res 54:1324–1330
4. Von Deimling A, Von Ammon K, Schoenfeld D, et al (1993) Subset of glioblastoma multiforme defined by molecular genetic analysis. Brain Pathol 3:19–26
5. Kamb A, Gruis NA, Weaver-Feldhaus J, et al (1994) A cell cycle regulator potentially involved in genesis of many tumor types. Science 264:436–440
6. Noburi T, Miura K, Wu DJ, et al (1994) Deletion of the cyclin-dependent kinase-4 inhibitor gene in multiple human cancers. Nature 368:753–756
7. Wong AJ, Bigner SH, Bigner DD, et al (1987) Increased expression of the epidermal growth factor receptor gene in malignant glioma is invariably associated with gene amplification. Proc Natl Acad Sci USA 84:6899–6903
8. Nister M, Liberman TA, Betsholtz C, et al (1988) Expression of messenger RNAs for platlet-derived growth factor and transforming growth factor-α and their receptors in human malignant glioma cell lines. Cancer Res 48:3910–3918
9. Sera V, Prisell P, Sjogren B, et al (1986) Enhancement of insulin-like growth factor 2 receptors in glioblastoma. Cancer Lett 32:229–234

10. Larsson I, Landstrom LE, Larner E, et al (1978) Interferon production in glia and glioma cell lines. Infect Immunol 22:786–789
11. Inoue I, Yoshida J, Nagata M, et al (1991) Superinduction of cytotoxic interferon-β in glioma cells. Neurol Med Chir (Tokyo) 31:485–487
12. Anderson F, Blaese RH, Culver K (1990) Treatment of severe combined immunodeficiency disease (SCID) due to adenosine deaminase (ADA) deficiency with autologous lymphocytes transduced with a human ADA gene. Hum Gene Ther 1:331–362
13. Mulligan RC (1993) The basic science of gene therapy. Science 26:926–932
14. Culver KW, Ram Z, Wallbridge S, et al (1992) In vivo gene transfer with retroviral vector-producer cells for treatment of experimental brain tumor. Science 256:1550–1552
15. Perez-Cruet MJ, Trask TW, Chen C-H, et al (1994) Adenovirus-mediated gene therapy of experimental gliomas. J Neurosci Res 39:506–511
16. Bangham AD, Hill MW, Miller NGA (1974) Preparation and use of liposomes as models of biological membrane. In: Korn ED (ed) Methods in membrane biology, Vol 1. Plenum, New York, pp 1–68
17. Schaefer-Ridder M, Wang Y, Hofschneider PH (1982) Liposomes as gene carriers: efficient transformation of mouse L cells by thymidine kinase gene. Science 215:166–168
18. Felgner PL, Gadek TR, Holm M, et al (1987) Lipofection: a highly efficient, lipid-mediated DAN-transfection procedure. Proc Natl Acad Sci USA 84:7413–7414
19. Yoshida J, Mizuno M (1994) Simple method to prepare cationic multilamellar liposomes for efficient transfection of human interferon-β gene to human glioma cells. J Neuro-Oncol 19:269–274
20. Wakabayashi T, Yoshida J, Seo H, et al (1988) Characterization of neuroectodermal antigen by a monoclonal antibody and its application in CSF diagnosis of human glioma. J Neurosurg 68:449–455
21. Yoshida J, Wakabayashi T, Mizuno M, et al (1992) Tumor-specific binding of radio-labeled G-22 monoclonal antibody in glioma patients. Neurol Med Chir (Tokyo) 32:125–129
22. Okada H, Yoshida J, Seo H, et al (1994) Anti-glioma surface antigen monoclonal antibody G-22 recognizes overexpressed CD44 in glioma cells. Cancer Immunol Immunother 39:313–317
23. Mizuno M, Yoshida J, Sugita K, et al (1990) Growth inhibition of glioma cells transfected with the human β-interferon gene by liposomes coupled with a monoclonal antibody. Cancer Res 50:7826–7829
24. Takiguchi M, Ting JPY, Buessow SC, et al (1985) Response of glioma cells to interferon-gamma: increase in class II RNA, protein and mixed lymphocyte reaction stimulating ability. Eur J Immunol 15:809–814
25. Mizuno M, Yoshida J, Takaoka T, et al (1994) Liposomal transfection of human γ-interferon gene into human glioma cells and adoptive immunotherapy using lymphokine-activated killer cells. J Neurosurg 80:510–514
26. Takaoka T, Yoshida J, Mizuno M, et al (1994) Transfection-induced tumor necrosis factor-α increases the susceptibility of human glioma cells to lysis by lymphokine-activated killer cells: continuous expression of intercellular adhesion molecule-1 on glioma cells. Jpn J Cancer Res 85:750–755
27. Nagai M (1983) Clinical trials of human fibroblast interferon (HuIFN-β) on malignant brain tumor. J Jpn Soc Cancer Ther 18:66–68
28. Yoshida J, Mizuno M, Yagi K (1992) Cytotoxicity of human β-interferon produced in human glioma cells transfected with its gene by means of liposomes. Biochem Int 28:1055–1061
29. Yoshida J, Mizuno M, Yagi K (1992) Antitumor effect of endogenous human β-interferon on malignant glioma and augmentation of the effect by tumor necrosis factor-α. J Clin Biochem Nutr 12:153–160
30. Hwu P, Yannelli J, Kriegler M, et al (1993) Functional and molecular characterization of tumor infiltrating lymphocytes transduced with the tumor necrosis factor-α cDNA for the gene therapy of cancer in man. J Immunol 150:4104–4115
31. Rosenberg SA (1992) Gene therapy for cancer [clinical conference]. JAMA 268:2416

32. Yannelli JR, Hyatt C, Johnson S, et al (1993) Characterization of human tumor cell lines transduced with the cDNA encoding either tumor necrosis factor-alpha or interleukin-2. J Immunol Meth 161:77

33. Vileck J, Lee TH (1991) Tumor necrosis factor. J Biol Chem 266:7313–7316

34. Yoshida J, Mizuno M, Yagi K (1991) Secretion of human β-interferon into the cystic fluid of glioma transfected with the interferon gene, J Clin Biochem Nutr 11:123–128

35. Harada K, Yoshida J, Mizuno M, et al (1994) Growth inhibition of subcutaneously transplanted human glioma by transfection-induced tumor necrosis factor-α and augmentation of the effect by γ-interferon. J Neuro-Oncol 22:221–225

36. Yagi K, Hayashi Y, Ishida N, et al (1994) Interferon-β endogenously produced by intratumoral injection of cationic liposome-encapsulated gene: cytocidal effect on glioma transplanted into nude mouse brain. Biochem Mol Biol Int 32:167–171

37. Eighth Report from the Brain Tumor Registry of Japan

Analysis of *sdi-1* Gene Functions in Human Malignant Gliomas

Kunyu Harada[1], Kaoru Kurisu[1], Kazuhiko Sugiyama[1],
Takashi Sadatomo[1], Ohtsura Niwa[2], and Tohru Uozumi[1]

Abstract. A senescent cell-derived inhibitor of DNA synthetase-1 (*sdi-1*) occurs in human senescent cells. *sdi-1* protein forms a complex with cyclin-dependent kinase 2 (cdk-2), and expression of *sdi-1* is regulated by the p53 suppressor gene. We investigated the molecular changes of the *sdi-1* gene in human gliomas and studied its effect on growth of glioma cells. DNA and mRNA were extracted from cultured human glioma cells and from clinical samples from patients with glioma and analyzed by Southern and northern blotting. The *sdi-1* gene was transfected into cultured human glioma cells by a novel liposome method, and its growth inhibitory effect was investigated.

Key words. sdi-1—Cell cycle-regulating gene—Glioma—Growth inhibition

Introduction

In research on malignant neoplasms, the role of cell cycle-regulating genes is worthy of note. Some recent reports [1–4] on the roles of p16, p21, p24, and p27 have indicated that these products of cell cycle-regulating genes are associated with a cyclin-dependent kinase (CDK) complex. *sdi-1* is expressed in human senescent cells; *sdi-1* protein forms a complex with cyclin-dependent kinase 2 (cdk-2), and expression of *sdi-1* is regulated by the p53 suppressor gene. In this chapter, we analyze the expression and the effect of forced expression of the *sdi-1* gene in human glioma cells.

Materials and Methods

Cell Lines and Clinical Materials

Cultured human glioma cell lines (U251-SP, U251-MG, A-7, U87-MG, and T98G) and clinical samples of malignant glioma were used. Glioma cell lines were grown in Eagle's minimum essential medium supplemented with 10% fetal calf serum, $2\,\mathrm{m}M$

[1] Department of Neurosurgery, Hiroshima University School of Medicine, Minami-ku, Hiroshima 734, Japan

[2] Department of Molecular Pathology, Hiroshima University, Research Institute for Nuclear Medicine and Biology, Minami-ku, Hiroshima 734, Japan

nonessential amino acids, 5 mM L-glutamine, and antibiotics (streptomycin, 100 μg/ml; penicillin, 100 units/ml).

Liposomes

An improved procedure of reverse-phase evaporation was used to entrap plasmids into the liposomes to avoid DNA damage from sonication. The reverse-phase micelles were prepared first by sonication, and plasmids were then added to form liposomes entrapping plasmids. Liposomes were charged positively and were composed of N-(α-trimethylammoioacetyl)-didodecyl-D-glutamate chloride (TMAG), dilauroyl phosphatidylcholine (DLPC), and dioleoyl-phosphatidylethanolamine (DOPE).

Plasmids

An *sdi-1* gene inserted into a simian virus 40-derived expression vector (pcDSRαδ) was used. The plasmid size was 5.5 kb, vector size 3.4 kb, and insert size 2.1 kb. Liposomes with entrapped plasmid were prepared as described previously [5].

Gene Transfection

One milliliter of cultured human glioma cells (A-7, U251-SP) suspended in culture medium (1×10^4/ml) was placed in each well of a Falcon plate (#3047) and incubated at 37°C for 24 h in a humidified atmosphere of 5% CO_2 and 95% air. After the liposomes (15 nmol lipids, 0.3 μg DNA) were added into the culture medium, the incubation was continued for up to 21 days.

Expression Efficiency by Transfection with Novel Liposomes

The expression efficiency by transfection with our novel liposomes was evaluated. Two milliliters of A-7 human glioma cell suspension in culture medium (1×10^4/ml) was placed in each well, and the cells were incubated at 37°C for 24 h in a humidified atmosphere at 5% CO_2 and 95% air. Liposomes (15 nmol lipids; 0.3 μg DNA per milliliter containing β-gal expression vector) were added to the medium and incubation continued. Cells were measured by counting the number of *x-gal*-excluding cells in a hemacytometer on the third day after transfection.

Southern and Northern Blotting

DNA was extracted from cultured human glioma cells and clinical samples, and 20 μg of DNA was applied on Southern blotting in the usual method. RNA was extracted from cultured human glioma cells and sarcoma cells by GTC methods and applied on northern blotting.

Detection of the Introduced *sdi-1* Gene in Transfected Glioma Cells by Polymerase Chain Reaction

DNA of the cultured human glioma cells (A-7) was extracted on the fourth day after transfection with the *sdi-1* gene and applied on polymerase chain reaction (PCR).

Growth Inhibition of Glioma by Transfection with *sdi-1* Gene

Two milliliters of glioma cell suspension in culture medium (1×10^4/ml) was placed in each well, and the cells were incubated at 37°C for 24h in a humidified atmosphere at 5% CO_2 and 95% air. Liposome (15nmol lipids; 0.3μg DNA/ml) were added to the medium and incubation was continued for an additional 24h. The medium was exchanged and replaced with fresh medium containing 500 mg/ml G418. The selected cells were designated pcDSRαδ-*sdi-1*. Human glioma cells that had been transfected with expression vector pcDSRαδ without the *sdi-1* cDNA insert were used as a control. The growth rates of pcDSRαδ-sdi 1 and pcDSRαδ were compared after 10 and 21 days. Cells were measured by counting the number of trypan blue-excluding cells using a hemacytometer.

Results

Expression Efficiency by Transfection with Novel Liposomes

The transfection efficiency was 15% as revealed by the marker of blue cells (Fig.1).

Southern and Northern Blotting

Southern blot analysis showed expression of *sdi-1* cDNA in all samples, although the density of the bands varied (Fig. 2). This result suggested loss of heterozygosity in the *sdi-1* coding region. In this research, mRNA of *sdi-1* was not detected in three of the cultured human glioma cell lines by northern blot analysis. On the contrary, the expression of mRNA of *sdi-1* was detected in some sarcoma cell lines.

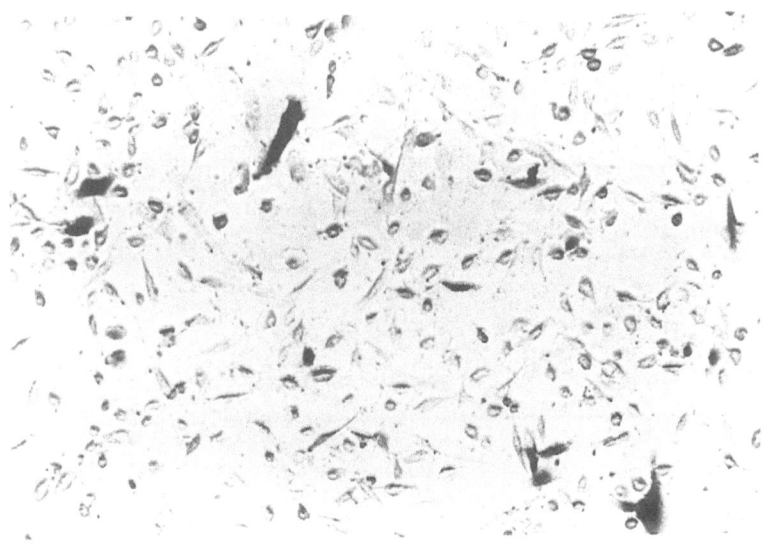

Fig. 1. Expression efficiency by transfection with novel liposomes is measured by counting the *x-gal*-excluding cells in a hemacytometen on the third day after transfection

Detection of the Introduced *sdi-1* Gene in Transfected Glioma Cells

The *sdi-1* expression vector was transferred into human glioma cells, and *sdi-1* cDNA in the transfectant was detected by the PCR method.

Growth Inhibition of Glioma by Transfection with *sdi-1* Gene

As shown in Fig. 3, the growth inhibition of human glioma cells was recognized in *sdi-1* transfectant. The cell numbers were (4.54 ± 0.85) × 10^4/ml on day 21 in A7

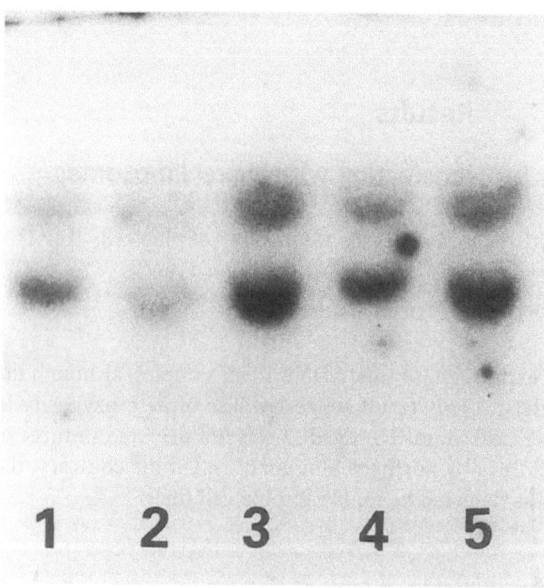

Fig. 2. Results of Southern blot analysis of cell lines. *Lane 1*, U251-SP; *lane 2*, U251-MG; *lane 3*, T98; *lane 4*, clinical sample 1; *lane 5*, clinical sample 2

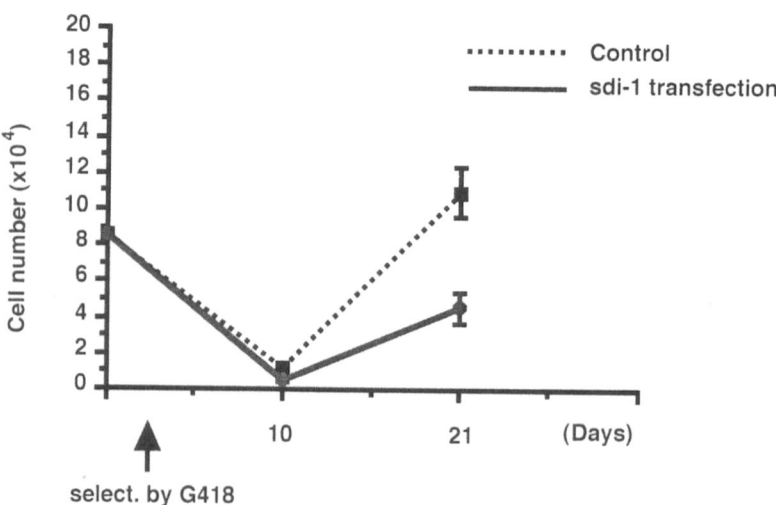

Fig. 3. Growth inhibition of A7 glioma cells by transfection with *sdi-1* gene

transfectant. In contrast, the cell numbers were $(10.98 \pm 1.41) \times 10^4$/ml on day 21 in the control (Fig. 3). Also the growth of U 251-SP transfectant was suppressed.

Discussion

Patients with malignant glioma have a poor prognosis, with an average survival time of less than 2 years even if extensive treatment with surgical resection, high-dose irradiation, and immunochemotherapy are undertaken [6–8]. With the progress of molecular biology and molecular genetics, a new approach in treating malignant tumor has been investigated using a gene modification technique [9–12]. In 1989, gene therapy for cancer was started by Rosenberg et al. [13–15], who improved immunotherapy by gene transfer in the following two ways: adding the TNF-α gene to the tumor-infiltrating lymphocytes (TIL) to make them more effective or adding TNF-α or the IL-2 gene to the tumor cells to induce the body's immune system to make more effective TIL.

In 1992, Culver et al. [16] proposed a new concept, molecular surgery for brain tumor. They reported using rats with a cerebral glioma. Murine fibroblasts that were producing a retroviral vector into which the herpes simplex thymidine kinase (HS-tk) gene had been inserted were injected stereotaxically into a tumor growing in the brain. After 5 days during which the HS-tk retroviral vectors that were produced in situ transduced neighboring proliferating glioma cells, the tumors were treated with the antiherpes drug ganciclovir. Gliomas in the ganciclovir- and vector-treated rats regressed completely.

We are now developing a new approach using the liposome-entrapped pcDSRαδ-adi-1 gene as the third approach. The product of *sdi-1* gene was revealed also as WAF-1 (wild-type p53-activated fragment-1) and cip-1 (cdk-interacting protein-1) [1–4, 17, 18]. These products combine with cdk-2 and also form a complex with cyclin A, D1, and E. This complex lost activity as kinase and histon H1 and RB protein were not phosphorylated.

This mechanism suggests that the growth of malignant neoplasms may be inhibited by transfection with the *sdi-1* gene. In this chapter, we confirmed its growth inhibition for malignant glioma cells. Although further investigation for the mechanism of the *sdi-1* gene is needed, this new approach may become one method of gene therapy for malignant glioma.

References

1. Pines J (1994) Arresting developments in cell-cycle control. Trends Biochem Sci 19:143–145
2. Nigg EA (1993) Cellular substrates of p34^{cdc2} and its companion cyclin-dependent kinase. Trends cell Biol 3:296–300
3. Ookata K, Hisanaga S, Okano T (1992) Relocation and distinct subcellular localization of p34^{cdc2} and its companion cyclin B complex at meiosis reinitiation in starfish oocytes. EMBO J 11:1763–1772
4. Satteerwhite LL, Lohka MJ, Wilson KL (1992) Phosphorylation of myosin-II regulatory light chain by cyclin-p34^{cdc2}. J Cell Biol 118:595–605
5. Mizuno M, Yosida J, Sugita K, Inoue I, Seo H, Hayashi Y, Koshizaka T, Yagi K (1990) Growth inhibition of glioma cells transfected with the human β-interferon gene by liposomes coupled with a monoclonal antibody. Cancer Res 50:7826–7829

6. Asher L, Mule JJ, Reichert CM (1989) Studies on the anti-tumor efficacy of systemically administered recombinant tumor necrosis factor against sereval murine tumors in vivo. J Immunol 138:963–974

7. Brem H, Mahaley MSJ, Vick NA (1991) Interstitial chemotherapy with drug polymer implants for the treatment of recurrent gliomas. J Neurosurg 74:441–446

8. Florell RC, Macdonald DR, Irish WD (1992) Selection bias, survival, and brachytherapy for glioma. J Neurosurg 76:179–183

9. Anderson WF (1992) Human gene therapy. Science 256:808–813

10. Cline MJ (1987) Gene therapy: current status. Am J Med 83:291–297

11. Collins VP, James CD (1990) Molecular genetics of primary intracranial tumors, Curr Opin Oncol 2:666–672

12. Eliyahu D, Michalovitz D, Eliyahu S (1989) Wild-type p53 can inhibit oncogene-mediated focus formation. Proc Natl Acad Sci USA 85:8763–8767

13. Rosenberg SA, Aebersold P, Cornetta K (1990) Gene transfer into humans—immunotherapy of patients with advanced melanoma, using tumor-infiltrating lymphocytes modified by retroviral gene transduction. N Engl J Med 323:570–578

14. Rosenberg SA (1990) Gene therapy of patients with advanced cancer using tumor infiltrating lymphocytes transduced with the gene coding for tumor necrosis factor. Hum Gene Ther 1:441–442

15. Rosenberg SA (1992) Immunization of cancer patients using autologous cancer cells modified by insertion of the gene for tumor necrodid factor. Hum Gene Ther 3:57–73

16. Culver KW, Ram Z, Wallbridge S (1992) In vivo gene transfer with retroviral vector-producer cells for treatment of experimental brain tumors. Science 256:1550–1552

Antisense DNA Approach to the Growth of Human Glioma Cells

Seiichi Yoshida, Ryuichi Tanaka, and Ryuya Yamanaka

Abstract. We were able to detect mRNA transcripts of transforming growth factor-alpha (TGF-α) in four of seven glioma cell lines. Transcripts of other oncogene products were not as clear as TGF-α. We then used four phosphorothioate oligonucleotides (S-oligo) complementary to the sense mRNA of erbB2, TGF-α, c-*fos*, and c-*myc* to investigate those effects on the growth of glioma cells. The antisense oligonucleotides complementary to TGF-α and epidermal growth factor receptor (EGFR) mRNA were efficiently incorporated into glioma cells within 48 h of incubation. Exposure of human glioma cells to S-oligo against TGF-α inhibited cell proliferation in a time- and dose-dependent fashion. These effects of the antisense TGF-α S-oligo were significant at 3 mM, and [³H]thymidine uptake by glioma cells was inhibited by 80%. The addition of anti TGF-α antibody (50 ng/ml) enhanced these antiproliferative effects. The antisense TGF-α S-oligo also suppressed completely the proliferation of the glioma cells throughout the extended culture period. These results clearly support a role of TGF-α protein in the proliferation process of glioma cells, which can be blocked by means of synthetic oligonucleotides complementary to their coding exons.

Key words. Antisense DNA—Oligonucleotides—TGF-α—S-Oligo—Glioma cells

Introduction

Elevated levels of growth factors and oncogene products have recently been described in several kinds of cancers. Transforming growth factor-α (TGF-α), which binds to the epidermal growth factor receptor (EGFR), is the first growth factor associated with tumorigenesis [1]. Partial inhibition of tumor growth has been obtained with anti-EGFR antibodies [2], anti-interleukin-6 antibodies [3], anti-b-fibroblast growth factor antibodies [4], and so on. Many studies have attempted to use antibodies to determine the role of these proteins in tumor growth [5]. Despite the difficulties with antibody studies, if the synthesis of these proteins could be disrupted [6,7] it should be possible

Department of Neurosurgery, Brain Research Institute, Niigata University, Asahimachi 1, Niigata 951, Japan

441

to determine whether a particular growth factor secreted by a tumor cell is required for proliferation.

Antisense oligonucleotides are able to enter cells relatively easily. Hybridization of the antisense molecules and the target genes is supposed to provide high specificity and binding affinity that is superior to that of antibody–ligand binding. Some antisense oligonucleotides have proven to be useful in selectively inhibiting the expression of specific genes and have been also used to disrupt the expression of a diverse range of oncogenic proteins [8]. In particular, phosphorothioate oligonucleotides (S-oligo) possess several unique properties that make them advantageous as antisense inhibition molecules: they are stable to cleavage by nucleases, have high aqueous solubility, and hybridize well to target sequence.

In this study, we investigated oncogene expression within cultured human glioma cell lines by using polymerase chain reaction (PCR) and similar techniques. After this investigation, we used four S-oligo complementary to the sense mRNA of erbB2, TGF-α, c-fos, and c-myc to investigate the effects of these oligonucleotides on the growth of glioma cells.

Materials and Methods

Cell Lines

Seven human glioma cells (NP-1, -2, -3, U251, Y51, O59, S28) were used as the experimental cell line. Cells were grown in RPMI 1640 with 10% fetal bovine serum (FBS) (GIBCO, Grand Island, NY, USA) in tissue culture dishes (Costar, Cambridge, MA, USA) and maintained at 37°C in an incubator with 5% CO_2.

PCR Analysis

Total RNA was isolated from glioma cells by in a single-step phenol extraction method; RNA was used as templates at 0.5 mg/reaction. Reverse transcription was performed at 22°C for 10 min and then at 42°C for 45 min. PCR was performed in 50-μl volumes with specific primers for each factor (PCR kit, Toyobo, Osaka, Japan). The amplification procedure involved denaturation at 94°C for 1 min, annealing at 60°C for 1 min, and extension at 72°C for 2 min during 30–45 PCR cycles in a DNA thermal cycler. The PCR products were resolved on a 2% agarose gel and visualized by ethidium bromide fluorescence. HindIII-digested λ DNA fragments served as the molecular weight markers in defining the size of the PCR products.

Oligonucleotide Preparation

Oligonucleotides were synthesized on an oligonucleotide synthesizer (model 380B, Applied BIO Systems, Foster City, CA, USA). These modified 18-mer phosphorothioate antisense oligonucleotides (S-oligo) are complementary to six bases starting at the translation initiation codon (ATG) (Fig. 1). The sense oligonucleotides of the complementary sequence were also synthesized as a control. Purity was verified by high performance liquid chromatography.

hu-c-neu/erbB2 : 5'-GGC TGC CAT GGT CCC-3'

hu-c-myc   : 5'-AAC GTT GAG GGG CAT-3'

hu-c-fos   : 5'-CTC CAT GGT GCC CAT-3'

hu-TGF-α   : 5'-TCC AGC CGA GGG CTA-3'

Fig. 1. Structures of antisense inhibition phosphorothioate antisense oligonucleotides (S-oligo)

Table 1. Summary of oncogene expression within human glioma cells.

	NP1	NP2	NP3	U251	Y51	O59	S28
neu/erbB2	−	+	−	+	−	±	ND
c-myc	−	−	+	+	±	ND	+
c-fos	±	−	ND	−	±	−	ND
TGF-α	±	+	ND	+	−	±	+

TGF-α, transforminy growth factor-alpha; ND, not done.

Oligonucleotide Uptake and Stability

S-oligo described previously were 5'-end labeled using Klenow enzyme with [^{32}P-α]ATP (3000 Ci/mmol, Amersham, Arlington Height, IL, USA) and added to the cells. After incubation for 2h, serum was added to the cultures to a final concentration of 10%. Cells were incubated for the appropriate times at 37°C. The reaction was interrupted by centrifugation at 4°C. The cells were transferred to tubes and washed three times with phosphate buffered saline (PBS), and radioactivity was measured as previously described [9].

Antisense Oligonucleotide Treatments

All cells were first plated at 1500 cells/well in 96-well microtiter plates and grown in 100 μl of RPMI 1640 medium, containing 10% fresh medium. Each S-oligo was added directly into the medium 1h after plating of cells at various concentrations. After these procedures, 0.15 μCi of [^{3}H]thymidine (80 Ci/mmol) was added to each well and incubated for 12h. Microtiter plates were frozen to lyse cells, and DNA was transferred to glass fiber filters using a cell harvester. [^{3}H]Thymidine incorporation was measured by liquid scintillation counting. The proliferative capacity of glioma cells was also verified by trypan blue exclusion. All the results reported here represent an average of three experiments, each experiment having been run in triplicate.

Results

We could detect mRNA transcripts of TGF-α in four of seven glioma cell lines. Transcripts of other oncogene products were not as clear as TGF-α (Table 1). Against these molecules, four kinds of 18 base-pair-modified phosphorothioate antisense oligonucleotides (S-oligo) were designed and tested for their effects on the growth of glioma cells. The antisense oligonucleotides complementary to TGF-α and EGFR mRNA were efficiently incorporated into glioma cells in vitro, and the kinetic study showed that maximum uptake occurred within 48h of incubation with antisense oligomers (Table 2).

Evaluation of the effects of these antisense oligonucleotides revealed that exposure of human glioma cell lines to TGF-α S-oligo inhibited cell proliferation in a time- and dose-dependent fashion. This effect was significant at 2mM, and by 5mM [³H]thymidine uptake by glioma cells was inhibited by 80% (Fig. 2). There were no nonspecific effects of these oligonucleotides. The addition of anti-TGF-α antibody (50ng/ml) enhanced this antiproliferative effect (Fig. 3). The random or other antisense oligonucleotides did not affect the proliferation of these cells.

It is also important to measure the effect of the antisense oligonucleotide on longer term cell proliferation, not just [³H]thymidine uptake. Consequently, cell counting was performed at several time points to test the effects of the antisense oligonucleotides. The antisense TGF-α oligonucleotides suppressed completely proliferation of the glioma cells throughout the extended culture period (Fig. 4). Glioma cells proliferating in the presence of those to which only the random sense

Table 2. Oligonucleotide uptake into glioma cells.

	24 h	48 h	72 h
U251			
neu/erbB	218 100	97 100	121 300
c-*myc*	800	1 200	700
TGF-α	27 300	141 400	87 200
NP-2			
neu/erbB2	110 300	100 900	90 500
c-*myc*	600	800	400
TGF-α	20 900	110 800	80 700

Data are scintillation counting.

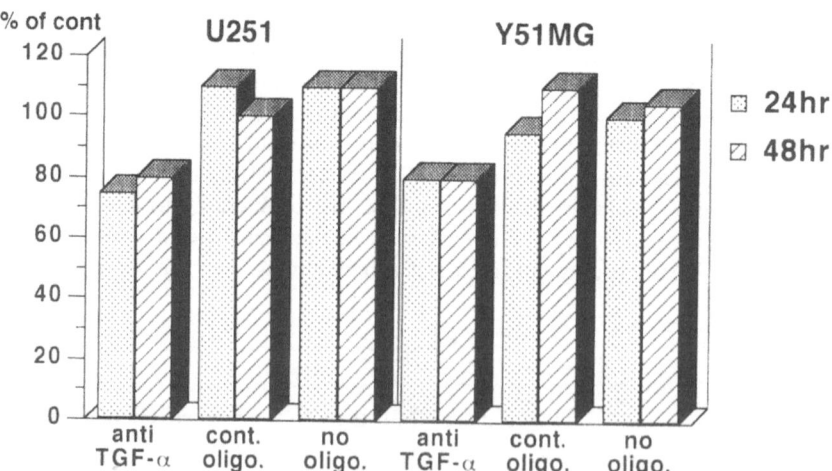

Fig. 2. Effects of antisense inhibition phosphorothioate antisense oligonucleotides against transforming growth factor-alpha (TGF-α) on the proliferation of glioma cells

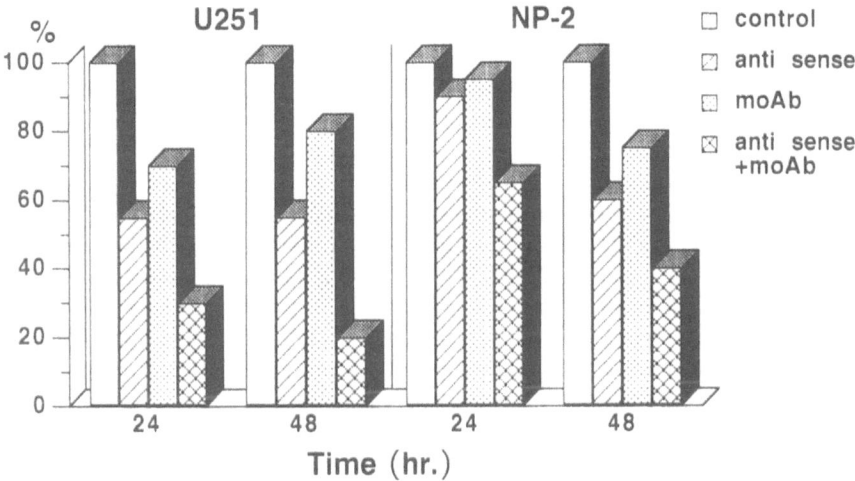

Fig. 3. Combination effects of antisense inhibition oligonucleotides against TGF-α and anti-TGF-α monoclonal antibody (moAb) on the proliferation of glioma cells

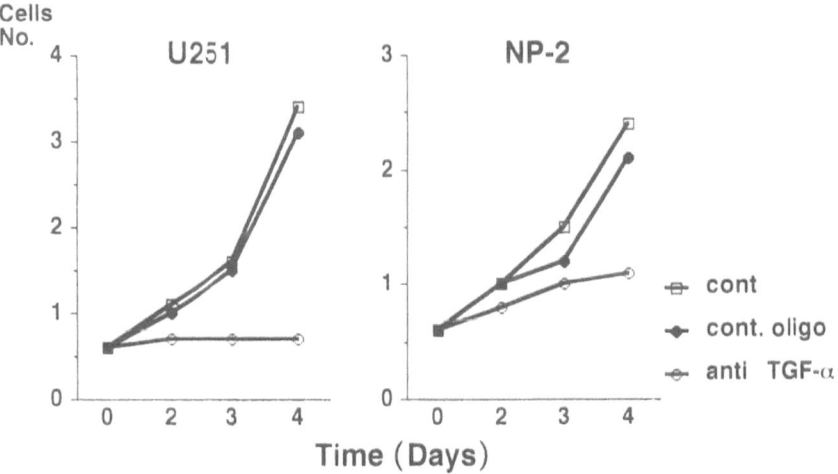

Fig. 4. Effects of antisense inhibition oligonucleotides against TGF-α on the proliferative capacity of glioma cells using trypan blue exclusion tests

oligonucleotide had been added proliferate at rates similar to untreated cells. These results clearly support a role of TGF-α protein in the proliferation process of glioma cells, which can be blocked by means of synthetic oligonucleotides complementary to their coding exons. Furthermore, we have reported previously that some glioma cells produced IL-8, which acted as a growth factor. Antisense DNA against IL-8 could also inhibit the growth of some glioma cells [10]. These results also indicated that antisense DNA against other autocrine factors for the glioma cells could suppress the glioma cell proliferation.

Discussion

Antisense oligonucleotides, which block the expression of a particular gene, have been proven useful in assessing the function of the product of the gene [11]. The antisense oligonucleotides seem to inhibit gene expression predominantly by hybridization arrest of mRNA translation [12]. We showed that several kinds of oncogene expression could be detected in human glioma cells in various degrees. Our results indicate that these oncogene products are important for proliferation of glioma cells. Our series of experiments revealed, especially, that S-oligo directed against TGF-α was capable of blocking the proliferation of glioma cells. It can be seen, in Figure 2, that glioma cells at a density of 10^5/ml undergo an inhibition of proliferation to 80% of control levels. The addition of anti-TGF-α antibody (50 ng/ml) 12 h after the addition of the antisense oligonucleotide, furthermore, enhanced this inhibitory effect against glioma cell proliferation (see Fig. 3).

The possibility of reversing the transformation of cancer cells may be a critical advantage of drugs targeted specifically against oncogenes. Most current drugs affect only replication nonspecifically. An antisense DNA able to reverse the transformation process may produce a reorganization of cellular genetic expression that affects a number of neoplastic and malignant attributes. Gilbert et al. [13] suggest that the c-Ha-*ras* oncogene may act only to trigger cellular changes initially, and it is these changes that subsequently served to maintain neoplastic behavior independent of the oncogene. Feramisco et al. [14] demonstrated that microinjection of anti-RAS p21 antibodies directly into c-Ha-*ras*-transformed cells reversed transformation as measured by morphology and growth rate. These results indicate that neoplastic growth is dependent on continued expression of oncogene.

Glioma cells also have identifiable oncogenes which may serve as targets for antisense DNA. Antisense DNA against these molecules has been shown here to be a very effective agent for in vitro treatment on the growth of human glioma cells. The high doses are necessary in vivo because of the susceptibility of normal DNA oligomers to rapid degradation by serum nucleases. More likely candidates for in vivo applications are modified oligonucleotides that are rendered resistant to nucleases by altering the nucleotide structure itself (e.g., alkylphosphonates, phosphorothioates, 2'-O-alkyl nucleotides) or by attaching protecting groups at the 3' and 5' ends of DNA oligomers [15].

Our findings here demonstrate the substantial potential of S-oligo as a new class of anticancer drugs against glioma cell proliferation. Although further studies (e.g., using antisense constructs or gene transfer technology) are necessary to analyze the complicated role of oncogenes on glioma cell proliferation, our results demonstrated direct evidence that antisense oligonucleotides directed against TGF-α could inhibit the proliferation of some glioma cells. In the future, antisense approach using these molecules may become useful in the treatment of glioma patients.

References

1. Todaro JG, Fryling C, De Larco JE (1980) Transforming growth factors produced by certain human tumor cells: polypeptides that interact with epidermal growth factor receptors. Proc Natl Acad Sci USA 77:5258–5262
2. Carpenter G, Stoscheck CM, Preston YA, De Larco JE (1983) Antibodies to the epidermal factor. Proc Natl Acad Sci USA 80:5627–5630

3. Kawano M, Hirano T, Matsuda T, Taga T, Horii Y (1988) Autocrine generation and requirement of BSF-2/IL-6 for human multiple myelomas. Nature 332:83–85
4. Sasada R, Kurokawa T, Iwane M, Igarashi K (1988) Transformation of mouse Balbc/3T3 cells with human basic fibroblast growth factor cDNA. Mol Cell Biol 8:588–594
5. Gewirtz AM, Anfossai G, Venturelli D, Valpreda S, Sims R, Calabretta B (1989) G1/S transition in normal human T lymphocytes requires the nuclear protein encoded by c-myb. Science 245:180–183
6. Derynck R, Roberets AB, Winkler ME, Chen EY, Goedel DV (1984) Human transforming growth factor-alpha: precursor structure and expression in *E. coli*. Cell 38:287–297
7. Keating MT, Williams LT (1988) Autocrine stimulation of intracellular PDGF receptors in v-sis-transformed cells. Cell 43:531–542
8. Heikila R, Schwab G, Wickstrom E, Loke SL, Pluznik DH, Watt R, Neckers LM (1987) A c-*myc* antisense oligodeoxynucleotide inhibits entry into S phase but not progress from G_0 to G_1. Nature 328:445–449
9. Wickstrom EL, Bacon TA, Gonzalez A, Freeman DL, Lyman GH, Wickstrom E (1988) Human promyelocytic leukemia HL-60 cell proliferation and c-myc protein expression are inhibited by an antisense pentadecadeoxynucleotide targeted against c-myc mRNA. Proc Natl Acad Sci USA 85:1028–1034
10. Yamanaka R, Tanaka R, Yoshida S (1993) Effects of irradiation on cytokine production in glioma cell lines. Neurol Med Chir (Tokyo) 33:744–748
11. Harel-Bellan A, Ferris DK, Vinocour M, Holt JT, Farrar WL (1988) Specific inhibition of c-myc protein biosynthesis using an antisense synthetic deoxyoligonucleotide in human T lymphocytes. J Immunol 140:2431–2435
12. Kawasaki ES (1985) Quantitative hybridization arrest of mRNA in *Xenopus* oocyte using single-strand complementary DNA or oligonucleotide probes. Nucleic Acids Res 13:4991–5004
13. Gilbert PX, Harris H (1988) The role of the *ras* oncogene in the formation of tumors. J Cell Sci 90:433–446
14. Feramisco JR, Clark R, Wong G, Arnheim N, Milley R, McCormic F (1985) Transient reversion of *ras* oncogene-induced cell transformation by antibodies specific for amino acid 12 of *ras* protein. Nature 314:639–641
15. Wickstrom E (1992) Strategies for administering targeted therapeutic oligodeoxynucleotides. Trends Biotechnol 10:281–287

Index

Acyclovir   412
Adoptive immunotherapy   364
Aggressive papillary tumor of the
    temporal bone   25
Allelic loss
  of 1p   190–196
    9p   194
    10   7, 8
    17p   7, 8, 194
    19q   190
1-(4-amino-2-methyl-5-pryrimidinyl)-3-
    (2-chloroethyl)-3-nitrosourea
    hydrochloride (ACNU)   128,
    206, 352–353, 365
Antibody
  antianti-idiotypic antibody
    (Ab3)   371–377, 381–386
  anti-Bcl-2   295
  anti-Fas   295, 296
  anti-idiotypic antibody (Ab2)   371–
    376
  antiparatope   384
  bispecific   365
  idiotypic   371
Antigen
  epithelial membrane   11
  Fas (APO-1)   284, 286, 293
  Ki-67, See Ki-67
  leucocyte common   13
  malignant-associated-(TA226)   371,
    374, 377
  melanoma (MAGE)   391
Antigen presenting cell (APC)   332
Antisense DNA   390, 398, 441
  – oligonucleotide   442–446

APC, See Antigen presenting cell
APO-1, See Fas antigen
Apoptosis   284–290, 400
Astroblastoma   10
Astrocytoma   30–35, 40–43, 120, 173,
    193, 239, 240, 256, 257, 264, 340,
    343, 344
  anaplastic   14, 40–43, 62, 142, 143,
    164, 173, 192, 195, 205, 222, 256,
    257, 264–268, 341, 365–378
  diffuse   180
  fibrillary   46
  gemistocytic   178, 260
  grade 4   249–251
  infantile desmoplastic   9
  low grade   48, 62, 142, 143, 178, 181,
    222, 242, 257–259, 341, 381, 383,
    424
  malignant   30–35, 350–360, 381, 383
  pilocytic   14, 173, 176
  protoplasmic   9, 46
  recurrent   47, 48
  subependymal giant cell   22
  WHO grade II   178
  WHO grade III   178

B7, See Costimulatory molecule
B70, See Costimulatory molecule
Basic fibroblast growth factor
    (bFGF)   203–207
BCNU   340–346
β-2-microglobulin   317–321
bFGF, See Basic fibroblast growth factor
Bispecific antibody   365

BrdU, *See* 5-Bromo-2-deoxyuridine
5-Bromo-2-deoxyuridine (BrdU,
        BUdR)   46–48, 142–145, 260
BUdR, *See* 5-Bromo-2-deoxyuridine
Bystander effect   392, 416

CAM, *See* Cell adhesion molecules
Capillary hemangioblastoma   12
Carbonic anhydrase C, 2'-3'-cyclic
        nucleotide-3'-phosphatase   190
Carmustine, *See* BCNU
Casein kinase II (CKII)   398, 399
CD3   364
CD4   328
CD8   328, 404
CD16   364
CD28   328, 397
CD44   427
CD68   331, 335
CDDP, *See* cis-Platinum
CDK4, *See* Cyclin-dependent kinase 4
CDK-4-proliferating cell nuclear
        antigen-cyclin D (CDK-4/PCNA/
        cyclin D) complex   168, 169,
        182, 195
Cell
   9L   110, 401, 403
   A172   284
   B104   404
   C6   110, 114, 294, 295, 399, 404
   GOTO (neuroblastoma)   110–115
   NB-1   324
   NB-V   322–324
   PC12   153
   T98G   110, 112, 264, 284, 435
   U251   264, 284, 399, 435, 442
   U373MG   110, 264
   U87MG   412, 435
   YAC-1   322
Cell adhesion molecules (CAM)   106
Cell migration assay   111
Cell proliferation assay   121
Central neurocytoma   9, 10, 21, 104,
        174
Chemoinvasion assay   121
Chemosensitizer   339–346
Chemotherapy   46, 56, 57, 62
Choroid plexus carcinoma   6

Choroid plexus tumor   6
Chromosome
   1   192
   1p   12
   9p   165, 174, 180
   9p21   179, 182, 190
   10   12, 176, 180
   12   11
   14q   12
   17p   164, 165, 176, 178, 180, 251, 424
   17q   176, 190
   19q   164, 176, 180, 190
   19q13.3–13.4   179
   22   11, 180
   22q12   12, 164
cis-Platinum [cisplatin; cis-diammine
        dichloroplatinum, CDDP]   61,
        64
CKII, *See* Casein kinase II
CLN-IgG   371–378, 381–386
Clonal expansion   390
   of p53   260
CNP, *See* Carbonic anhydrase C   2'-3'-
        cyclic nucleotide-3'-phosphatase
Combination therapy
   with IFN, ACNU, and radiation   352,
        353
Costimulatory molecule
   B7, B70   328–335, 391
Craniopharyngioma   12
CRK protein   153–157
CTL, *See* Cytotxic-T-lymphocyte
Cyclin-dependent kinase 4
        (CDK4)   182, 266, 424
Cytotxic-T-lymphocyte (CTL)   317,
        322, 323, 335, 364, 429

Desmoplastic infantile
        ganglioglioma   9, 24, 25
DIG, *See* Desmoplastic infantile
        ganglioglioma
Dimethyl sulfoxide (DMSO)   317, 340,
        342
DMSO, *See* Dimethyl sulfoxide
DNA fragmentation   285
   ladder of DNA fragments   287
DNA index   130
DNA-ligase 1 (LIG1)   192

DNT, *See* Dysembryoplastic
    neuroepithelial tumor
Dysembryoplastic neuroepithelial
    tumor   9, 23

EGFR, *See* Epidermal growth factor
    receptor gene
EMA, *See* Epithelial membrane antigen
Embryonal tumor   10
Ependymoblastoma   10
Ependymoma   10, 164, 174
  myxopapillary   14
Epidermal growth factor   273
Epidermal growth factor receptor
    (EGFR) gene   7, 8, 166–168, 174,
    175, 177, 180–182, 195, 424
Epithelial membrane antigen
    (EMA)   11, 13
Epitope   373, 374, 376
Ezrin   271

Fas antigen   284, 286
Fas monoclonal antibody   284–289
FGF, *See* Fibroblast growth factor
Fibroblast growth factor (FGF) 221
  FGF1   222–229
  FGF2   222–229
Fibronectin type III   104, 105
Flow cytometry   127
Flu-like symptoms   342, 345

GADPDH, *See* Glyceraldehyde
    phosphate dehydrogenase
Gamma-enolase   189
Gamma-knife surgery   46
Gancyclovir (GCV)   391, 392, 412, 413,
    417–420
Ganglioglioma   9, 104
GAP, *See* Glyceraldehyde-3-phosphate
Gemistocyte   257, 259, 260
Gene
  bcl-2   293, 300
  bFGF   390
  C3G   154
  CDC25   157
  CDK2 (p16/MTS1)   194

CDK4   174
class I interfereon   165
c-myc   401
c-Myc   398
c-sis   390
c-src   318
cytokine   428
disptk   410–412
EGFR, *See* EGFR
flg   203–207
flk-1   242
flt-l   242
G3PDH   264
HSV-tk   391, 392
HTK   416–420
L1   111–115
lacZ   411, 412, 417
mdm-2   174
mdr   390
MDM2   8, 166–168
MTS1   190
MYC   195
N-myc   318, 398, 405
p53, *See* p53
RB, *See* RB
SAS   174
sdi-1   438, 439
s-Myc   398–405
s-myc   398–405
thymidine kinase   391
trk   211–219
Gene alteration   161–168
Gene amplification
  of EGFR   165, 166
Gene therapy   390–393, 397, 415, 424–
    432
  Cytokine –   428–432
Gene transfection   436
Genomic hybridization   8
GFAP, *See* Glial fibrillary acidic protein
Glial differentiation   10
Glial fibrillary acidic protein
    (GFAP)   7, 8, 24, 25, 53, 54, 57,
    189, 190
Glioblastoma (multiforme)   7, 8, 14,
    30–37, 40–43, 62, 104, 120, 122–
    124, 128, 142–146, 163, 164, 173,
    193, 195, 205, 207, 222, 240, 241,
    242, 259, 264–268, 289, 308, 329–

Glioblastoma (multiforme) (*cont.*):
    335, 350, 351, 364, 366–368, 381,
    383
  de novo   180, 268
  heterogeneity of   7, 182
  primary   8, 255
  secondary   8
  type 1   8, 180
  type 2   8, 180
  type 3   8
  type 4   8
  WHO grade IV   179–182
Glioma   163, 241, 340, 350
  anaplastic   128, 242
  anaplastic mixed   14
  benign   310
  high grade   340, 343
  low grade   128, 341
  malignant   123, 299, 307, 310, 352,
    364–368, 423, 435
  malignant progression of   164
  mixed   6, 41, 190, 195
  recurrent   340, 367
Glioma-derived motility factor
    (GMF)   109
Glioma score   143
Gliomatosis cerebri   10
Gliosarcoma   41
Glutathione S-transferase (GST)   153,
    270–272, 274
Glyceraldehyde-3-phosphate   177
Glyseraldehyde phosphate
    dehydrogenase (GAPDH)   239,
    240
GM-CSF, *See* Granulocyte-macrophage
    colony-stimulating factor
GMF, *See* Glioma-derived motility
    factor
Grading system   40–43
  Burger   41
  Daumas-Duport   42
  Kernohan   41
Granulocyte-macrophage colony-
    stimulating factor (GM-
    CSF)   390, 391
GST, *See* Glutathione S-transferase

Hemangioblastoma   241, 278–281
Hemangiopericytoma   240

Herpes simplex thymidine kinase
    (HS-tk)   425, 439
Herpes simplex virus type 1 (HSV-tk)
    391, 392, 410–413, (HTK),   416–
    420
Heterozygosity
  at the DIZ2 locus (1p36.3)   193
    DIS57   193
    DIZ2   193
Homozygous deletion   264, 265
HS-tk, *See* Herpes simplex thymidine
    kinase
HSV-tk, *See* Herpes simplex virus type 1
HTK gene, *See* Herpes simplex virus
    tyep 1

IAR (Interferon-ACNU-radiation)
    therapy   352, 353, 381
ICAM-1, *See* Intercellular molecule-1
ICP, *See* Infected cell protein
Idiotope   374
Idiotype network   371, 376, 384
IFN, *See* Interferon
Image cytometry   130
Immunocytochemistry   330
Immunodot analysis   110
Immunohistochemistry   331
Immunoglobulin C   104, 105
Immunoliposome   427
Immunosurveillance (Immune
    surviellance)   316, 324, 328, 335
Infected cell protein (ICP)   411, 412
Intercellular molecule-1   428
Interferon (IFN)   339, 350
  Interferon-α   339–346
  Interferon-β   46, 128, 351–360, 428–
    431
  Interferon-γ   175, 331
  Lymphoblastoid   340
  Recombinant   340
Isopropyl [125I]iodoamphetamine
    (IMP)   46

Ki-67   12, 56, 70, 91, 94, 97, 142–146,
    257

LAK, *See* Lymphokine activatied killer
    cell

– therapy   364, 366
L1CAM (Neuronal cell adhesion
      molecule)   104–106, 109–116
LCA, *See* Leucocyte common antigen
Leucocyte common antigen   13
Li-Fraumeni   163, 165
Lipofectin   399, 401
Liposome   392, 428–430, 436, 437
   cationic –   428
   immuno-   427
Local injection
   of IFN   351
LOH, *See* Loss of heterozygosity
Loss of heterozygosity   163, 176
   LOH 1p   193, 196
   LOH 9   164
   LOH 9p21   424
   LOH 10   164, 165, 178–182, 195, 196,
      424
   LOH 17p   164, 178–182, 194, 251, 424
   LOH 17q   178
   LOH 19   165
   LOH 19p   196
   LOH 19q   164, 178–180, 191, 196
   LOH 22q   164
   of VHL gene   278–280
Lymphokine activatied killer cell (LAK)
      364, 365
Lymphoma
   malignant   13
   non-Hodgkin   13

Macrophage
   infiltration   306, 309
MAG, *See* Myelin associated
      glycoprotein
Maintenance therapy   353, 358, 384
Major histocompatibility complex
      (MHC)   316, 327, 364, 391, 397,
      405, 428
   H-2 class I   316–321
   MHC class I   398
   MHC class II   335
Malignant peripheral nerve sheath
      tumors   11
MBP, *See* Myelin basic protein
MCP-1, *See* Monocyte-chemoattractant
      protein-1
MDM2   8, 166–168

mdm2   174
Mean survival time   357
Median survival   56, 343, 344
Median time to tumor progression   343
Medulloblastoma   10, 104, 193, 211–
      219, 242, 350, 352, 411
   desmoplastic variant   22
Medulloepithelioma   10
Meningioma,   69–77, 89–97, 120, 242,
      275, 308
   anaplastic (malignant)   11, 75, 76
   angiomatous   82, 87, 91
   atypical   11, 12, 70–76, 91, 94, 95
   chordoid   11
   clear cell   11
   fibrous   82
   hemangiblastic   91
   hemangiopeicytic   11, 91
   incidental   79–87
   lymphocyte rich   11
   malignant   11, 97, 128, 132, 411
   meningothelial   82, 91, 93, 240
   metaplastic   11
   microcystic   11
   papillary   11, 91
   psammomatous   82, 87
   secretory   11
   transitional   82
Meningoangiomatosis   23
Mesenchymal non-meningothelial
      tumors   12
Metallothionein   61–66, 398
Metastasis   240
Metastatic brain tumor   120, 123
Merlin   271, 273
Merlin-ezrin-radixin-moesin   271–274
MERM, *See* Merlin-ezrin-radixin-
      moesin
MHC, *See* Major histocompatibility
      complex
MIB-1   12, 56, 59, 70–77, 82, 142–146,
      256–258
Moesin   271
Molecular genetics   187
Monoclonal antibody
   AD2   153
   against rat macrophage   307
   anti-CD3   365, 368
   anti-CD68   329
   anti-Fas   284–289

Monoclonal antibody (*cont.*):
  antiglioma (NE150)   365
  anti-idiotypic   371–377
  anti-Leu-7 (CD57)   189
  G22   427–429, 432
  human (CLN-IgG)   371–378, 381–
    386
  TGK-1   213–218
Monocyte-chemoattractant protein-1
    (MCP-1)   306–310
Morphometry   133
MPNST, *See* Malignant peripheral nerve
    sheath tumors
MTS1   8
Multinuclear giant cell   257, 259
Myelin associated glycoprotein
    (MAG)   190
Myelin basic protein (MBP)   53, 416
Myelosuppression   342, 344

Natural killer (NK) cell   322–324
NCAM (Neural cell adhesion molecule)
    115
Nerve growth factor (NGF)   211, 293
  low affinity (LANGF) –   211–219
Neurilemmoma   10
Neurinoma   10, 120, 240
Neuroblastoma   10, 270, 316
  cerebellar-   22
Neuroepithelial tumor   5, 6, 104
Neurofibrillary tangle   24
Neurofibroma   10
Neurofibromatosis
  type 1 (NF1)   163
    von Recklinghausen's
      neurofibromatosis   177
  type 2 (NF2)   12, 163, 275
Neurofibrosarcoma   411
Neuron specific enolase (NSE)   53
Neuronal differentiation   22, 317, 318
NGF, *See* Nerve growth factor
NK cell, *See* Natural killer cell
NORS, *See* Nucleolar organizer regions
Nucleolar organizer regions (NORSs)
    84

Olfactory neuroblastoma   104, 106
Oligoastrocytomas   6, 9, 52–59, 164,

188–196, 340, 341, 343
  anaplastic (malignant)   6
Oligodendrolcyte   187, 190
Oligodendrocytoma   341
Oligodendroglioma   6, 9, 36, 104, 142,
    174, 187–197, 240, 340
  anaplastic (malignant)   14, 188–192
Oligonucleotide
  antisense-   442–448
Oncogene   152, 162, 174, 425
  amplification of   196
  overexpression of   390
  supressor-   425

p15   174, 179
p16   165, 166, 174, 179, 264–267
p21   168
p53   256–260
p53   7, 8, 165, 167, 174, 179, 180, 248,
    250–252, 256–260
p85   274
p107   405
p125   270–274
p145   271, 272
p165   270–274
PAI, *See* Plasminogen activator
    inhibitor
Paratope   373–376
PC12 cell   212, 214
pCEPcmyc   401–404
pCEPp53   401–404
PCI, *See* Proliferating cell index
PCNA, *See* Proliferating cell nuclear
    antigen
PDGF, *See* Platelet-derived growth
    factor
PET, *See* Positron emission tomography
Phosphothioate oligonucleotide (S-
    oligo)   442–448
Pineal parencynal tumor   6
Pineoblastoma   6, 10
Pineocytoma   6
Plasminogen activator inhibitor
    (PAI)   119–124
Platelet-derived growth factor
    (PDGF)   273, 309
Pleomorphic xanthoastrocytoma
    (PXA)   8, 9, 41

PNET, *See* Primitive neuroectodermal
     tumor
Point mutation   249
    of p53   257
Polar spongioblastoma   10
Polymerase chain reaction   175, 249,
     264, 270, 278, 438, 442
Positron emission tomography
     (PET)   46-48
Primitive neuroectodermal tumor
     (PNET)   10, 104, 107, 174, 242
Primitive polar spongioblastoma   10
Prognostic factors   30, 32
Programmed cell death   398
Progression   251, 256
    Malignant progression of astrocytic
    glioma   178, 179
    Tumor progression   342
Proliferating cell index   143, 144, 257,
     259
Proliferating cell nuclear antigen
     (PCNA)   82-86, 90, 94, 97

Radiation (therapy)   46, 58, 65, 343-
     346, 352, 353, 365
Radxin   271-273
Rb gene   249, 251
Recklinghausen's disease   23
Regression tree analysis   35
Response rate
    of IFN-α   342
    of IFN-β   351-353, 355
Restiction fragment length
     polymorphis   163, 178, 190
Retroviral vector   391, 393, 416, 420
Reverse transcriptase-polymerase chain
     reaction (RT-PCR)   62, 66, 106,
     110, 204, 222
RFLP, *See* Restiction fragment length
     polymorphism
Rhabdomyosarcoma   11
Ribonucleotide reductase (RR)   412
RR, *See* Ribonucleotide reductase
RT-PCR, *See* Reverse transcriptase-
     polymerase chain reaction
     (RT-PCR)

S100 protein   7, 53

Sarcoma amplified sequence
     (SAS)   182, 195
SAS, *See* Sarcoma amplified sequence
Schwannoma   174, 275
SH, *See* Src homology
Side effects
    of IFN-β   351, 353
    of STT   367
Single photon computed tomography
     (SPECT)   46-48
Single strand conformation
     polymorphism (SSCP)   177,
     249, 278, 279
S-oligo, *See* Phosphorothioate oligo-
     nucleotides
Specific targeting therapy (STT)   363-
     366
SPECT, *See* Single photon computed
     tomography
Sphingomyelin   284, 285, 287
Src homology (SH)   153-156
SSCP, *See* Single strand conformation
     polymorphism
STT, *See* Specific targeting therapy
Subependymoma   14, 22
Survival rate
    of IFN therapy   355-359
    of STT therapy   366
Survival time   58, 357
    Long-   357
    Mean-   357
    Median-   343, 344
Synaptophysin   22, 25

TAM, *See* Tumor associated
     macrophage
TGF-α, *See* Transforming growth
     factor-α
Thymidine kinase gene-deficient HSV-1
     dlsptk   410-413
TIL, *See* Tumor infiltrating lymphocyte
Time to recurrence   367
Time to tumor progression   128, 144,
     354
TNF, *See* Tumor necrosis factor
Toxicity
    of gene therapy   392
    of IFN-α   342-346

TP53   190, 194
Transforming growth factor-α   441,
    443–445
TSG, *See* Tumor suppressor gene
Tuberous sclerosis   22, 24
Tumor associated macrophage
    (TAM)   307
Tumor infiltrating lymphocyte
    (TIL)   335
Tumor necrosisi factor (TNF)   284,
    293, 428–430
Tumor progression   341
Tumor regression   341
Tumor suppressor gene   162–165, 193,
    195
  p53   258–260
  RB   166, 167
  replacement of   390
  VHL   13, 278–281
Tyrosine kinase receptor family   242

u-PA, *See* Urokinase-type plasminogen

activator
Urokinase-type plasminogen activator
    (u-PA)   119–124

Vascular endothelial-derived growth
    factor   13, 238–242
VDEP, *See* Viral directed enzyme
    prodrug therapy
VEGF, *See* Vascular endothelial-derived
    growth factor
VHL, *See* von Hippel-Lindau
Viral directed enzyme prodrug therapy
    (VDEP)   391–393
von Hippel-Lindau (VHL)   12, 277–281
  -gene   277–281
VP-16 (etoposide)   46

WHO classification
    of tumors of the central nervous
    system   4, 5, 69, 70, 75, 80, 90
WHO grading system   14, 15